Spinal Control: The Rehabilitation of Back Pain
State of the art and science

Spinal Control: The Rehabilitation of Back Pain
State of the art and science

Content Strategist: *Rita Demetriou-Swanwick*
Content Development Specialist: *Ewan Halley, Catherine Jackson*
Project Manager: *Anne Collett*
Designer/Design Direction: *Christian Bilbow*
Illustration Manager: *Jennifer Rose*
Illustrator: *Kinesis*

Spinal Control: The Rehabilitation of Back Pain

State of the art and science

Edited by

Paul W. Hodges PhD

Professor and NHMRC Senior Principal Research Fellow, NHMRC Centre of Clinical Research Excellence in Spinal Pain, Injury and Health, School of Health and Rehabilitation Sciences, University of Queensland, Brisbane, Australia

Jacek Cholewicki PhD

Walter F. Patenge Professor, Department of Osteopathic Surgical Specialties, College of Osteopathic Medicine, Michigan State University, East Lansing, Michigan, USA

Jaap H. van Dieën PhD

Professor of Biomechanics, MOVE Research Institute Amsterdam, Faculty of Human Movement Sciences, VU University Amsterdam, Amsterdam, The Netherlands

CHURCHILL LIVINGSTONE ELSEVIER

Edinburgh   London   New York   Oxford   Philadelphia   St Louis   Sydney   Toronto   2013

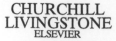

ISBN 978-0-7020-4356-7

British Library Cataloguing in Publication Data
A catalogue record for this book is available from the British Library

Library of Congress Cataloging in Publication Data
A catalog record for this book is available from the Library of Congress

Contents

Contents

Contributors

Michael A. Adams BSc PhD
Professor of Biomechanics,
Centre for Comparative and Clinical Anatomy,
University of Bristol,
Bristol, UK

Simon Brumagne PhD PT
Professor,
Department of Rehabilitation Sciences,
University of Leuven,
Leuven, Belgium

Jack P. Callaghan PhD CK CCPE
Professor and Canada Research Chair in Spine Biomechanics
and Injury Prevention,
Faculty of Applied Health Sciences,
University of Waterloo,
Waterloo, Ontario, Canada

Jacek Cholewicki PhD
Walter F. Patenge Professor,
Department of Osteopathic Surgical Specialties,
College of Osteopathic Medicine,
Michigan State University,
East Lansing, Michigan, USA

Kurt Claeys MSc MT
PhD student,
Catholic University College of Bruges – Ostend (KHBO),
Department of Health Care;
Research Assistant,
Musculoskeletal Research Unit,
Department of Rehabilitation Sciences and Physiotherapy,
University of Leuven,
Leuven, Belgium

Patricia Dolan BSc PhD
Reader in Biomechanics,
Centre for Comparative and Clinical Anatomy,
University of Bristol, Bristol, UK

Julie A. Hides PhD MPhytSt BPhytSt BPhyt FACP
Professor and Head of School,
School of Physiotherapy,
Australian Catholic University,
McAuley Campus,
Banyo, Queensland, Australia

Paul W. Hodges PhD MedDr DSc BPhty(Hons) FACP
Professor and NHMRC Senior Principal Research Fellow,
NHMRC Centre of Clinical Research Excellence in Spinal Pain,
Injury and Health,
School of Health and Rehabilitation Sciences,
University of Queensland,
Brisbane, Queensland, Australia

Lotte Janssens MSc
PhD student,
Department of Rehabilitation Sciences,
University of Leuven,
Leuven, Belgium

Gregory Neil Kawchuk BSc DC MSc PhD
Associate Professor,
Canada Research Chair in Spinal Function,
Faculty of Rehabilitation Medicine,
University of Alberta,
Edmonton, Alberta, Canada

Idsart Kingma PhD
Associate Professor,
MOVE Research Institute Amsterdam,
Faculty of Human Movement Sciences,
VU University Amsterdam,
Amsterdam, The Netherlands

Bart W. Koes PhD
Professor of General Practice,
Department of General Practice,
Erasmus Medical Centre,
Rotterdam, The Netherlands

Stuart McGill PhD
Professor of Spine Biomechanics,
Department of Kinesiology,
Faculty of Applied Health Sciences,
University of Waterloo,
Waterloo, Ontario, Canada

Contributors

G. Lorimer Moseley PhD
NHMRC Senior Research Fellow,
Professor of Clinical Neurosciences and
Chair in Physiotherapy,
Sansom Institute for Health Research,
University of South Australia, Adelaide,
and Neuroscience Research Australia,
Sydney, Australia

Erika Nelson-Wong PT DPT PhD
Assistant Professor,
Rueckert–Hartman College of Health Professions,
School of Physical Therapy,
Regis University,
Denver, Colorado, USA

Barbara J. Norton PT PhD FAPTA
Professor of Physical Therapy and Neurology,
Associate Director for Postprofessional Studies,
Program in Physical Therapy and Department of Neurology,
Washington University School of Medicine at Washington
University Medical Center,
St Louis, Missouri, USA

Raymond Ostelo PhD PT
Associate Professor of Evidence Based Musculoskeletal
Health,
Department of Epidemiology and Biostatistics,
Department of Health Sciences and EMGO Institute for
Health and Care Research, VU University Medical Centre,
Amsterdam, The Netherlands

Mohamad Parnianpour PhD
Professor,
Department of Information and Industrial Engineering,
Hanyang University, Ansan, Republic of Korea,
and Adjunct Professor,
Department of Mechanical Engineering
Sharif University of Technology,
Tehran, Iran

**Mark Pearcy BSc PhD DEng FIEAust
CPEng(Biomed)**
Professor of Biomedical Engineering,
Institute of Health and Biomedical Innovation,
Queensland University of Technology,
Brisbane, Queensland, Australia

Joel G. Pickar DC PhD
Professor,
Palmer Center for Chiropractic Research,
Palmer College of Chiropractic,
Davenport, Iowa, USA

Madelon Pijnenburg
PhD student,
Department of Rehabilitation Sciences,
University of Leuven,
Leuven, Belgium

N. Peter Reeves PhD
Assistant Professor,
Department of Osteopathic Surgical Specialties,
College of Osteopathic Medicine,
Michigan State University,
East Lansing, Michigan, USA

Sidney M. Rubinstein DC, PhD
Senior Researcher,
Department of Epidemiology and Biostatistics
and EMGO Institute for Health and Care Research,
VU University Medical Centre,
Amsterdam, The Netherlands

Shirley A. Sahrmann PT PhD FAPTA
Professor,
Program in Physical Therapy,
Department of Cell Biology and Physiology
and Department of Neurology and Neurophysiology,
Washington University School of Medicine at Washington
University Medical Center,
St Louis, Missouri, USA

Jaap H. van Dieën PhD
Professor of Biomechanics,
MOVE Research Institute Amsterdam,
Faculty of Human Movement Sciences,
VU University Amsterdam,
Amsterdam, The Netherlands

Linda R. Van Dillen PT PhD
Associate Director,
Musculoskeletal Research, Research Division,
Program in Physical Therapy;
Associate Professor,
Program in Physical Therapy
and Department of Orthopaedic Surgery,
Washington University School of Medicine at Washington
University Medical Center,
St Louis, Missouri, USA

Marienke van Middelkoop PhD
Assistant Professor,
Department of General Practice,
Erasmus Medical Centre,
Rotterdam, The Netherlands

Maurits van Tulder
Professor of Health Technology Assessment,
Department of Epidemiology and Biostatistics,
Department of Health Sciences
and EMGO Institute for Health and Care Research,
VU University Medical Centre,
Amsterdam, The Netherlands

Arianne Verhagen PhD
Associate Professor, Department of General Practice,
Erasmus Medical Centre,
Rotterdam, The Netherlands

Preface: A meeting of minds on spine control

Paul W. Hodges[1]; Jaap H. van Dieën[2]; Jacek Cholewicki[3]
1. NHMRC Centre of Clinical Research Excellence in Spinal Pain, Injury and Health, School of Health and Rehabilitation Sciences, University of Queensland, Brisbane, Queensland, Australia
2. MOVE Research Institute Amsterdam, Faculty of Human Movement Sciences, VU University Amsterdam, Amsterdam, The Netherlands
3. Department of Osteopathic Surgical Specialties, College of Osteopathic Medicine, Michigan State University, East Lansing, Michigan, USA

There are many different views about how the spine is controlled, how this is changed in spinal pain, whether these changes are relevant to a patient's presentation, and the best options for rehabilitation. The field is evolving rapidly, as are the different opinions. This has led to considerable confusion in both research and clinical practice, and there have been widely publicised debates in the literature and media about the best ways to approach exercise interventions in low back and pelvic pain.

The rapid expansion of knowledge, and the apparent divergence in interpretation of the available data, provided the impetus to convene a meeting of experts in the field. The aims of this meeting were to summarize what is known about the field, to identify areas of convergence and divergence of understanding and interpretation, and to consider the clinical implications. In the context of this meeting and book, 'motor control' has been broadly defined as the combination of neurophysiological and biomechanical mechanisms that contribute to control of the spine.

A summit meeting of international experts was hosted in November 2009 by the Centre of Clinical Research Excellence in Spinal Pain Injury and Health, which is competitively funded by a grant from the National Health and Medical Research Council of Australia. The organizing team of PH, JvD and JC devised a list of international experts who represent different disciplines (Biomechanics, Chiropractic, Clinical Trials, Engineering, Ergonomics, Kinesiology/Exercise Physiology, Medicine, Neuroscience, Pain Science, Physiotherapy/Physical Therapy), different research methods, and different views. Of the nominated invitees, 83% agreed to participate and ultimately 70% attended the meeting. The invitees were expert basic scientists and expert clinicians. The meeting was structured to involve presentations by all attendees and each was requested to nominate the areas of convergence and divergence within the field. These areas were reviewed by the organizing team and moderator who then divided them thematically into five topics based on prevalence of nominations for each specific area. The five topics were presented to the group and each was discussed with the ultimate aim of generating a statement that best described the theme. Each theme was allocated time for discussion based on the identification of:

- What is known?
- What are the main issues?
- What are the areas of convergence and divergence of opinion?
- What are the key questions that need to be answered?

During each session, discussants were nominated for each theme, who provided a list of their responses to the above questions, and the group discussed the list. There was opportunity to remove, combine or add issues based on consensus of the group. This was followed by presentation by each discussant to address the issues and moderated discussion. The discussion was followed and thematically organized under each of the issues. At the end of the session the major themes were reviewed and additional discussion was undertaken as required. After the session a summary of the thematically arranged discussion of each issue within each theme was sent to the attendees for comments and clarification. No attempt was made to prioritize the order of importance of the issues, as each was considered to add value to the understanding of motor control of the spine. The final result was a list of key themes and issues that were considered necessary to address in order to progress understanding in the field. The ultimate goal was to identify important areas of study, without providing an exhaustive list. A critical aspect was consideration of relevance for clinical management (or prevention) of low back and pelvic pain. Each topic was then formulated into a summary chapter for inclusion in this volume in Part 5. During 2010–2011 these chapters were reviewed, revised and updated, culminating in the versions included here.

The field is at an exciting phase of expansion, but there remains the challenge to prove the relevance of consideration of motor control issues in the management of spinal pain. This volume provides a review of the current state-of-the-art in understanding on the topic of spine control, and a wealth of research and clinical questions that are ripe for picking. We hope readers of the book will be challenged and excited by the information, and ultimately stimulated to think deeply about the relevance of motor control to low back and pelvic pain and opportunities for clinical and laboratory research.

PH, JvD, JC

Chapter | 1 |

Introduction: convergence and divergence of opinions on spinal control

Paul W. Hodges*, Jaap H. van Dieën† and Jacek Cholewicki‡
*NHMRC Centre of Clinical Research Excellence in Spinal Pain, Injury and Health, School of Health and Rehabilitation Sciences, University of Queensland, Brisbane, Queensland, Australia, †MOVE Research Institute Amsterdam, Faculty of Human Movement Sciences, VU University Amsterdam, Amsterdam, The Netherlands and ‡Department of Osteopathic Surgical Specialties, College of Osteopathic Medicine, Michigan State University, East Lansing, Michigan, USA

CHAPTER CONTENTS

It is well defended and accepted that control of the spine and pelvis depends on the contribution of active, passive and control systems (Panjabi 1992). In this interpretation of spine physiology, ideal control relies on the appropriate passive support, supplemented with muscle forces that are coordinated by the nervous system. Conversely, changes in any of these systems can lead to less than optimal control and this has formed the basis of a range of rehabilitation strategies that aim to restore control and reduce pain and disability or the potential for further pain or injury. Although the theoretical underpinning is relatively straightforward, there is variable evidence for the many assumptions that underlie the understanding of 'spine control' and the way in which it may be modified with pain and/or injury or the manner in which aspects of spine control may be a precursor to development of pain and/or injury. An area of considerable variation in opinion is how this model can be applied to clinical practice for the treatment of people with low back and pelvic pain.

Low back and pelvic pain is a major issue facing the modern world. The economic burden of musculoskeletal pain is second only to cardiovascular disease (Australian Bureau of Statistics 2001) and of that burden, spinal complaints contribute the greatest percentage due to long-term disability. Low back pain (LBP) is the most common chronic pain in Australia (Blyth et al. 2001), and the most common work-related condition in Western society. Recurrence and persistence of symptoms are major issues in LBP and are associated with the majority of its health care and social costs. Persistent LBP is increasing and its prevalence has doubled in the last 14 years (Freburger et al. 2009). Although clinical guidelines promote the view that acute LBP has a favourable prognosis with most people recovered in 6 weeks (Koes et al. 2001), systematic reviews of prospective trials suggest that 73% of people experience at least one recurrence in 12 months of an acute episode, and pain and disability have only recovered by 58% at one month (Pengel et al. 2003). Further recovery is slow (Pengel et al. 2003; Henschke et al. 2009). Identification of modifiable factors associated with LBP is a key objective in the international research agenda. However, reviews of risk factors provide less than encouraging results (Linton 2000; Pincus et al. 2002). Even factors that have been purported to have the strongest relationship to outcome, such as psychosocial aspects of distress (Pincus et al. 2002) and job satisfaction (Linton 2000), can only account for a small proportion of the variability (Linton 2000; Young Casey et al. 2008). There is no evidence for an association between biological factors such as trunk muscle strength or endurance, or range of motion and LBP outcome (Hamberg-van Reenen et al. 2007). However, in clinical practice and many fields of research, it has been proposed that 'spine control' is related to low back and pelvic pain and investigation of this promising notion is worthy of a concerted research effort.

There are considerable promising data of changes in spine control as a potential candidate factor underpinning the development and persistence of low back and pelvic pain from cross-sectional studies (Hodges and Richardson 1996; MacDonald et al. 2009) and some longitudinal studies (Cholewicki et al. 2005). Positive outcomes from clinical trials, that have been summarized and subjected to meta-analyses in a number of systematic reviews (Ferreira et al. 2006; Macedo et al. 2009), provide additional strength to the argument that consideration of 'spine control' in the management of low back and pelvic pain is worthwhile and promising.

The counter argument is that biological aspects are less important than psychosocial aspects of pain, and that compromised spine control may be present but neither sufficient nor necessary for the perpetuation of pain. Criticism of the biological model of pain has come from a number of sources. For instance, the lack of a one-to-one relationship between indications of structural damage on diagnostic imaging and pain is commonly used as an argument against the importance of mechanical injury in its origin. However, such argumentation could be used similarly to deny the relation between smoking and lung cancer; not every person with lung cancer is or was a smoker, nor does every smoker develop lung cancer. A probabilistic model is more appropriate here and structural abnormalities are strong risk factors for LBP.

Current evidence suggests we cannot reject the contribution of biological issues to development and persistence of pain. The quality of 'spine control' which determines the nature and magnitude of loading on spinal structures is likely to be a key factor in this equation. However, within the consideration of spine control there are different interpretations and opinions. There are differing opinions regarding the most appropriate theoretical models to understand the systems; this extends to biomechanical/ engineering models, neurophysiological models of control of motor output and sensory input, and clinical models extrapolating from research and clinical practice to formulate effective treatments for back pain. This book aims to provide a state-of-the-art review of the current understanding of these issues, the areas where opinions converge and diverge, and a road map for consideration of how to resolve the critical questions in the field.

MODELS OF SPINE CONTROL AND EXPERIMENTAL APPROACHES

There are fundamental differences in how people define and model spine control leading to different interpretations of what is optimal. Although early models relied on *static* methods, more recent approaches propose *dynamic*

models and consideration of systems engineering aimed at understanding the mechanisms by which the spine is controlled to meet the demands of everyday activities. A key issue is that different models rely on different assumptions and lead to different conclusions about the optimal mechanisms for spine control and about the consequences of changes in control for the health of the system and, therefore, lead to different extrapolations from science to clinical practice. The first part of this book (Chapters 2–4) takes a look at the state-of-the-art research in terms of modelling and novel experimental approaches that aim to provide insight into the mechanisms for control of this complex system.

MOTOR CONTROL

Motor control is a term that can be used to refer to all aspects of control of movement. This can extend from the motivation within the frontal and other regions of the brain related to the decision to move, the sensory inputs to the system that provide information of the body segments' current location and movement, the various levels of the nervous system that integrate inputs and plan outputs (from simple spinal cord mechanisms to complex supraspinal integration and decision making), the motor output to the muscles (the effector organs of the system), and down to the mechanical properties of the tissues (including muscle mechanics and passive tissues that influence joint mechanics) that influence the manner in which motor commands to muscles relate to movement.

There are many views of how consideration of motor control can be applied to the issue of spine control, and how the nervous system meets the challenge to control the spine and pelvis when considered in the context of the entire human body function. Drawing on the developments in modelling of spine biomechanics highlighted in Chapters 2–4, this view of spine control involves not only control of the spine movement and position that is specific to the demands of the task, but also the contribution of the spine to other physiological functions such as breathing and maintaining whole body equilibrium, to name but a few functions that the nervous system must consider concurrently.

Perhaps the most debated aspect of motor control, as it relates to spine control, is how and why motor control is altered in people with pain and injury. Fundamental questions remain unresolved. Are there issues in motor control that can predispose an individual to development of pain and/or injury? Does motor control adapt in response to pain and injury or is this a factor in the persistence and recurrence of pain? Which aspects of motor control are the most critical for low back and pelvic pain, if at all? Which aspects of motor control, if any, should be addressed in patients with low back and pelvic pain? Part 2 of this book

(Chapters 5–11) tackles these fundamental issues to provide a comprehensive view of the current state of knowledge.

PROPRIOCEPTIVE SYSTEMS

Although sensation is a critical element of motor control, there are issues related to sensory function that require specific consideration. Deficits in proprioception have been described for many conditions related to pain and injury in the musculoskeletal system. From deficits in the acuity to detect input (Lee et al. 2010), to changes in the organization of cortical areas associated with sensory function (Flor et al. 1997). A glaring issue in the low back and pelvic pain literature is why do some studies report differences in sensory function between patients with low back pain and healthy control subjects, whereas others do not? This could be explained by many reasons: differences between patient subgroups, differences between specific parameters of sensory function that have been studied, or other methodological issues (e.g. sample size and reliability/validity of measures). Resolution of this issue and other issues (such as the question of which sources of sensory information are used in the control of the spine, and how this is used) requires deeper understanding of sensory function as it relates to the spine and pelvis. Any extrapolation from research to clinical practice necessitates an understanding of the state-of-the-art of this field. This discussion forms the basis of Part 3 (Chapters 12–14).

SPINAL CONTROL AS A BASIS FOR DESIGN OF CLINICAL TREATMENTS FOR LOW BACK AND PELVIC PAIN

Perhaps the biggest point of apparent divergence of opinion arises when the findings of research and the observations from clinical practice are translated into clinical interventions for the management of low back and pelvic pain. Many clinical programs have been proposed. On the surface, these approaches have often been viewed as divergent and the unique aspects of each are often emphasized to amplify points of difference. But how different are they really? Do they share a common foundation with some specific distinctions based on different interpretations of the literature and clinical observations? Or are they diametrically opposed, mutually exclusive and incapable of being amalgamated into a single broader approach? The debate has often been fuelled by presentation of simplified/reductionist views of an approach to a single element (e.g. activation of deep abdominal muscles in a lying position) rather than presentation of an entire concept, and work that misinterprets the literature and

perpetuates misunderstanding of the scope of some phenomena (e.g. Levin 2002; Lederman 2010). In some ways it may be considered that the indirect debate and criticism within the field is its own worst enemy.

We have reached a critical point in time at which it is necessary to consider where the divergence and convergence of opinions lie in order to move the field forward. Points of convergence require clarification and where divergence remains, studies must be planned to test the relative merits of the different ideas. It is possible that one hypothesis is correct, that several are correct (but it depends on the individual patient as to which alternative approach applies to them) or the research may lead to generation of new hypotheses.

A major aim of this book is to present the arguments and consider the areas for divergence and convergence in opinions. The state-of-the-art evidence on efficacy of exercise interventions for low back and pelvic pain is outlined in Part 4 (Chapter 15), whereas the foundations for different clinical ideas is presented throughout Chapters 2–14 with references to research and the justification for the extrapolations that have been made from basic science to clinical practice.

CONVERGENCE AND DIVERGENCE OF OPINIONS IN 'SPINE CONTROL'

The chapters that make up Part 5 (Chapters 16–20) forge new territory in the debate regarding spine control and its relevance for low back and pelvic pain. These chapters are prepared by collaboration between key players in each area of consideration in the book, and draw the line between the convergence and divergence of viewpoints. These five chapters help resolve some of the misunderstanding within the field and provide a unique insight into what is known, what is unknown and what are the priorities for the future. Key issues that are addressed include:

1. Biomechanical modelling and engineering approaches provide considerable promise to understand the relevance of spine control to low back and pelvic pain. But can this information be used to understand the individual patient and design treatment? Chapter 16 considers this and other areas of convergence and divergence of opinion in modelling of spinal control.
2. Multiple groups are working on the challenge to subgroup individuals with low back and pelvic pain for the targeting of interventions (Chapter 17). Although this approach is logical, different approaches exist, it cannot *a priori* be assumed that subgrouping improves outcomes, and there are many pitfalls and challenges for the development of clinical methods and the subsequent validation of these approaches.

3. Whether differences in motor control between patients and healthy controls are a cause or consequence of low back and pelvic pain requires consideration (Chapter 18). This is not a trivial question to resolve as it requires complex experimental methods, and the fact that changes in motor control could be either, neither or both cause and consequence.

4. If and how sensory function is affected in low back pain and injury, if this is relevant for development or persistence of symptoms, and how this could be addressed in low back and pelvic pain is far from resolved. This issue is debated in Chapter 19.

5. An issue of considerable discussion in the literature and a topic of surprising convergence of fundamental concepts – but also considerable divergence of opinions – is how experimental and

clinical observations can be extrapolated to effective clinical interventions. Chapter 20 makes a major contribution by highlighting where the views converge and diverge and presents a road map for how to progress knowledge in this sometimes-contentious issue.

Finally, Part 6 of the book (Chapter 21) highlights all that has been gained from identification of the state-of-the-art of understanding across the field of spine control and discusses ways that this has been applied to the design and implementation of treatment for people with low back and pelvic pain. The result is a multifaceted approach to optimization of motor control that considers individual differences within a multi-dimensional framework that includes consideration of the bio-psycho-social model of pain.

REFERENCES

Australian Bureau of Statistics, 2001. Musculoskeletal Conditions in Australia: a snapshot.

Blyth, F.M., March, L.M., Brnabic, A.J., Jorm, L.R., Williamson, M., Cousins, M.J., 2001. Chronic pain in Australia: a prevalence study. Pain 89, 127–134.

Cholewicki, J., Silfies, S., Shah, R., Greene, H., Reeves, P., Alvi, K., et al., 2005. Delayed trunk muscle reflex responses increase the risk of low back pain injuries. Spine 30, 2614–2620.

Ferreira, P.H., Ferreira, M.L., Maher, C.G., Herbert, R.D., Refshauge, K., 2006. Specific stabilization exercise for spinal and pelvic pain: a systematic review. Aust J Physiother 52, 79–88.

Flor, H., Braun, C., Elbert, T., Birbaumer, N., 1997. Extensive reorganization of primary somatosensory cortex in chronic back pain patients. Neurosci Lett 224, 5–8.

Freburger, J.K., Holmes, G.M., Agans, R.P., Jackman, A.M., Darter, J.D., Wallace, A.S., et al., 2009. The rising prevalence of chronic low back pain. Arch Intern Med 169, 251–258.

Hamberg-van Reenen, H.H., Ariëns, G.A., Blatter, B.M., van Mechelen, W., Bongers, P.M., 2007. A systematic review of the relation between physical capacity and future low back and neck/shoulder pain. Pain 130, 93–107.

Henschke, N., Maher, C., Refshauge, K., Herbert, R.D., Cumming, R., Bleasel, J. et al., 2009. Prognosis in patients with recent onset low back pain in Australian primary care: inception cohort study. BMJ 337, a171.

Hodges, P.W., Richardson, C.A., 1996. Inefficient muscular stabilization of the lumbar spine associated with low back pain: a motor control evaluation of transversus abdominis. Spine 21, 2640–2650.

Koes, B.W., van Tulder, M.W., Ostelo, R., Kim Burton, A., Waddell, G., 2001. Clinical guidelines for the management of low back pain in primary care: an international comparison. Spine 26, 2504–2513; discussion 13–14.

Lederman, E., 2010. The myth of core stability. J Bodywork Movement Ther [review]. 14, 84–98.

Lee, A.S., Cholewicki, J., Reeves, N.P., Zazulak, B.T., Mysliwiec, L.W., 2010. Comparison of trunk proprioception between patients with low back pain and healthy controls. Arch Phys Med Rehabil 91, 1327–1331.

Levin, S.M., 2002. The tensegrity-truss as a model for spine mechanics: biotensegrity. J Mech Med Biol 2, 375–388.

Linton, S.J., 2000. A review of psychological risk factors in back and neck pain. Spine 25, 1148–1156.

MacDonald, D., Moseley, G.L., Hodges, P.W., 2009. Why do some patients

keep hurting their back? Evidence of ongoing back muscle dysfunction during remission from recurrent back pain. Pain 142, 183–188.

Macedo, L.G., Maher, C.G., Latimer, J., McAuley, J.H., 2009. Motor control exercise for persistent, nonspecific low back pain: a systematic review. Phys Ther 89, 9–25.

Panjabi, M.M., 1992. The stabilizing system of the spine. Part I. Function, dysfunction, adaptation, and enhancement. J Spinal Disorders 5, 383–389.

Pengel, L.H., Herbert, R.D., Maher, C.G., Refshauge, K.M., 2003. Acute low back pain: systematic review of its prognosis. BMJ 327 (7410), 323.

Pincus, T., Burton, A.K., Vogel, S., Field, A.P., 2002. A systematic review of psychological factors as predictors of chronicity/disability in prospective cohorts of low back pain. Spine. 27, E109–E120.

Young Casey, C., Greenberg, M.A., Nicassio, P.M., Harpin, R.E., Hubbard, D., 2008. Transition from acute to chronic pain and disability: a model including cognitive, affective, and trauma factors. Pain 134, 69–79.

Part | 1 |

Models of the spine

Chapter | 2 |

Spine systems science: a primer on the systems approach

N. Peter Reeves and Jacek Cholewicki
Department of Osteopathic Surgical Specialties, College of Osteopathic Medicine, Michigan State University, East Lansing, Michigan, USA

THE RATIONALE FOR THE SYSTEMS APPROACH

The prevalent method for studying clinical conditions is based on a reductionist approach in which the problem is broken down into smaller and smaller parts to isolate elements of the condition. This type of approach is well suited for containable diseases such as local infection, but less helpful when the problem is multi-factorial and more dispersed. Reductionism becomes less helpful when the process of dividing a problem into its parts leads to a loss of important information necessary to solve the problem (Ahn et al. 2006). The loss of information stems from the omission of the interaction effect between these smaller

parts and how these interactions affect the behaviour of the system as a whole. For instance, predicting the behaviour of a new aeroplane design would be impossible by designing the parts of the system in isolation and not considering how these individuals parts would interact with one another.

Starting in the twentieth century, it became apparent that society and modern technology was becoming increasingly more complex, and as a result, a new approach was required to analyze and resolve problems. Out of necessity, the branch of science known as systems science emerged. With a systems approach, it was now possible to study complex systems in a way that not only included their parts, but also how these parts interacted to affect the behaviour of the entire system. Over time, the application of systems science spawned the field of systems medicine, and with this, expanded medicine beyond the realm of reductionism. Systems medicine is defined as the application of the systems approach to the prevention of, understanding and modulation of, and recovery from developmental disorders and pathological processes in human health (Clermont et al. 2009). It adopts principles of systems science to focus on uniquely human attributes, such as genetics, environment and behaviour (Federoff and Gostin 2009). Benefits of the systems approach include individualized, multi-dimensional treatment that is both time- and space-sensitive, and which can explore synergistic effects (Ahn et al. 2006).

Depending on the nature of the clinical condition, both reductionist and systems approaches can be advantageous. Which approach is better suited for studying low back pain (LBP)? One of the landmark hypotheses in spine research is Panjabi's proposed stability-based model of spine dysfunction leading to chronic pain (Panjabi, 1992a, 1992b). As he stated, the behaviour of the spine system is affected by the interaction between various subsystems:

the passive subsystem representing the spinal column, the active subsystem representing the spinal muscles, and the control subsystem representing the neural elements. He suggested that impairment in one or more subsystems can be accommodated by the other systems, but only up to a certain level. Inability to adequately compensate leads to chronic dysfunction and pain. This hypothesis has gained popularity and has led to a paradigm shift in LBP treatment. Unfortunately, this hypothesis has not been rigorously tested. This is partly because the reductionist approach we currently employ cannot be used to test such a hypothesis. To do so requires a systems approach since the focus of the problem is not on isolated subsystems, but instead on the interactions between these subsystems.

Although systems medicine uses the general principles of the systems approach to study clinical conditions, it typically does not adopt mathematical systems theory, which represents the formal end of the approach. This theory is useful in framing the problem and developing models to study general properties of systems such as stability, performance, robustness and goal-directedness. Model validity is always a concern with this type of approach. But if models can be developed that accurately reflect the spine system, significant insight can be gained. Moreover, given the interdisciplinary nature of systems science, this type of framework could help integrate data from the spine research community thus leveraging our expertise and resources.

The goal of this chapter is to serve as a primer to develop a common understanding regarding the systems approach. Given that all systems must be stable to fulfil their intended goal, the first part of the chapter will use systems theory to address the questions: what is stability, and how is it achieved? Other characteristics of systems such as performance and robustness will also be described. Later in the chapter, we will use a stick-balancing task to describe concepts of control, which will then be used to elucidate possible spine system impairments. Finally, we will present a possible roadmap, which can be used to integrate future spine research efforts in the community.

SPINE (IN)STABILITY: AN UNSTABLE TERM

As a community, we have the right to develop our own set of definitions that we deem 'useful'. However, if these definitions lead to confusion and unnecessary debate, or are not stable with time, then the community may deem them 'not useful'. A case can be made that the term spine (in) stability has not been enlightening, as illustrated by the lack of consensus about its definition (Nachemson 1985, Reeves et al. 2007a). Other disciplines have struggled with

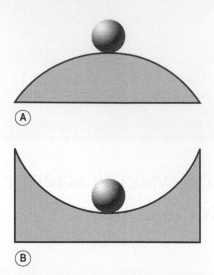

Figure 2.1 (A) Unstable and (B) stable ball position.

the concept of stability, and in the process have developed more rigorous definitions (Reeves and Cholewicki 2003). Using concepts from systems science, we will describe what stability is and how it is achieved.

What is stability?

Stability of a system, whether it is stationary or moving, is tested by applying a small perturbation and observing the new behaviour. If the new behaviour is approximately the same as the old, the system is stable. If the new behaviour becomes indistinguishable from the old behaviour, the system is asymptotically stable. Finally, if the new behaviour differs significantly from the old behaviour, the system is unstable.

Using a ball on a hill as an example (Fig. 2.1a), there is no size of perturbation that can be applied that will keep the ball in the original undisturbed position; hence this system is unstable. Whereas a ball in a valley (Fig. 2.1b), following a perturbation, will oscillate and settle in the undisturbed position – assuming that there is some friction in the system.

This definition of stability is generic and applicable to any system. It is important to point out that stability is context dependent, which may explain some of the confusion when applying it in the context of the spine system (Reeves et al. 2007b). For instance, are we interested in mechanical stability of the spine, such as controlling the displacement of individual vertebrae following a perturbation, or are we interested in performing tasks without injuring spinal tissue or experiencing pain? At this point, it is much easier to address mechanical stability of the spine, but the same framework could be applied to address injury and pain. For this chapter, we will primarily focus on mechanical stability.

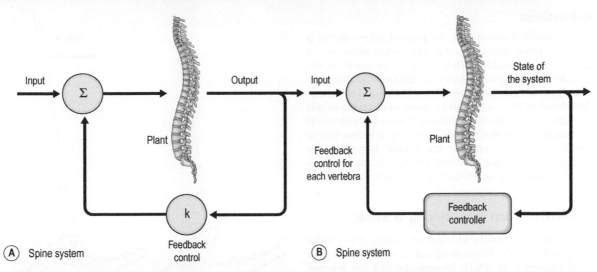

Figure 2.2 (A) Simple and (B) complex examples of feedback control of the spine. *Reproduced from, Reeves, P.N., Narenda, K.S., Cholewicki, J., 2007b. Spine stability: the six blind men and the elephant. Clinical Biomechanics 22, 266–274, with permission from Elsevier.*

How is stability achieved?

Given that the spine has similar characteristics to an inverted pendulum, it can be shown to be unstable; therefore some form of control must be applied to ensure that it is behaving in a stable manner. The principal approach for stabilizing any system is feedback control. With feedback control, information concerning the output of the system is fed back and used to modify the input (Fig. 2.2a,b). Using systems terminology, the isolated system is called the *plant*, which represents the osteoligamentous spine. The logic by which the control input is generated from the output is the *controller*, which represents a feedback controller. The plant (osteoligamentous spine) together with the controller (feedback control) is the overall system (spine system). A simple example of a feedback control spine system is shown in Figure 2.2a.

In Figure 2.2a, the control input to the plant is proportional to its output. This is indicated by the feedback gain denoted by k. Feedback can be positive or negative. If positive, the system is unstable since the force applied to the system is in the same direction as the displacement (i.e. ball on top of the hill). For stability, negative feedback is used so that the force is applied in the opposite direction to the displacement (i.e. ball in the valley). Therefore, the goal of feedback control for the inherently unstable spine is to give it stable behaviour. To do this, the controller's negative feedback must be larger than the positive feedback of the unstable spine. Stated differently, the overall system (spine and feedback controller) must have negative feedback.

Figure 2.2a shows the simplest form of feedback control for the spine system. In reality, the spine system is significantly more complex. Multiple feedback signals come from sensory receptors that convey information about the state of the entire system (Fig. 2.2b). These signals are processed by the feedback controller (CNS), which in turn, generates many control signals to be applied to the different segmental levels. Unlike the feedback gain represented by k in the simple system, the controller consists of a sophisticated network of neural connections, which applies the logic for transferring sensory information into control input.

There are a number of feedback pathways for the spine system: intrinsic properties of the joint and muscles, which apply resistive forces to the spine instantaneously; reflexes, which apply their control input after short, medium and long delays following a disturbance; and voluntary corrections, which also take time to respond. It is important to note that delays in feedback control can destabilize the system. The longer the delay the more problematical it is. This will be discussed in more detail later.

Performance

Once the stability of a system is established, the interest shifts to its performance. *Performance* reflects how closely and rapidly the disturbed position of the system tends to the undisturbed position. Accuracy and speed are important attributes of any control system. Following a perturbation, a system performing well will have behaviour that resembles the undisturbed behaviour, indicating that the error between a disturbed and undisturbed system is minimal. For asymptotically stable systems, a system performing well will also converge to the undisturbed position in a short time interval.

Robustness

From a practical standpoint, the issue of spine stability is probably not a major concern. The overall spine system appears to be stable. What is more pertinent is the question, is the spine robust? For instance, is the spine sufficiently robust to recover from both small and large disturbances? Or is a person's control of the spine robust enough to accommodate various types of impairment? *Robustness* reflects the level of tolerance a system has to disturbances or changes in the system properties. For example, some individuals may be less tolerant to degenerative disc disease or whole body vibration than others.

Lessons from balancing a stick

There are many subtle nuances of control that can be explained with the example of balancing a stick in your hand (Reeves et al. 2011). Because the stick has inverted pendulum characteristics (like the spine), it is unstable and requires some form of feedback control to keep it upright.

We can test stability of the upright stick by basically doing nothing. If you keep your hand in the same position, the stick will eventually fall over. Therefore, to stabilize the stick, you need to move your hand in a controlled fashion in order to keep the centre-of-pressure (COP) acting on the hand under the centre-of-mass (COM) of the stick. Although it may not be obvious, how you move your hand is based on feedback control.

As discussed earlier, feedback control uses information about the state of the system to apply control. For stick balancing, this means you must track the stick and use this information to determine where to move your hand. Therefore, if you cannot track the stick, say for instance you close your eyes, than it becomes impossible to keep the stick upright. Or stated in a more general sense, if we cannot track the state of the system, we cannot stabilize it.

When we apply feedback control, there is a minimum amount of information that must be obtained to stabilize the system. For instance, it is obvious that we use our visual system to track the position of the stick, but what is less obvious is the fact that we must also track the velocity of the stick. To demonstrate, we will present two stick-balancing scenarios (Fig. 2.3a,b). In the first scenario, the stick is positioned to the right of the hand and is stationary (velocity = 0). In this situation, you would want to move your hand to the right to bring the COM under the COP. In the second scenario, the stick is in the same position, but is moving to the left. It is unclear in this case which direction to move the hand and it depends on the velocity of the stick. If the stick is moving slowly, you would want to move your hand to the right. But if the stick is moving really fast, to catch the stick would require moving your hand to the left. This simple experiment shows that two independent sets of data, referred to as *states*, are used for

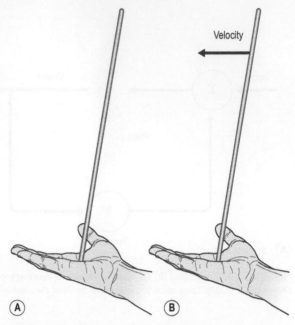

Figure 2.3 (A) Stick is positioned to the right of the hand with zero velocity. (B) Stick is positioned to the right of the hand, but is moving to the left. *Reproduced from Reeves, N.P., Cholewicki, J., 2010. Expanding our view of the spine system.* European Spine Journal 1, *with kind permission of Springer Science and Business Media.*

feedback control. We use position-related feedback, referred to as stiffness, and velocity-related feedback, referred to as damping, to control and stabilize a system with mass. This is an important observation that has significant ramifications for how we study the spine system.

To demonstrate our limited view of the spine system, we recently performed two PubMed searches using the following terms: (i) 'stiffness' AND 'spine' AND 'stability' and (ii) 'damping' AND 'spine' AND 'stability'. Searches (i) and (ii) yielded 234 and 5 hits respectively. If you exchange 'stability' with 'instability' you will obtain similar results. This exercise shows that we have an incomplete picture of the spine system. We need to expand our definition of stability from the current static representation to include dynamics. This transition will be essential if we plan to investigate control aspects of LBP (Reeves and Cholewicki 2010).

Another necessary condition for stability is *controllability*. Now let us consider the task of balancing two sticks, one set in series (Fig. 2.4a) and another in parallel (Fig. 2.4b). In these examples, all sticks are identical, having the same mass and length. Which of these two conditions can be controlled? It is not obvious, but only the sticks in series can be controlled. Even though we cannot apply

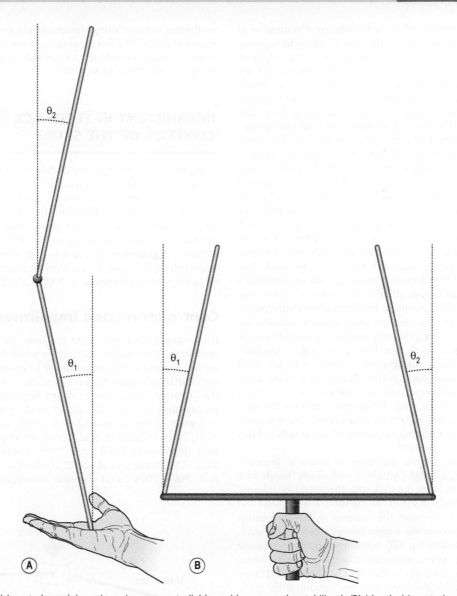

Figure 2.4 (A) Inverted pendulums in series are controllable and hence can be stabilized. (B) Identical inverted pendulums in parallel are not controllable and cannot be stabilized. *Reproduced from Reeves, N.P., Narenda, K.S., Cholewicki, J., 2011, Spine stability: lessons from balancing a stick. Clinical Biomechanics 26, 325–330, with permission from Elsevier.*

control directly to the top stick, by moving the hand, we can change the states of the bottom stick, which in turn can change the states of the top stick. What is important is that movement of the hand will change the position and velocity of the bottom stick in a way that is different than the upper stick. This means we have independent control over the two sticks. Thus, we can use the system's states to generate feedback control to bring both sticks upright, whereas the states of the two sticks in parallel cannot be

independently changed. Consequently, if one stick is bumped or has a different starting position, there is no possible way to bring both sticks to the upright position. If, however, one stick is slightly longer than the other, it now becomes possible to control both sticks. This is because the sticks will have different natural frequencies, meaning they will tend to move at different speeds, which then allows for independent control over the states of the system. One point to note: the closer in lengths the two sticks are, the faster and more forceful control must be to stabilize the system. Also in the case of the sticks in series, we would need fast and forceful control. Can a human balance two sticks? Most likely not. The dynamics of the plant (two sticks) are such that it may require more power than a human controller can apply. This is an issue of force saturation. Also, timing of control becomes an issue. The human controller may not be able to respond fast enough.

Next, we would like to spend some time discussing performance issues. Recall that how we move our hand to keep the stick upright is determined by the position and velocity of the stick. This also implies that the force applied to the stick through the hand will be proportional to the size and rate of stick movement. Consequently, any impairment in control that causes larger and faster stick movement also requires more stabilizing force. This can be demonstrated by balancing the stick and focusing either at the top or near the bottom of the stick. You should notice that focusing higher on the stick makes it easier to balance. You should also notice that focusing lower on the stick results in larger and faster stick movements, which in turn, requires more effort to stabilize the stick. What is causing this impairment? It stems from differences in visual resolution. For a given angular displacement, more linear displacement occurs at higher focal points than lower focal points. Therefore, you are more sensitive to displacement of the stick when you focus at a higher point on the stick. When you can track the stick more precisely, less *noise* enters the system, and the precision of hand positioning improves, which in turn reduces effort to balance the stick.

We will next discuss the issue of *delays* in feedback control. Using a weight attached with elastic bands to a stick, you can balance the stick with the weight in different positions. Which is easier to balance, a stick with the weight at the top or near the bottom? You should find it harder to balance as the weight moves closer to the hand, and in fact, balancing will become impossible at some critical height. As you move the weight closer to the hand, you should notice that the stick will have larger and faster oscillations. With the mass near the bottom of the stick, the stick will tend to fall faster, reflecting a higher natural frequency of the system. Conversely, with the mass at the top of the stick, it will take longer to fall, reflecting a lower natural frequency.

So what causes the stick to become unstable? Force saturation may be a culprit. It is possible that the large and fast movements of the stick require stabilizing forces that are greater than your arm and shoulder muscles can generate. But in this case, instability most likely stems from delays in feedback control. Because your controller has inherent delays, as the stick (plant) moves faster, the CNS (controller) does not have enough time to register the states of the system, process this information and then send commands to move the hand. Controllers with longer delays respond slower, which in turn means they

are limited to controlling slower moving systems. And as demonstrated with a fast moving stick, once the dynamics of the plant are outside the bandwidth of the controller, the system will become unstable.

IMPAIRMENT IN FEEDBACK CONTROL OF THE SPINE

Using lessons from balancing a stick, we can now discuss the issue of impairment in feedback control of the spine. As shown in Figure 2.5, there are a number of sources for impairment. In terms of the controller, these include poor proprioception, faulty control logic, longer delays and decreased resolution in the regulation of muscle force. In addition, degenerative changes to the osteoligamentous spine (plant) can also be considered as impairments in feedback control (Reeves et al. 2007a, 2007b).

Controller-related impairment

If we cannot track the spine precisely, the information used by the CNS will contain noise, which in turn means control applied to the spine will not be precise. Do people with LBP have impaired proprioception? It is unclear from the literature. Some studies report impairment in trunk proprioception with LBP (Field et al. 1997; Gill and Callaghan, 1998; Brumagne et al. 2000; Leinonen et al. 2002, 2003; O'Sullivan et al. 2003), while others find no such impairment (Lam et al. 1999; Koumantakis et al. 2002; Descarreaux et al. 2005; Åsell et al. 2006; Silfies et al. 2007). This could represent heterogeneity in study

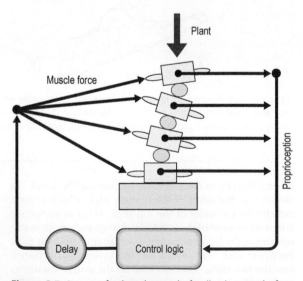

Figure 2.5 Sources for impairment in feedback control of the spine.

populations (O'Sullivan et al. 2003), meaning some subjects in some proprioception studies have impairment while subjects in other studies do not.

Another source of impairment may stem from faulty control logic. For instance, when balancing the stick, there are a number of possible control strategies that belong to a stable set of solutions. For instance, you can balance the stick with short, fast hand movements, or you could use larger, slower hand movements. If the goal is to improve the performance, meaning keeping the stick more upright closer to the equilibrium position, you may choose short, fast hand movements. If you are required to balance the stick for longer periods and fatigue may be an issue, you may choose a less aggressive control strategy, using larger, slower hand movements. We suspect that goals may be different between people with and without LBP, which in turn leads to different control strategies. This may explain some of the muscle recruitment differences between healthy and LBP populations (van Dieën et al. 2003b; Reeves et al. 2006a). Furthermore, there is growing belief that people with LBP may have non-optimal control, which predisposes them to future injury (Brumagne et al. 2008; Hodges et al. 2009). It appears that people with LBP have less variety in control strategies and it is believed that this lack of flexibility in applying the appropriate control strategy leads to impaired spine performance (Hodges and Cholewicki 2007).

Delays may also be relevant to LBP. There are a number of studies that have linked longer trunk muscles' latencies to LBP (Magnusson et al. 1996; Wilder et al. 1996; Radebold et al. 2000, 2001; Reeves et al. 2005; Thomas et al. 2007), although there is also a study showing no link between pain and trunk muscle responses (Hjortskov et al. 2005). Again, this could be an LBP heterogeneity issue or a reflection of experimental nuances. There is also some evidence to suggest that delays may be predisposing to LBP (Cholewicki et al. 2005), although it could be specific to the study group, which was composed of varsity athletes. As shown with stick balancing, delays become more problematical when the dynamics are faster. Therefore, it is possible that the competitive arena could accentuate the problems of delays in this specific population. But it is also possible that other groups could also be vulnerable if their control systems are too slow (e.g. nurses during patient transfers).

Aside from proprioception, noise can also originate from force variability in muscle activation. It is well established that force variability increases with activation (Sherwood et al. 1988; Hamilton et al. 2004), including trunk muscles activation (Sparto et al. 1997; Reeves et al. 2008). There is some speculation that increased coactivation associated with LBP (Marras et al. 2001; van Dieën et al. 2003a) impairs postural performance. We have shown that over-activation of trunk muscles affects postural control during a seated balancing task (Reeves et al. 2006b), which supports this hypothesis. In addition to muscle

force variability, there is some evidence to suggest that people with LBP also experience muscle wasting (Hides et al. 1994), which does not appear to resolve following pain recovery (Hides et al. 1996). This could be problematical by limiting the force capacity of the paraspinal muscles. This is the issue of force saturation. If a disturbance requires a large restorative force to control the spine, it is possible in a person with muscle wasting that the required force exceeds their capacity. The problem becomes what size perturbations the person can withstand. This is an issue of spine robustness.

Plant-related impairment

Based on the static notion of stability that was predominant in the past, *in vitro* work assessing properties of the spine was focussed on flexibility (Panjabi et al. 1984; Crisco et al. 1992; Oxland et al. 1992; Mimura et al. 1994; Oxland et al. 1996; Yingling et al. 1997; Fujiwara et al. 2000b; Krismer et al. 2000; Tanaka et al. 2001), or its reciprocal, stiffness (Schmidt et al. 1998; Haughton et al. 1999; Brown et al. 2002; Stokes et al. 2002) (as noted already, stiffness, which represents position-dependent feedback, by itself does not ensure stability in the dynamic sense). There is considerable evidence that stiffness of a spine is decreased following disc injury (Panjabi et al. 1984; Crisco et al. 1992; Oxland et al. 1992; Schmidt et al. 1998) and in degenerative disc disease (DDD) (Haughton et al. 1999; Fujiwara et al. 2000a; Krismer et al. 2000; Tanaka et al. 2001). The effects of DDD may produce mixed results depending on the specific types and grade of degenerative changes. In terms of degeneration severity, the most advanced stage of DDD characterized by disc space collapse, has been shown to decrease spine motion (Fujiwara et al. 2000a), suggesting the spine becomes stiffer (Fujiwara et al. 2000b). These findings support the notion that the severely degenerate spine regains some of its stabilizing potential (Kirkaldy-Willis and Farfan 1982), which may explain why LBP prevalence grows steadily with age, peaks at 60, and then declines rapidly (Andersson 1999; Loney and Stratford 1999).

In terms of damping properties of the spine, information in the literature is sparse. Most of the work has investigated the response of the disc to various loading rates in compression (Yingling et al. 1997; Race et al. 2000; Nuckley et al. 2005; Elias et al. 2006; Kemper et al. 2007). These studies found that 'compressive stiffness' in the spine increased with higher strain rates, which suggests that a damping component exists. Surprisingly, the use of such improper nomenclature is common throughout the literature, illustrating a lack of understanding of the characterization of dynamic systems. Only recently has *in vitro* testing quantified damping of a lumbar spine segment in the axial direction (Izambert et al. 2003) and more recently in the sagittal plane (Crisco et al. 2007). To our knowledge, there are no studies investigating the effects of disc injury or DDD on the spine's damping properties. Given that fluid flow is likely altered in a degenerated disc, it is also likely that the viscous properties of a spine with DDD would be different from a healthy spine.

THE SYSTEMS APPROACH APPLIED TO LBP

Currently in our lab, we are developing methods to integrate data obtained from *in vitro* testing of human cadaveric spines and *in vivo* testing of live subjects' control of the spine. With *in vitro* testing, we will define the plant for the spine system by assessing its stiffness and damping. With *in vivo* testing, we will define the controller for the spine system, which includes aspects such as feedback gains, delays and noise. The basic methods for defining the plant and the controller are the same. We apply perturbations to the system of interest and record the response of the system. Because we have knowledge of the input and output signals, we can identify parameters of the system. With the right type of perturbations, we can define the system completely – meaning we can predict the response of the system to any type of disturbance. This is what makes systems science so powerful. We now have the ability to manipulate elements of the system to assess their effect on the overall systems behaviour. For instance, we could change the osteoligamentous spine to reflect degenerative changes and determine if the controller is still capable of stabilizing the spine. We began performing some simulations like this and found that some individuals have more robust control than others. In some, degenerative changes make no difference in the performance of the spine, while in others the system is significantly affected (although not unstable in the true sense). With these models of the spine system, we can also simulate degraded control. We recently investigated the effects of delays of postural control using a dynamic model and found that longer delays associated with LBP impaired spine performance, leading to more trunk displacement and trunk muscle effort (Reeves et al. 2009). The idea with this type of approach is that possible sources of impairment documented in the literature can now be assessed to determine if they are clinically relevant in isolation or in combination. Moreover, we can also assess how the different subsystems of the spine interact and adapt to accommodate different types of impairments. Such knowledge is necessary to target various impairments through specific and individualized rehabilitation programmes. These are key features of the systems approach mentioned in the introduction.

FINAL REMARKS

The spine is extremely complex. Two approaches can be applied to deal with complexity: the reductionist approach and the systems approach. Reductionism has been used in the past to study various subsystems of the spine and helped us understand how those individual parts function. Using a systems approach, it will now be possible to integrate these data, leveraging the expertise and resources of the research community, to understand how various parts of the system interact to affect the behaviour of the entire spine system. With this type of approach, it will be possible to address some long-standing research questions, such as Panjabi's stability-based model of spine dysfunction leading to chronic pain. Benefits of the systems approach include a new framework for identification of impairment, which in turn can be used to target rehabilitation. The first step in this effort is to present the concepts inherent to systems science, so that a common understanding can be formed within the spine community – the purpose of our chapter.

ACKNOWLEDGEMENTS

The authors would like to thank Professor Narendra from Yale University for his insight into systems science.
Part of this chapter is reprinted from *Clinical Biomechanics*, 22(3), 266–274, N. Peter Reeves, Kumpati S. Narendra, Jacek Cholewicki, 2007; Spine stability: the six blind men and the elephant, with permission from Elsevier.

REFERENCES

Ahn, A.C., Tewari, M., Poon, C.S., Phillips, R.S., 2006. The clinical applications of a systems approach. PLoS Med 3, e209.

Andersson, G.B., 1999. Epidemiological features of chronic low-back pain. Lancet 354, 581–585.

Åsell, M., Sjölander, P., Kerschbaumer, H., Djupsjöbacka, M., 2006. Are lumbar repositioning errors larger among patients with chronic low back pain compared with asymptomatic subjects? Arch Phys Med Rehabil 87, 1170–1176.

Brown, M.D., Holmes, D.C., Heiner, A.D., 2002. Measurement of cadaver lumbar spine motion segment stiffness. Spine (Phila Pa 1976) 27, 918–922.

Brumagne, S., Cordo, P., Lysens, R., Verschueren, S., Swinnen, S., 2000. The role of paraspinal muscle spindles in lumbosacral position sense in individuals with and without low back pain. Spine 25, 989–994.

Brumagne, S., Janssens, L., Knapen, S., Claeys, K., Suuden-Johanson, E., 2008. Persons with recurrent low back pain exhibit a rigid postural control strategy. European Spine J 17, 1177–1184.

Cholewicki, J., Silfies, S.P., Shah, R.A., Greene, H.S., Reeves, N.P., Alvi, K., et al., 2005. Delayed trunk muscle reflex responses increase the risk of low back injuries. Spine 30, 2614–2620.

Clermont, G., Auffray, C., Moreau, Y., Rocke, D.M., Dalevi, D., Dubhashi, D., et al., 2009. Bridging the gap between systems biology and medicine. Genome Med 1, 88.

Crisco, J., Fujita, L., Spenciner, D., 2007. The dynamic flexion/extension properties of the lumbar spine in vitro using a novel pendulum system. J Biomech 40, 2767–2773.

Crisco, J.J., Panjabi, M.M., Yamamoto, I., Oxland, T.R., 1992. Euler stability of the human ligamentous lumbar spine. Part II: experiment. Clin Biomech 7, 27–32.

Descarreaux, M., Blouin, J.S., Teasdale, N., 2005. Repositioning accuracy and movement parameters in low back pain subjects and healthy control subjects. Eur Spine J 14, 185–191.

Elias, P.Z., Nuckley, D.J., Ching, R.P., 2006. Effect of loading rate on the compressive mechanics of the immature baboon cervical spine. J Biomech Eng 128, 18.

Federoff, H.J., Gostin, L.O., 2009. Evolving from reductionism to holism: is there a future for systems medicine? JAMA 302, 994–996.

Field, E., Abdel-Moty, E., Loudon, J., 1997. The effect of back injury and load on ability to replicate a novel posture. J Back Musculoskel Rehabil 8, 199–207.

Fujiwara, A., Lim, T.H., An, H.S., Tanaka, N., Jeon, C.H., Andersson, G.B., et al., 2000a. The effect of disc degeneration and facet joint osteoarthritis on the segmental flexibility of the lumbar spine. Spine (Phila Pa 1976) 25, 3036–3044.

Fujiwara, A., Tamai, K., An, H.S., Kurihashi, T., Lim, T.H., Yoshida, H., et al., 2000b. The relationship between disc degeneration, facet joint osteoarthritis, and stability of the degenerative lumbar spine. J Spinal Disord 13, 444–450.

Gill, K.P., Callaghan, M.J., 1998. The measurement of lumbar proprioception in individuals with and without low back pain. Spine 23, 371–377.

Hamilton, A., Jones, K., Wolpert, D., 2004. The scaling of motor noise with muscle strength and motor unit number in humans. Exp Brain Res 157.

Haughton, V.M., Lim, T.H., An, H., 1999. Intervertebral disk appearance correlated with stiffness of lumbar spinal motion segments. Am J Neuroradiol 20, 1161–1165.

Hides, J.A., Stokes, M.J., Saide, M., Jull, G.A., Cooper, D.H., 1994. Evidence of lumbar multifidus muscle wasting ipsilateral to symptoms in patients with acute/subacute low back pain. Spine (Phila Pa 1976) 19, 165–172.

Hides, J.A., Richardson, C.A., Jull, G.A., 1996. Multifidus muscle recovery is not automatic after resolution of acute, first-episode low back pain. Spine (Phila Pa 1976) 21, 2763–2769.

Hjortskov, N., Essendrop, M., Skotte, J., Fallentin, N., 2005. The effect of delayed-onset muscle soreness on stretch reflexes in human low back muscles. Scand J Med Sci Sports 15, 409–415.

Hodges, P.W., Cholewicki, J., 2007. Functional control of the spine. In: Vleeming, A., Mooney, V., Stoeckart, R. (eds), Movement, Stability and Lumbopelvic Pain: integration of research and therapy, 2nd edn. Churchill Livingstone/Elsevier, Edinburgh.

Hodges, P., Van Den Hoorn, W., Dawson, A., Cholewicki, J., 2009. Changes in the mechanical properties of the trunk in low back pain may be associated with recurrence. J Biomech 42, 61–66.

Izambert, O., Mitton, D., Thourot, M., Lavaste, F., 2003. Dynamic stiffness and damping of human intervertebral disc using axial oscillatory displacement under a free mass system. Eur Spine J 12, 562–566.

Kemper, A.R., Mcnally, C., Duma, S.M., 2007. The influence of strain rate on the compressive stiffness properties of human lumbar intervertebral discs. Biomed Sci Instrum 43, 176–181.

Kirkaldy-Willis, W.H., Farfan, H.F., 1982. Instability of the lumbar spine. Clin Orthop Relat Res 110–123.

Koumantakis, G.A., Winstanley, J., Oldham, J.A., 2002. Thoracolumbar proprioception in individuals with and without low back pain: intratester reliability, clinical applicability, and validity. J Orthop Sports Phys Ther 32, 327–335.

Krismer, M., Haid, C., Behensky, H., Kapfinger, P., Landauer, F., Rachbauer, F., 2000. Motion in lumbar functional spine units during side bending and axial rotation moments depending on the degree of degeneration. Spine (Phila Pa 1976) 25, 2020–2027.

Lam, S.S., Jull, G., Treleaven, J., 1999. Lumbar spine kinesthesia in patients with low back pain. J Orthop Sports Phys Ther 29, 294–299.

Leinonen, V., Maatta, S., Taimela, S., Herno, A., Kankaanpaa, M., Partanen, J., et al., 2002. Impaired lumbar movement perception in association with postural stability and motor- and somatosensory-evoked potentials in lumbar spinal stenosis. Spine 27, 975–983.

Leinonen, V., Kankaanpaa, M., Luukkonen, M., Kansanen, M., Hanninen, O., Airaksinen, O., et al., 2003. Lumbar paraspinal muscle function, perception of lumbar position, and postural control in discherniation-related back pain. Spine 28, 842–848.

Loney, P.L., Stratford, P.W., 1999. The prevalence of low back pain in adults: a methodological review of the literature. Phys Ther 79, 384–396.

Magnusson, M.L., Aleksiev, A., Wilder, D.G., Pope, M.H., Spratt, K., Lee, S.H., et al., 1996. Unexpected load and asymmetric posture as etiologic factors in low back pain. Eur Spine J 5, 23–35.

Marras, W.S., Davis, K.G., Maronitis, A.B., 2001. A non-MVC EMG normalization technique for the trunk musculature: Part 2, Validation and use to predict spinal loads. J Electromyogr Kinesiol 11, 11–18.

Mimura, M., Panjabi, M.M., Oxland, T.R., Crisco, J.J., Yamamoto, I., Vasavada, A., 1994. Disc degeneration affects the multidirectional flexibility of the lumbar spine. Spine (Phila Pa 1976) 19, 1371–1380.

Nachemson, A., 1985. Lumbar spine instability. A critical update and symposium summary. Spine (Phila Pa 1976) 10, 290–291.

Nuckley, D., Hertsted, S., Eck, M., Ching, R., 2005. Effect of displacement rate on the tensile mechanics of pediatric cervical functional spinal units. J Biomech 38, 2266–2275.

O'Sullivan, P.B., Burnett, A., Floyd, A.N., Gadsdon, K., Logiudice, J., Miller, D., et al., 2003. Lumbar repositioning deficit in a specific low back pain population. Spine, 28, 1074–1079.

Oxland, T.R., Crisco, J.J., 3rd, Panjabi, M.M., Yamamoto, I., 1992. The effect of injury on rotational coupling at the lumbosacral joint. A biomechanical investigation. Spine (Phila Pa 1976) 17, 74–80.

Oxland, T.R., Lund, T., Jost, B., Cripton, P., Lippuner, K., Jaeger, P., et al., 1996. The relative importance of vertebral bone density and disc degeneration in spinal flexibility and interbody implant performance. An in vitro study. Spine (Phila Pa 1976) 21, 2558–2569.

Panjabi, M.M., 1992a. The stabilizing system of the spine. Part I. Function, dysfunction, adaptation, and enhancement. J Spinal Disord 5, 383–389.

Panjabi, M.M., 1992b. The stabilizing system of the spine. Part II. Neutral zone and instability hypothesis. J Spinal Disord 5, 390–396.

Panjabi, M.M., Krag, M.H., Chung, T.Q., 1984. Effects of disc injury on mechanical behaviour of the human spine. Spine (Phila Pa 1976) 9, 707–713.

Race, A., Broom, N.D., Robertson, P., 2000. Effect of loading rate and hydration on the mechanical properties of the disc. Spine (Phila Pa 1976) 25, 662–669.

Radebold, A., Cholewicki, J., Panjabi, M.M., Patel, T.C., 2000. Muscle response pattern to sudden trunk loading in healthy individuals and in patients with chronic low back pain. Spine 25, 947–954.

Radebold, A., Cholewicki, J., Polzhofer, G.K., Greene, H.S., 2001. Impaired postural control of the lumbar spine is associated with delayed muscle response times in patients with chronic idiopathic low back pain. Spine 26, 724–730.

Reeves, N.P., Cholewicki, J., 2003. Modeling the human lumbar spine for assessing spinal loads, stability, and risk of injury. Crit Rev Biomed Eng 31, 73–139.

Reeves, N.P., Cholewicki, J., 2010. Expanding our view of the spine system. Eur Spine J 19, 331–332.

Reeves, N., Cholewicki, J., Milner, T., 2005. Muscle reflex classification of low-back pain. J Electromyogr Kinesiol 15, 53–60.

Reeves, N., Cholewicki, J., Silfies, S., 2006a. Muscle activation imbalance and low-back injury in varsity athletes. J Electromyogr Kinesiol 16, 264–272.

Reeves, N.P., Everding, V.Q., Cholewicki, J., Morrisette, D.C., 2006b. The effects of trunk stiffness on postural control during unstable seated balance. Exp Brain Res 174, 694–700.

Reeves, N., Cholewicki, J., Narendra, K., 2007a. Reply. Clin Biomech 22, 487–488.

Reeves, N.P., Narendra, K.S., Cholewicki, J., 2007b. Spine stability: The six blind men and the elephant. Clin Biomech 22, 266–274.

Reeves, N.P., Cholewicki, J., Milner, T., Lee, A.S., 2008. Trunk antagonist co-activation is associated with impaired neuromuscular performance. Exp Brain Res 188, 457–463.

Reeves, N., Cholewicki, J., Narendra, K., 2009. Effects of reflex delays on postural control during unstable seated balance. J Biomech 42, 164–170.

Reeves, N.P., Narendra, K.S., Cholewicki, J., 2011. Spine stability: lessons from balancing a stick. Clin Biomech 26, 325–330.

Schmidt, T.A., An, H.S., Lim, T.H., Nowicki, B.H., Haughton, V.M., 1998. The stiffness of lumbar spinal motion segments with a high-intensity zone in the anulus fibrosus. Spine (Phila Pa 1976) 23, 2167–2173.

Sherwood, D.E., Schmidt, R.A., Walter, C.B., 1988. The force/force-variability relationship under controlled temporal conditions. J Mot Behav 20, 106–116.

Silfies, S.P., Cholewicki, J., Reeves, N.P., Greene, H.S., 2007. Lumbar position sense and the risk of low back injuries in college athletes: a prospective cohort study. BMC Musculoskel Disorders 8, 129.

Sparto, P.J., Parnianpour, M., Marras, W.S., Granata, K.P., Reinsel, T.E., Simon, S., 1997. Neuromuscular trunk performance and spinal loading during a fatiguing isometric trunk extension with varying torque requirements. J Spinal Disorders 10, 145–156.

Stokes, I.A., Gardner-Morse, M., Churchill, D., Laible, J.P., 2002. Measurement of a spinal motion segment stiffness matrix. J Biomech 35, 517–521.

Tanaka, N., An, H.S., Lim, T.H., Fujiwara, A., Jeon, C.H., Haughton, V.M., 2001. The relationship between disc degeneration and flexibility of the lumbar spine. Spine J 1, 47–56.

Thomas, J.S., France, C.R., Sha, D., Vander Wiele, N., Moenter, S., Swank, K., 2007. The effect of chronic low back pain on trunk muscle activations in target reaching movements with various loads. Spine (Phila Pa 1976) 32, E801–E808.

Van Dieën, J.H., Cholewicki, J., Radebold, A., 2003a. Trunk muscle recruitment patterns in patients with low back pain enhance the stability of the lumbar spine. Spine 28, 834–841.

Van Dieën, J.H., Selen, L.P., Cholewicki, J., 2003b. Trunk muscle activation in low-back pain patients, an analysis of the literature. J Electromyogr Kinesiol 13, 333–351.

Wilder, D.G., Aleksiev, A.R., Magnusson, M.L., Pope, M.H., Spratt, K.F., Goel, V.K., 1996. Muscular response to sudden load. A tool to evaluate fatigue and rehabilitation. Spine 21, 2628–2639.

Yingling, V.R., Callaghan, J.P., Mcgill, S.M., 1997. Dynamic loading affects the mechanical properties and failure site of porcine spines. Clin Biomech (Bristol, Avon) 12, 301–305.

Chapter | 3 |

Computational models for trunk trajectory planning and load distribution: a test-bed for studying various clinical adaptation and motor control strategies of low back pain patients

Mohamad Parnianpour
Department of Information and Industrial Engineering, Hanyang University, Ansan, Republic of Korea and Department of Mechanical Engineering, Sharif University of Technology, Tehran, Iran

Nomenclature

Θ = angular position vector in the inertial coordinate system
W = angular velocity vector in the body coordinate system
$G(\Theta)$ = moment vector arising from gravity
J_1 = moment of inertia matrix about the centre of rotation
N_{input} = net muscular torque about L5–S1 in the body coordinate system
N_R = resistance torque about L5–S1 in the body coordinate system
WW = skew symmetric matrix corresponding to W
B = transformation matrix between the body and inertial coordinate systems

$\dfrac{\partial L}{\partial \Theta}^{\mathrm{T}}$ = matrix of moment arm of muscles (3×48)

F = vector of muscle forces (48×1)
K = stiffness matrix of the linearized system (3×3)
V = viscosity matrix of the linearized system (3×3)
A = linearized system state matrix (6×6)
N_p = perturbation torque
$PCSA$ = muscle physiological cross-sectional area
σ_{max} = maximum muscle stress
a_m = muscle activation level of each muscle (m = 1 to 48)
f_{max} = maximum muscle force
l = muscle length
$\dot{l}$ = muscle velocity
q = is the constant of proportionality
$f(l)$ = force – length relationship of muscle
$f(\dot{l})$ = force – velocity relationship of muscle
$f_p(l)$ = passive force relationship of muscle

Abbreviations for muscle fascicle names

EO = external oblique
IL = iliocostalis lumborum
IO = internal oblique
LD = latissimus dorsi
LT = longissimus thoracis
PL = pars lumborum
PS = psoas
QL = quadratus lumborum
RA = rectus abdominus

The role of motor control in the development of low back pain is the subject of much speculation and intense research both in experimental and theoretical fields (Thorstensson et al. 1985). The neuromusculoskeletal system of the spine represents a mechanically redundant system with ostensibly an over-actuated motor system and endowed with multiple sensory mechanisms (to estimate the state of the skeletal and actuators in the system). However perhaps at closer scrutiny it may have just about the right number of muscles (i.e. nothing to spare as redundant), given the system's requirement of providing both structural stability and tremendous flexibility in an unpredictable and changing environment (Hodges and Richardson 1996; Hodges 1999; Cholewicki et al. 2000; Stokes et al. 2000, 2006; Cholewicki and VanVliet 2002; Shirazi-Adl 2006; Arjmand et al. 2008). The additional degree of freedom in our linkage system, theoretically allows us to maintain a given spinal posture with many different configurations of intersegmental motions. However, certain invariant features emerge as coordinative structure with remarkable consistency. According to Professor Panjabi's classic description of interactions of active motor, passive osteoligamentous and neural control subsystems, any overload or overuse of the mechanical system (by large forces at low repetitions or low forces at high repetition) or inappropriate neural command may cause strain and sprain of many elements of the spine that are endowed by nociceptors (Panjabi 2003, 2006). Given the time and load history dependency of all three subsystems, the prolonged loading affects their functional responses in the short term and cellular responses over longer timescales. The former is characterized by recoverable fatigue of muscles, excitation/inhibition of sensory and reflexive autonomic responses and creep/stress relaxation of discs or ligaments. The latter may lead to nutritionally mediated degenerative processes of the disc that could alter mechanical responses, which could lead to various stages of instability and re-stabilization of the spine as explained by others (Cholewicki and McGill 1996; Gardner-Morse and Stokes 1998; Stokes and Gardner-Morse 2001, 2003).

Hence, there are compensatory and/or maladaptation responses to the altered functional capacity and status of three aforementioned subsystems. Without delineating the normal strategies, it is difficult to assess and distinguish the compensatory or maladaptation responses. Without assuming that the central nervous system is using any optimal control strategies, although many suggest such an approach, the paradigm is capable of shedding light on solutions of a number of ill-posed problems (Flash and Hogan 1985; Scott 2004).

A number of our recent computational model studies that illustrate the biomechanical rationale to various behaviour, such as co-activation of muscles during static and dynamic trunk exertions, is reviewed.

The equation of motion is developed for the simplest 3D model of the spine, assuming that the spine is constrained at L5/S1 and multiple muscles are attaching the pelvis to the spine and generating the torque for purposeful flexion/extension movement. The spinal motion against constant resistance to simulate trunk performance against iso-resistive dynamometers (Zeinali-Davarani et al. 2007, 2008) is modelled; also asymmetrical movements are modelled (Shahvarpour et al. 2008; Zeinali-Davarani et al. 2008). The equation of motions and the details of the Hill-based muscle model with a non-linear spindle model (representing the stretch reflex feedbacks) and the stability analysis are presented in the Appendix. For full details of the model, earlier publications can be consulted (Zeinali-Davarani et al. 2008, 2011). Figure 3.1 gives an overall description of the control strategy. There are both an inverse-dynamic model and a stability-based optimization algorithm in the feed-forward control, which predicts the set of muscle activations needed to realize the desired movement trajectory of the spine. The activation values based on the current muscle length, velocity and moment arm (based on an anatomical-geometrical model of the musculoskeletal system) drive the forward dynamic model of the spine while the equations of motions are integrated forward to provide the future states of the system. These sensed/estimated states are fed back to the spindle model and any deviation between the desired length and actual length of muscle will generate appropriate $a_{feedback}$ that is added to feed-forward activation. Hence, any inaccuracy in modelling or external perturbation will be rejected to maintain the desired trajectory. The gain and time delay of the feedback system were parametrically studied and it was concluded that the higher time delays would require a lower gain to maintain the stability of the system (Franklin and Granata 2007). We have shown that co-activation of muscles close to upright position must be augmented to satisfy the stability condition in addition to equilibrium conditions (Fig. 3.2). Hence, intrinsic impedance of muscle mechanics besides neural strategy (increase the co-activation) provides the system with instantaneous impedance to ensure stability (Bergmark 1989; Dariush et al. 1998; Granata and Orishimo 2001; Van Dieen et al. 2003). The added predicted compression and shear forces due to higher co-activation justifies the existing theory that the observed co-activation of low back pain patients should be considered a compensation mechanism which must be addressed by proper rehabilitation, since the higher rate of fatigue and higher risk of disc degeneration accompanying co-activation are undesirable (Brown and Potvin 2005; El-Rich and Shirazi-Adl 2005). Hence, we call this a maladaptation which must be considered in rehabilitation protocols. While we have modelled the reflex loops by simple muscle spindle model, the more advanced approach calls for identifying the synergistic automatic response to the sudden loading or postural perturbations (Ting 2007).

This study also confirmed the earlier prediction that we may have two biomechanical phenomena when modelling spinal injury: one is the structural instability which

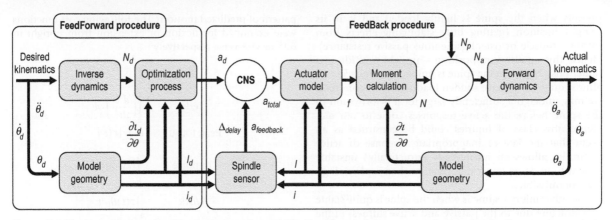

Figure 3.1 The computation algorithm is shown schematically. Feed-forward process: muscle neural activations are computed based on the desired kinematics with or without application of the stability constraint in the optimization routine. Feedback process: effects of muscle spindles on total muscle activations and the kinematics profiles of the movement are evaluated with or without application of the perturbation moment. θ_a, $\dot{\theta}_a$, $\ddot{\theta}_a$ are the actual kinematics and θ_d, $\dot{\theta}_d$, $\ddot{\theta}_d$ are the desired kinematics, α_d is the desired activation, N_d, N_a, N_p are the desired, actual and perturbation moments. A delay of 20 ms is applied in the transmission of feedback signals. *Reproduced courtesy of Zeinali-Davarni, et al., 2008. IEEE TNSRE. 16 (1), 106–118.*

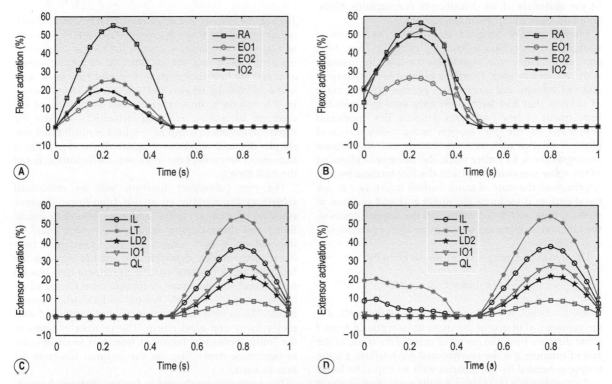

Figure 3.2 Forward flexion of the spine is simulated from upright to 60° of flexion against no resistance for 1 second duration without any perturbation. Muscle activation profiles without (A,C) and with (B,D) application of the stability constraint without the effects of spindle feedback. Top panels show flexor muscles and the bottom panels illustrate the extensor muscles. Additional activation of flexors and co-activation of extensors are seen at upright position when satisfaction of the stability constraint is required. *Reproduced courtesy of Zeinali-Davarni, et al., 2008. IEEE TNSRE. 16 (1), 106–118.*

prevails when the spine is lightly loaded and is in its upright position (getting little stabilizing effects from intrinsic muscle or osteoligamentous passive resistance). Hence, this equilibrium position – upright position – is rather unstable when the spine is unloaded or muscles are almost quiet. If we have sudden loading in this condition we may undergo a sufficiently large local deformation in the spine before the active responses come to our aid. Hence, this class of injuries could be construed as an event that the late or inappropriate response of active controller allows an intrinsically (structurally) unstable system to undergo larger deformation than is physiologically permissible.

The other injury regime is when the spine is quite stable as a structure due to the passive and active stiffness of the spine, and its musculature is sufficient to resist the perturbations. However, the large magnitudes of loads are eliciting large strains approaching the tolerance limits of sub-elements of the spine. In this mode, spinal constituents are failing due to material failure from high magnitude of load and motion characteristic of the task. Simply, we are overexerting the spine and exceeding the strength of the materials of its constituents (i.e. annulus fibres, endplate, ligaments) (Parnianpour 2000).

Clinical studies designed to find the risk factors of workplace tasks characteristically leading to low back pain and classification algorithms for detecting patients with various low back disorders, pointed to more importance of velocity and acceleration profiles than the range of motion that had been previously used to assess the impairment of low back pain patients. That motivated evaluation of the the motion using well-understood physical metrics such as work, energy and smoothness amongst others. In earlier work, the movement planning of the spine was considered and the Ritz method used to approximate the state of trunk motion trajectory – to ask the question: if we knew the initial and final position of motion, how well could we predict the angular position, velocity and acceleration trajectory of spine (Parnianpour et al. 1999)?

The dynamic equation of motion is given by:

$$J\frac{d^2\theta}{dt^2} - B\sin\theta = \tau \quad L \leq \tau \leq U$$

where $J = I + ml^2$, $B = mgl$, m is the mass of the trunk, I is the moment of inertia of the trunk at its centre of mass, l is the distance from the centre of mass of the trunk to the axis of rotation, g is the gravitational acceleration, τ is the torque generated by the muscles with its respective lower and upper bounds (L, U), and θ is the angle of trunk about the vertical upright position. The anthropometric data for an individual with height and weight of 1.7 m and 80 kg were used in these simulations.

Various cost functions were looked at and in one particular case tested – if there is a strength constraint due to impairment, would there be any significant difference in pattern of predicted motion? The following cost functions were examined for flexion or extension from upright to 60° or vice versa respectively:

Energy	$\frac{1}{2}\int_0^T \tau^2(t)dt$
Jerk	$\frac{1}{2}\int_0^T \left(\frac{d^3\theta}{dt^3}\right)^2 dt$
Peak torque	$\max_{t\in(0,T)}\|\tau(t)\|$
Impulse	$\int_0^T \|\tau(t)\|dt$
Work	$\int_0^T \|\tau(t)\dot{\theta}\|dt$

The initial and final velocity and acceleration was considered to be nil. The optimal trajectory $\theta(t)$ is approximated by a fifth degree polynomial plus a linear combination of Fourier terms with weight coefficients (Nagurka and Yen 1990):

$$\theta(t) = p(t) + \sum_{i=1}^k a_i \cos\left(\frac{2i\pi t}{t_f}\right) + \sum_{i=1}^k b_i \sin\left(\frac{2i\pi t}{t_f}\right)$$

The angular velocity and acceleration can be obtained analytically using the above approximation of $\theta(t)$. Based on an equation of motion, we obtain the torque corresponding to the given trajectory as function of the coefficients a_i, b_i and the final time t_f set to 1 second (the coefficients of the polynomial are also functions of a_i, b_i and t_f). Hence, in this approach, instead of forward integration of the equation of motion (forward dynamics), we use the inverse dynamics to compute τ, which is much faster and simpler due to its algebraic structure. The cost function is then also a function of the unknown coefficients a_i, b_i and the final time t_f.

The cost (objective) function will be minimized subject to the equality constraint (non-linear dynamic equation of motion; initial and final boundary conditions) and the inequality constraints (which could be imposed on τ, θ, $\dot{\theta}$, and/or $\ddot{\theta}$). The constrained non-linear programming algorithm was used to simulate the following trunk movements. The movement time was set to 1 second and the range of motion used for the simulation was 60° for both flexion and extension movements. The motion started from rest and terminated with zero velocity and acceleration. The number of terms in the Fourier series was increased from two to six in order to determine their effect on the optimal trajectory for various costs.

The predicted trunk profile for unconstrained conditions for both 60° trunk flexion and extension tasks are depicted in Figure 3.3. The velocity profile and the time to peak velocity were used to distinguish the different cost functions.

The results of all simulations are summarized in Table 3.1. When the energy was minimized, there was 13.48

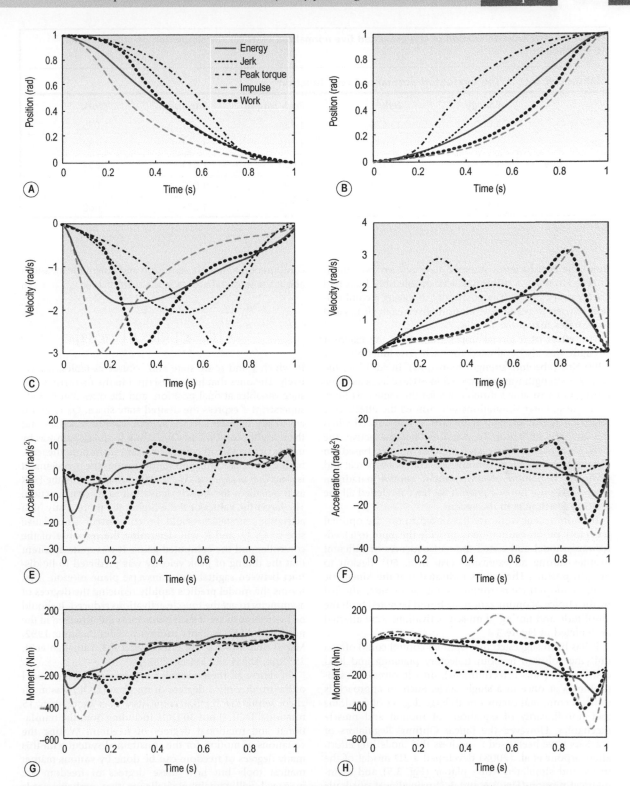

Figure 3.3 The optimized unconstrained trunk flexion and extension trajectories are shown for the five cost functions. The magnitude and timing of velocity and acceleration are significantly different based on the different cost functions. The anthropometric data for an individual with height of 1.7 m and weight of 80 kg were used in these simulations. *Reproduced courtesy of Parnianpour, et al., 1999. Biomed Eng App Bas C. 11, 27–38.*

Table 3.1 The cross-tabulation of the evaluated five normalized costs for the simulation of unconstrained trunk flexion

Minimum cost	The evaluated normalized cost function				
	Energy	Jerk	Peak torque	Impulse	Work
Energy	1.000	13.476	1.734	1.427	1.035
Jerk	1.199	1.000	1.201	1.811	1.164
Peak torque	1.712	10.126	1.000	2.511	1.652
Impulse	1.461	54.624	2.791	1.000	1.007
Work	1.323	24.456	2.322	1.098	1.000

times the cost in jerk compared to when jerk was minimized. However, a minimum jerk profile only increased energy cost by 20%. The possibility of having a combination of costs to predict the motion observed in clinics and workplaces may prove fruitful.

The effect of a global upper bound for the extensor strength was also evaluated for each cost function $-L = -200$ Nm (absolute strength reduction). In addition, the extensor strength was constrained to 80% of its peak value during unconstrained simulations for the same cost function. These latter simulations determined the effects of a relative extensor strength reduction. It was noticed when the strength limitation (constraints) become active, the difference between predicted motion profiles based on different cost functions diminished. That is a very real and alarming limitation of the optimal control paradigm, since we do not know *a priori* if we have modelled all the existing constraints in the system.

In more recent work, we have tried to use the optimal trajectory profile estimation to provide the input to a feed-forward model and tested the consequences of different profiles during an extension task from 60° flexion to upright posture. The results indicated that the kinematic profiles and muscle recruitments are significantly affected by the choice of optimization. It should be noted both the amplitude and timing of muscle activations were affected as depicted in Figure 3.4.

It has been suggested that optimal control could offer a unifying solution to both trajectory planning and load distribution (muscle recruitment), since it solves both sub-problems at once in a single stage. Such an approach is difficult computationally due to large degrees of freedoms and non-linearity of equations of motion and muscle mechanics. However, the Linear Optimal Regulators or Trackers have been used to address this modelling effort. Shahvarpour et al. (2008) developed a 3D model of the trunk and simulated trunk planar (Fig. 3.5) and asymmetrical motion (Figs 3.6 and 3.7) using linear quadratic regulators. The cost function that was used included a combination of muscle activation and kinematic measures about the terminal accuracy as shown below:

$$Cost = \left[\underline{x}_f - \underline{x}_f^d\right]^T Q_f \left[\underline{x}_f - \underline{x}_f^d\right]$$
$$+ \int_0^{t_f} \left\{ \left[\underline{x} - \underline{x}^d\right]^T Q \left[\underline{x} - \underline{x}^d\right] + \underline{\alpha}^T R \underline{\alpha} \right\} dt$$

in which $\underline{x}$ and $\underline{\alpha}$ are state and control variables, respectively. The ones that have subscript f in the first term show state variables at final position; and the ones that include superscript d express the desired state space. Q_f, Q and R are weighting matrices. The system was linearized around the upright position and calculating feedback gain was by means of two Riccati equations. Then we impose the feedback control law with this gain on non-linear systems. It is clear that there is no co-activation predicted by the LQR as it penalizes the muscle activation in its cost function. The larger the values of R the higher the more costly high activations strategies would be considered. The relative size of Q, Q_f and R will determine the response of the controller and the computed gains. It was quite apparent that the timing of peak velocity was predicted to be distinct between sagittal and transverse plane motion. That means the model predicts rapidly reducing the degrees of asymmetry to get the muscle activations reduced. It should be interesting to see if such behaviours are observed in the normal and LBP patients' motion profiles (Schmitz 1992; Marras and Mirka 1993; Ross et al. 1993; Fathallah et al. 1998a,b; Davis and Marras 2000).

Of course all these models use a very simplistic model of the trunk, only 3 degrees of freedom (DOF) was modelled, while the lumbar spine itself has more than 15 rotational DOF, if not 30 DOF including both the translational and rotational degrees of freedom. Writing the equations of motion for the constrained system with this many degrees of freedom can be done by various mathematical tools but how these degrees of freedom are managed will remain a challenge that perhaps needs further investigation from neuroscientific paradigms. The

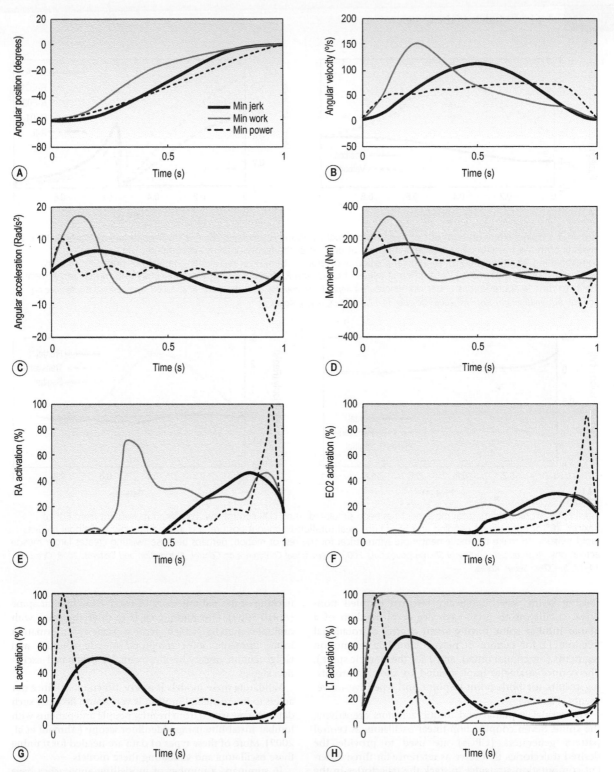

Figure 3.4 Extension movement of the spine is performed in 1 second from 60° flexion to upright with optimal profiles for angular position (A), velocity (B) and acceleration (C) based on different cost functions (minimizing jerk, work and power) and corresponding net joint moments at L5/S1 (D) and muscle activation profiles of flexors rectus abdominis (RA) (E) and external oblique (EO2) (F) and extensors iliocostalis lumborum (IL) (G) and longissimus thoracis (LT) (H) with the stability constraint included (no external resistance $R=0$ Nm and $q=2$). *Reproduced from Shahrokh Zeinali-Davarini, Aboulfazl Shirazi-Adl, Behzad Dariush, et al., 2011. The effects of resistance level and stability demands on recruitment patterns and internal loading of spine in dynamic flexion and extension using a simple truck model. Computer Methods in Biomechanics and Bioengineering 14 (7), reprinted by permission of Taylor & Francis Ltd,* http://tandf.co.uk/journals

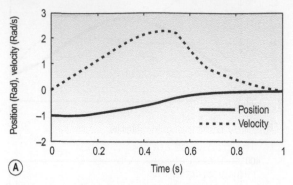
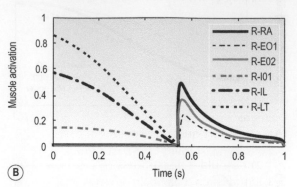

Figure 3.5 Spine extension from 60° of flexion into upright position is simulated using a linear quadratic regulator (LQR) that predicts both the trajectory and muscle recruitment at once after the feedback gains are computed via solving the corresponding Ricatti equations: (A) angular position and velocity; (B) muscles recruitment patterns of right side of body. (R-RA: right-rectus abdominis.) With different values of Q, Q_f and R, one will get different trajectory and muscle recruitment. (Refer to muscle abbreviations under Nomenclature.) *Reproduced courtesy of Shahvarpour, et al., 2008. International Conference on Control, Automation and Systems. 2008, October 14–17, in COEX, Seoul, Korea.*

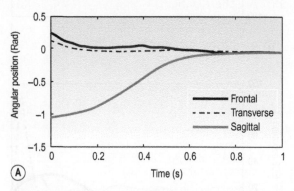
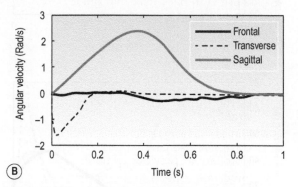

Figure 3.6 Trunk asymmetrical movement has been simulated using LQR control law: combined movement from 60° of flexion, 10° of right lateral bending and 5° of right axial rotation to upright posture. It is interesting how the model predicts rapid twisting to make the movement more symmetrical for the rest of motion, perhaps because twisting creates larger muscle activations. *Reproduced courtesy of Shahvarpour, et al., 2008. International Conference on Control, Automation and Systems. 2008, October 14–17, in COEX, Seoul, Korea.*

starting point was biologically inspired coupled non-linear oscillators to drive each degree of freedom of a planar lumbar spine having seven degrees of rotational freedom (1 for sacrum or pelvis, 5 for lumbar motion segments (functional units), and 1 for the thoracic spine). The control strategies implemented are showing promising results for both point-to-point and repetitive movements (Fig. 3.8).

The model is planar and torque actuators are driving the spine. Seven coupled non-linear oscillators as central pattern generators (CPGs) are used to provide the desired trajectories that serve as reference for three different computation strategies to track the trajectories in the face of perturbation: (i) inverse model used with proportional-derivative (PD) controller; (ii) feedback linearization controller; and (iii) the combined feedback linearization and PD controllers were used to ensure

tracking of desired trajectory of the 7 DOF lumbar spine (Abedi 2009). Our future goal is to drive the spine with multiple muscles which receive sensory information from ligaments, joint receptors, muscle spindles and Golgi tendon organs besides centrally originated excitation signals.

Validating these models is a very difficult task, since our access to intervertebral motion is very scant. Recently such data were measured from healthy people and patients with lumbar instability using videofluoroscopy (Ahmadi et al. 2009). More of these types of data are needed for training these oscillators and validating these models.

In summary, a number of modelling approaches have been provided to gradually capture the complexity of interaction of the three subsystems making up the neuromusculoskeletal spine. Future development of experimental and theoretical paradigms may allow us to use

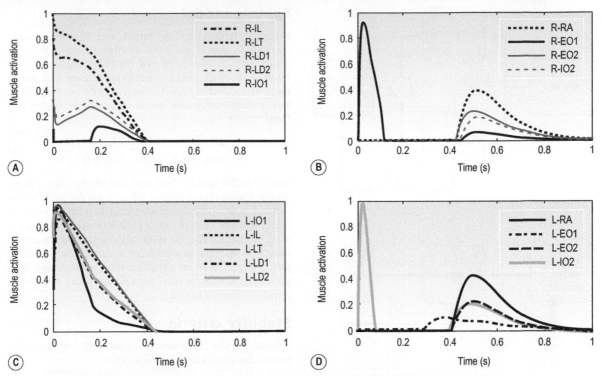

Figure 3.7 Trunk asymmetrical movement has been simulated using LQR control law: combined movement from 60° of flexion, 10° of right lateral bending and 5° of right axial rotation to upright posture. (Refer to muscle abbreviations under Nomenclature.) It would be extremely difficult to identify if these muscle activities were due to co-activation or not, if it was not for the fact that co-activation is non-existent due to consideration of the penalty of muscle activations, *α*, in the cost function. *Reproduced courtesy of Shahvarpour, et al., 2008. International Conference on Control, Automation and Systems. 2008, October 14–17, in COEX, Seoul, Korea.*

these models to test the feasibility of certain strategies for control of healthy or injured spines. There is a need to carry out more interdisciplinary research to understand this complex system (Todorov and Jordan 2002; Granata et al. 2004).

APPENDIX

Biomechanical model

The model used here is slightly different from the one presented previously (Zeinali-Davarani et al. 2008) as it represents external resistance as a Coulomb friction. The dynamic equations of motion of the inverted pendulum were derived in a compact form:

$$J_1 \dot{W} = -WWJ_1 W + N_{input} + G(\Theta) + N_R + N_P \quad (1)$$

in which, W is the angular velocity vector, Θ is the angular position vector, $G(\Theta)$ is the moment vector arising from

gravity, J_1 is the matrix of moment of inertia and N_{input} is the net muscular torque about L5/S1 in body coordinate system, $WWJ_1 W$ represents the torque due to the Coriolis forces, N_p and N_R are the perturbation torque and the constant resistance torque opposing the direction of motion, respectively, defined as:

$$N_R = -R \cdot Sign(\dot{\theta}) \quad (2)$$

where, R is the magnitude of resistance and N_p and θ are in Newton-meter and degree, respectively.

Muscle model

$$f - f_{max} \cdot \{a \cdot f(l) \cdot f(\dot{l}) + f_p(l)\} \quad (3)$$

where $f(l)$, $f(\dot{l})$, $f_p(l)$ are force – length, force – velocity and passive force relations and a is the muscle activation level. f_{max} is the maximum muscle force based on maximum muscle stress σ_{max} taken as 0.55 MPa which is within the range reported in literature (El-Rich and Shirazi-Adl 2005; Arjmand and Shirazi-Adl 2006).

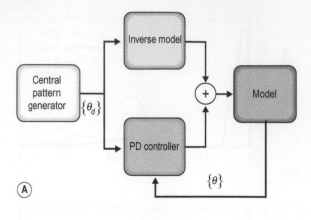

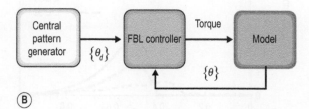

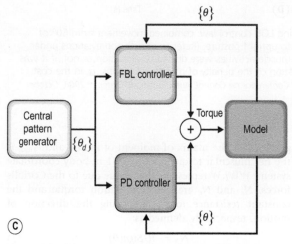

Figure 3.8 Using seven coupled non-linear oscillators as central pattern generators (CPGs) to provide the desired trajectories that are used as reference for three different computation strategies to track the trajectories in face of perturbation: inverse model used with proportional-derivative (PD) controller (A), feedback linearization controller (FBL) (B), and the combined feedback linearization and PD controller (c) to ensure tracking of desired trajectory of the 7 DOF lumbar spine. The model is planar and torque actuators are driving the spine. The future goal is to drive the spine with multiple muscles. *Reproduced courtesy of Maryam Abedi, 2009. Master's Thesis, Sharif University of Technology.*

Spindle model

Regulatory behaviour of the muscle spindle in response to the muscle stretch has been studied in many research works. Stretch reflex is one of the most important neuromuscular functions in controlling posture and movement. The model of stretch reflex invoked in our algorithm was derived from earlier works (Stark 1968; Gielen and Houk 1987):

$$r = g(l - l_d)\dot{l}^3 \quad \text{when} \quad l - l_d > 0, \dot{l} > 0$$
$$r = 0.1g(l - l_d) \quad \text{when} \quad l - l_d \geqslant 0, \dot{l} \leqslant 0 \quad (4)$$

where r is the spindle discharge rate (firing rate), l is the muscle length, $\dot{l}$ is the muscle velocity, g is the spindle gain factor, l_d is set to be the desired muscle length computed from the desired kinematics at each instance of simulation time. Physiologically, the value of gain may vary from one muscle to another and even for a single muscle during different tasks. A linear transformation was adopted from the earlier studies to map the spindle firing rate to the muscle activation level $a_{feedback}$.

Stability criteria

Substituting the net muscular torque with corresponding muscle forces and their moment arms:

$$J_1\dot{W} + WWJ_1W + G(\Theta) - N_R - N_P = -B^T\frac{\partial L}{\partial \Theta}^T F \quad (5)$$

where, B is the transformation matrix between the body coordinate system and that of the inertial coordinate system, $\frac{\partial L}{\partial \Theta}^T$ is the matrix of moment arm of muscles and F is the vector of muscle forces.

Assuming static equilibrium condition about an equilibrium point, Θ_e, and following linearization of the equation of motion around the equilibrium point yields, we obtained:

$$J_1\dot{W}\big|_e + \left(-\frac{\partial G(\Theta)}{\partial \Theta}\bigg|_e + B^T\frac{\partial L}{\partial \Theta}^T\bigg|_e \frac{\partial F}{\partial L}\bigg|_e \frac{\partial L}{\partial \Theta}\bigg|_e\right)(\Theta - \Theta_e)$$
$$+ \left(B^T\frac{\partial L}{\partial \Theta}^T\bigg|_e \frac{\partial F}{\partial \dot{L}}\bigg|_e \frac{\partial L}{\partial \Theta}\bigg|_e B\right)W = 0. \quad (6)$$

In compact form, the linearized equation of motion can be rewritten as:

$$J_1\dot{W}\big|_e + K(\Theta - \Theta_e) + VW = 0, \quad (7)$$

where, $J_1\dot{W}\big|_e$ is the inertial torque about the equilibrium point, K is the stiffness matrix that arises from conservative forces (gravitational and muscle stiffness), V is the viscosity matrix that arises from non-conservative forces due to muscle viscosity. In state space form, we can write:

$$\begin{bmatrix}\dot{\Theta}\\\dot{W}\end{bmatrix}_{6\times 1} = A_{6\times 6}\begin{bmatrix}\Theta - \Theta_e\\W\end{bmatrix}_{6\times 1}, \quad (8)$$

where

$$A = \begin{bmatrix} zeros_{3\times3} & B_{3\times3} \\ -J_1^{-1}K_{3\times3} & -J_1^{-1}V_{3\times3} \end{bmatrix}_{6\times6}. \qquad (9)$$

To ensure stability of the linearized system, eigenvalues of A should have negative real parts (Hemami and Katbab 1982; Dinneen and Hemami 1993; Dariush et al. 1998):

$$REAL\ (Eig(A)) < 0, \qquad (10)$$

where the stiffness of each muscle is computed by a linear equation $\partial F/\partial L \cong qF/L$.

Computation algorithm

The 'geometry' process in the solution algorithm (see Fig. 3.1) involved the computation of instantaneous muscle lengths (based on the angular position and the origin-insertion coordinates of muscles in the upright posture (Katbab 1989)), muscle velocities (based on the derivative of muscle lengths with respect to time) and the moment arm of muscles (based on the derivative of muscle lengths with respect to each degree of freedom). The program ran in MATLAB 12, and Optimization Toolbox was used for the optimization process.

Feed-forward process

The first stage involved a feed-forward process, where the static optimization was used to derive a set of neural excitation of muscles under steady-state conditions. Based on the prescribed kinematics, the needed joint torque, which should be provided by trunk muscles, was computed using inverse dynamics. The performance criterion (P) was taken as the sum of the squared muscle activations (Kaufman et al. 1991; Thelen et al. 2003). The optimization problem was set by the following equations:

$$Min\quad P = \sum_{m=1}^{48} (a_m)^2$$

subject to:

$$J_1\dot{W} + WWJ_1W - G(\Theta) - N_R - N_P = -B^T\frac{\partial L}{\partial\Theta}^T F$$

$$\left.\begin{array}{l} f_{max_m} = \sigma_{max} \times PCSA_m \\ 0 \le a_m \le 1 \end{array}\right\};\quad m = 1\ to\ 48 \qquad (11)$$

$$REAL\ (Eig(A)) < 0.$$

Feedback process

The second stage, as depicted in Figure 3.1, involved a feedback process in which kinematics parameters were computed through forward dynamics subject to neural excitation of muscles. In order to evaluate the performance of spindles in providing the reflexive stiffness, a perturbation moment was added to the existing moment. Having the net muscular moment, resulting kinematics parameters were obtained by numerical integration (depicted as forward dynamics in Fig. 3.1). It has been shown that the equations of motion are ill-posed. Spindles were responsible to compensate any deviation of the predicted kinematics and the desired one which could be due to neural noise, numerical errors or the perturbation. In view of the neural transmission delay, a delay of 20 ms was applied in the transmission of feedback signals which lies within the range of reported spinal muscle reflex latencies (Zedka et al. 1999; Granata et al. 2004).

ACKNOWLEDGEMENT

This chapter is a summary of work over the past 20 years with many invaluable contributions: Professors A. Shirazi-Adl, H. Hemami, K. Barin, M. Nordin, W.S. Marras, A. Ahmadi, J.L. Wang, G. Lafferriere, J. Mousavi, Drs B. Dariush, and Mr. S. Zeinali and A. Shahvarpour, B. Nasseroleslami, A. Sanjari, E. Rashedi and Miss M. Abedi. Partial support was provided by Hanyang University Research Foundation grant HY 2009-N9.

REFERENCES

Abedi, M., 2009. Control of lumbar spine using central pattern generators by using nonlinear biologically inspired oscillators. Master Thesis. Sharif University of Technology, Tehran, Iran.

Ahmadi, A., Maroufi, N., Behtash, H., Zekavat, H., Parnianpour, M., 2009. Kinematic analysis of dynamic lumbar motion in patients with lumbar segmental instability using digital videofluoroscopy. Eur Spine J 18, 1677–1685.

Arjmand, N., Shirazi-Adl, A., 2006. Model and in vivo studies on human trunk load partitioning and stability in isometric forward flexions. J Biomech 39, 510–521.

Arjmand, N., Shirazi-Adl, A., Parnianpour, M., 2008. Relative efficiency of abdominal muscles in spine stability. Comput Meth Biomech Biomed Eng 11, 291–299.

Bergmark, A., 1989. Stability of the lumbar spine. A study in mechanical

engineering. Acta Orthop Scand 230, 1–54.

Brown, S.H., Potvin, J.R., 2005. Constraining spine stability levels in an optimization model leads to the prediction of trunk muscle cocontraction and improved spine compression force estimates. J Biomech 38, 745–754.

Cholewicki, J., McGill, S.M., 1996. Mechanical stability of the in vivo lumbar spine: implications for injury and chronic low back pain. Clin Biomech 11, 1–15.

Cholewicki, J., VanVliet, J.J., 2002. Relative contribution of trunk muscles to the stability of the lumbar spine during isometric exertions. Clin Biomech 17, 99–105.

Cholewicki, J., Simons, A.P., Radebold, A., 2000. Effects of external trunk loads on lumbar spine stability. J Biomech 33, 1377–1385.

Dariush, B., Parnianpour, M., Hemami, H., 1998. Stability and control strategy of a multilink musculoskeletal model with applications in FES. IEEE T Bio-Med Eng 45, 3–14.

Davis, K.G., Marras, W.S., 2000. The effects of motion on trunk biomechanics. Clin Biomech 15, 703–717.

Dinneen, J.A., Hemami, H., 1993. Stability and movement of a neuromusculoskeletal sagittal arm. IEEE T Bio-Med Eng 40, 541–548.

El-Rich, M., Shirazi-Adl, A., 2005. Effect of load position on muscle forces, internal loads and stability of the human spine in upright postures. Comput Meth Biomech Biomed Eng 8, 359–368.

Fathallah, F.A., Marras, W.S., Parnianpour, M., 1998a. An assessment of complex spinal loads during dynamic lifting tasks. Spine 23, 706–716.

Fathallah, F.A., Marras, W.S., Parnianpour, M., 1998b. The role of complex, simultaneous trunk motions in the risk of occupation-related low back disorders. Spine 23, 1035–1042.

Flash, T., Hogan, N., 1985. The coordination of arm movements: an experimentally confirmed mathematical model. J Neurosci 5, 1688–1703.

Franklin, T.C., Granata, K.P., 2007. Role of reflex gain and reflex delay in spinal stability– a dynamic simulation. J Biomech 40, 1762–1767.

Gardner-Morse, M., Stokes, I.A., 1998. The effects of abdominal muscle co-activation on lumbar spine stability. Spine 23, 86–91.

Gielen, C.C., Houk, J.C., 1987. A model of the motor servo: incorporating nonlinear spindle receptor and muscle mechanical properties. Biol Cybern 57, 217–231.

Granata, K.P., Orishimo, K.F., 2001. Response of trunk muscle co-activation to changes in spinal stability. J Biomech 34, 1117–1123.

Granata, K.P., Slota, G.P., Bennett, B.C., 2004. Paraspinal muscle reflex dynamics. J Biomech 37, 241–247.

Hemami, H., Katbab, A., 1982. Constrained inverted pendulum model for evaluating upright postural stability. J Dyn Syst-T ASME 104, 343–349.

Hodges, P.W., 1999. Is there a role for transverse abdominis in lumbo-pelvic stability? Man Ther 4, 74–86.

Hodges, P.W., Richardson, C.A., 1996. Inefficient muscular stabilization of the lumbar spine associated with low back pain. A motor control evaluation of transverse abdominis. Spine 21, 2640–2650.

Katbab, A., 1989. Analysis of human torso motion with muscle actuators. Ann Biomed Eng 17, 17–91.

Kaufman, K.R., An, K.N., Litchy, W.J., Chao, E.Y., 1991. Physiological prediction of muscle forces – I. Theoretical formulation. Neuroscience 40, 781–792.

Marras, W.S., Mirka, G.A., 1993. Electromyographic studies of the lumbar trunk musculature during the generation of low-level trunk acceleration. J Orthop Res 11, 811–817.

Nagurka, M.L., Yen, V., 1990. Fourier-based optimal control of nonlinear dynamic systems. J Dyn Syst-T ASME 112, 17–26.

Panjabi, M.M., 2003. Clinical spinal instability and low back pain. J Electromyogr Kines 13, 371–379.

Panjabi, M.M., 2006. A hypothesis of chronic back pain: ligament subfailure injuries lead to muscle control dysfunction. Eur Spine J 15, 668–676.

Parnianpour, M., 2000. The Biomedical Engineering Handbook. CRC Press, Boca Raton, Florida, Application of quantitative assessment of human performance in occupational medicine. 55, 1–17.

Parnianpour, M., Wang, J.L., Shirazi-Adl, A., Khayatian, B., Lafferriere, G., 1999. A computational method for simulation of trunk motion: towards a theoretical based quantitative assessment of trunk performance. Biomed Eng-App Bas C 11, 27–38.

Ross, E.C., Parnianpour, M., Martin, D., 1993. The effects of resistance level on muscle coordination patterns and movement profile during trunk extension. Spine 18, 1829–1838.

Schmitz, T.J., 1992. The effects of direction and resistance on iso-inertial trunk movement profiles, motor outputs and muscle coordination patterns during unidirectional trunk motion [dissertation]. New York University, New York (NY).

Scott, S.H., 2004. Optimal feedback control and the neural basis of volitional motor control. Nat Rev Neurosci 5, 532–546.

Shahvarpour, A., Pourtakdoust, H., Vossoughi, G.R., Kim, J.Y., Parnianpour, M., 2008. Muscles force patterns prediction and joint reactions determination during 3D spine movements by means of optimal control theory. International Conference on Control, Automation and Systems. Oct. 14–17, 2008, pp. 100–106, Seoul, Korea.

Shirazi-Adl, A., 2006. Analysis of large compression loads on lumbar spine in flexion and in torsion using a novel wrapping element. J Biomech 39, 267–275.

Stark, L., 1968 Neurological Control Systems. Plenum Press, New York.

Stokes, I.A., Gardner-Morse, M., 2001. Lumbar spinal muscle activation synergies predicted by multi-criteria cost function. J Biomech 34, 733–740.

Stokes, I.A., Gardner-Morse, M., 2003. Spinal stiffness increases with axial load: another stabilizing consequence of muscle action. J Electromyogr Kinesiol 13, 397–402.

Stokes, I.A., Gardner-Morse, M., Henry, S.M., Badger, G.J., 2000. Decrease in trunk muscular response to perturbation with preactivation of lumbar spinal musculature. Spine 25, 1957–1964.

Stokes, I.A., Fox, J.R., Henry, S.M., 2006. Trunk muscular activation patterns and responses to transient force perturbation in persons with self-reported low back pain. Eur Spine J 15, 658–667.

Thelen, D.G., Anderson, F.C., Delp, S.L., 2003. Generating dynamic simulation of movement using computed muscle control. J Biomech 36, 321–328.

Thorstensson, A., Oddsson, L., Carlson, H., 1985. Motor control of voluntary trunk movements in standing. Acta Physiol Scand 125, 309–321.

Ting, L.H., 2007. Dimensional reduction in sensorimotor systems: a framework for understanding muscle coordination of posture. Prog Brain Res 165, 299–321.

Todorov, E., Jordan, M.I., 2002. Optimal feed-back control as a theory of motor coordination. Nat Neurosci 5, 1226–1235.

Van Dieen, J.H., Cholewicki, J., Radebold, A., 2003. Trunk muscle recruitment patterns in patients with low back pain enhance the stability of the lumbar spine. Spine 28, 834–841.

Zedka, M., Prochazka, A., Knight, B., Gillard, D., Gauthier, M., 1999. Voluntary and reflex control of human back muscles during induced pain. J Physiol 520, 591–604.

Zeinali-Davarani, S., Shirazi-Adl, A., Hemami, H., Mousavi, S.J., Parnianpour, M., 2007. Dynamic iso-resistive trunk extension simulation: contributions of the intrinsic and reflexive mechanisms to spinal stability. Technol Health Care 15, 415–431.

Zeinali-Davarani, S., Hemami, H., Barin, K., Shirazi-Adl, A., Parnianpour, M., 2008. Dynamic Stability of spine using stability-based optimization and muscle spindle reflex. IEEE T Neur Sys Reh 16, 106–118.

Zeinali-Davarani, S., Shirazi-Adl, A., Dariush, B., Hemami, H., Parnianpour, M., 2011. The effect of resistance level and stability demands on recruitment patterns and internal loading of spine in dynamic trunk flexion and extension movements. Comput Methods Biomech Biomed Eng 14, 645–656.

Chapter | 4 |

Mechanical changes in the spine in back pain

Gregory Neil Kawchuk
Faculty of Rehabilitation Medicine, University of Alberta, Edmonton, Alberta, Canada

INTRODUCTION

When it comes to studying motor control, there are an endless number of techniques used to stimulate the system as well as to measure its response.

On the stimulation side, the possibilities range from isometric voluntary contraction to magnetic stimulation of the human brain (Fig. 4.1). On the response side, a wide spectrum of tools exist, ranging from tissue biopsy to direct visualization of muscle behaviour in real time (Fig. 4.1).

While the number of techniques to stimulate the motor system and measure its behaviour are many, not all of these techniques are employed regularly. Arguably, the majority of spinal motor control studies utilize traditional, well-established approaches such as surface-based EMG; likely a reflection of its cost, ease of use, non-invasive nature and the existence of abundant information on its implementation and interpretation. But is everything about spinal motor control revealed with these common approaches? While they may not yet be evolved fully, alternative technologies for studying spinal motor control may have potential value in revealing the mechanisms that underlie and influence spinal motor control. This chapter is devoted to highlighting just a few of these possibilities.

VIBRATION

Engineers are often faced with the problem of testing an object to determine if it is structurally and functionally sound. While mathematical models can be used to predict these behaviours, at some point, there is no replacement for physically testing the object of interest. While physical testing can be achieved easily with smaller objects, it is difficult to assess larger structures like bridges and aeroplanes in a controlled laboratory setting. How do you test a bridge before traffic is allowed to pass or an aeroplane before it takes flight?

One well-established technique is vibration analysis. In this approach, vibration is passed into the structure by something as crude as an instrumented sledgehammer or as sophisticated as a computer-controlled electromechanical shaker. The response to that vibration is then recorded in real time by a variety of devices including accelerometers. Data from the sensors can then be analyzed with various techniques to assess the structural and functional integrity of the object under consideration.

Recently, this approach has been adapted to evaluate surgical disruptions of normal spinal anatomy (Kawchuk et al. 2008a, 2009). Specifically, bone pins installed in cadaveric pig spines can be used with a cable-tie system that stiffens spinal segments in discrete increments (Fig. 4.2). In addition, stiffness of the spine can be reduced by creating disc injuries of increasing stab-depth (Fig. 4.2).

With this investigative platform, vibration responses from individual vertebrae can be collected when vertebrae are stiffened, returned to normal, and following progressive disc injury. By using a neural network to analyze the resulting data, it was found that each of the applied conditions had a unique vibration signature (Fig. 4.2). Not only were signatures unique, they could be used to determine if the system was healthy or compromised, the location of the compromise, as well as the magnitude of the compromise. In 5040 decisions made by the neural network in six

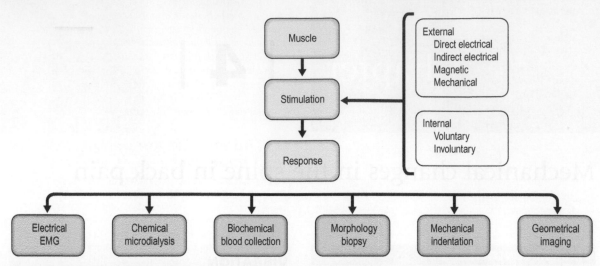

Figure 4.1 Examples of different ways to stimulate the motor system as well as to quantify its response.

different cadavers having over 20 different conditions, the network made only 10 errors.

The resulting data from this approach provides information about the structural integrity of the spine. But like bridge and aeroplane testing, response data can be obtained not only in a 'non-functional' state, but also when the object is engaged in its usual activity (the bridge supporting traffic or the aeroplane in flight).

Given that one function of the motor control system is to create muscular contraction of a sufficient magnitude to allow static and dynamic loading without buckling, the spine can be tested for its vibration response during defined motor activities. Specifically, muscular contractions can be created voluntarily or through direct electric stimulation to activate specific spinal muscles to contract. During this process, the spine can be vibrated and the resulting accelerations from skin-based accelerometers recorded (Fig. 4.3). From this information, the functionality of the motor control system may be assessed. While testing of the unloaded, neutral spine is of great interest in detecting structural problems, vibration testing during additional static or dynamic loading may be the equivalent of a cardiac stress test where specific pathologies are revealed during exertion.

INDENTATION TESTING AND TISSUE STIFFNESS

If we assume that an important function of spinal motor control is to create, and/or respond to, spinal loading, then perhaps one way to assess the performance of the motor control system is to measure its end product – spinal stiffness. While the electrical activity of muscle is a valuable entry point for motor control evaluation, it does not allow us to understand the context for why the muscle was activated.

Fortunately, the measurement of tissue stiffness has been evolving over several decades. Historically, a change in tissue stiffness has been associated with increased tissue pathology. Whether it be lax ligaments or hardening of the arteries, clinicians have used tissue stiffness as a way to evaluate tissue health. Up until recently, these assessments have occurred manually. Only decades ago, clinicians pushed gently into a closed eye to detect a decrease in compliance – a harbinger of glaucoma. In manual stiffness assessment, resulting deformations and displacements created by the force of the fingertips generates a subjective impression in the clinician who then makes a judgement as to the tissue being too soft, too hard or just right (a.k.a. the three bears school of diagnosis).

Obviously, there are restrictions to this approach. While tissues do indeed change their force–displacement properties with certain disease processes, there are limits to the sensitivity with which humans can detect these changes. In addition, use of an internal scale of reference to ascertain the magnitude of stiffness is subject to many problems in addition to the inability of a clinician to communicate their impression of stiffness as a quantity.

As a result, various probes have been devised which are capable of measuring applied force and the resulting deformations and displacements of tissues. With these tools, it is possible to quantify the bulk tissue stiffness underneath the indentation probe (Stanton and Kawchuk 2009). By recording these features throughout the application of indentation loading, an entire force–displacement curve can be created (Stanton and Kawchuk 2008). Building on this, if various internal landmarks are followed with ultrasound during the indentation process (Fig. 4.4), bulk

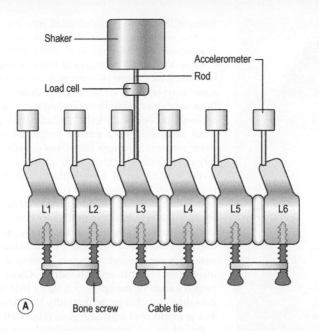

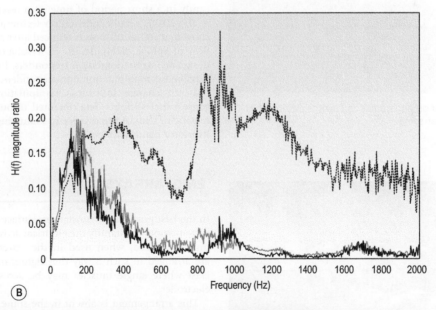

Figure 4.2 Example of an experimental setup (A) and the resulting frequency response functions (B) showing a healthy state (dark line), L1–2 linkage (light line) and a L1–2 disc stab (dashed line). *Reproduced from Kawchuk, G.N., Decker, C., Dolan, R., Carey, J., 2009. Structural health monitoring to detect the presence, location and magnitude of structural damage in cadaveric porcine spines.* Journal of Biomechanics *42 (7), 109–115, with permission from Elsevier.*

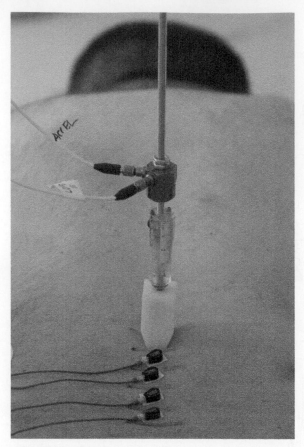

Figure 4.3 Vibration application and sensor placement in the human lumbar spine.

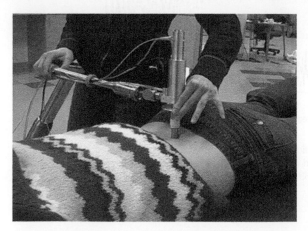

Figure 4.4 Indentation loading applied to the human spine with concurrent quantification of soft tissue deformation and vertebral displacement via onboard ultrasound.

tissue stiffness can be subdivided into regional measures or even measures specific to discrete anatomical features (e.g. vertebrae) (Kawchuk et al. 2001, 2006).

Most often, bulk measures of tissue stiffness are used to evaluate how passive stiffness may be altered as a result of some intervention. Unfortunately, these techniques have been used most often in the resting spine. As a result, bulk stiffness measures typically exclude muscular contributions other than their passive properties. In some cases, tissue stiffness measures have been collected when voluntary or involuntary contraction states are created thereby giving a glimpse of how stiffness can be used as an outcome for assessing motor control.

In some incarnations, indentation devices can be used to track the vertebrae themselves to estimate the stability of the system during a given loading scenario. This technique is particularly well suited to evaluations where stiffness data are needed from one particular region during quasi-static, simple spine loading. Given the interconnected nature of the spine, it is likely that segmental stiffness does not change dramatically from level to level, but as a gradient over a given region (Hu et al. 2009a).

Recent use of indentation technologies have generated data which suggest that spinal stiffness can change significantly in a short period of time. In a recent trial by Fritz et al. (2011), a bulk indentation technique was used to show that spinal stiffness is reduced after a single application of spinal manipulation in a subgroup of subjects designated as manipulation responders. In those subjects classified as manipulation non-responders, spinal stiffness did not change following manipulation. These data suggest that stiffness data obtained through indentation may be of clinical importance in evaluating the spine and its motor control system.

EMG ARRAYS

In the best possible circumstances, surface electromyography attempts to quantify the electrical activity of a specific muscle. Indeed, when used in the extremities, muscles are arranged in such a way that significant areas of skin exist where single muscles may be accessed by surface electrodes.

This arrangement is absent in the spine where muscles are not arranged in singular tracks, but in numerous layers. Because of short interarticular distances, many muscles of the spine are extremely short in length making their electrical isolation difficult at best. Combined with longer, multi-segmental muscles, the muscles of the spine are arranged more as layers with multiple points of attachment suggesting a need for something greater than gross control of segmental movements. This spatial arrangement also suggests that the spine does not move with

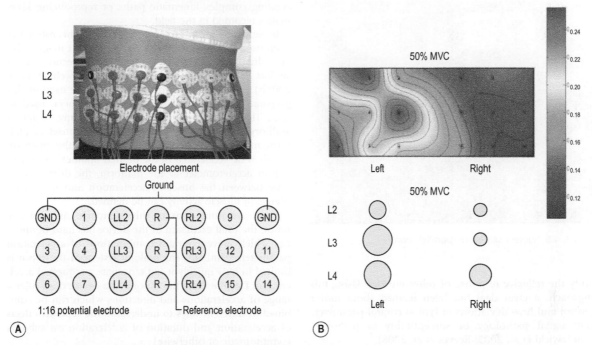

Figure 4.5 Surface EMG electrode array (A), resulting isobar map of electrical activity at 50% maximal voluntary contraction (MVC) (B) and map of indentation stiffness. *Reproduced from Hu, Y., Wong, Y.L., Wu, W.L., Kawchuk, G.N., 2009. Creation of an asymmetrical gradient of back muscle activity and spinal stiffness during asymmetrical hip extension. Clinical Biomechanics 24 (10), 799–806, with permission from Elsevier.*

activation of distinct muscles (as is more the case in the extremities), but that the spine creates regional activation to manage the tremendous moments that can be generated within it.

Given this arrangement, it is unlikely that a single set of electrodes placed off the midline of the spine can represent the activity of any single muscle, yet this approach remains the status quo in spinal EMG assessment. In reality, surface EMG signals recorded from the spine are an amalgam of activity from various muscles in various spinal layers. If the goal of motor control is to manage the static or dynamic force demands of the spine, there would be value in assessing the regional activation of muscle in the spine to better reflect the activity of the requested muscular activation patterns.

With the use of EMG arrays, this possibility exists (Fig. 4.5). Rather than use the traditional pair of electrodes to span the region of interest, a two-dimensional array of multiple electrodes is used. Analogous to a radiotelescope made up of multi-receiver dishes, an array of surface electrodes can paint a picture of spinal EMG activity in geographical terms (Hu et al. 2009b). As a result, regional maps of EMG activity resembling isobar weather maps can be created (Fig. 4.5). With current computing power, these maps can be updated with sufficient speed to display changes in regional muscular activity over time.

Already, this technique has been used to demonstrate how regional muscle activity changes with simple spinal movements and how regional activity changes with increasing task intensity (Hu et al. 2009a).

Another benefit of this approach is that for clinicians and patients, the resulting output is easy to understand and conveys intuitive information about the intensity and location of muscular activity.

STIMULATION – ROBOT PLATFORM

A number of stimulation techniques exist for generating reflexive muscle contractions in the spine. One of the more common techniques uses gravity to stimulate a self-righting reflex. In this technique, subjects are seated then flexed or extended at the trunk and held in that position by a cable restraint. If the cable is released suddenly, specific muscles will be activated in an attempt to right the trunk against gravity. Similarly, the technique can be used to suspend subjects in extension or lateral bending to

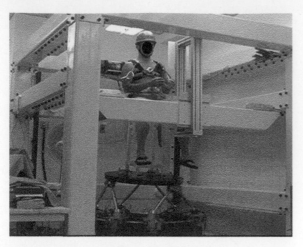

Figure 4.6 Subject seated on parallel robot.

study the reflexive response of other muscles. Using this approach, a great deal has been learned about motor control and how deviations in typical control parameters may signal pathology or susceptibility to pathology (Cholewicki et al. 2005; Reeves et al. 2008).

While the value of this technique is obvious, it does have limitations. Namely, the amount of 'gravity' cannot be controlled – the stimulus is always the same, just applied with the subject beginning in different postures. If the effect of gravity could be controlled, it may be possible to look at motor control with various parameters of acceleration.

Specifically, gravitational acceleration is a constant. If the magnitude, direction and exposure time of the acceleration could be manipulated, then the reflex control of the system may be better defined and other pathological circumstances identified. Manipulation of this type is possible with a number of devices, but most commonly with flight simulators or common facsimiles that are used in arcades and amusements rides. Instead of using these devices to recreate jet flight over the Grand Canyon, the device can move a seated subject in a variety of directions while controlling the acceleration magnitude and the duration of acceleration exposure (Fig. 4.6).

Essentially a small flight simulator, the robot pictured in Figure 4.6 consists of a platform supported by six fixed-length struts mounted on a circular track. By controlling the position of the struts along the track, the platform can be moved in any combination of translation and rotation within a defined volume. Because each strut is controlled independently by computer, the robot is capable of creating complex kinematic paths or reproducing kinematics recorded in the field.

In studying the motor control system, the robot has been used to apply accelerations of different magnitudes and durations in single or multiple directions to a subject seated on the robot's platform (Kawchuck et al. 2008b). Although any form of EMG can be used in this preparation, traditional surface EMG has been used to date. The subject is then shielded from any visual or auditory cues that may alert them to the onset of platform movement. After these precautions, the platform can then be accelerated in the desired manner. By attaching an accelerometer to the platform, the difference in time between the onset of acceleration and the onset/silence of muscle activity can be defined.

There are limitations to this approach. As with any robot, the total excursion of the device has hard boundaries which prevent certain combinations of acceleration parameters. Similarly, the braking system of the robot is limited in how quickly it can terminate a requested acceleration. Despite these limitations, the device does offer a range of accelerations and directions which can be combined in different ways to understand the separate effects of acceleration and duration of acceleration on subjects (symptomatic or otherwise).

To date, we have used this approach to collect data over a range of accelerations and acceleration magnitudes in four different directions of translation. While these preliminary data await further analysis, it is apparent that this technique may be of use in controlling stimulation of reflexive spinal contractions while separating out the influence of acceleration versus velocity etc. This approach has the potential to further explore the role of the reflex response in motor control, spinal injury and back pain.

CONCLUSIONS

While few would deny the importance of the muscular system and its control with respect to back pain, one pressing issue we face is trying to investigate this system within the context of its end product; development of sufficient load in a timely manner. While approaches used toward understanding other aspects of spinal motor control are bound to be of use and importance, we must remember that the system is designed to produce a specific load in a specific timeframe. Being able to measure deviations of that function may best illuminate the underlying mechanisms of the system itself.

REFERENCES

Cholewicki, J., Silfies, S.P., Shah, R.A., Greene, H.S., Reeves, N.P., Alvi K., et al., 2005. Delayed trunk muscle reflex responses increase the risk of low back injuries. Spine 30, 2614–2620.

Fritz, J.M., Koppenhaver, S.L., Kawchuk, G.N., Teyhen, D.S., Hebert, J.J., Childs, J.D., 2011. Preliminary investigation of the mechanisms underlying the effects of manipulation: exploration of a multivariate model including spinal stiffness, multifidus recruitment, and clinical findings. Spine 36, 1772–1781.

Hu, Y., Wong, Y.L., Lu, W.W., Kawchuk, G.N., 2009a. Creation of an asymmetrical gradient of back muscle activity and spinal stiffness during asymmetrical hip extension. Clin Biomech 24, 799–806.

Hu, Y., Siu, S.H., Mak, J.N., Luk, K.D., 2009b. Lumbar muscle electromyographic dynamic topography during flexion-extension. J Electromyogr Kinesiol.

Kawchuk, G.N., Kaigle, A.M., Holm, S.H., Rod Fauvel, O., Ekström, L., Hansson, T., 2001. The diagnostic performance of vertebral displacement measurements derived from ultrasonic indentation in an in vivo model of degenerative disc disease. Spine 26, 1348–1355.

Kawchuk, G.N., Liddle, T.R., Fauvel, O.R., Johnston, C., 2006. The accuracy of ultrasonic indentation in detecting simulated bone displacement: a comparison of three techniques. J Manipulative Physiol Ther 29, 126–133.

Kawchuk, G.N., Decker, C., Dolan, R., Fernando, N., Carey, J., 2008a. The feasibility of vibration as a tool to assess spinal integrity. J Biomech 41, 2319–2323.

Kawchuk, G.N., Clayholt, L., Douglas, S., Fitzgerald, S., Willis, A., 2008b. Trunk muscle activity caused by 360 degree robotic tilting. Proceedings of the International Society for the Study of the Lumbar Spine, Geneva, p. 126.

Kawchuk, G.N., Decker, C., Dolan, R., Carey, J., 2009. Structural health monitoring to detect the presence, location and magnitude of structural damage in cadaveric porcine spines. J Biomech 42, 109–115.

Reeves, N.P., Cholewicki, J., Milner, T., Lee, A.S., 2008. Trunk antagonist co-activation is associated with impaired neuromuscular performance. Exp Brain Res 188, 457–463.

Stanton, T., Kawchuk, G., 2008. The effect of abdominal stabilization contractions on posteroanterior spinal stiffness. Spine 33, 694–701.

Stanton, T.R., Kawchuk, G.N., 2009. Reliability of assisted indentation in measuring lumbar spinal stiffness. Man Ther 14, 197–205.

Part | 2 |

Motor control of the spine

Chapter | 5 |

Spine function and low back pain: interactions of active and passive structures

Jaap H. van Dieën and Idsart Kingma
MOVE Research Institute Amsterdam, Faculty of Human Movement Sciences, VU University Amsterdam, Amsterdam, The Netherlands

INTRODUCTION

Both clinicians and researchers involved with disorders of the human musculoskeletal system and especially of the spine frequently use the terms stability and instability. It is however questionable whether the same concepts are implied whenever these terms appear. In a recent paper, Peter Reeves (Reeves et al. 2007) phrased it as follows: 'Stability … is a term that appears to change depending upon the context, and as such, appears to have unstable definitions.' Obviously this inconsistent use of terminology may lead to confusion and is undesirable. Within mechanics, stability is clearly defined and Reeves argued that such a strict definition should be adopted for use in the clinical context as well.

A simple example could be the stability of patient X in standing. The question might be: is patient X stable when standing in tandem stance? Mechanical stability refers to a state of a system in which a perturbation of that state does not cause an unbounded change in the state. An unstable system cannot function, since perturbations will always occur. According to this definition, X is stable when he can stand, in spite of the unavoidable perturbations (postural sway). Vice versa, a patient who is unstable will not remain standing. A system is either stable or unstable, there is no degree of stability and the unstable system is actually quite uninteresting. The unstable patient cannot stand and investigating his ability to stand will cause a guaranteed fall. While such conditions do occur, it is not what clinicians and researchers generally mean by instability.

If we were to investigate the stability of X while standing in a decelerating bus, we might consider X stable when he steps forward. X moves away from the state before the perturbation even further than the displacement caused by the perturbation itself and does not return to his initial state, but the change in the state is clearly bounded. However, when X falls flat on his face, the change in state is also bounded (by the contact with the floor of the bus). So it is important to consider the question whether the bounds fall within a desirable operating range. While it may be trivial to exclude lying flat on the floor from the desirable operating range in this case, the question whether a patient is stable when he or she takes a step upon a perturbation illustrates that there is a degree of subjectivity in the definition, when it is to be applied to real-world problems.

White and Panjabi (1990) proposed a definition of clinical instability, specifically for the spine, defining instability as the loss of the spine's ability to limit its movements under physiological loads such that neurological disturbances (e.g. through nerve root compression), deformation (e.g. scoliosis, spondylolisthesis) or pain are prevented. The strength of this definition is that the bounds to the state of the spine are defined in view of resulting disorders and symptoms and not relative to some non-existent ideal movement pattern (as appears common in clinical practice). Perhaps, the definition should be expanded by adding the criterion that long-term tissue damage should be avoided. Think for example of the increased probability of osteoarthritis after an injury of the anterior cruciate ligament (Hertel et al. 2005; Salmon et al. 2006), which may result from altered joint kinematics (Stergiou et al. 2007). However, inclusion of adverse long-term health effects as a criterion for stability assumes that such long-term effects are predictable, and that is in general far from sure.

A weakness of the proposed definition, which Panjabi corrected in later work (Panjabi 1992), is that it describes stability as a capacity of the spine itself. Maintaining stability is not a capacity of the spine alone, but requires muscular contribution (Crisco et al. 1992b; Wilder et al. 1988). In his seminal paper (Panjabi 1992), Panjabi emphasized that spinal stability depends on the contributions of three sub-systems: the passive sub-system, i.e. the osteoligamentous spine; the active sub-system, i.e. the muscles surrounding the spine; and the control sub-system, i.e. those parts of the nervous system that are involved with sensorimotor control of the spine, which exert effect through the active sub-system.

These above considerations may allow a sufficiently strict yet usable definition of spinal stability, however, stability is only a minimum requirement for a system to function. In that sense using the concept of stability in itself does not do justice to – for clinical practice highly relevant – nuances. When patient X can stand, many relevant questions remain, like how far and for how long does his posture deviate from the original position after a perturbation of a certain magnitude, how large a perturbation can X accommodate without falling and how much effort does X have to invest to stand? These three questions address crucial aspects of the function of any system. The first addresses the response to a perturbation or the system's performance, which is usually characterized by the time it takes to return to the planned state, or by the rate at which the system returns to this state. The second question can be generalized to: under how large a range of conditions will the system be stable, which is referred to as the robustness the system. While robustness is often positively related to performance, this is not necessarily the case. For example, when X deals with the deceleration of the bus by stiffening through co-contraction of muscles, this may provide very good performance when dealing with limited perturbations. However, if the bus driver hits the brakes very hard, this response may no longer be adequate and stepping may prove to be more robust. Finally, the third question is usually taken to relate to the control effort required to stabilize a system. To stay with the example of patient X, maintaining upright stance may require substantial cognitive effort in pathology. However, from a physiological perspective other costs also need to be considered. Co-contraction for example will stiffen joints, which may enhance performance, but it obviously requires metabolic energy and will increase joint loading.

We will use the term spine function instead of spinal stability, to encompass all these aspects (stability, performance, robustness, control effort and control costs). In this chapter, we will discuss the interaction of the sub-systems in relation to spine function and low back pain (LBP) and attempt to build a conceptual framework for the analysis of spine function in the clinical context.

MAINTAINING STABLE EQUILIBRIUM IN THE LUMBAR SPINE

To analyze spine function, it is useful to start with a very simple task, for which we will choose maintaining upright posture. To control spinal alignment, first of all, attaining mechanical equilibrium for all degrees of freedom is required. In addition, this equilibrium needs to be stable. Figure 5.1A presents a simplified model of the osteoligamentous lumbar spine, connecting the thorax and pelvis, which will be considered as rigid segments. To simplify this analysis even further we will consider the intervertebral joints as ball-in-socket joints that allow rotation around three axes only (no translations). To maintain a posture, equilibrium of moments around all joints needs to be present. In Figure 5.1A, gravity on the upper body (indicated by the arrow) acts vertically through the centres of the joints and hence causes no moments. Therefore the spine is in equilibrium. Theoretical modelling and experimental data, however, show that the equilibrium would in this situation be unstable. The stiffness provided by ligaments and discs would be too small to provide stability. A force as small as 90 N would cause the spine to buckle (Crisco et al. 1992a, 1992b) and deformation and potentially injurious compression and tension stresses would result (Fig. 5.1B). It has been shown that the additional stiffness provided by a low level of contraction of trunk muscles would suffice to provide stability (Cholewicki et al. 1997). To maintain equilibrium, muscles on both sides of the spine would need to produce equal moments to achieve zero net moments around all joints (Fig. 5.1C).

Next, let's assume that the spine is equilibrated by muscle activity only and consider the case where the upright posture needs to be maintained under an external force, for example the force exerted by a dog on a leash. The external force will produce moments around the lumbar joints that need to be equilibrated by muscles (Fig. 5.2A). However, when the direction of the pull on the leash changes with the dog stepping forward and the leash extending, muscle activity needs to be adjusted to provide totally different muscle moments around the joints (Fig. 5.2B). This suggests that control over the lumbar spine would be highly complicated and independently working muscle fascicles inserting on the vertebrae would be needed to fine-tune the moments produced at

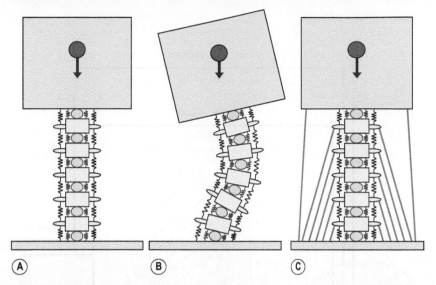

Figure 5.1 A simplified model of the osteoligamentous lumbar spine, connecting the thorax and pelvis, which are represented as rigid segments (A). Loaded with a mass equivalent to the mass of the upper body, the spine will be unstable and buckle (B). Muscles, when active, can provide sufficient stiffness to stabilize the spine in an upright posture (C).

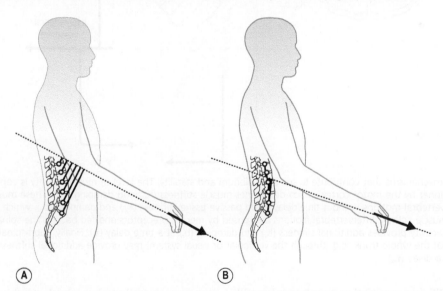

Figure 5.2 The effect of the force caused by a dog pulling on a leash (arrow) on the moments around the lumbar intervertebral joints (circles). The moment around each joint is equal to the length of the moment arm, i.e. the black lines representing the shortest distance from the joint to the working line of the force, multiplied by the magnitude of the force. (A) Equilibrating the pulling force requires extensor moments around all joints, increasing in magnitude in the caudal direction. (B) The differences between required moments at the different levels are larger, flexor moments are required at T12/L1 and L1/L2 and increasing extensor moments between L2/L3 and L5/S1.

each level. While several muscle fascicles insert on each lumbar vertebra (Bognuk et al. 1992), it is unclear whether these fascicles can be controlled independently by the nervous system and to what extent they can function independently in a mechanical sense, in view of interconnecting connective tissues (Huijing 2003). The complexity of the required motor control also contrasts sharply with the limited size of the area of the motor cortex that is involved with trunk muscle control.

Fortunately several mechanisms may facilitate control (Fig. 5.3). These mechanisms have in common that they are driven by displacements occurring as a consequence

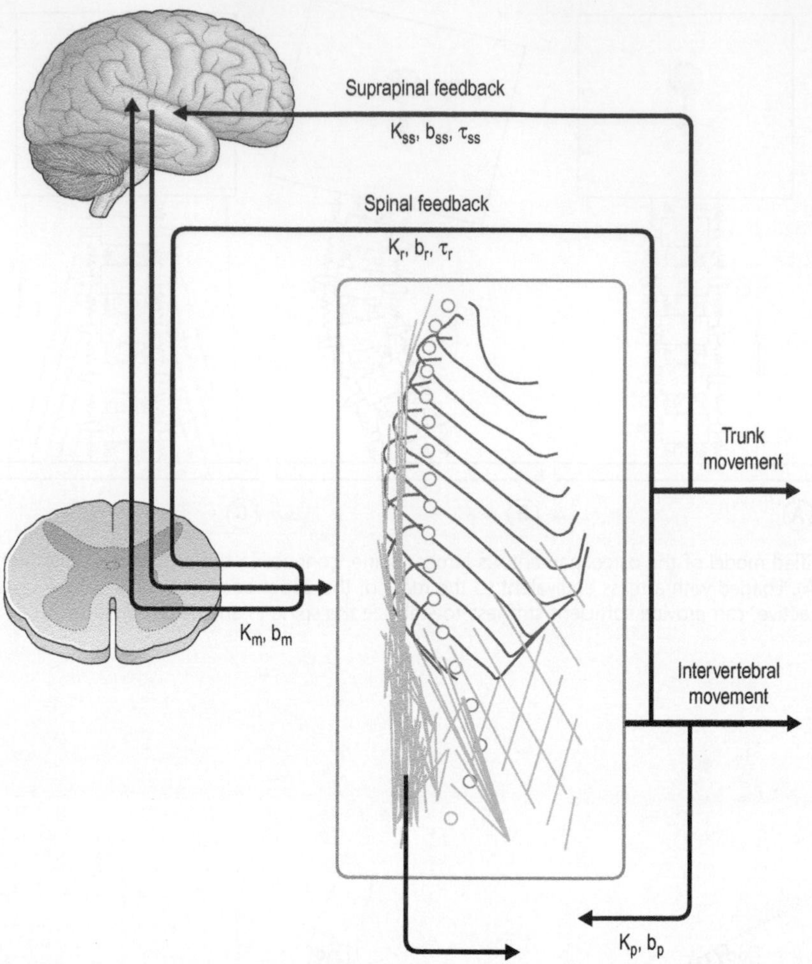

Figure 5.3 The mechanisms that contribute to spine equilibrium and stability. The level of muscle activity is controlled in a feed-forward manner by the motor cortex, which determines muscle stiffness (K_m) and damping (b_m). These muscle properties counteract intervertebral motions without time delay as do passive tissue stiffness (K_p) and damping (b_p), which are in turn determined by muscle activity. Intervertebral motions are sensed by mechanoreceptors and fed back to the spinal cord where reflexive muscle activity provides additional stiffness (K_r) and damping (b_r) at a time delay (τ_r). Finally, supraspinal feedback of sensed motions of the whole trunk (e.g. through the vestibular or visual system) may provide additional stiffness (K_{ss}) and damping (b_{ss}) at a delay (τ_{ss}).

of lack of equilibrium and in that sense can be considered feedback mechanisms. The first mechanism is the resistance against movement of the osteoligamentous spine itself. This resistance has two components: stiffness, which is dependent on the length of passive tissues and hence on the displacement between vertebrae, and damping, which is dependent on the rate of lengthening of the tissues. The second mechanism is the stiffness and damping provided by muscles. Muscles, when active, produce more force at higher length (within the range of muscle lengths typically encountered in normal movement) and when stretched. Hence active muscles also provide stiffness and damping (Young et al. 1992), which

appear to contribute importantly to the robustness of trunk movements (van der Burg et al. 2005a). The magnitude of muscle stiffness and damping increases with the level of muscle activity and hence these can be modulated by co-contraction (Selen et al. 2005). In addition, the axial forces that trunk muscles exert on the spine appear to increase the passive stiffness of the intervertebral discs (Gardner-Morse and Stokes 2003), which would make the spine more robust (Stokes and Gardner-Morse 2003). The third mechanism is based on neural feedback of length and rate of length change of passive tissues and muscles. These afferent signals can trigger reflex muscle activity that counteracts the signalled length change. In contrast with the first two mechanisms, reflex control occurs at a delay, which has important drawbacks for control as it may cause undesirable oscillations. Finally, as a fourth mechanism, central control is adjusted based on afferent feedback, including visual and vestibular feedback, but this involves even longer delay times and the dependence of long-delay responses on movement amplitude suggests that these only contribute when movements of the trunk as a whole do occur (Goodworth and Peterka 2009).

In modelling work, it has been assumed that passive tissue stiffness might be responsible for fine-tuning moment equilibrium around the intervertebral joints (Stokes et al. 1995). The assumption is that some intervertebral movement occurs, because muscles do not provide equilibrium. Consequently, passive tissues would be compressed or lengthened until they provide sufficient resistance to attain equilibrium. To test the validity of this assumption we performed an experiment, which simulated the dog on a leash (Kingma et al. 2007). We studied trunk muscle activity and lumbar curvature in subjects who were standing upright with their pelvis fixed to a frame. A marker was placed at C7 and the subject was given feedback of the position of this marker and was instructed to keep that position constant. Forward horizontal forces were applied at the thorax at three levels: the spinous processes of either Th3, Th6 or Th9 (Fig. 5.4). At each point of application the force yielded a moment of 30 or 50 Nm around the L3 spinous process. Like the dog

on a leash, this causes a different distribution of moments around the lumbar intervertebral joints. When applied at Th9, the moments between caudal and cranial levels differ strongly, while for forces applied at Th3, the moments are much more similar between levels. The task was static, i.e. we did not suddenly apply the forces, and recorded data only whethe subject had reached a steady state. The results showed that the lower the point of application of the force, the higher the activity in 8 of 11 muscles studied. More importantly spinal curvature also changed systematically with the point of application (Fig. 5.4C). The lower the point of application, or the larger the difference between moments at the adjacent intervertebral joints, the more kyphotic the spine was.

Although these data showed that muscle activation was adjusted to deal with different external loads, these changes in muscle activity did not prevent vertebral rotations. Instead, passive structures appeared to be strained until these produced moments that equilibrated the externally imposed moments or until feedback resulting from these strains caused sufficiently tuned muscle activity. This implies that the brain controls spinal posture only approximately and delegates part of the control to the periphery. It also suggests that the exact mutual orientation of the vertebrae is relatively unimportant and a substantial margin is used in the control of the spine, without necessarily causing problems. The results of this study emphasize the interaction between the passive and active structures.

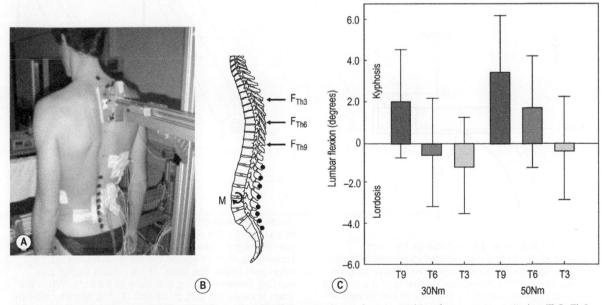

Figure 5.4 Photograph (A) and schematic illustration (B) of the experimental setup. Pushing forces were applied at Th3, Th6 and Th9 to produce equal moments of 30 and 50 Nm around L3. Resulting moment distributions with larger differences in moments between cranial and caudal intervertebral joints, i.e. a more caudal point of application of the external force, coincided with a significantly more kyphotic lumbar curvature (C), both at 30 and 50 Nm average moments.

DISORDERS OF THE PASSIVE SUB-SYSTEM

The way in which passive tissues interact with musculature to control spinal equilibrium will depend on the mechanical properties of the intervertebral joints and when stiffness of these joints is low, relatively large changes in spinal curvature can be expected in an experiment as described above, while for a stiffer spine, small rotations may suffice to reach the required moments (Fig. 5.5). From this perspective, the effects of degeneration and injury on spine stiffness are of particular interest.

Early work by Panjabi et al. (1984) showed that disc degeneration, simulated by inducing annulus injuries and nucleus resection, increased the intervertebral range of motion for a given moment. More recent work confirmed this for biological degeneration of the intervertebral disc, showing a larger range of motion for a given moment, a lower tangent stiffness and an increased neutral zone (NZ, i.e. the range of joint motion for which stiffness is minimal) (Gay et al. 2008; Hasegawa et al. 2008; Quint and Wilke 2008). Interestingly, one of these studies showed that the relationship between disc degeneration and stiffness, with disc degeneration graded based on histology, was much stronger than for degeneration graded based on imaging (Quint and Wilke 2008).

Ligament ruptures, not surprisingly, also decrease spinal stiffness, although the effects for some ligaments are very limited (Adams et al. 1980; Panjabi et al. 1982), especially after sustained loading (Busscher et al. 2011). Recently, Zhao et al (2005) showed that endplate failure due to compression likewise decreases stiffness and increases the NZ magnitude.

When equilibrium around the intervertebral joints is controlled by active structures only approximately, as we suggested above, the effects of a loss of stiffness of an intervertebral joint will be that more rotation will occur before equilibrium is reached (see θ_1 and θ_2 in Fig. 5.5). This might lead to excessive rotations, which could cause impingement of structures and as such provoke pain. From a control perspective, such a change in stiffness can quite easily be dealt with, if it occurs as a homogeneous change over the whole lumbar spine. A small overall increase in muscle activity for a given moment would suffice to compensate for the reduced moment generated by the spine and limit the rotations to within acceptable boundaries. However, if a single intervertebral joint is degenerated while adjacent joints are healthy, the heterogeneous stiffness may lead to instability, as the local deflection will tend to increase the bending moment at that level (Fig. 5.6).

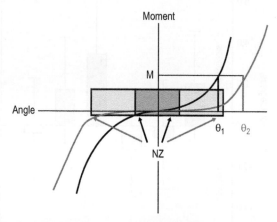

Figure 5.5 Moment–angle relationships for a non-degenerated (black) and degenerated (grey) intervertebral joint. The slope to the curve is the intervertebral (tangent) stiffness, which increases with an increasing joint angle and is lower in degenerated joints. The area of low stiffness is called the neutral zone (NZ), and is increased in degenerated joints. At a given moment (M) a smaller angle (θ_1) will occur for the non-degenerated joint than for the degenerated joint (θ_2).

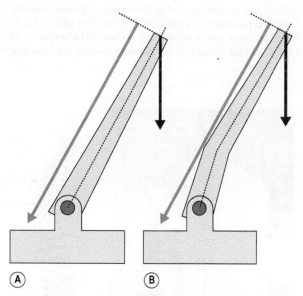

Figure 5.6 Loading of the spine can be compared to loading of a crane (A). The black arrow represents the load due to gravity, the grey arrow represents the muscle force that provides equilibrium around the center of rotation at the hinge joint below. The beam of the crane is loaded by a bending moment causing it to bend to the right. When the beam is locally less stiff, it will kink (B). The bending moment in the beam is maximal at the kink and consequently the kink tends to increase. When the bending moment at the kink increases faster with increasing angle than the tangent stiffness, the beam is unstable and will fail.

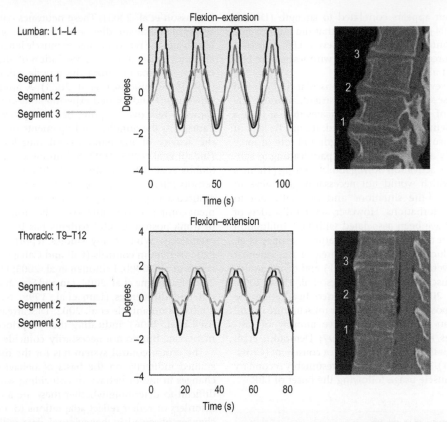

Figure 5.7 Bending angles of the three adjacent segments in one lumbar and one thoracic section of a single human spine as a function of time during a 4-point bending test and CT scans of the same spine sections.

To investigate whether heterogeneity in stiffness of the spine occurs, we investigated human cadaver spines from six 55–84-year-old donors. The spines were dissected in sections each comprising three motion segments. Pure moments were applied to each section in flexion-extension, lateral bending and axial rotation, ensuring constant moments throughout the whole spine section. Figure 5.7 gives an illustration of the results. The plots show the bending angles of the three adjacent segments in one lumbar and one thoracic section of a single human spine as a function of time. The differences in range of motion between adjacent segments in the lumbar section, which occur while the same moments (ranging from −4 to +4 Nm) are applied to these segments, clearly illustrate that stiffness is quite heterogeneous, with stiffness in segment 1 under positive bending moments being almost 50% of the stiffness in segment 2. Heterogeneity was less pronounced in thoracic spine sections. In addition, heterogeneity was much more pronounced in human spines than in spines of young pigs. All in all, these data suggest that degeneration can cause substantial heterogeneity in lumbar spine stiffness, which would complicate control over the spine.

DISORDERS OF THE ACTIVE SUB-SYSTEM

Given the fact that spine function relies on the interaction of the passive system with the active sub-system, i.e. muscles, instability might arise from disorders in the active sub-system as well as from disorders of the passive sub-system. To control the spine, muscles need sufficient strength. In most motor tasks, muscle force required will not be very high. However, especially in case of mechanical perturbations, muscle strength and especially the rate at which muscle forces can be generated may be limiting. The muscular disorders described below may affect strength and contraction velocity of the trunk muscles. Indeed several studies have shown differences between LBP patients and controls in muscle strength (Cassisi et al. 1993; Lee et al. 1995; Takemasa et al. 1995; Kankaanpaa et al. 1998; Thomas et al. 2008). Other studies, however, reported negative results (Ng et al. 2002; Lariviere et al. 2003). Rate of force rise, which is likely more important from the point of view of spine function, has been much less studied, but appears correlated to strength (Descarreaux et al. 2004). In the one study that did address rate of force rise controls, patients with severe LBP showed a faster rate of force rise than patients with less severe LBP (Descarreaux et al. 2004).

All in all, the evidence for loss of muscular strength and rate of force rise with LBP is not consistent, although the large number of positive results indicates that at least a part of the patients' strength is reduced. It must be kept in mind that measures of muscle strength and rate of force may be strongly affected by (fear of) pain leading to submaximal muscle activation during muscle testing (Thomas et al. 2008), which would not necessarily generalize to activation in real-life situations and especially not to responses to perturbations. However, several disorders of muscle tissue have been associated with LBP. Infiltration of fatty tissue in the extensor musculature (Mooney et al. 1997) and reduced cross-sectional area of the extensor musculature overall (Kaser et al. 2001) and of the multifidus (MU) muscle specifically (Hides et al. 1994, 2008; Wallwork et al. 2009) have been reported. In addition, the fibre type composition of the extensor musculature in LBP patients appears to indicate selective atrophy of fastglycolytic fibres (Mannion et al. 1997; Demoulin et al. 2007), although these findings were not consistent (Crossman et al. 2004). These changes are presumably secondary to decreased muscle usage following the onset of LBP.

DISORDERS OF THE CONTROL SUB-SYSTEM

The contribution of the active sub-system to spine function is regulated by the nervous system – loss of control and eventually instability might thus also arise from disorders of the control sub-system. For spine function, sensory information providing information on the state of the system needs to be integrated and used to generate adequate control of the active sub-system. Thus both disorders of the sensory system and the motor control system need to be considered here.

The sensory system comprises mechanoreceptors in ligaments, which have been suggested to have an important sensory function in feedback control of joint position (Johansson and Sjölander 1993; Sjölander et al. 2002). The annulus fibrosus of the intervertebral disc most likely serves a similar function, as it is richly supplied with mechanoreceptors (Yoshizawa et al. 1980; Roberts et al. 1995). Sensory afference from spinal ligaments and the annulus is likely to be corrupted when passive tissue injuries occur either due to damage to afferents or to changes in length of structures following a loss of disc height (Panjabi 2006). In addition, nociceptive afference from muscle and joint tissue has been shown to affect the activity of the gamma motor neurones (Pedersen et al. 1998;

Johansson et al. 2003). These neurones control the excitability of muscle spindles, sensory organs signalling muscle length and the rate of change of muscle length. Nociceptive afference causes a reduced resolution of afferent, proprioceptive information from the muscle spindles (Pedersen et al. 1998; Johansson et al. 2003). A number of animal experiments and limited experimentation in humans has shown a reflexive coupling between provocation of and damage to the annulus and ligaments on one hand and the activity of the paravertebral muscles on the other (Indahl et al. 1995, 1997; Solomonow et al. 1998, 2003; Stubbs et al. 1998; Holm et al. 2002). If proprioceptive sensory afference is affected in LBP, patients should have a reduced acuity of perception of trunk posture and movement compared to healthy controls. Proprioceptive acuity of trunk posture in LBP patients has been studied quite extensively. While many studies report lower acuity in patients than in controls (Gill and Callaghan 1998; Newcomer et al. 2000b; Leinonen et al. 2003; O'Sullivan et al. 2003; Brumagne et al. 2004; Lin and Sun 2006), others did not find differences (Lam et al. 1999; Newcomer et al. 2000a; Koumantakis et al. 2002; Descarreaux et al. 2005; Asell et al. 2006), indicating that proprioceptive impairments can, but do not necessarily, coincide with LBP.

The motor control system has for the major part been studied indirectly on the basis of behavioural data, i.e. changes in motor behaviour coinciding with LBP. As it is difficult to determine whether these are a direct result of disorders or rather reflect adaptations to a disorder, such changes observed in behavioural data will be discussed separately in the next section. In this section, we will focus on changes that have been observed in the motor control system itself, i.e. the nervous system, with only a brief excursion into behavioural consequences that may result.

Experimentally induced pain has been shown to change the gain of motor reflex loops to other muscles, with either inhibitory (Graven-Nielsen et al. 1997), or excitatory (Matre et al. 1998, 1999), effects, possibly through effects on the gamma-loop as discussed above. However, experimentally induced LBP specifically did not have an effect on stretch reflexes in the erector spinae (ES) (Young et al. 1992; Zedka et al. 1999). In line with this, a review of the literature on ES activity in LBP concluded that the changes observed with LBP cannot be explained by hard-wired, deterministic reflex responses (van Dieën et al. 2003c).

Changes upstream in the motor control system have rarely been studied in relation to LBP. Tsao et al. (2008), showed with transcranial magnetic stimulation that the motor cortical map of the transverse abdominus muscle (TA) is shifted in patients with recurrent LBP. This muscle shows delayed activation in LBP patients (see 'Motor behaviour in low back pain' below) that might thus be attributable to this cortical re-organization, although cortical motor thresholds appeared decreased rather than increased. In addition, Strutton et al. (2005), showed higher thresholds for both facilitory and inhibitory responses of the ES to transcranial magnetic stimulation compared to healthy individuals. The functional consequences of these findings remain unclear, but the results may suggest problems in modulating ES activity.

MOTOR BEHAVIOUR IN LOW BACK PAIN

There is evidence that control over trunk posture and movement is degraded in LBP patients. Patients have been shown to be less able to precisely grade force of the trunk extensor muscles (Grabiner et al. 1992; Descarreaux et al. 2004), and to perform less well in making goal-directed trunk movements (Descarreaux et al. 2005). In addition, Radebold et al. (2001) reported increased trunk sway with LBP in seated balancing. In a recent study, we found no increase in sway amplitude in subjects with less severe LBP during seated balancing. However, a decrease in the sway frequency was found, which was taken to be indicative of an increase in spine stiffness due to changes in trunk muscle recruitment (van Dieën et al. 2010).

Stiffening the spine in a feed-forward manner would create robust control over the spine at limited control effort. Therefore, we had previously hypothesized that LBP would coincide with compensatory changes in trunk muscle activity, aimed at stiffening the spine. To test this hypothesis, we first studied the feasibility of such adaptive strategies using model simulations and next we investigated whether such changes in recruitment were present in patients with LBP.

To investigate whether muscular compensation for a loss of spine function is possible, we used model simulations to test the effect of potential trunk muscle recruitment strategies (van Dieën et al. 2003a). First, co-contraction of antagonistic muscles was expected to increase spine stiffness (strategy 1). Second, Bergmark (1989), using a strongly simplified model of the lumbar trunk, indicated that so-called local muscles, i.e. muscles that insert on the lumbar vertebrae, would contribute more to stiffening the spine than so-called global muscles, which insert on pelvis and thorax only. We chose to test the effect of recruiting the lumbar part of the ES (LES) preferentially over its synergist, the thoracic part of the ES (TES; strategy 2), as this was a recruitment pattern that could later be studied using surface electromyography. For the same reason we studied the effect of preferential recruitment of the internal oblique muscle (IO) relative to the rectus abdominus (RA; strategy 3).

Using a detailed musculoskeletal trunk model (Cholewicki et al. 1996), we simulated slow movements around the upright posture in the sagittal, transverse and frontal planes separately. Furthermore, we investigated maintenance of upright posture against an external force applied to the thorax in the sagittal and frontal planes. EMG data were obtained for these tasks from two healthy subjects. Data from the two subjects were averaged to create a data set representative of a healthy subject and fed into the model. In short, EMG amplitudes were used to estimate muscle force and stiffness for each of the 90 muscles represented in the model. The model output summarizes the stiffness in each of the 18 degrees of freedom (6 lumbar intervertebral joints times 3 rotations) in a single number. Subsequently, the EMG data were manipulated to simulate each of three strategies separately. For strategy 1, antagonistic activity was increased by 20%. To test strategies 2 and 3, the activity of TES and RA was decreased by 50% in separate simulations for the two strategies. The activity of the other muscles was increased to keep the lumbar moment equal.

The model predicted that for all tasks each of the three strategies would increase lumbar spine stiffness. The effect generally was strongest for the preferential recruitment of the LES over the TES. Simulation of all three strategies simultaneously had an additive effect and resulted in the largest enhancement of spine stiffness.

As a next step, we investigated whether patients with aspecific, chronic LBP use these compensatory strategies (van Dieën et al. 2003a). Sixteen patients were compared to 16 matched healthy volunteers. They performed the same tasks as used for the simulations described above, while surface EMG was measured from selected trunk muscles. The ratio of EMG amplitudes of antagonistic over agonistic muscles was calculated. For example, when the subject was bending forward, the sum of the abdominal muscles' EMG amplitudes was divided by the sum of the extensors' EMG amplitudes. In addition, the ratios of LES over TES EMG amplitude and of IO over RA EMG amplitude were calculated.

It was found that over all conditions, LBP patients showed a higher ratio of antagonistic over agonistic EMG activity and a higher LES/TES ratio than the healthy subjects. While IO/RA activity was also higher on average in the LBP patients, this effect was not significant.

In a second study (van der Hoorn et al. 2012), involving another group of patients and controls, similar measurements were made during gait at a range of velocities. Again, the ratio of LES over TES was significantly higher and antagonistic activity tended to be higher in the patient group. Moreover, the magnitude of the ratios appeared to be related to the level of pain reported by the patients.

More detailed analysis of the data of the two studies showed that some patients did consistently use preferential recruitment of the LES over the TES, while others were found to consistently use increased co-contraction of antagonistic muscles. Moreover, discriminant analysis showed that a sub-group of patients could be discerned with an increased IO/RA ratio, even though this ratio was not significantly increased over the group as a whole.

Finally, in some patients no compensatory strategies were revealed, and in some patients evidence was found for a potentially counter-productive strategy, i.e. preferential recruitment of the TES, in line with findings by Reeves et al. (2006).

In contrast with the line of reasoning advanced above, other authors have emphasized motor control changes in LBP that they interpret as ineffective in stabilizing the spine. Expected mechanical perturbations of the trunk, which occur for example when rapidly raising an arm, are usually preceded by activation of deep trunk muscles such as the TA (Cresswell et al. 1994; Hodges and Richardson 1997) and the MU (Moseley et al. 2002, 2003). This anticipatory activity is delayed in patients with LBP (Hodges 2001; Hodges and Richardson 1996, 1998, 1999). This delayed onset of deep muscle activity was hypothesized to negatively affect spinal stabilization and it has been suggested that while the delay appears to be a result rather than the cause of pain (Hodges et al. 2003; Moseley et al. 2004b), this could play a role in recurrence of LBP (Hodges and Moseley 2003; Moseley and Hodges 2006; MacDonald et al. 2009). Also reactive control after unexpected perturbations of the trunk appears to be different between LBP patients and controls in a way that appears to indicate reduced spine function. Delayed responses of the ES in LBP patients were found both in a sudden release experiment (Radebold et al. 2000) and a sudden loading experiment (Magnusson et al. 1996). The amplitude of the ES response to sudden loading also was reduced (Magnusson et al. 1996). Short latency reflexes in the ES in response to sudden upper limb loading appeared unaffected, but in contrast to controls the latency was not shortened when subjects anticipated the perturbation (Leinonen et al. 2001).

In our opinion, an alternative explanation can be offered for the reported findings. Anticipatory muscle activity may be less necessary in LBP patients, because they stiffen their spine by recruitment of superficial muscles as described above, which provides robustness against ensuing perturbations (Hodges and Richardson 1999; van Dieën et al. 2003b). Increased spine stiffness by feed-forward strategies could also account for the delayed and reduced responses after a perturbation, since prior activation of muscles reduces the magnitude of the displacement resulting from a given perturbation and the amplitude of the responses in these muscles to the perturbation (Stokes et al. 2000). We thus hypothesize that the stabilizing strategies described above may account for the disappearance of anticipatory muscle activation and the consequent anticipatory postural adjustments in back pain patients preceding fast limb movements, as well as the delay and decrease in feedback responses after perturbations. Observations of increased activity in other trunk muscles coinciding with delayed anticipatory activity of deep muscles (Moseley et al. 2004a) would be in line with this hypothesis.

Patients with LBP may rely less on anticipation for the very reason of wanting to avoid spinal instability. If the possibilities for corrections are limited, anticipation might impose a risk. For this reason, patients might prefer a simple and robust strategy, such as co-contraction, like healthy subjects do when specific anticipation is impossible (Lavender et al. 1993; van Dieën et al. 2003b) and anticipatory postural adjustments might be suppressed, as was found in healthy subjects when the risk associated with balance loss was high (Adkin et al. 2002) and in patient groups with problems in maintaining whole-body equilibrium (Latash and Anson 1996).

In conclusion, patients with LBP appear to use muscle recruitment strategies that increase trunk stiffness, possibly as a compensatory strategy to counteract impaired spine function. However not all patients used these compensatory strategies. Control can also be enhanced by optimizing active feedback control. Increasing reflex gains can provide increased perturbation resistance. However, as discussed above, no consistent indications for an increase in reflex gains with LBP have been found. Moreover, increasing reflex gains is effective only provided that the sensory information driving these reflexes is adequate, whereas it can be questioned whether feedback from injured or degenerated spinal structures is accurate and, as discussed above, proprioceptive acuity is often reduced in LBP. In addition, when reflex delays are too long, increased gains can actually cause instability, while reflex delays may actually be increased in LBP. These considerations suggest that feedback control may be less efficient in LBP.

The data presented, which indicate that most subjects with LBP use muscle recruitment strategies that may be simple feed-forward compensatory strategies for a loss of spine function, should be interpreted with care. LBP definitely entails more than a loss of spine function. Fear of pain or re-injury, which is associated with LBP (Vlaeyen et al. 1995), may emphasize the importance of a robust control strategy. Whenever the perceived probability of and/or the risk attached to a loss of control is large, compensatory strategies can be expected to be used, whether warranted or not. Experimentally induced fear of pain in the back indeed appeared to trigger changes in motor control comparable to those described above (van Dieën et al. 1999; Newcomer et al. 2000a). Moreover, several studies have shown that trunk muscle activation patterns preceding an expected perturbation are less variable in patients with LBP (Moseley and Hodges 2006; Jacobs et al. 2009), and that the prefrontal cortex is more strongly involved in preparing these actions than in controls (Jacobs et al. 2009). These findings appear to indicate more conscious spinal control in LBP patients. Also in goal-directed trunk movements, an indication for more cognitive involvement in the control was found in the form of longer deceleration times, suggesting closed-loop control to enhance movement accuracy in spite of impairments (Descarreaux et al. 2005). In conclusion, the trigger for changes in motor behaviour may be aspecific and it can be questioned whether control effort is indeed reduced. Nevertheless, we hypothesize that the control strategies used by LBP patients make spine function more robust.

COSTS OF BEHAVIOURAL ADAPTATIONS

Since motor control must compromise between various criteria, increasing robustness of spine function will likely have negative consequences regarding other criteria, such as efficiency. Increased trunk muscle co-contraction comes at the cost of increased spinal loading. Indeed, LBP patients lifting loads have been reported to expose their spine to higher forces than controls, although patient and control groups were poorly matched in these studies (Marras et al. 2001, 2004, 2005). These adverse effects appeared most pronounced during the least heavy tasks (Marras et al. 2005). This would imply that the risk of acute overloading of the spine is not much increased, but nevertheless risks related to cumulative loading may be elevated. Furthermore, low-level co-contraction of trunk muscles may occur in LBP patients even at rest (van Dieën et al. 2003c), implying that compression of the spine is sustained during rest. Animal models implicate sustained low-level compression as a cause of disc degeneration, allegedly due to disrupted fluid flow into and out of the intervertebral disc (Hutton et al. 2000, 2001, Lotz and Chin 2000, Stokes and Iatridis 2004, Strutton et al. 2005). Suppressed flow of fluid into the disc, due to sustained compression, would hamper recovery of disc height. Therefore, reduced recovery of stature in LBP patients during rest after exercise, which is correlated to trunk muscle activity during rest (Healey et al. 2005a, 2005b), indeed suggests that fluid inflow may be impaired by sustained muscle contractions in these patients. The different muscle recruitment strategies found in LBP as described above will likely differ in terms of these costs. For example, some LBP patients used increased antagonistic co-contraction to stiffen the lumbar spine, whereas others used preferential recruitment of LES over TES. The latter strategy appeared more effective in stabilizing the spine (van Dieën et al. 2003a), and is probably less costly in terms of spinal compression. Such differences in cost–benefit ratio may well have clinical relevance.

Sustained low-level muscle activity, as was found in some patients (van Dieën et al. 2003c), may have harmful effects, when local circulation is compromised, or when the same motor units are continuously active (Visser and van Dieën 2006). Recently, we showed that trunk extensor contractions at intensities as low as 2% of maximum activation can cause fatigue manifestation over the course of half an hour (van Dieën et al. 2009). Patients that do show

sustained trunk muscle activation may thus incur fatigue and discomfort (Jorgensen et al. 1988; van Dieën et al. 2009), or even back pain of muscular origin (Visser and van Dieën 2006).

It has been shown that LBP patients have poor balance in standing compared to healthy controls (Alexander and LaPier 1998; Luoto et al. 1998; Hamaoui et al. 2002; Grimstone and Hodges 2003), especially when postural control is challenged by manipulation of visual (Takala et al. 1997; Alexander and LaPier 1998; Mientjes and Frank 1999; Brumagne et al. 2004, 2008; Hamaoui et al. 2004; della Volpe et al. 2006) or vestibular (Nies and Sinnott 1991; Mientjes and Frank 1999) information, or by manipulations of the support surface (Nies and Sinnott 1991; Takala et al. 1997; Mientjes and Frank 1999; Hamaoui et al. 2002; della Volpe et al. 2006; Popa et al. 2007; Brumagne et al. 2008). When poor balance control leads to balance loss, the ensuing strong muscular responses may be a cause of (aggravation of) LBP (Oddsson et al. 1999; Burg et al. 2005b). Furthermore, when balance loss results in a fall, this can be a cause of serious injury, especially in the elderly (Tideiksaar 1997). In fact, fall risk is increased by LBP in young adults (Hollowell et al. 2007) and the elderly (unpublished analysis of data in the LASA (Pluijm 2001) cohort). Degraded postural control with LBP can of course be a direct consequence of the impairments discussed above. However, interestingly it has also been attributed to a reduced use of lumbar motion to correct balance, due to the stiffening effect of trunk muscle co-contraction (Mok et al. 2004, 2007). Recent data from our lab, on postural sway in sitting on an unstable surface, show that subjects with current LBP display postural sway with low-frequency content (van Dieën et al. 2010). This is consistent with stiffening of the lumbar spine, which leads to sway of the body as a whole instead of pelvic and thoracic counter movements (Burg et al. 2006). Thus it appears that enhanced spine function obtained by stiffening the spine may occur at the cost of balance control.

DISCUSSION AND CONCLUSIONS

LBP is frequently associated with 'instability' of the spine. As discussed above, one path towards spinal instability might be a loss of mechanical stiffness of the passive tissues of the spine or a single spinal motion segment due to injury or degeneration. However, the relationship between LBP and loss of spinal stiffness due to injury or degeneration is not proven. In most cases of LBP, no specific diagnosis is made. Injury to the spine may well be a cause of LBP and may in fact be the underlying cause of many LBP cases that presently go undiagnosed (van Dieën et al. 1999). Also it has been shown that the presence of disc degeneration as diagnosed with X-ray, increases the probability of having LBP by a factor higher than 3 (van

Tulder et al. 1997a). The literature on patho-anatomical findings in relation to LBP however clearly shows that the relationship between such findings and pain is stochastic. Some people may have substantial degeneration, without symptoms, others may have severe symptoms with no or negligible degeneration. In fact, the data described above may explain this disparity. First, the relationship between imaging-based gradations of degeneration and spinal stiffness is not perfect and moreover non-linear (Quint and Wilke 2008). Second, when active compensation for loss of spinal stiffness is possible, such a loss does not necessarily lead to symptoms.

A second route towards spinal instability might be through muscular disorders. The literature reviewed above, however, suggests that muscular changes may usually be secondary to LBP. Also the third route towards instability, through disorders of the control sub-system, appears a secondary phenomenon rather than a primary cause. In the case of a loss of proprioceptive acuity, this would appear to be due to nociception or injury to structures containing mechanoreceptors. For disorders of the motor control system, evidence based on behavioural measures also indicates a secondary phenomenon, since similar behavioural changes are usually found in induced pain experiments. Furthermore, the functional implications of changes in motor behaviour remain as yet unclear as these have been interpreted as adaptive but also as maladaptive.

One could argue that the question as to primary cause or secondary phenomenon is not very relevant in a dynamic system with compensatory interactions between sub-systems. Reduced capacity of any of the sub-systems, whether pathological or within the normal range, could set the stage for a loss of spine function and eventually instability. Moreover, secondary phenomena may be the primary cause of recurrence.

Low back pain is widely prevalent, entails major costs, and can severely compromise quality of life (van Tulder et al. 1995; Andersson 1999). Invariably, LBP affects motor behaviour, which to a large extent accounts for its disabling effects. Unfortunately, the relationship between musculoskeletal disorders and motor behaviour is poorly understood and the literature lacks a theoretical framework to guide the development of a more appropriate understanding. Consequently, the (para-)medical disciplines involved lack a basis for treatment and outcome evaluation with respect to motor function. This severely hampers clinical practice. For disorders with major tissue damage, treatment aims at reconstruction or replacement of structures, without a follow-up to optimize functional outcome. For disorders without major tissue damage, (conservative) treatment options often lack a clear rationale that can be translated into a successful approach. In the case of LBP, different therapeutic interventions, for example exercise therapies, abound, often based on mutually contradictive principles, while overall clinical success is marginal (van Tulder et al. 1997b, 2000). Although clinical guidelines emphasize that patients with musculoskeletal disorders should remain physically active, these usually pay no attention to the quality of motor behaviour. In the context of loss of spine function in LBP, the above suggests a role for motor training to enhance the use of compensatory motor strategies, to counteract muscle atrophy and possibly to de-learn compensatory changes when these occur at high costs, especially when the underlying problem has been resolved. However, to make this possible, future research will need to provide the methods to allow clinicians to assess the adaptive and maladaptive aspects of motor behaviour that may be present in a specific patient or sub-group of patients. Such research will need to address motor control changes (feedforward as well as feedback) in relation to mechanical integrity of the spine (e.g. based on MRI grading of disc degeneration) and address the relationship of these factors to recurrence and prognosis in LBP, to differentiate between adaptive and maladaptive changes in motor behaviour.

REFERENCES

Adams, M.A., Hutton, W.C., Stott, J.R.R., 1980. The resistance to flexion of the lumbar intervertebral joint. Spine 5:245–253.

Adkin, A.L., Frank, J.S., Carpenter, M.G., Peysar, G.W., 2002. Fear of falling modifies anticipatory postural control. Exp Brain Res 143:160–170.

Alexander, K.M., LaPier, T.L., 1998. Differences in static balance and weight distribution between normal subjects and subjects with chronic unilateral low back pain. J Orthop Sports Phys Ther 28:378–383.

Andersson, G.B.J., 1999. Epidemiological features of chronic low-back pain. Lancet 354:581–585.

Asell, M., Sjolander, P., Kerschbaumer, H., Djupsjobacka, M., 2006. Are lumbar repositioning errors larger among patients with chronic low back pain compared with asymptomatic subjects? Arch Phys Med Rehabil 87:1170–1176.

Bergmark, A., 1989. Stability of the lumbar spine. A study in mechanical engineering. Acta Orthop Scand Suppl 230:1–54.

Bogduk, N., Macintosh, J.E., Pearcy, M.J., 1992. A universal model of the lumbar back muscles in the upright position. Spine 17:897–913.

Brumagne, S., Cordo, P., Verschueren, S., 2004a. Proprioceptive weighting changes in persons with low back pain and elderly persons during upright standing. Neurosci Lett 366:63–66.

Brumagne, S., Cordo, P., Verschueren, S., 2004b. Proprioceptive weighting changes in persons with low back pain and elderly persons during upright standing. Neurosci Lett 366:63–66.

Brumagne, S., Janssens, L., Knapen, S., Claeys, K., Suuden-Johanson, E., 2008. Persons with recurrent low back pain exhibit a rigid postural control strategy. Eur Spine J 17:1177–1184.

Busscher, I., van Dieën, J.H., van der Veen, A.J., Kingma, I., Meijer, G.J.M., Verkerke, G.J., et al., 2011. The effects of creep and recovery on the in-vitro biomechanical behaviour of human multi-level thoracolumbar spinal segments. Clin Biomech 26: 438–444

Cassisi, J.E., Robinson, M.E., O'Conner, P., MacMillan, M., 1993. Trunk strength and lumbar paraspinal muscle activity during isometric exercise in chronic low-back pain patients and controls. Spine 18:245–251.

Cholewicki, J., McGill, S.M., 1996. Mechanical stability of the in-vivo lumbar spine – implications for injury and chronic low-back-pain. Clin Biomech 11:1–15.

Cholewicki, J., Panjabi, M.M., Khatchatryan, A., 1997. Stabilizing function of trunk flexor/extensor muscles around a neutral spine posture. Spine 22:2207–2212.

Cresswell, A.G., Oddson, L., Thorstensson, A., 1994. The influence of sudden perturbations on trunk muscle activity and intra-abdominal pressure while standing. Exp Brain Res 98:336–341.

Crisco, J.J., Panjabi, M.M., 1992a. Euler stability of the human ligamentous spine. Part I Theory. Clin Biomech 7:19–26.

Crisco, J.J., Panjabi, M.M., 1992b. Euler stability of the human ligamentous spine. Part II Experiment. Clin Biomech 7:27–32.

Crossman, K., Mahon, M., Watson, P.J., Oldham, J.A., Cooper, R.G., 2004. Chronic low back pain-associated paraspinal muscle dysfunction is not the result of a constitutionally determined 'adverse' fiber-type

composition. Spine (Phila Pa 1976) 29:628–634.

della Volpe, R., Popa, T., Ginanneschi, F., Spidalieri, R., Mazzocchio, R., Rossi, A., 2006. Changes in coordination of postural control during dynamic stance in chronic low back pain patients. Gait Posture 24:349–355.

Demoulin, C., Crielaard, J.M., Vanderthommen, M., 2007. Spinal muscle evaluation in healthy individuals and low-back-pain patients: a literature review. Joint Bone Spine 74:9–13.

Descarreaux, M., Blouin, J.S., Teasdale, N., 2004. Force production parameters in patients with low back pain and healthy control study participants. Spine 29:311–317.

Descarreaux, M., Blouin, J.S., Teasdale, N., 2005. Repositioning accuracy and movement parameters in low back pain subjects and healthy control subjects. Eur Spine J 14:185–191.

Gardner-Morse, M.G., Stokes, I.A.F., 2003. Physiological axial compressive preloads increase motion segment stiffness, linearity and hysteresis in all six degrees of freedom for small displacements about the neutral posture. J Orthop Res 21:547–552.

Gay, R.E., Ilharreborde, B., Zhao, K., Bournediene, E., An, K.A., 2008. The effect of loading rate and degeneration on neutral region motion in human cadaveric lumbar motion segments. Clin Biomech 23:1–7.

Gill, K.P., Callaghan, M.J., 1998. The measurement of lumbar proprioception in individuals with and without low back pain. Spine 23:371–377.

Goodworth, A.D., Peterka, R.J., 2009. Contribution of sensorimotor integration to spinal stabilization in humans. J Neurophysiol 102:496–512.

Grabiner, M.D., Koh, T.J., El Ghazawi, A., 1992. Decoupling of bilateral paraspinal excitation in subjects with low back pain. Spine 17:1219–1223.

Graven-Nielsen, T., Svensson, P., Arendt-Nielsen, L., 1997. Effects of experimental muscle pain on muscle activity and co-ordination during static and dynamic motor function. Electroencephalogr Clin Neurophysiol 105:156–164.

Grimstone, S.K., Hodges, P.W., 2003. Impaired postural compensation for respiration in people with recurrent low back pain. Exp Brain Res 151:218–224.

Hamaoui, A., Do, M., Poupard, L., Bouisset, S., 2002. Does respiration perturb body balance more in chronic low back pain subjects than in healthy subjects? Clin Biomech (Bristol, Avon) 17:548–550.

Hamaoui, A., Do, M.C., Bouisset, S., 2004. Postural sway increase in low back pain subjects is not related to reduced spine range of motion. Neurosci Lett 357:135–138.

Hasegawa, K., Kitahara, K., Hara, T., Takano, K., Shimoda, H., Homma, T., 2008. Evaluation of lumbar segmental instability in degenerative diseases by using a new intraoperative measurement system. J Neurosurg Spine 8:255–262.

Healey, E.L., Fowler, N.E., Burden, A.M., McEwan, I.M., 2005a. Raised paraspinal muscle activity reduces rate of stature recovery after loaded exercise in individuals with chronic low back pain. Arch Phys Med Rehabil 86:710–715.

Healey, E.L., Fowler, N.E., Burden, A.M., McEwan, I.M., 2005b. The influence of different unloading positions upon stature recovery and paraspinal muscle activity. Clin Biomech (Bristol, Avon) 20: 365–371.

Hertel, P., Behrend, H., Cierpinski, T., Musahl, V., Widjaja, G., 2005. ACL reconstruction using bone-patellar tendon-bone press-fit fixation: 10-year clinical results. Knee Surg Sports Traumatol Arthrosc 13:248–255.

Hides, J.A., Stokes, M.J., Saide, M., Jull, G.A., Cooper, D.H., 1994. Evidence of lumbar multifidus muscle wasting ipsilateral to symptoms in patients with acute/subacute low back pain. Spine 19:165–172.

Hides, J., Gilmore, C., Stanton, W., Bohlscheid, E., 2008. Multifidus size and symmetry among chronic LBP and healthy asymptomatic subjects. Man Ther 13:43–49.

Hodges, P.W., 2001. Changes in motor planning of feedforward postural responses of the trunk muscles in low back pain. Exp Brain Res 141:261–266.

Hodges, P.W., Moseley, G.L., 2003. Pain and motor control of the lumbopelvic region: effect and possible mechanisms. J Electromyogr Kinesiol 13:361–370.

Hodges, P.W., Richardson, C.A., 1996. Inefficient muscular stabilization of the lumbar spine associated with low back pain. A motor control evaluation of transversus abdominis. Spine 21:2640–2650.

Hodges, P.W., Richardson, C.A., 1997. Feedforward contraction of transversus abdominis is not influenced by the direction of arm movement. Exp Brain Res 114:362–370.

Hodges, P.W., Richardson, C.A., 1998. Delayed postural contraction of transversus abdominis in low back pain associated with movement of the lower limb. J Spinal Disord 11:46–56.

Hodges, P.W., Richardson, C.A., 1999. Altered trunk muscle recruitment in people with low back pain with upper limb movement at different speeds. Arch Phys Med Rehabil 80:1005–1012.

Hodges, P.W., Moseley, G.L., Gabrielsson, A., Gandevia, S.C., 2003. Experimental muscle pain changes feedforward postural responses of the trunk muscles. Exp Brain Res 151:262–271.

Hollowell, J., Kerry, R., Walsh, D., 2007. Static balance confidence and falls in chronic low back pain sufferers and healthy controls. 6th Interdisciplinary World Congress on Low Back and Pelvic Pain. Barcelona, p. 389.

Holm, S., Indahl, A., Solomonow, M., 2002. Sensorimotor control of the spine. J Electromyogr Kinesiol 12:219–234.

Huijing, P.A., 2003. Muscular force transmission necessitates a multilevel integrative approach to the analysis of function of skeletal muscle. Exerc Sport Sci Rev 31:167–175.

Hutton, W.C., Ganey, T.M., Elmer, W.A., Kozlowska, E., Ugbo, J.L., Doh, E.S., et al., 2000. Does long-term compressive loading on the intervertebral disc cause degeneration? Spine 25:2993–3004.

Hutton, W.C., Elmer, W.A., Bryce, L.M., Boden, S.D., Kozlowski, M., 2001. Do the intervertebral disc cells respond to different levels of hydrostatic pressure? Clin Biomech (Bristol, Avon) 16:728–734.

Indahl, A., Kaigle, A., Reikeras, O., Holm, S., 1995. Electromyographic response of the porcine multifidus musculature after nerve stimulation. Spine 20:2652–2658.

Indahl, A., Kaigle, A.M., Reikeras, O., Holm, S.H., 1997. Interaction betweeen the porcine lumbar intervertebral disc, zygapophysial joints, and paraspinal muscles. Spine 22:2834–2840.

Jacobs, J., Henry, S., Nagle, K., 2009. Low back pain associates with altered activity of the cerebral cortex prior to amr movements that require anticipatory postural adjustments of the trunk. In: Chiari, L., Nardone A. (eds),. XIX Conference of the International Society for Posture & Gait Research. DEIS – Universita di Bolhna, Bologna, p. 184.

Johansson, H., Sjölander, P., 1993. Neurophysiology of joints. In: Wright, V., Radin E.L. (eds), Mechanics of Human Joints. Marcel Dekker, New York, pp. 243–290.

Johansson, H., Arendt-Nielsen, L., Bergenheim, M., Djupsjöbacka, M., Gold, J.E., Ljubisavljevic, M., Passatore, M., 2003. Epilogue: an integrative model. In: Johansson, H., Windhorst, U., Djupsjöbacka, M., Passatore, M., et al. (eds), Chronic Work-related Myalgia. Neuromuscular mechanisms behind work-related chronic muscle syndromes. Gävle University Press, Gävle, Sweden, pp. 291–300.

Jorgensen, K., Fallentin, N., Krogh-Lund, C., Jensen, B., 1988. Electromyography and fatigue during prolonged, low-level static contractions. Eur J Appl Physiol Occup Physiol 57:316–321.

Kankaanpaa, M., Taimela, S., Laaksonen, D., Hanninen, O., Airaksinen, O., 1998. Back and hip extensor fatigability in chronic low back pain patients and controls. Arch Phys Med Rehabil 79:412–417.

Kaser, L., Mannion, A.F., Rhyner, A., Weber, E., Dvorak, J., Muntener, M., 2001. Active therapy for chronic low back pain: part 2. Effects on paraspinal muscle cross-sectional area, fiber type size, and distribution. Spine 26:909–919.

Kingma, I., Staudenmann, D., van Dieën, J.H., 2007. Trunk muscle activation and associated lumbar spine joint shear forces under different levels of external forward force applied to the trunk. J Electromyogr Kinesiol 17:14–24.

Koumantakis, G.A., Winstanley, J., Oldham, J.A., 2002. Thoracolumbar proprioception in individuals with and without low back pain: intratester reliability, clinical applicability, and validity. J Orthop Sports Phys Ther 32:327–335.

Lam, S.S.K., Jull, G., Treleaven, J., 1999. Lumbar spine kinesthesia in patients with low back pain. J Orthop Sports Phys Ther 29:294–299.

Lariviere, C., Arsenault, A.B., Gravel, D., Gagnon, D., Loisel, P., 2003. Surface electromyography assessment of back muscle intrinsic properties. J Electromyogr Kinesiol 13:305–318.

Latash, M.L., Anson, J.G., 1996. What are 'normal movements' in atypical populations? Behav Brain Sci 19:55–106.

Lavender, S.A., Marras, W.S., Miller, R.A., 1993. The development of response strategies in preparation for sudden loading to the torso. Spine 18:2097–2105.

Lee, J.H., Ooi, Y., Nakamura, K., 1995. Measurement of muscle strength of the trunk and the lower-extremities in subjects with history of low-back-pain. Spine 20:1994–1996.

Leinonen, V., Kankaanpaa, M., Luukkonen, M., Hanninen, O., Airaksinen, O., Taimela, S., 2001. Disc herniation-related back pain impairs feed-forward control of paraspinal muscles. Spine 26:E367–372.

Leinonen, V., Kankaanpaa, M., Luukkonen, M., Kansanen, M., Hanninen, O., Airaksinen, O., 2003. Lumbar paraspinal muscle function, perception of lumbar position, and postural control in disc herniation-related back pain. Spine 28:842–848.

Lin, Y.H., Sun, M.H., 2006. The effect of lifting and lowering an external load on repositioning error of trunk flexion-extension in subjects with and without low back pain. Clin Rehab 20:603–608.

Lotz, J.C., Chin, J.R., 2000. Intervertebral cell death is dependent on the magnitude and duration of spinal loading. Spine 25:1477–1483.

Luoto, S., Aalto, H., Taimela, S., Hurri, H., Pyykko, I., Alaranta, H., 1998. One-footed and externally disturbed two-footed postural control in patients with chronic low back pain and healthy control subjects. A controlled study with follow-up. Spine 23:2081–2089; discussion 9–90.

MacDonald, D., Moseley, G.L., Hodges, P.W., 2009. Why do some patients keep hurting their back? Evidence of ongoing back muscle dysfunction during remission from recurrent back pain. Pain 142:183–188.

Magnusson, M.L., Aleksiev, A.R., Wilder, D.G., Pope, M.H., Spratt, K.F., Lee, S.H., et al., 1996. Unexpected load and asymmetric posture as etiologic factors in low back pain. Eur Spine J 5:23–35.

Mannion, A.F., Weber, B.R., Dvorak, J., Grob, D., Muntener, M., 1997. Fibre type characteristics of the lumbar paraspinal muscles in normal healthy subjects and in patients with low back pain. J Orthop Res 15:881–887.

Marras, W.S., Davis, K.G., Ferguson, S.A., Lucas, B.R., Gupta, P., 2001. Spine loading characteristics of patients with low back pain compared with asymptomatic individuals. Spine 26: 2566–2574.

Marras, W.S., Ferguson, S.A., Burr, D., Davis, K.G., Gupta, P., 2004. Spine loading in patients with low back pain during asymmetric lifting exertions. Spine J 4:64–75.

Marras, W.S., Ferguson, S.A., Burr, D., Davis, K.G., Gupta, P., 2005. Functional impairment as a predictor of spine loading. Spine 30:729–737.

Matre, D.A., Sinkjaer, T., Svensson, P., Arendt-Nielsen, L., 1998. Experimental muscle pain increases the human stretch reflex. Pain 75:331–339.

Matre, D.A., Sinkjaer, T., Knardahl, S., Andersen, J.B., Arendt-Nielsen, L., 1999. The influence of experimental muscle pain on the human soleus stretch reflex during sitting and walking. Clin Neurophysiol 110:2033–2043.

Mientjes, M.I.V., Frank, J.S., 1999. Balance in chronic low back pain patients compared to healthy people under various conditions in upright standing. Clin Biomech 14: 710–716.

Mok, N.W., Brauer, S.G., Hodges, P.W., 2004. Hip strategy for balance control in quiet standing is reduced in people with low back pain. Spine 29:E107–112.

Mok, N.W., Brauer, S.G., Hodges, P.W., 2007. Failure to use movement in postural strategies leads to increased spinal displacement in low back pain. Spine (Phila Pa 1976) 32:E537–543.

Mooney, V., Gulick, J., Perlman, M., Levy, D., Pozos, R., Leggett, S., et al., 1997. Relationships between myoelectric activity, strength, and MRI of lumbar extensor muscles in back pain patients and normal subjects. J Spinal Disord 10:348–356.

Moseley, G.L., Hodges, P.W., 2006. Reduced variability of postural strategy prevents normalization of motor changes induced by back pain: a risk factor for chronic trouble? Behav Neurosci 120:474–476.

Moseley, G.L., Hodges, P.W., Gandevia, S.C., 2002. Deep and superficial fibers of the lumbar multifidus muscle are differentially active during voluntary arm movements. Spine 27:E29–36.

Moseley, G.L., Hodges, P.W., Gandevia, S.C., 2003. External perturbation of the trunk in standing humans differentially activates components of the medial back muscles. J Physiol 547:581–587.

Moseley, G.L., Nicholas, M.K., Hodges, P.W., 2004a. Does anticipation of back pain predispose to back trouble? Brain 127:2339–2347.

Moseley, G.L., Nicholas, M.K., Hodges, P.W., 2004b. Pain differs from non-painful attention-demanding or stressful tasks in its effect on postural control patterns of trunk muscles. Exp Brain Res 156:64–71.

Newcomer, K., Laskowski, E.R., Yu, B., Larson, D.R., An, K.N., 2000a. Repositioning error in low back pain. Comparing trunk repositioning error in subjects with chronic low back pain and control subjects. Spine 25:245–250.

Newcomer, K.L., Laskowski, E.R., Yu, B., Johnson, J.C., An, K.N., 2000b. Differences in repositioning error among patients with low back pain compared with control subjects. Spine 25:2488–2493.

Ng, J.K., Richardson, C.A., Parnianpour, M., Kippers, V., 2002. EMG activity of trunk muscles and torque output during isometric axial rotation exertion: a comparison between back pain patients and matched controls. J Orthop Res 20:112–121.

Nies, N., Sinnott, P.L., 1991. Variations in balance and body sway in middle-aged adults. Subjects with healthy backs compared with subjects with low-back dysfunction. Spine (Phila Pa 1976) 16:325–330.

O'Sullivan, P.B., Burnett, A., Floyd, A.N., Gadsdon, K., Logiudice, J., Miller, D., et al., 2003. Lumbar repositioning deficit in a specific low back pain population. Spine 28:1074–1079.

Oddsson, L.I.E., Persson, T., Cresswell, A.G., Thorstensson, A., 1999. Interaction between voluntary and postural motor commands during perturbed lifting. Spine 24:545–552.

Panjabi, M.M., 1992. The stabilizing system of the spine. Part, I. Function, dysfunction, adaptation, and enhancement. J Spinal Disord 5:383–389; discussion 97.

Panjabi, M.M., 2006. A hypothesis of chronic back pain: ligament subfailure injuries lead to muscle control dysfunction. Eur Spine J 15:668–676.

Panjabi, M.M., Goel, V.K., Takata, K., 1982. Physiologic strains on the lumbar spinal ligaments. Spine 7:192–203.

Panjabi, M.M., Krag, M.H., Chung, T.Q., 1984. Effects of disc injury on mechanical behavior of the human spine. Spine 9:707–713.

Pedersen, J., Ljubisavljevic, M., Bergenheim, M., Johansson, H., 1998. Alterations in information transmission in ensembles of primary muscle spindle afferents after muscle fatigue in heteronymous muscle. Neuroscience 84:953–959.

Pluijm, S.M.F., 2001. Predictors and Consequences of Falls and Fractures in the Elderly. Vrije universiteit, Amsterdam, the Netherlands, p. 165.

Popa, T., Bonifazi, M., Della Volpe, R., Rossi, A., Mazzocchio, R., 2007. Adaptive changes in postural strategy selection in chronic low back pain. Exp Brain Res 177:411–448.

Quint, U., Wilke, H.J., 2008. Grading of degenerative disk disease and functional impairment: imaging versus patho-anatomical findings. Eur Spine J 17:1705–1713.

Radebold, A., Cholewicki, J., Panjabi, M.M., Patel, T.C., 2000. Muscle response pattern to sudden trunk loading in healthy individuals and in patients with chronic low back pain. Spine 25:947–954.

Radebold, A., Cholewicki, J., Polzhofer, G.K., Greene, H.S., 2001. Impaired postural control of the lumbar spine is associated with delayed muscle response times in patients with chronic idiopathic low back pain. Spine 26:724–730.

Reeves, N.P., Cholewicki, J., Silfies, S.P., 2006. Muscle activation imbalance and low-back injury in varsity athletes. J Electromyogr Kinesiol 16:264–272.

Reeves, N.P., Narendra, K.S., Cholewicki, J., 2007. Spine stability: the six blind men and the elephant. Clin Biomech 22:266–274.

Roberts, S., Eisenstein, S.M., Menage, J., Evans, E.H., Ashton, K., 1995. Mechanoreceptors in intervertebral discs. Morphology, distribution, and neuropeptides. Spine 20:2645–2651.

Salmon, L.J., Russell, V.J., Refshauge, K., Kader, D., Connolly, C., Linklater, J., et al., 2006. Long-term outcome of endoscopic anterior cruciate ligament reconstruction with patellar tendon autograft: minimum 13-year review. Am J Sports Med 34:721–732.

Selen, L.P.J., Beek, P.J., van Dieën, J.H., 2005. Can co-activation reduce kinematic variability? A simulation study. Biol Cybernetics 93: 373–381.

Sjölander, P., Johansson, H., Djupsjö-backa, M., 2002. The sensory function of ligaments. J Electromyogr Kinesiol 12:167–176.

Solomonow, M., Zhou, B.H., Harris, M., Lu, Y., Baratta, R.V., 1998. The ligamento-muscular stabilizing system of the spine. Spine 23:2552–2562.

Solomonow, M., Baratta, R.V., Zhou B.-H., Burger, E., Zieske, A., Gedalia, A., 2003. Muscular dysfunction elicited by creep of lumbar viscoelastic tissues. J Electromyogr Kinesiol 13:381–396.

Stergiou, N., Ristanis, S., Moraiti, C., Georgoulis, A.D., 2007. Tibial rotation in anterior cruciate ligament (ACL)-deficient and ACL-reconstructed knees: a theoretical proposition for the development of osteoarthritis. Sports Med 37:601–613.

Stokes, I.A.F., Gardner-Morse, M., 1995. Lumbar spine maximum efforts and muscle recruitment patterns predicted by a model with multijoint muscles and joints with stiffness. J Biomech 28:173–186.

Stokes, I.A.F., Gardner-Morse, M., 2003. Spinal stiffness increases with axial load: another stabilizing consequence of muscle action. J Electromyogr Kinesiol 13:397–402.

Stokes, I.A.F., Iatridis, J.C., 2004. Mechanical conditions that accelerate intervertebral disc degeneration: overload versus immobilization. Spine 29:2724–2732.

Stokes, I.A.F., Gardner-Morse, M., Henry, S.M., Badger, G.J., 2000. Decrease in trunk muscular response to perturbation with preactivation of lumbar spinal musculature. Spine 25:1957–1964.

Strutton, P.H., Theodorou, S., Catley, M., McGregor, A.H., Davey, N.J., 2005. Corticospinal excitability in patients with chronic low back pain. J Spinal Disord Tech 18:420–424.

Stubbs, M., Harris, M., Solomonow, M., Zhou, B.Y., Lu, Y., Baratta, R.V., 1998. Ligamento-muscular protective reflex in the lumbar spine of the feline. J Electromyogr Kinesiol 8:197–204.

Takala, E.P., Korhonen, I., Viikarijun-tura, E., 1997. Postural sway and stepping response among working population – reproducibility, long-term stability, and associations with symptoms of the low back. Clin Biomech 12:429–437.

Takemasa, R., Yamamoto, H., Tani, T., 1995. Trunk muscle strength in and effect of trunk muscle exercises for patients with chronic low-back-pain – the differences in patients with and without organic lumbar lesions. Spine 20:2522–2530.

Thomas, J.S., France, C.R., Sha, D., Wiele, N.V., 2008. The influence of pain-related fear on peak muscle activity and force generation during maximal isometric trunk exertions. Spine (Phila Pa 1976) 33:E342–348.

Tideiksaar, R., 1997. Falling in Old, Age. Springer Publishing Company, New York.

Tsao, H., Galea, M.P., Hodges, P.W., 2008. Reorganization of the motor cortex is associated with postural control deficits in recurrent low back pain. Brain 131:2161–2171.

van der Burg, J.C.E., Casius, L.J.R., Kingma, I., van Dieën, J.II., van Soest, A.J., 2005a. Factors underlying the perturbation resistance of the trunk in the first part of a lifting movement. Biol Cybernetics 93, 54–62.

van der Burg, J.C.E., Pijnappels, M., van Dieën, J.H., 2005b. Out-of-plane trunk movements and trunk muscle activity after a trip during walking. Exp Brain Res 165, 407–412.

van der Burg, J.C.E., van Wegen, E.E.H., Rietberg, M.B., Kwakkel, G., van Dieën, J.H., 2006. Postural control of the trunk during unstable sitting in Parkinson's disease. Parkinsonism Rel Disorders 12, 492–498.

van der Hoorn, W., Bruijn, S.M., Meijer, O.G., Hodges, P.W., van Dieën, J.H., 2012. Mechanical coupling between the pelvis and the thorax in the transverse plane during gait is higher in people with low back pain. J Biomech 45:342–347.

van Dieën, J.H., Weinans, H., Toussaint, H.M., 1999. Fractures of the lumbar vertebral endplate in the etiology of low back pain. A hypothesis on the causative role of spinal compression in a-specific low back pain. Med Hypoth 53:246–252.

van Dieën, J.H., Cholewicki, J., Radebold, A., 2003a. Trunk muscle recruitment patterns in patients with low back pain enhance the stability of the lumbar spine. Spine 28:834–841.

van Dieën, J.H., Kingma, I., van der Burg, J.C.E., 2003b. Evidence for a role of antagonistic contraction in controlling trunk stiffness during lifting. Journal of Biomechanics 36:1829–1836.

van Dieën, J.H., Selen, L.P.J., Chole-wicki, J., 2003c. Trunk muscle activation in low-back pain patients, an analysis of the literature. J Electromyogr Kinesiol 13:333–351.

van Dieën, J.H., Westebring–van der Putten, E., Kingma, I., d Looze, M.P., 2009. Low-level activity of trunk extensor muscles causes electromyographic manifestations of fatigue in absence of decreased oxygenation. J Electromyogr Kinesiol 19:398–406.

van Dieën, J.H., Koppes, L., Twisk, J., 2010. Low-back pain history and postural sway in unstable sitting. Spine 35:812–817.

van Tulder, M.W., Koes, B.W., Bouter, L.M., 1995. A cost-of-illness study of back pain in The Netherlands. Pain 62:233–240.

van Tulder, M.W., Assendelft, W.J., Koes, B.W., Bouter, L.M., 1997a. Spinal radiographic findings and nonspecific low back pain. A systematic review of observational studies. Spine 22:427–434.

van Tulder, M.W., Koes, B.W., Bouter, L.M., 1997b. Conservative treatment of acute and chronic nonspecific low back pain. A systematic review of

randomized controlled trials of the most common interventions [see comments]. Spine 22:2128–2156.

van Tulder, M., Malmivaara, A., Esmail, R., Koes, B., 2000. Exercise therapy for low back pain: A systematic review within the framework of the cochrane collaboration back review group [In Process Citation]. Spine 25:2784–2796.

Visser, B., van Dieën, J.H., 2006. Pathophysiology of upper extremity muscle disorders. J Electromyogr Kinesiol 16:1–16.

Vlaeyen, J.W.S., Kole-Snijders, A.M.J., Boeren, R.G.B., van Eek, H., 1995. Fear of movement/(re)injury in chronic low back pain and its relation to behavioral performance. Pain 62:363–372.

Wallwork, T.L., Stanton, W.R., Freke, M., Hides, J.A., 2009. The effect of chronic low back pain on size and contraction of the lumbar multifidus muscle. Man Ther 14:496–500.

White, A.A., Panjabi, M.M., 1990. Clinical Biomechanics of the

Spine, 2nd edn. J.B. Lippincott, Philadelphia.

Wilder, D.G., Pope, M.H., Frymoyer, J.W., 1988. The biomechanics of lumbar disc herniation and the effect of overload and instability. J Spinal Dis 1:16–32.

Yoshizawa, H., O'Brien, J.P., Smith, W.T., Trumper, M., 1980. The neuropathology of intervertebral discs removed for low-back pain. J Pathol 132:95–104.

Young, R.P., Scott, S.H., Loeb, G.E., 1992. An intrinsic mechanism to stabilize posture – joint-angle-dependent moment arms of the feline ankle muscles. Neurosci Lett 145:137–140.

Zedka, M., Prochazka, A., Knight, B., Gillard, D., Gauthier, M., 1999. Voluntary and reflex control of human back muscles during induced pain. J Physiol 520:591–604.

Zhao, F.D., Pollintine, P., Hole, B.D., Dolan, P., Adams, M.A., 2005. Discogenic origins of spinal instability. Spine 30:2621–2630.

Chapter | 6 |

Adaptation and rehabilitation: from motoneurones to motor cortex and behaviour

Paul W. Hodges
NHMRC Centre of Clinical Research Excellence in Spinal Pain, Injury and Health, School of Health and Rehabilitation Sciences, University of Queensland, Brisbane, Queensland, Australia

INTRODUCTION

There is no doubt that movement is changed in pain. Whether these changes precede or follow the onset of pain is not always clear. Although some changes may be protective and potentially beneficial (at least in the short term), others are not. It is our contention that adapted strategies are not ideal and clinical benefit can be derived from rehabilitation of motor control to either reduce pain and disability, prevent recurrence of symptoms, or prevent the first onset of back pain. There are differing views of the methods that can be used to change motor control and differing views of what the clinical objective should be when aiming to change motor control. It makes sense that the response to both these issues will vary when applied to individual patients as a function of differences in their strategy of adaptation, their pain presentation and their functional demands. Attempts to restore optimal spine control will require consideration of multiple aspects; from strategies of muscle activation to the patient's posture and movement patterns, and consideration of the interaction between motor control and psychological aspects. This chapter discusses new ideas about the basis for adaptation in the motor system with pain and injury (Hodges and Tucker 2011), the challenge to determine the clinical goal for the individual patient, and considerations regarding application of this information for rehabilitation.

CHANGES IN MOTOR CONTROL IN LUMBOPELVIC PAIN

Many factors may be responsible for adaptation in motor control. Although nociceptor discharge and associated pain is a major stimulus, other stimuli are likely to be responsible for changes in movement (e.g. anticipation/threat of pain, postural habits, competition between the multiple physiological functions of the trunk muscles such as contributions to breathing and continence, in addition to spine control). Regardless of the stimulus for adaptation, not all components of the muscle system are affected in the same way, nor are the changes identical between individuals or between tasks. When individual parts of the trunk muscles system are considered in isolation this can lead to incomplete interpretation of the net effect on lumbopelvic control. A key issue is that although some changes suggest compromised control, others suggest augmented or even excessive control. It is our contention that rehabilitation should aim to optimize control to match the individual's abilities to their functional demands and this may require augmentation or reduction of muscle activity, or both.

Motor control changes that suggest compromised lumbopelvic control

Acute and chronic lumbopelvic pain are associated with changes in morphology and behaviour of a number of muscles, this commonly includes the deep trunk muscles such as transversus abdominis and multifidus (Fig. 6.1). Atrophy and fatty infiltration of the multifidus muscle have been common observations since the 1960s (Knutsson, 1961; Hides et al. 1994; Danneels et al. 2000). These changes are present at multiple spinal levels in people with persistent problems (Danneels et al. 2000), but are more localized in acute pain, can occur within days of an acute episode (Hides et al. 1994) and has been replicated in an animal model of intervertebral disc lesion (Hodges et al. 2006). Behaviour of multifidus is also modified with reduced (Sihvonen et al. 1997; Kiesel et al. 2008; MacDonald et al. 2010) or delayed (MacDonald et al. 2009) activity in people with persistent problems. Activity of transversus abdominis is compromised in a number of ways including delayed activity (Hodges and Richardson 1996), reduced activity (Hodges et al. 2003a; Ferreira et al. 2004) and a change from persistent to phasic activity (Saunders et al. 2004a). The deep location of these muscles means that invasive measures of activity (e.g. intramuscular electromyography electrodes) are required. This has precluded widespread investigation of these muscles. Ultrasound and MRI provide a non-invasive measure of changes in morphology. Yet, although changes in muscle morphology are related to activity and can be used to infer activation of the muscle (Misuri et al. 1997; Hodges et al. 2003c), the relationship is affected by many issues such as contraction type (eccentric, concentric, isometric), contraction intensity and activation of adjacent muscles (Hodges et al. 2003b).

Compromised deep trunk muscle morphology and behaviour occurs in many individuals with lumbopelvic

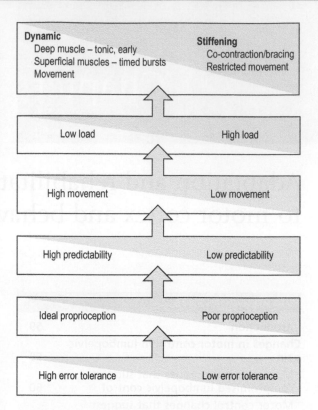

Figure 6.1 Dynamic control of the spine involves a spectrum of control strategies that range from co-contraction stiffening to more dynamic control strategies that involve carefully timed muscle activity and movement. Multiple factors such as load, movement, predictability, proprioceptive function and error tolerance are likely to influence the selection of the appropriate dynamic control strategy.

pain. There is also evidence of compromised activity of other muscles, but this is generally restricted to specific patient subgroups. Examples include delayed/reduced gluteal muscle activation in people with sacroiliac joint dysfunction (Hungerford et al. 2003) and Janda's 'distal cross syndrome' (Janda 1978), reduced cross-sectional area of psoas in sciatica (Dangaria and Naesh 1998) and reduced/delayed activity of superficial trunk muscles in some individuals (Hodges et al. 2013).

Compromised muscle morphology and behaviour have been interpreted to imply the spine is 'unstable'. There is good evidence that deep muscles, such as transversus abdominis and multifidus, contribute to lumbopelvic control (Tesh et al. 1987; Kaigle et al. 1995; Wilke et al. 1995; Hodges et al. 2003a; Barker et al. 2005). However, their mechanical contribution is not straightforward. For instance, although the contribution of transversus abdominis has been modelled in terms of torque generation (Kavcic et al. 2004), it is likely to have a greater effect on the spine via its contribution to intra-abdominal pressure (Cresswell et al. 1992; Hodges et al. 2001a, 2003a) and tension of the thoracolumbar fascia (Barker et al. 2005). As these muscles attach to individual spine segments they have an advantage to 'fine-tune' control at the level of intervertebral motion. Another advantage is that these muscles appear to improve the quality of control, without compromising range of motion; i.e. they enhance control within the range of motion (Kaigle et al. 1995). Considering the potential of deep muscles to contribute to spine control it is reasonable to conclude that if this contribution is reduced, then spine control will be impaired. Hypothetically this impairment would be likely to change spinal loading. Yet the net effect will depend on adaptation in the other parts of the system.

Several questions remain to be answered. First, it is necessary to determine whether reduced activity of muscles, including the deep muscles, changes the quality of control of the spine and pelvis, and second, it is necessary to establish whether such changes contribute to the development of pain or recurrence of pain and/or injury. These questions are currently under investigation in large-scale longitudinal experiments.

Motor control changes that suggest augmented lumbopelvic control

In contrast to observations of compromised activity of deep muscles, other work suggests that lumbopelvic control is enhanced/augmented in pain. When pain is induced experimentally by injection of hypertonic saline into the lumbar longissimus, in addition to a relatively uniform effect on the timing (delayed) and amplitude (reduced) of activity of transversus abdominis, activity of one or more of the more superficial trunk muscles is augmented, but uniquely for each individual (Hodges et al. 2003a). This observation of individual variation is supported by other work. Radebold et al. (2000) showed delayed reduction of activity of the trunk muscle in response to removal of a trunk load, i.e. muscles remained active for longer, which can be interpreted as overactivity. Close inspection of the data shows not all participants in the study adapted in the same manner. Whereas the offset of activity of obliquus externus abdominis was delayed in the group analysis, this was not the case for all individuals, and those with unchanged activity of this muscle commonly had changes in one of the other trunk flexors. Further, a comprehensive review by van Dieën et al. (2003) highlighted augmented activity, but with variation between individual subjects and studies.

Recent work has tested the hypothesis more directly in response to acute experimental pain. Recordings were made from multiple superficial trunk muscles with surface electromyography electrodes during slow trunk movements (Hodges et al. 2013). In the mid upright position, minimal activity is required to maintain the body against gravity, and trunk muscle activity in this position is maintained to contribute to spine stability (i.e. to ensure maintenance or return to the position if perturbed) (Cholewicki et al. 1997). During the period of pain, net trunk muscle activity increased in the mid position to augment stability. However, the most interesting and clinically relevant observation was that every subject used a different strategy to achieve the increase in activity, and theses strategies involved unique patterns of increased and decreased muscle activity. There were some similarities between groups/clusters of individuals. Many factors may influence the selected strategy, such as body anthropometrics, postural parameters, habitual strategies, and functional demands (e.g. involvement in sports with high rotational demand). Similarities between clusters of individuals may relate to the subgroups that present in back pain patients that have been described by other authors (Kendall and McCreary 1983; Sahrman 2002; O'Sullivan 2005).

Why does the nervous system adapt by augmentation of muscle activity? Increased activity is likely to be a strategy to protect the body region from further pain or injury, or the perceived potential for further pain or injury. It is important to note that not all people adapt with increased activity and the adaptation is not always consistent with protection, but this is a common presentation.

Data of augmented activity of superficial trunk muscles provide an alternative picture of the motor control strategies adopted in people with lumbopelvic pain. Although compromised activity of deep muscles implies reduced robustness of the system, augmented activity of the more superficial muscles implies increased protection. This solution can be better understood by consideration of lumbopelvic control along a continuum from more static strategies at one end to more dynamic solutions at the other (Fig. 6.1). Stability of the spine has often been considered only from a static perspective with respect to the potential to maintain position when perturbed (McGill et al. 2003). The contemporary view is that the spine must be considered dynamically; optimal function of the spine requires control during movement (e.g. moving the spine through a range of motion) (Hodges and Cholewicki 2007; Reeves and Cholewicki 2010), and movement also provides a solution to maintain stability (e.g. movement in preparation for reactive moments from arm movement (Hodges et al. 1999)). At the static end of the spectrum the spine is controlled primarily by stiffening strategies such as co-contraction of large flexor and extensor muscles, such as occurs when the load is high (Cholewicki et al. 1991) or the forces are unpredictable (van Dieën and de Looze 1999). At the other end of the spectrum, the spine is controlled in a more dynamic manner with carefully timed alternating bursts of activity of superficial muscles with underlying tonic and early activity of deep muscles, such as occurs during arm movements (Hodges and Richardson 1997a, 1997b) and walking (Saunders et al.

2004b). At the dynamic end of the spectrum muscle activity must be carefully matched to the demands of the task. Both ends of the spectrum are important and the nervous system selects strategies from along this spectrum based on demands of an individual task or the perceived demands/risks (Fig. 6.1). One interpretation of the changes in control in pain and injury is that the nervous system either resorts to a simpler, 'one-size-fits-all' strategy at the more static end of the spectrum with the intention to increase spine stiffness (as a result of the perceived/real increased risk to the spine) or makes errors in the selection of strategies along the spectrum of choices of strategies for spine control. In the latter case errors may be made either because afferent input is inaccurate (as is commonly reported in low back and pelvic pain (see Chapter 12 for review)) or because the consequences of making an inaccurate strategy selection are not immediately realized: that is, the effect of the error may not be immediately apparent as it may take time for suboptimal loads to have a negative impact on spine health, and as such the nervous system is unlikely to perceive the need to make any correction.

How is the new understanding of the complex adaptation in the presence of pain and injury, which includes augmented activity, reconciled with the assumption that low back and pelvic pain is associated with 'instability'? There is some evidence of poor control of intervertebral motion in association with specific groups with back pain (e.g. spondylolisthesis (Schneider et al. 2005)), and reduced activity of deep muscles implies reduced robustness of trunk control. However, if the system adapts to use a more protective strategy then the net effect will be increased stiffness. Whether a protective strategy such as this should be enhanced, removed or reduced and whether the deep muscle control should be enhanced or encouraged requires consideration, and is discussed below.

NEW IDEAS ABOUT THE MECHANISMS FOR ADAPTATION WITH PAIN

What is the mechanism for the diffuse and apparently contrasting (increased vs. decreased activity) changes in control of the trunk muscles in the presence of pain and injury? The answer is likely to involve multiple discrete and inter-related mechanisms that may have complementary, additive or competing effects on the system. These mechanisms are likely to affect control/coordination of muscle control/movement at multiple levels of the nervous system (e.g. spinal cord; motor and sensory cortices; subcortical regions).

Existing theories of motor adaptation to pain are relatively simplistic. Clinical observations and experiments involving simple systems led to the development of the

'vicious cycle' theory and the 'pain adaptation' theory. The vicious cycle theory proposed a uniform increase in muscle activity to splint the painful body segment and subsequent further pain due to accumulation of metabolites (Roland 1986). The pain adaptation model proposed more flexibility in response to pain and injury with facilitation of antagonist muscle activity and inhibition of agonist muscle activity with the intention to reduce the amplitude and velocity of voluntary movement of the painful segment (Lund et al. 1991). Although data support these relatively straightforward theories (e.g. Arendt-Nielsen et al. 1996), their predictions cannot explain the variable nature of adaptation observed in lumbopelvic pain (van Dieën et al. 2003). New theories are required. Observations from people with back pain, as described in the preceding section, provide the foundation for a new comprehensive theory to understand and explain the complex changes in motor control in back pain (Hodges and Tucker 2011).

The new theory hypothesizes that the motor adaptation to acute pain:

1. leads to 'protection' from further pain or injury, or threatened pain or injury;
2. involves redistribution of activity *within* and *between* muscles;
3. changes the *mechanical behaviour* such as modified movement and stiffness;
4. is not explained by simple changes in excitability of elements of the nervous system, but involves changes at *multiple levels of the motor system* and these changes may be complementary, additive or competitive;
5. has short-term benefit, but with potential *long-term consequences*.

Adaptation to acute pain leads to 'protection' of the region/part from real or perceived risk of further pain and/or injury

The first element of the new theory is that the nervous system adopts a new strategy during pain to protect the painful or injured part. This is consistent with the augmented activity of superficial muscles described earlier. Why does the spine and pelvis system need protection? There are several reasons why the nervous system may 'choose' to adopt a new strategy during pain and injury (Fig. 6.2). First, this could be explained by an attempt to splint the injured, painful or potentially painful part. However, it does so in a more variable, individual-specific and, perhaps, task-specific manner than predicted by the pain adaptation or vicious cycle theories. A key feature is that the adaptation occurs both when there is a real injury (Hodges et al. 2009c), real pain (Hodges and Richardson 1996; Hodges et al. 2003c) or simply the anticipation that the task may be painful (Moseley et al. 2004; Moseley and Hodges 2005; Tucker et al. 2012). Thus, adoption of the

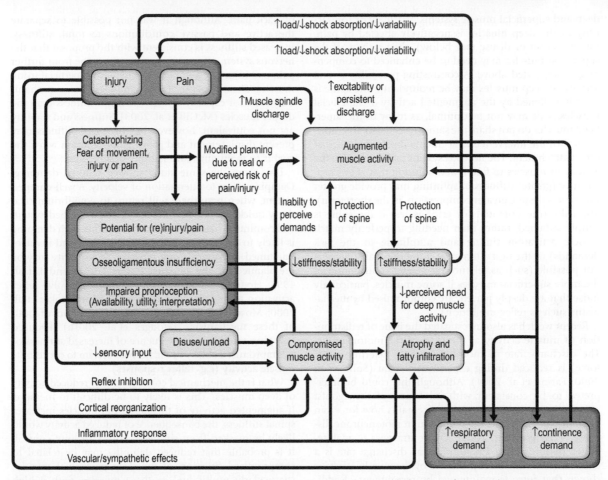

Figure 6.2 Possible mechanisms and consequences of changes in morphology and behaviour of the trunk muscles.

adapted strategy is not dependent on actual risk to the spine and pelvis.

There are other reasons that the nervous system may adopt a protective strategy. First, increased muscle activity may be required to compensate for injury to osseoligamentous structures (Panjabi 1992). In this case some adaptation may be necessary for function. Second, muscle activity may be increased to provide a simplified solution to protect the spine if sensory information is not available, corrupted (Panjabi 2006) or ignored (Brumagne et al. 2004) by the nervous system. If the consequence of movements or loads cannot be sensed or predicted accurately (as a result of a compromised internal representation of the body built up on faulty sensory information) then a simple protective strategy may be the best solution. Third, adaptation to augment activity of the more superficial muscles of the trunk may be necessary to compensate for compromised activity of the deeper trunk muscles (MacDonald et al. 2010). Fourth, in the presence of peripheral

sensitization of nociceptors from local inflammatory changes in the tissues, it may be necessary to engage greater quality/accuracy of spine control to prevent irritation of the sensitized neurons.

Adaptation to pain involves redistribution of activity *within* and *between* muscles in an individual-specific manner

One issue that is difficult to reconcile is that if we accept that deep muscles provide an important contribution to lumbopelvic control, why is their activity reduced rather than increased in response to pain and injury? Although compromised activity of deep muscles seems counterintuitive to the goal of protecting the injured part from further pain/(re)injury, there are several possible explanations. First, it may represent redistribution of activity between deep and superficial muscle systems. If activity or contractility of the deep muscles is negatively affected by pain, inflammation or disuse (see below), then activity of the superficial muscles may need to be enhanced to compensate, as suggested above. A contrasting possibility is that activity of deep muscles may be redundant if the spine is already stiffened by the augmented activity of superficial muscles. This may not be optimal, as many of the superficial muscles do not share the same potential to 'fine-tune' control of the intervertebral segments due to their lack of direct attachment. The nervous system may reorganize the activity of muscles to find a new solution that is less provocative (greater stiffness or splinting may provide greater protection despite greater compression, in the short term), less risky (the potential for error is less if the spine is simply stiffened, rather than needing to perfectly match muscle activation timing and amplitude to the task demands) or the best alternative if the optimal strategy is not possible (such as reliance on greater contribution of the more superficial muscles if some muscles, particularly those that are deeply placed, are compromised by mechanisms such as reflex inhibition).

Recent work has also investigated the issue of redistribution of muscle activity at the level of the motoneurone. The discharge rate of motoneurones (a determinant of force) is reduced during experimental pain (Sohn et al. 2000; Farina et al. 2004). Although this could be interpreted to be consistent with inhibition of the agonist muscle during pain, the question remains how force can be maintained, despite the reduction in motoneurone discharge (Hodges et al. 2008). Other strategies to maintenance of force must be adopted, as discharge rate is a determinant of the force produced by the muscle. We have shown that force is maintained by recruitment of additional motoneurones that were not active prior to the presence of pain (Tucker et al. 2009) with redistribution of activity between regions of the painful muscle and its synergist (Tucker and Hodges 2009). The new strategy leads to a slightly different direction of force, potentially to reduce pain provocation (Tucker and Hodges 2010). This implies that even at the smallest level of the motor system there is reorganization to protect the painful segment, and in this case, reorganization occurs *within* a muscle.

Adaptation changes the *mechanical behaviour* of the spine

Other recent work has investigated the mechanical consequences of adapted muscle responses. One such study involved estimation of trunk stiffness and damping in response to a small perturbation in a semi-seated position with the pelvis fixed (Hodges et al. 2009b). In contrast to the assumption that people with recurrent episodes of back pain are 'unstable', this study identified increased trunk stiffness in those with episodic/recurring episodes of back pain. Although it was not possible to separate the active and passive contributions to trunk stiffness, increased stiffness is consistent with the proposal that the nervous system attempts to protect the spine from further pain and injury by augmented activity of superficial trunk muscles. These superficial trunk muscles have a mechanically superior capacity to increase trunk stiffness than the deeper muscles (McGill et al. 2003). Stiffness and stability are not equivalent, however, but increased stiffness may prevent displacement and provide one solution when the goal is to maintain static stability of a posture.

Data from the same study showed reduced damping. Damping refers to attenuation of velocity. A well-damped system, when perturbed, will return to equilibrium relatively quickly when perturbed. A poorly damped system will continue to oscillate. In many functions, high damping is likely to reflect more ideal spinal control and involves fine-tuned activity of trunk muscles. This activity may be pre-planned by the nervous system (Aruin and Latash 1995; Hodges and Richardson 1997a) or involve reflex activation to an unpredictable perturbation (Stokes et al. 2000; Moseley et al. 2003), or a combination of both of these mechanisms (Hodges et al. 2001b). Reduced damping could be a consequence of increased stiffness or a compromised ability of the nervous system to coordinate muscle activity (e.g. reflex responses).

What is the mechanical consequence of reduced activity of deep muscles? This is likely to be difficult to measure. If augmented activity of the superficial muscles increases spinal stiffness, the consequence of reduced activity would likely be masked from simple measures of joint control. It is probable that reduced damping may be related to compromised function of the deep paraspinal muscles (particularly multifidus) as these muscles, with a high density of muscle spindles (Nitz and Peck 1986), are likely to be the ones that are most sensitive to small motions (Chapter 12) and have the anatomical arrangement with the optimal potential to fine-tune control of individual segments (Moseley et al. 2002). Other work using radiographic methods (including fluoroscopy) have shown changes in coordination between translation and rotation (Schneider et al. 2005) that may be related to changes in deep muscle activity. This requires clarification.

Adaptation involves changes at *multiple levels* of the motor system

As alluded to in the preceding sections, the complex nature of motor control changes in lumbopelvic pain involves the interplay of multiple mechanisms that may be complementary, additive or competitive (Fig. 6.2). A first consideration is the mechanisms for augmented activity of the more superficial muscles. This adaptation could represent a modified solution to meet functional demands (e.g. increased gain of postural responses and/or a new simplified solution to stiffen the body part rather than use the carefully tuned response of trunk muscles). Alternatively, augmented activity could be mediated by spinal or peripheral mechanisms such as increased sensitivity of muscle spindles (Pedersen et al. 1997); activation of persistent inward currents to support sustained discharge of motoneurones, as has been shown in other conditions; (McPherson et al. 2008) or changes in motoneurone excitability (Lund et al. 1991).

Although peripheral mechanisms cannot be excluded, modified motor planning to adopt a new strategy provides a viable explanation for augmented superficial muscle activity for several reasons. First, adaptation occurs in the absence of nociceptor discharge. That is, activity of the superficial muscles is augmented during an arm movement task in the absence of nociceptor discharge when pain is anticipated (Moseley et al. 2004). This implies that simple nociceptor-dependent events in the periphery are not required and changes to descending inputs from supraspinal centres of the nervous system must be involved. Second, the 'gain' of postural adjustments is increased during pain. When people step down from steps of increasing height, activity of the gluteal muscles increases in amplitude and is earlier. However, when they step from a small step, but anticipate that they will experience pain on contact with the floor, they use a strategy that is normally reserved for a high step (Hodges et al. 2009a). That is, the gain of the postural adjustment is increased. Third, although data from several studies show increased response of the back muscles (or lower threshold for activation) to transcranial magnetic stimulation of the motor cortex (Strutton et al. 2003; Hodges et al. 2009c; Tsao et al. 2011b), when excitability of the cortical and spinal networks is studied separately in pigs after intervertebral disc lesion, the results show increased cortical excitability and reduced excitability of the spinal networks (Hodges et al. 2009c). Augmented activity is more consistent with the supraspinal changes. Recent data also show differential effects of experimental pain on corticospinal inputs to trunk muscles; although the size of responses evoked in obliquus externus abdominis and erector spinae were increased with pain, those evoked in transversus abdominis were reduced (Tsao et al. 2011b). Taken together, these data suggest changes in higher motor function and motor planning contribute to the adaptation to motor control of the spine, including aspects that aim to protect the spine.

Contrasting changes of compromised morphology and behaviour, generally of the deeper muscles, have different underlying mechanisms. Although reduced activity could be secondary to increased spinal stiffness, other mechanisms are likely. Atrophy and fatty infiltration of the multifidus muscle occurs within days of onset of acute spinal pain or injury (Hides et al. 1994; Hodges et al. 2006). Several mechanisms have been mooted. Rapid atrophy of limb muscles follows disuse/immobilization (Appell 1990), tenotomy (McLachlan 1981; Meyer et al. 2005), inflammation (Herbison et al. 1979), and muscle (Weber et al. 1997) or joint injury (Okada 1989); can occur rapidly (Max et al. 1971; Fitts et al. 2000); and is mediated by changes in neural drive (Fitts et al. 2001). This could explain rapid changes in multifidus. Greater effect on the deeper muscles is consistent with the argument that atrophy from disuse (e.g. hindlimb suspension in rats) or microgravity is not uniformly distributed across a muscle (Meyer et al. 2005). Greater changes have been shown in slow muscles (i.e. more type I muscle fibres) (Haggmark et al. 1981; Jiang et al. 1992; Fitts et al. 2000) and data from human cadavers provide some evidence of a greater density of type I fibres in the deeper portion of multifidus (Sirca and Kostevc 1985). This may explain the localization of the atrophy to a single segment. This may also explain the localization of reduced cross-sectional area to a single spinal level, as the shortest fibres have their greatest bulk adjacent to the single spinous process below the level of origin, and if these are the fibres that are most profoundly affected this would be where greatest atrophy is identified (Hodges et al. 2009c).

An inhibitory process, such as reflex inhibition, may reduce neural drive to multifidus. Reflex inhibition is the reduction in alpha motoneurone excitability due to afferent discharge from joint structures (Stokes and Young 1984). Activity of knee extensor muscles is reduced in response to mechanical stimuli such as pinching the joint capsule (Ekholm et al. 1960), joint effusion (Spencer et al. 1984; Indahl et al. 1997) and joint injury/surgery (Stokes and Young 1984). In pigs, the amplitude of response of the multifidus muscle to electrical stimulation of an intervertebral disc is reduced by injection of saline into the facet joint (Indahl et al. 1997). Furthermore, the response of multifidus to electrical stimulation of the cortex is increased after intervertebral disc lesion, but excitability of spinal networks is reduced. This latter observation suggests inhibitory mechanisms localized to the spinal cord (Hodges et al. 2009c). Other evidence comes from the failure of some experimental pain studies (Rother et al. 1996; Hodges et al. 2003c; but not all (Kiesel et al. 2008)) to replicate changes in multifidus that have been identified in clinical pain. As reflex inhibition is mediated by input related to injury rather than pain and nociception (Stokes and Young 1984), it follows that experimental pain should not necessarily change activity of multifidus if reflex inhibition is the mechanism that underlies changes in this muscle. Taken together these data support the mediation of multifidus atrophy by disuse/reduced neural input due to reflex inhibitory mechanisms.

Other mechanisms require consideration. Due to the rate of atrophy, changes in muscle components that can be readily modified such as water volume, may be responsible. Changes in intra-muscular water have been studied after injury (Hayashi et al. 1997). However this did not explain rapid atrophy in pigs after disc lesion (Hodges et al. 2006). Vasoconstriction (e.g. due to changes in sympathetic activity) may reduce muscle volume. Furthermore, changes could also be related to inflammatory effects. Pro-inflammatory cytokines such as tumour necrosis factor-alpha (TNF-α) and IL-6 (Jackman and Kandarian 2004) are linked to muscle atrophy. Human studies show expression of TNF-α, IL-1β, IL-6 and IL-8 following disc lesion (Burke et al. 2002; Weiler et al. 2005) and facet disease (Igarashi et al. 2004). The proximity of the posterior branch of the dorsal ramus (innervation of the multifidus) to the intervertebral disc and facet joints places it at particular risk for the effects of a local inflammatory response with injury to either structure.

Intramuscular fat is also increased in multifidus in chronic back pain (Alaranta et al. 1993) and begins to develop rapidly after injury (Hodges et al. 2006). The origin of the fat cells is not completely understood, but may be adipoplastic or myoblastic in origin (Dulor et al. 1998). Fibroblasts and preadipocytes are present in connective tissue around muscle fibres and may differentiate in response to inflammation (Dulor et al. 1998). Adipocytes also increase after sympathetic denervation (Cousin et al. 1993), which is likely after nerve lesion. Alternatively, there is a dramatic increase in DNA synthesis after injury leading to secretion of factors such as pro-inflammatory cytokines which may in turn stimulate fibroblasts, preadipocytes and muscle precursor cells (Lefaucheur et al. 1996; Floss et al. 1997) potentially leading to proliferation of adipocytes (Dulor et al. 1998).

Although reflex inhibition may explain changes in multifidus, this is unlikely to explain delayed or reduced activity of transversus abdominis for several reasons. First, reflex inhibition involves mechanisms at a single spinal segment, yet the innervation for transversus abdominis is derived from the thoracic spinal segments (Williams et al. 1989). Second, changes in transversus abdominis can be induced by anticipation of pain, in the absence of local injury and in response to experimental pain (Moseley et al. 2004). These issues suggest changes in transversus abdominis may be mediated by changes in motor planning. Recent studies of people with recurring episodes of back pain have shown reorganization of the networks in the motor cortex that input onto the cortical cells that synapse onto transversus abdominis motoneurones (Tsao et al. 2008). The amplitude of shift of the cortical networks was correlated with the delay in timing of transversus abdominis activation during an arm movement task. Although it is impossible to infer causality, this suggests that timing and cortical organization are related, again suggesting a supraspinal mechanism for the change in control of transversus abdominis. Other recent data have also highlighted changes in cortical organization of neural networks with inputs onto the back muscles. People with no history of back pain have two areas of motor cortex that evoke responses in the back muscles when stimulated with transcranial magnetic stimulation (O'Connell et al. 2007; Tsao et al. 2011c), and these areas are thought to relate to separate representations of the deep/short back muscles and the superficial/long back muscles (Tsao et al. 2011c). However, people with low back pain have a single area of motor cortex that evokes responses in both muscle groups (Tsao et al. 2011a). This change has been referred to as 'smudging' (Tsao et al. 2011a), and this appears to be related to a loss of differential behaviour of the muscles that is observed in this patient group (e.g. simultaneous onset of activity of deep and superficial multifidus in low back pain (MacDonald et al. 2009)), unlike pain-free individuals (Moseley et al. 2002). The apparent link between behaviour and cortex physiology again appears to suggest a possible physiological underpinning of the change in spine control strategy.

It is also important to consider the role of the sensory system in changes in motor control. Planning of movement and the response to perturbations requires accurate sensory input and accurate interpretation of the sensory input. It has been argued that corrupted input from injury to receptors may underlie sensory deficit (Panjabi, 2006). However, as a limited proportion of the population of receptors that provide information about motion and position of a segment are likely to be affected by an injury, it is perhaps more likely that compromised utility of sensory information from the spine (Brumagne et al. 2004) and the reorganization of sensory representation in the brain (Flor et al. 1997) have a greater impact on coordination of movement. Inaccurate sensory information or interpretation of sensory information may underlie errors in selection of motor strategies or a shift of movement control to the more static end of the spectrum of solutions to control movement and stability of the spine, whereby the nervous system uses a simplified stiffening strategy rather than a flexible and fine-tuned solution that is perfectly matched to the demands of the movement.

A final consideration is the interaction between biological and psychosocial factors in back pain. First, there is important interaction between multiple biological changes in pain that range from the response of the inflammatory system to spinal loading and biological changes in nervous system changes including peripheral and central sensitization. Second, psychosocial aspects interact with motor control. For instance, anticipation of pain is sufficient to change motor control (Moseley et al. 2004) and the resolution of motor adaptation is related to an individual's beliefs about pain (Moseley and Hodges 2006). With respect to the latter observation, there is preliminary evidence that people with unhealthy attitudes regarding pain may have a lesser capacity to resolve adaptations in the motor system after the resolution of pain (Moseley and Hodges 2006). These interactions may influence the changes in motor control in pain and are likely to require attention to optimize recovery. Biology, psychology, and for that matter social issues, cannot be considered in isolation and the interaction between them must also be addressed.

Time-course of changes in motor control

The preceding discussion has emphasized the role of pain and injury in the initiation of adapted motor control. There are two issues to consider. First, stimuli other than pain and injury may lead to changes in motor control and potentially contribute to the development of pain. Several factors have been identified. Disuse from bed rest leads to greater atrophy of the multifidus muscle than the other paraspinal muscles or psoas (Hides et al. 2007). Breathing disorders (Smith and Hodges, unpublished data) and incontinence (Smith et al. 2007a, 2007b) are associated with changes in control of the trunk muscles in a similar manner to back pain and longitudinal studies of people with these disorders provide evidence of a link to future development of lumbopelvic pain (Smith et al. 2009). Other examples may be habitual movement patterns or postures.

Second, there are likely to be differences between the adaptation in the acute and chronic phases. Acute pain is likely to be associated with more predictable adaptations in control. Changes in chronic pain are more variable. For instance, morphological changes in multifidus differ between acute and chronic pain; changes are localized in acute pain (Hides et al. 1994; Hodges et al. 2006) but more diffuse in chronic pain (Danneels et al. 2000)). Furthermore, the relevance of psychosocial factors (Boersma and Linton 2005) changes over time and their interaction with biological variables is likely to change also.

Regardless of the initial mechanism for modification in motor control, once a person is in the cycle it is likely to be self-perpetuating. When a patient presents with pain, the challenge is to break the cycle. It is also likely that motor control changes may contribute to the recurrence of pain. Numerous studies have shown that changes in trunk muscles' morphology and behaviour (Hodges and Richardson 1996; MacDonald et al. 2009) and the mechanical properties of the spine (Hodges et al. 2009b) are present during remission from symptoms. Whether these changes are related to recurrence and how they interact with other biological, psychological and social factors is a topic of ongoing longitudinal research.

Adaptation has short-term benefit, but with potential *long-term* consequences

It follows that compromised activity, particularly of the deep muscles, would have negative consequences for the spine, but does augmentation of trunk muscles' activity have consequences for the spine? At first glance, and in the short term, an attempt to increase spine protection seems logical but this may have long-term consequences. Consider the example of the protective strategy adopted after ankle sprain. After ankle sprain it is common to adopt an adaptation to walk with an externally rotated leg to avoid ankle dorsiflexion, which would stress the injured anterior talo-fibular ligament. This short-term adaptation to walking is likely to be a successful short-term solution, but with long-term consequences. To continue to walk with an externally rotated leg after ankle sprain would compromise shock absorption through the leg as knee flexion would be compromised on foot strike, and fail to load the ligament, which is necessary to aid collagen healing. In a similar manner the protective strategy adopted to protect the spine is likely to have consequences due to increased load, decreased movement, decreased movement variability, and the potential to compromise other functions such as balance, breathing and continence. Load from augmented activity of superficial muscles is increased during lifting in people with low back pain (LBP) (Marras et al. 2004). Movement of the spine is required for shock absorption and is used to prepare for and respond to perturbations (Hodges et al. 1999; Mok et al. 2007). Some variability in movement is also important for tissue health in order to vary the structures that are loaded and the load amplitude. Although too much variation is likely to be problematical, so too is too little variation (Hamill et al. 1999). Increased stiffness from a protective muscle activation strategy is likely to impact on variation.

Finally, movement and control of the spine is important for other functions. Strategies that increase trunk stiffness are likely to compromise these functions. For instance, increased trunk stiffness reduces balance performance (Reeves et al. 2006; Mok et al. 2007), and increased superficial abdominal muscle activity is likely to affect chest wall expansion for breathing (Smith, unpublished data) and place greater demand on the continence system as a result of increased intra-abdominal and, therefore, bladder pressure (Smith et al. 2007a, 2007b).

If the adaptation has negative consequences, why is it adopted by the nervous system? One alternative is that the adaptation develops over time as a result of a search for a new alternative that is less provocative of pain and/or injury and this is likely to involve trial and error (Hodges and Tucker 2011). Searching such as this is thought to be one of the outcomes of variability in movement performance (Moseley and Hodges 2006; Madeleine et al. 2008), although the adaptation may have long-term consequences that are not immediately apparent, as they take time to develop. Thus the link between the adaptation and consequence would not be obvious to the nervous system, and the adaptation may become entrenched.

REHABILITATION OF MOTOR CONTROL IN LUMBOPELVIC PAIN

In view of the complexity of the motor control changes in lumbopelvic pain rehabilitation, control of lumbopelvic

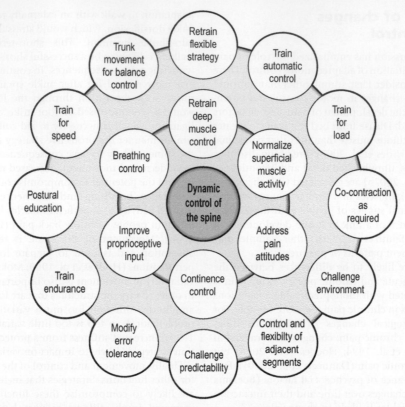

Figure 6.3 Components that require consideration in order to reach optimal dynamic control of the spine in the management of patients with low back pain.

pain requires a comprehensive approach to restore dynamic control that addresses the multiple muscle systems and multiple levels of the nervous system (Fig. 6.3).

Motor control training approach

A key aspect is the requirement for thorough assessment to determine the elements of the system that require rehabilitation. Assessment involves determination of the aspects of motor control that: may be provocative; may compromise the robustness of stability; and may be necessary to compensate for osseoligamentous injury. Training then aims to optimize spinal loading, reduce irritation, encourage normal movement and provide appropriate sensory input. This involves the training of controlled compliance of the spine rather than training of rigidity. This is achieved by correction of identified changes in deep muscle activation, changes in superficial muscle control (whether this requires increased or decreased activity), and optimization of posture and movement. Training of deep muscles may initially involve training their activation independently from the other trunk muscles, not to encourage activation of these muscles alone in function,

but rather as a training stimulus to encourage improved use of these muscles in function.

Training of dynamic control must be individualized for the patient. If a protective stiffening strategy has been adopted it is likely to be beneficial for this to be reduced. This may initially involve reduction of activity of superficial muscles. However, it would be critical to find a balance between what is needed to meet functional demands, what is needed to compensate for any osseoligamentous insufficiency and what exceeds the demands of function. On the basis of evidence of the role of the deep muscles in spinal control and the changes in this system (see above), rehabilitation involves training of deep muscle activation as a component of dynamic control of the spine.

Many other aspects require consideration to optimize function, yet their relevance depends on the individual patient. Such issues include training of dynamic control of more superficial torque producers, rehabilitation of proprioceptive function, modification of real/perceived error tolerance, retraining of static control as one strategy, and rehabilitation of dynamic strategies. An additional goal is to manage the attitudes and beliefs about pain that may be associated with poor recovery and non-resolution of symptoms.

Effectiveness of motor control training

Does motor control training change the control of the trunk muscles? There is increasing evidence that motor control training can change control of deep and superficial trunk muscles. These studies show that a single session of learning to independently activate the deep trunk muscles improves their activity in an untrained functional task (Tsao and Hodges 2007, 2008). This can be improved further and maintained in the long term by repeated training (Tsao and Hodges 2008). Activity of superficial muscles can also be reduced (Tsao et al. 2010). Activity of the deep muscles, as a marker of motor control, cannot be changed simply by activating the muscles (such as during a sit up (Tsao and Hodges 2007) or other tasks (Hall et al. 2009)) and is dependent on the quality of practice (Tsao and Hodges 2007). Although some studies and case reports suggest activity of the deep muscles can be improved with manipulative therapy (Marshall and Murphy 2006; Brenner et al. 2007; Gill et al. 2007), this does not appear to be the case in the long term (Ferreira et al. 2007). There is also evidence that activation of the deep muscles at baseline can be used to identify those who respond best to motor control training (Ferreira et al. 2009, Unsgaard-Tøndel et al. 2012) and changes in coordination of transversus abdominis is linked to the clinical outcomes of the intervention, such as pain and disability (Ferreira et al. 2009, Vasseljen and Fladmark 2010).

A number of clinical trials and systematic reviews have highlighted the efficacy of motor control training for the management of lumbopelvic pain (Macedo et al. 2009, Ferreira et al. 2006). A basic conclusion is that when the intervention is applied to specific subgroups (e.g. spondylolisthesis (O'Sullivan et al. 1997), acute unilateral low back pain (Hides et al. 2001), pregnancy-related pelvic girdle pain (Stuge et al. 2004)) the approach has a large effect size. However, when the intervention is used on a generic population the effect size is smaller. Although it has been argued that motor control training is no better than other interventions (Macedo et al. 2009), these studies have only been undertaken on generic back pain populations where the effect size is expected to be smaller. A recent study showed that even in a group of people who are difficult to treat (i.e. those from low socio-economic areas with co-morbidities and a long duration of pain), they do better with this intervention than graded activity in the short term (Ferreira et al. 2007), and they do better than treatment with a placebo (Costa et al. 2009).

The clear challenge for the future is to identify those who respond best to motor control interventions and target them. Some attempts have been made to identify groups who have 'clinical instability' (Kiesel et al. 2007). However, it is our view that motor control interventions have a place in many individuals who have adapted the way that they move in pain, across a spectrum from those with too little control to those with too much. A clear goal in people with chronic symptoms is to identify the appropriate balance between strategies to manage movement and strategies to manage beliefs and attitudes about pain; both of which must be addressed. This is a topic of current clinical trials.

CONCLUSION

In summary, it is our contention that benefit can be gained in many individuals with back pain by addressing their motor control in rehabilitation. There is sufficient evidence from clinical trials and basic physiology and biomechanics to consider that motor control is relevant for a person's pain presentation. However, it is also clear that all patients must be considered as individuals to identify the components of their motor control strategies (including posture, movement and muscle activation) that may or may not be relevant to their outcome. The challenge for the future is to identify who should be treated, how and when, and how it should be combined with or replaced by other interventions (e.g. cognitive behavioural therapy). It is likely that many individuals need a combination of education on how to move and attempts to change their attitudes and beliefs about pain and their abilities.

REFERENCES

Alaranta, H., Tallroth, K., Soukka, A., Heliaara, M., 1993. Fat content of lumbar extensor muscles in low back disability: a radiographic and clinical comparison. J Spinal Dis 6, 137–140.

Appell, H.J., 1990. Muscular atrophy following immobilization. A review. Sports Med 10, 42–58.

Arendt Nielsen, L., Graven Nielsen, T., Svarrer, H., Svensson, P., 1996. The influence of low back pain on muscle activity and coordination during gait: a clinical and experimental study. Pain 64, 231–240.

Aruin, A.S., Latash, M.L., 1995. Directional specificity of postural muscles in feed-forward postural reactions during fast voluntary arm movements. Exp Brain Res 103, 323–332.

Barker, P., Guggenheimer, K., Grkovic, I., Briggs, C., Jones, D., Thomas, C., et al., 2005. Effects of tensioning the lumbar fasciae on segmental stiffness during flexion and extension. Spine 31, 397–405.

Boersma, K., Linton, S.J., 2005. How does persistent pain develop? An analysis of the relationship between psychological variables, pain and function across stages of chronicity. Behaviour Res Ther 43, 1495–1507.

Brenner, A.K., Gill, N.W., Buscema, C.J., Kiesel, K., 2007. Improved activation of lumbar multifidus following spinal manipulation: a case report applying rehabilitative ultrasound imaging. J Orthop Sports Phys Ther 37, 613–619.

Brumagne, S., Cordo, P., Verschueren, S., 2004. Proprioceptive weighting changes in persons with low back pain and elderly persons during upright standing. Neurosci Lett 366, 63–66.

Burke, J.G., Watson, R.W., McCormack, D., Dowling, F.E., Walsh, M.G., Fitzpatrick, JM., 2002. Intervertebral discs which cause low back pain secrete high levels of proinflammatory mediators. J Bone Joint Surg 84, 196–201.

Cholewicki, J., McGill, S.M., Norman, R.W., 1991. Lumbar spine loading during the lifting of extremely heavy weights. Med Sci Sports Exercise 23, 1179–1186.

Cholewicki, J., Panjabi, M.M., Khachatryan, A., 1997. Stabilizing function of trunk flexor-extensor muscles around a neutral spine posture. Spine 22, 2207–2212.

Costa, L.O., Maher, C.G., Latimer, J., Hodges, P.W., Herbert, R.D., Refshauge, K.M., et al., 2009. Motor control exercise for chronic low back pain: a randomized placebo-controlled trial. Phys Ther 89, 1275–1286

Cousin, B., Casteilla, L., Lafontan, M., Ambid, L., Langin, D., Berthault, M.F., et al., 1993. Local sympathetic denervation of white adipose tissue in rats induces preadipocyte proliferation without noticeable changes in metabolism. Endocrinology 133, 2255–2262.

Cresswell, A.G., Grundstrom, H., Thorstensson, A., 1992. Observations on intra-abdominal pressure and patterns of abdominal intra-muscular activity in man. Acta Physiol Scand 144, 409–418.

Dangaria, T.R., Naesh, O., 1998. Changes in cross-sectional area of psoas major muscle in unilateral sciatica caused by disc herniation.

Spine [Clinical Trial Comparative Study] 23, 928–931.

Danneels, L.A., Vanderstraeten, G.G., Cambier, D.C., Witvrouw, E.E., De Cuyper, H.J., 2000. CT imaging of trunk muscles in chronic low back pain patients and healthy control subjects. Eur Spine J 9, 266–272.

Dulor, J.P., Cambon, B., Vigneron, P., Reyne, Y., Nougues, J., Casteilla, L., et al., 1998. Expression of specific white adipose tissue genes in denervation-induced skeletal muscle fatty degeneration. FEBS Lett 439, 89–92.

Ekholm, J., Eklund, G., Skoglund, S., 1960. On the reflex effects from the knee joint of the cat. Acta Physiol Scand 50, 167–174.

Farina, D., Arendt-Nielsen, L., Merletti, R., Graven-Nielsen, T., 2004. Effect of experimental muscle pain on motor unit firing rate and conduction velocity. J Neurophysiol 91, 1250–1259.

Ferreira, P., Ferreira, M., Hodges, P., 2004. Changes recruitment of the abdominal muscles in people with low back pain: ultrasound measurement of muscle activity. Spine 29, 2560–2566.

Ferreira, P.H., Ferreira, M.L., Maher, C.G., Herbert, R.D., Refshauge, K., 2006. Specific stabilisation exercise for spinal and pelvic pain: a systematic review. Aust J Physiother 52, 79–88.

Ferreira, M.L., Ferreira, P.H., Latimer, J., Herbert, R.D., Hodges, P.W., Jennings, M.D., et al., 2007. Comparison of general exercise, motor control exercise and spinal manipulative therapy for chronic low back pain: a randomized trial. Pain 131, 31–37.

Ferreira, P., Ferreira, M., Maher, C., Refshauge, K., Herbert, R., Hodges, P., 2009. Changes in recruitment of transversus abdominis correlate with disability in people with chronic low back pain. Br J Sports Med. 55, 153–169.

Fitts, R.H., Riley, D.R., Widrick, J.J., 2000. Physiology of a microgravity environment invited review: microgravity and skeletal muscle. J Appl Physiol 89, 823–839.

Fitts, R.H., Riley, D.R., Widrick, J.J., 2001. Functional and structural adaptations of skeletal muscle to

microgravity. J Exp Biol 204, 3201–3208.

Flor, H., Braun, C., Elbert, T., Birbaumer, N., 1997. Extensive reorganization of primary somatosensory cortex in chronic back pain patients. Neurosci Lett 224, 5–8.

Floss, T., Arnold, H.H., Braun, T., 1997. A role for FGF-6 in skeletal muscle regeneration. Genes Dev 11, 2040–2051.

Gill, N.W., Teyhen, D.S., Lee, I.E., 2007. Improved contraction of the transversus abdominis immediately following spinal manipulation: a case study using real-time ultrasound imaging. Man Ther 12, 280–285.

Haggmark, T., Jansson, E., Eriksson, E., 1981. Fiber type area and metabolic potential of the thigh muscle in man after knee surgery and immobilization. Int J Sports Med 2, 12–17.

Hall, L., Tsao, H., MacDonald, D., Coppieters, M., Hodges, P.W., 2009. Immediate effects of co-contraction training on motor control of the trunk muscles in people with recurrent low back pain. J Electromyogr Kinesiol 19, 763–773.

Hamill, J., van Emmerik, R.E., Heiderscheit, B.C., Li, L., 1999. A dynamical systems approach to lower extremity running injuries. Clin Biomech 14, 297–308.

Hayashi, Y., Ikata, T., Takai, H., Takata, S., Ishikawa, M., Sogabe, T., et al., 1997. Effect of peripheral nerve injury on nuclear magnetic resonance relaxation times of rat skeletal muscle. Invest Radiol 32, 135–139.

Herbison, G.J., Jaweed, M.M., Ditunno, J.F., 1979. Muscle atrophy in rats following denervation, casting, inflammation, and tenotomy. Arch Phys Med Rehabil 60, 401–404.

Hides, J.A., Stokes, M.J., Saide, M., Jull, G.A., Cooper, D.H., 1994. Evidence of lumbar multifidus muscle wasting ipsilateral to symptoms in patients with acute/subacute low back pain. Spine 19, 165–177.

Hides, J.A., Jull, G.A., Richardson, C.A., 2001. Long term effects of specific stabilizing exercises for first episode low back pain. Spine 26, E243–238.

Hides, J.A., Belavy, D.L., Stanton, W., Wilson, S.J., Rittweger, J., Felsenberg, D., et al., 2007. Magnetic resonance imaging assessment of trunk muscles during prolonged bed rest. Spine. 32, 1687–1692.

Hodges, P., Cholewicki, J., 2007. Functional control of the spine. In: Vleeming, A., Mooney, V., Stoeckart, R. (Eds.), Movement., Stability and Lumbopelvic Pain. Elsevier, Edinburgh.

Hodges, P.W., Richardson, C.A., 1996. Inefficient muscular stabilization of the lumbar spine associated with low back pain: A motor control evaluation of transversus abdominis. Spine 21, 2640–2650.

Hodges, P.W., Richardson, C.A., 1997a. Feedforward contraction of transversus abdominis is not influenced by the direction of arm movement. Exp Brain Res 114, 362–370.

Hodges, P.W., Richardson, C.A., 1997b. Contraction of the abdominal muscles associated with movement of the lower limb. Phys Ther 77, 132–144.

Hodges, P., Tucker, K., 2011. Moving differently in pain: A new theory to explain the adaptation to pain. Pain 152, S90–98.

Hodges, P.W., Cresswell, A.G., Thorstensson, A., 1999. Preparatory trunk motion accompanies rapid upper limb movement. Exp Brain Res 124, 69–79.

Hodges, P.W., Cresswell, A.G., Daggfeldt, K., Thorstensson, A., 2001a. In vivo measurement of the effect of intra-abdominal pressure on the human spine. J Biomech 34, 347–353.

Hodges, P.W., Cresswell, A.G., Thorstensson, A., 2001b. Perturbed upper limb movements cause short-latency postural responses in trunk muscles. Exp Brain Res 138, 243–350.

Hodges, P., Kaigle Holm, A., Holm, S., Ekstrom, L., Cresswell, A., Hansson, T., et al., 2003a. Intervertebral stiffness of the spine is increased by evoked contraction of transversus abdominis and the diaphragm: in vivo porcine studies. Spine 28, 2594–2601.

Hodges, P., Pengel, L., Herbert, R., Gandevia, S., 2003b. Measurement of muscle contraction with ultrasound imaging. Muscle Nerve 27, 682–692.

Hodges, P.W., Moseley, G.L., Gabrielsson, A., Gandevia, S.C., 2003c. Experimental muscle pain changes feedforward postural responses of the trunk muscles. Exp Brain Res 151, 262–271.

Hodges, P.W., KaigleHolm, A., Hansson, T., Holm, S., 2006. Rapid atrophy of the lumbar multifidus follows experimental disc or nerve root injury. Spine 31, 2926–2933.

Hodges, P.W., Ervilha, U.F., Graven-Nielsen, T., 2008. Changes in motor unit firing rate in synergist muscles cannot explain the maintenance of force during constant force painful contractions. J Pain 9, 1169–1174.

Hodges, P., Simms, K., Tsao, H. (eds), 2009a. Gain of postural responses is increased in anticipation of pain. Australian Physiotherapy Association Conference Week, Sydney.

Hodges, P., van den Hoorn, W., Dawson, A., Cholewicki, J., 2009b. Changes in the mechanical properties of the trunk in low back pain may be associated with recurrence. J Biomech 42, 61–66.

Hodges, P.W., Galea, M.P., Holm, S., Holm, A.K., 2009c. Corticomotor excitability of back muscles is affected by intervertebral disc lesion in pigs. Eur J Neurosci 29, 1490–1500.

Hodges, P.W., Coppieters, M.W., Macdonald, D., Cholewicki, J., 2013. New insight into motor adaptation to pain revealed by a combination of modelling and empirical approaches. Eur J Pain, 2013 Jan 25. doi: 10.1002/j.1532-2149.2013.00286.x. [Epub ahead of print]

Hungerford, B., Hodges, P., Gilleard, W., 2003. Evidence of altered lumbopelvic muscle recruitment in the presence of sacroiliac joint pain. Spine 28, 1593–1600.

Igarashi, A., Kikuchi, S., Konno, S., Olmarker, K., 2004. Inflammatory cytokines released from the facet joint tissue in degenerative lumbar spinal disorders. Spine 29, 2091–2095.

Indahl, A., Kaigle, A.M., Reikeras, O., Holm, S.H., 1997. Interaction between the porcine lumbar intervertebral disc, zygapophysial joints, and paraspinal muscles. Spine 22, 2834–2840.

Jackman, R.W., Kandarian, S.C., 2004. The molecular basis of skeletal muscle atrophy. Am J Physiol Cell Physiol 287, C834–843.

Janda, V., 1978. Muscles, central nervous motor regulation and back problems. In: Korr, I.M. (Ed.), The Neurobiologic Mechanisms in Manipulative Therapy, first ed. Plenum Press, New York, pp. 27–41.

Jiang, B., Ohira, Y., Roy, R.R., Nguyen, Q., Ilyina-Kakueva, E.I., Oganov, V., et al., 1992. Adaptation of fibers in fast-twitch muscles of rats to spaceflight and hindlimb suspension. J Appl Physiol 73, 58S–65S.

Kaigle, A.M., Holm, S.H., Hansson, T.H., 1995. Experimental instability in the lumbar spine. Spine 20, 421–430.

Kavcic, N., Grenier, S., McGill, S.M., 2004. Determining the stabilizing role of individual torso muscles during rehabilitation exercises. Spine 29, 1254–1265.

Kendall, F.P., McCreary, E.K., 1983. Muscles: testing and function, third ed. Williams and Wilkins, Baltimore.

Kiesel, K.B., Underwood, F.B., Mattacola, C.G., Nitz, A.J., Malone, T.R., 2007. A comparison of select trunk muscle thickness change between subjects with low back pain classified in the treatment-based classification system and asymptomatic controls. J Orthop Sports Phys Ther 37, 596–607.

Kiesel, K.B., Uhl, T., Underwood, F.B., Nitz, A.J., 2008. Rehabilitative ultrasound measurement of select trunk muscle activation during induced pain. Man Ther 13, 132–138.

Knutsson, B., 1961. Comparative value of electromyographic, myelographic and clinical-neurological examinations in diagnosis of lumbar root compression syndrome. Acta Orthop Scand 49, 1–135.

Lefaucheur, J.P., Gjata, B., Lafont, H., Sebille, A., 1996. Angiogenic and inflammatory responses following skeletal muscle injury are altered by immune neutralization of endogenous basic fibroblast growth factor, insulin-like growth factor-1 and transforming growth factor-beta 1. J Neuroimmunol 70, 37–44.

Lund, J.P., Donga, R., Widmer, C.G., Stohler, C.S., 1991. The pain-adaptation model: a discussion of the relationship between chronic musculoskeletal pain and motor activity. Can J Physiol Pharmacol 69, 683–694.

MacDonald, D., Moseley, G.L., Hodges, P.W., 2009. Why do some patients keep hurting their back? Evidence of ongoing back muscle dysfunction during remission from recurrent back pain. Pain 142, 183–188.

MacDonald, D., Moseley, G.L., Hodges, P.W., 2010. People with recurrent low back pain respond differently to trunk loading despite remission from symptoms. Spine 35, 818–824.

Macedo, L.G., Maher, C.G., Latimer, J., McAuley, J.H., 2009. Motor control exercise for persistent, nonspecific low back pain: a systematic review. Phys Ther 89, 9–25.

Madeleine, P., Mathiassen, S.E., Arendt-Nielsen, L., 2008. Changes in the degree of motor variability associated with experimental and chronic neck-shoulder pain during a standardized repetitive arm movement. Exp Brain Res 185, 689–698.

Marras, W.S., Ferguson, S.A., Burr, D., Davis, K.G., Gupta, P., 2004. Spine loading in patients with low back pain during asymmetric lifting exertions. Spine J 4, 64–75.

Marshall, P., Murphy, B., 2006. The effect of sacroiliac joint manipulation on feed-forward activation times of the deep abdominal musculature. J Manipulative Physiol Ther 29, 196–202.

Max, S.R., Mayer, R.F., Vogelsang, L., 1971. Lysosomes and disuse atrophy of skeletal muscle. Arch Biochem Biophys 146, 227–232.

McGill, S.M., Grenier, S., Kavcic, N., Cholewicki, J., 2003. Coordination of muscle activity to assure stability of the lumbar spine. J Electromyogr Kinesiol 13, 353–359.

McLachlan, E.M., 1981. Rapid atrophy of mouse soleus muscles after tenotomy depends on an intact innervation. Neurosci Lett 25, 269–274.

McPherson, J.G., Ellis, M.D., Heckman, C.J., Dewald J.P., 2008. Evidence for increased activation of persistent inward currents in individuals with chronic hemiparetic stroke. J Neurophysiol 100, 3236–3243.

Meyer, D.C., Pirkl, C., Pfirrmann, C.W., Zanetti, M., Gerber, C., 2005. Asymmetric atrophy of the supraspinatus muscle following tendon tear. J Orthop Res 23, 254–258.

Misuri, G., Colagrande, S., Gorini, M., Iandelli, I., Mancini, M., Duranti, R., et al., 1997. In vivo ultrasound assessment of respiratory function of abdominal muscles in normal subjects. Eur Respir J 10, 2861–2867.

Mok, N.W., Brauer, S.G., Hodges, P.W., 2007. Failure to use movement in postural strategies leads to increased spinal displacement in low back pain. Spine 32, E537–543.

Moseley, G.L., Hodges, P.W., 2005. Are the changes in postural control associated with low back pain caused by pain interference? Clin J Pain 21, 323–329.

Moseley, G.L., Hodges, P.W., 2006. Reduced variability of postural strategy prevents normalization of motor changes induced by back pain – a risk factor for chronic trouble? Behav Neurosci 120, 474–476.

Moseley, G.L., Hodges, P.W., Gandevia, S.C., 2002. Deep and superficial fibers of lumbar multifidus are differentially active during voluntary arm movements. Spine 27, E29–36.

Moseley, G.L., Hodges, P.W., Gandevia, S.C., 2003. External perturbation of the trunk in standing humans differentially activates components of the medial back muscles. J Physiol 547, 581–587.

Moseley, G.L., Nicholas, M.K., Hodges, P.W., 2004. Does anticipation of back pain predispose to back trouble? Brain 127, 2339–2347.

Nitz, A.J., Peck, D., 1986. Comparison of muscle spindle concentrations in large and small human epaxial muslces acting in parallel combinations. Am Surgeon 52, 273–277.

O'Connell, N.E., Maskill, D.W., Cossar, J., Nowicky, A.V., 2007. Mapping the cortical representation of the lumbar paravertebral muscles. Clin Neurophysiol 118, 2451–2455.

O'Sullivan, P., 2005. Diagnosis and classification of chronic low back pain disorders: maladaptive movement and motor control impairments as underlying mechanism. Man Ther 10, 242–255.

O'Sullivan, P.B., Twomey, L.T., Allison, G.T., 1997. Evaluation of specific stabilizing exercise in the treatment of chronic low back pain with radiologic diagnosis of spondylolysis or spondylolisthesis. Spine 22, 2959–2967.

Okada Y., 1989. Histochemical study on the atrophy of the quadriceps femoris muscle caused by knee joint injuries of rats. Hiroshima J Med Sci 38, 13–21.

Panjabi, M., 2006. A hypothesis of chronic back pain: ligament subfailure injuries lead to muscle control dysfunction. Eur Spine J 15, 668–676.

Panjabi, M.M., 1992. The stabilizing system of the spine. Part I. Function, dysfunction, adaptation, and enhancement. J Spinal Dis 5, 383–389.

Pedersen, J., Sjolander, P., Wenngren, B.I., Johansson, H., 1997. Increased intramuscular concentration of bradykinin increases the static fusimotor drive to muscle spindles in neck muscles of the cat. Pain 70, 83–91.

Radebold, A., Cholewicki, J., Panjabi, M.M., Patel, T.C., 2000. Muscle response pattern to sudden trunk loading in healthy individuals and in patients with chronic low back pain. Spine 25, 947–954.

Reeves, N.P., Cholewicki, J., 2010. Expanding our view of the spine system [letter]. Eur Spine J 19, 331–332.

Reeves, N.P., Everding, V.Q., Cholewicki, J., Morrisette, D.C., 2006. The effects of trunk stiffness on postural control during unstable seated balance. Exp Brain Res 174, 696–700.

Roland, M., 1986. A critical review of the evidence for a pain-spasm-pain cycle in spinal disorders. Clin Biomech 1, 102–109.

Rother, P., Löffler, S., Dorschner, W., Reibiger, I., Bengs, T., 1996. Anatomic basis of micturition and urinary continence. Muscle systems in urinary bladder neck during ageing. Surgical and radiologic anatomy. SRA 18, 173–177.

Sahrman, S., 2002. Diagnosis and Treatment of Movement Impairment Syndromes. Mosby, St Louis.

Saunders, S., Coppieters, M., Hodges, P. (Eds.), 2004a. Reduced Tonic Activity of the Deep Trunk Muscle During Locomotion in People with Low Back Pain. World Congress of Low Back and Pelvic Pain, Melbourne.

Saunders, S.W., Rath, D., Hodges, P.W., 2004b. Postural and respiratory activation of the trunk muscles changes with mode and speed of locomotion. Gait Posture 20, 280–290.

Schneider, G., Pearcy, M.J., Bogduk, N., 2005. Abnormal motion in spondylolytic spondylolisthesis. Spine 30, 1159–1164.

Sihvonen, T., Lindgren, K.A., Airaksinen, O., Manninen, H., 1997. Movement disturbances of the lumbar spine and abnormal back muscle electromyographic findings in recurrent low back pain. Spine 22, 289–295.

Sirca, A., Kostevc, V., 1985. The fibre type composition of thoracic and lumbar paravertebral muscles in man. J Anat 141, 131–137.

Smith, M.D., Coppieters, M.W., Hodges, P.W., 2007a. Postural activity of the pelvic floor muscles is delayed during rapid arm movements in women with stress urinary incontinence. Int Urogynecol J Pelvic Floor Dysfunct 18, 901–911.

Smith, M.D., Coppieters, M.W., Hodges, P.W., 2007b. Postural response of the pelvic floor and abdominal muscles in women with and without incontinence. Neurourol Urodyn 26, 377–385.

Smith, M.D., Russell, A., Hodges, P.W., 2009. Do incontinence, breathing difficulties, and gastrointestinal symptoms increase the risk of future back pain? J Pain 10, 876–886.

Sohn, M.K., Graven-Nielsen, T., Arendt-Nielsen, L., Svensson, P., 2000. Inhibition of motor unit firing during experimental muscle pain in humans. Muscle Nerve 23, 1219–1226.

Spencer, J.D., Hayes, K.C., Alexander, I.J., 1984. Knee joint effusion and quadriceps reflex inhibition in man. Arch Phys Med Rehabil 65, 171–177.

Stokes, I.A., Gardner-Morse, M., Henry, S.M., Badger, G.J., 2000. Decrease in trunk muscular response to perturbation with preactivation of lumbar spinal musculature. Spine 25, 1957–1964.

Stokes, M., Young, A., 1984. The contribution of reflex inhibition to arthrogenous muscle weakness. Clin Sci (Lond) 67, 7–14.

Strutton, P.H., Catley, M., Theodorou, S., McGregor, A.H., Davey, N.J., 2003. A transcranial magnetic stimulation study of back muscles in patients with low back pain. J Physiol, 647P.

Stuge, B., Laerum, E., Kirkesola, G., Vollestad, N., 2004. The efficacy of a treatment program focusing on specific stabilizing exercises for pelvic girdle pain after pregnancy: a randomized controlled trial. Spine 29, 351–359.

Tesh, K.M., ShawDunn, J., Evans, J.H., 1987. The abdominal muscles and vertebral stability. Spine 12, 501–508.

Tsao, H., Hodges, P.W., 2007. Immediate changes in feedforward postural adjustments following voluntary motor training. Exp Brain Res 181, 537–546.

Tsao, H., Hodges, P.W., 2008. Persistence of changes in postural control following training of isolated voluntary contractions in people with recurrent low back pain. J Electromyogr Kinesiol 18, 559–567.

Tsao, H., Galea, M.P., Hodges, P.W., 2008. Reorganization of the motor cortex is associated with postural control deficits in recurrent low back pain. Brain 131, 2161–2171.

Tsao, H., Danneels, L.A., Hodges, P.W., 2011a. ISSLS prize winner: Smudging the motor brain in young adults with recurrent low back pain. Spine 36, 1721–1727.

Tsao, H., Druitt, T.R., Schollum, T.M., Hodges, P.W., 2010. Motor training of the lumbar paraspinal muscles induces immediate changes in motor coordination in patients with recurrent low back pain. J Pain 11, 1120–1128.

Tsao, H., Tucker, K.J., Hodges, P.W. 2011b. Changes in excitability of corticomotor inputs to the trunk muscles during experimentally-induced acute low back pain. Neuroscience 181, 127–133.

Tsao, H., Danneels, L., Hodges, P.W., 2011c. Individual fascicles of the paraspinal muscles are activated by discrete cortical networks in humans. Clin Neurophysiol 122, 1580–1587.

Tucker, K., Larsson, A., Oknelid, S., Hodges, P., 2012. Similar alteration of motor unit recruitment strategies during the anticipation and experience of pain. Pain 153, 636–643.

Tucker, K., Butler, J., Graven-Nielsen, T., Riek, S., Hodges, P., 2009. Motor unit recruitment strategies are altered during deep-tissue pain. J Neurosci 29, 10820–10826.

Tucker, K.J., Hodges, P.W., 2009. Motoneurone recruitment is altered with pain induced in non-muscular tissue. Pain 141, 151–155.

Tucker, K.J., Hodges, P.W., 2010. Changes in motor unit recruitment strategy during pain alters force direction. Eur J Pain 14, 932–938.

Unsgaard-Tøndel, M., Lund Nilsen, T.I., Magnussen, J., Vasseljen, O., 2012. Is activation of transversus abdominis and obliquus internus abdominis associated with long-term changes in chronic low back pain? A prospective study with 1-year follow-up. British Journal of Sports Medicine 46, 729–734.

van Dieën, J.H., de Looze, M.P., 1999. Directionality of anticipatory activation of trunk muscles in a lifting task depends on load knowledge. Exp Brain Res 128, 397–404.

van Dieën, J.H., Selen, L.P., Cholewicki, J., 2003. Trunk muscle activation in low-back pain patients, an analysis of the literature. J Electromyogr Kinesiol 13, 333–351.

Vasseljen, O., Fladmark, A.M., 2010. Abdominal muscle contraction thickness and function after specific and general exercises: a randomized controlled trial in chronic low back pain patients. Man Ther 15, 482–489.

Weber, B.R., Grob, D., Dvorak, J., Muntener, M., 1997. Posterior surgical approach to the lumbar spine and its effect on the multifidus muscle. Spine 22, 1765–1772.

Weiler, C., Nerlich, A.G., Bachmeier, B.E., Boos, N., 2005. Expression and distribution of tumor necrosis factor alpha in human lumbar intervertebral discs: a study in surgical specimen and autopsy controls. Spine 30, 44–53.

Wilke, H.J., Wolf, S., Claes, L.E., Arand, M., Wiesend, A., 1995. Stability increase of the lumbar spine with different muscle groups: a biomechanical in vitro study. Spine 20, 192–198.

Williams, P.L., Warwick, R., Dyson, M., Bannister, L.H. (Eds.), 1989. Grays Anatomy, thirtyseventh ed. Churchill Livingstone, London.

Chapter | 7 |

Opinions on the links between back pain and motor control: the disconnect between clinical practice and research

Stuart McGill
Department of Kinesiology, Faculty of Applied Health Sciences, University of Waterloo, Waterloo, Ontario, Canada

Research needs more clinical practice
And
Clinical practice needs more research

Dr Steven Rose, St Louis

INTRODUCTION

This chapter contributes answers to the question, 'What are your opinions on the links between back pain and motor control?' Opinions are listed in no particular order of importance. The format of stating them as a list is intended to focus discussion. They are intentionally provocative to serve this purpose.

The opinions in this chapter have been formed from clinical experience with patients, through my work as a consultant to governmental and non-governmental health organizations, industry and athletic organizations, and working as a professor/scientist. It cannot be stated which perspective was most influential but each was certainly important.

Finally, the term 'motor control' means different things to different people. To some it means very specific activation control of some selected muscles at low amplitudes without regard to the mechanical consequence of the contraction. To me, motor control is a much larger entity that includes not only the activation patterns and subsequent force magnitudes of both muscle and supporting tissues, but also the influence of the forces that result in body segment linkage motion, the motion of the various spine components, and controlled variables such as spine stiffness, stability, mobility and compliance. After all, the muscles are controlled to create purposeful movement in a way to enhance performance and avoid injury. Of course there are links between 'motor control' and biomechanics, psychology and physiology. The biomechanist must be concerned with the controllers of force to understand their consequences. The physiologist needs to understand the reason for contraction to fully grasp the dynamics of muscle cell protein involvement in force production. And the psychologist appreciates that controlled motion starts as a thought to move (not conscious focus on activation of specific muscles) that is modulated by many variables such as personality and arousal state, to name only two.

OPINIONS

1. Dr Rose's quote is true

Some back pain scientists have stated, 'If it can't be proved with experimental hypothesis testing then I will dismiss the concept'. But then give them 10 patients that present with a wide spectrum of back disorders with the directive to treat them. Most would not be able to conduct an assessment, interpret the results, prescribe a plan to eliminate the cause, prescribe a plan to address the deficits and prevent further pain and disability. But this is the clinical reality that clinicians must face and their impressions after helping or failing with patients builds their perspective. On the other hand, some clinicians may state, 'my treatment approach works because XXX'. Is the effect real and did it produce the best outcome? A wise clinician once stated, 'Nothing ruins clinical efficacy like patient follow-up'. I believe a scientist exposed to clinical reality and a clinician exposed to the scientific process produces a discourse that fosters both better science and clinical practice.

2. Is spine 'stability' the best term – or should it be 'stiffness'?

Spine stability has many meanings and interpretations. In my conversations with Professor Hodges he lamented that the term 'hollowing' was not the best choice while I lamented that 'stability' falls into the same category. The stability needed to prevent falling off a bike or when walking is different from Euler column stability needed to prevent buckling under load. Being stable is a similar state to being pregnant – one is or is not. However, stiffness is a variable. Stiffness is increased or decreased through muscle activation and joint position to modulate vertebral motion from applied load. In the spine, stiffness is created to allow the joints to withstand anticipated load that could be in a compressive, shear or bending mode. Insufficient stiffness would allow micromovements that cause pain. This is what happens during provocative testing of a patient by a clinician, where load is applied that causes pain, and the clinician works to find co-contraction patterns that produce enough stiffness so that the pain disappears. This description accommodates shear loads and microdisplacements while typical descriptions of stability do not. It also helps to address static verses dynamic stability. Reflex activity is reflected in the muscle electromyography (EMG) and is captured in the instantaneous estimates of stiffness which can be compared to the applied load, from whatever direction or mode, to determine if micromovements will be arrested. Thus determining the stiffness state of the system, and testing it with dynamic load to see if micromovements are contained, is probably a better description of what is needed for analysis of spine 'stability'.

3. Studies on 'back pain' are not helpful – particularly RCTs

Consider the claim: 'Recent randomized controlled trial (RCT) on "leg pain" shows "taking pills" or "doing exercise" to be ineffective'. A trained clinician or scientist would think this to be absurd. RCTs are important and provide insight when an intervention has a chance of being effective, or not. They make great sense when the mechanism of action is understood. But in this example, what was the leg disorder and what was the pill or exercise? Thus I am left with the opinion that studies on 'back pain' have obscured the links that exist between those with pain and motor control issues. Back pain is not a homogeneous malady. There have been all kinds of RCTs and meta-analyses comparing treatments that have shown nothing works, or at least works well. This is an artefact due to the lack of classification of patients. For example, a study comparing spine mobilization approaches (e.g. chiropractic) with approaches for stabilization (e.g. a form of physical therapy) on a back pain group is not helpful for several reasons. There are some 'back pain' patients who will do better with mobilization while stabilization is contraindicated and vice versa in other patients. Without pre-classification of the patients the results show an average effect – which is zero. Then some readers of the 'back pain' RCT will assume that it does not matter which approach is chosen, or may simply use no approach at all and do nothing. Some will use this interpretation for political gain as it may suit their purpose if exercise did not help. However, if the 'back pain' patients were assessed and subclassified using a system appropriate for the clinical question, a different conclusion is reached. Such a trial was performed in a study by Fritz and colleagues (2005). The results showed that the 'stiff backs' did better with mobilizing interventions while the unstable backs did better with stabilizing approaches. Subclassifying the patients facilitated the identification of those who would benefit from a specific approach. Perhaps just as valuable was the insight obtained into which patients would do worse. The point is that a better impression is obtained with categorized homogeneous study groups than a heterogeneous 'low back pain' group.

The type of intervention also needs consideration. Consider a skilled clinician who conducts an assessment that may involve the utilization of some 'clinical prediction rules' to classify patients into treatment clusters. However, even within a cluster different exercises may be tuned for dosage, starting challenge, and combined with prevention efforts etc. Thus given the spectrum of patients' responses to any 'exercise progression', RCTs of singular treatments are of little use. Skilled clinicians would not use a controlled therapy consisting of a continual 'dose' throughout the process of treatment. They would begin perhaps with removing the physical loads that continue to exacerbate the painful tissues. They would choose appropriate corrective exercise, while combining strategies for avoidance of painful movement, perhaps use some passive muscle manual therapy, perhaps transition to endurance and stability/mobility training, and perhaps strength training. Then they would refine the transference of the corrected movement patterns to the activities of daily and occupational life. Until controlled trials incorporate such therapeutic progressions they will not represent how effective treatments are, and will continue to retard development of clinical practice guidelines.

As a case in point, consider a cohort of back pain patients with radiating symptoms. One patient may become pained when lying in bed. The next patient gets relief from lying but experiences sharp pain when rolling over. There must be a different genesis to their pain. Is the pain from a bulging disc or from stenosis linked to arthritic bone changes? Each one would benefit from a quite different intervention, and further, the intervention that would help one would worsen the other. Another impediment to consuming the results of the RCT is that the clinicians themselves are not equal just as car mechanics or policemen or professors are not equivalent performers. The skill level of the clinician must be high to obtain understanding of the genesis of the pain, to obtain immediate reduction in pain through modification of specific loads and postures, to assess the personality and learning style of the patient etc. Excellent clinical skill and practice tends to reveal more details of the pathology resulting in clinicians/scientists categorizing patients into smaller and finer detailed treatment cluster groups. Recalling the previous example of Fritz et al. (2005), even within the group benefitting from stabilization, there would have been a spectrum of starting dosages of exercise and even different exercises matched to the pain-free tolerance and capacity of the patient, the location of the instability, etc. The most challenging patients, those with intransigent pain, deserve to form a cluster group with an N of 1 to best match the specific treatment to their specific presentation. Excellent practice with difficult patients implies that the most logical investigative methodology is the case study. Thus there is a time and place for RCTs on those with back pain if they are subclassified with schemes best suited to the nature of the treatment. RCTs of non-specific 'back pain' are not helpful, or perhaps even counterproductive when they are used to push agendas that are oblique to getting patients better with a specific approach.

Having worked with some outstanding clinicians I have given thought to how an RCT could be conducted on the clinical approach that we follow. With each patient an assessment is performed that takes approximately 2 hours to identify motions, postures and loads that are both tolerable and problematical. Tests of specific muscle function may be conducted depending on whether any suspicious signs were observed in the provocative testing. Then corrective and therapeutic exercises would be devised to address the specific movement disorder which includes both whole body movements with muscle activation patterns and with joint- and muscle-specific focus. Then exercise progressions would be formulated to address issues of muscle endurance, followed by strength and power development should this be warranted in a particular patient. This is the way many elite clinicians practice, which begs the question, 'How can a controlled trial be conducted when every single patient has a different treatment?' The option is that the entire approach could be compared to another approach yet there would be no insight provided about a controlled variable or mechanism of action.

Given the number of reports that state they studied 'exercise' interventions, two more issues come to light: What was the exercise therapy and what classification scheme could be helpful? Hence the next opinion.

4. Exercise is not a generic intervention – studies must give sufficient detail of the 'exercise'

Some studies report 'exercise' as a controlled independent variable and intervention. But any individual can be exacerbated with exercise that is excessive or not appropriate. Similarly, challenges that are well below the tolerance of the patient have little effect. The type of exercise, dosage, posture and motion, and intervals of training are a few variables that determine whether the exercises cause relief or more pain. The solution is to expect much more description of the reported exercise intervention to ferret out the link in those with back pain and motor control disturbances. Further, within a clinical practitioners group such as physical therapists, there are many philosophies and approaches such that scientific manuscripts that report 'physical therapy exercises were conducted' are not helpful. Full description of the patients and the exercise intervention, together with the criteria for progression within the programme, greatly enhances the clinical relevance and utility of the study.

5. Establish classification schemes for those with back pain that guide the conservative treatment

There are several patient classification schemes that exist. Some are based on the tissue suspected to be causing pain, for example 'discogenic pain' or 'facet pain'. This is helpful for the surgeon, for example, who seeks to cut out the pain. In contrast, this scheme is not very helpful for those in physical medicine. It is proposed that classifying patients using motion, postures and loads that provoke pain will result in a classification scheme that would guide the clinician/patient on what to avoid, and what to do. For example, a compression-intolerant and flexion-bending intolerant patient would not do well with a therapy that increased compression on their spine nor would they experience relief with flexion bending. Probably they would have to avoid spine-bending postures such as when tying their shoe and adopt alternate movement strategies such as the hip hinge lunge to unload their back. Further, specific exercises would have to be selected that spare the painful spine from provocative

compression loads. Using another example, a shear-intolerant patient would prosper with another set of exercises and avoidance strategies. This proposal would draw specific links to the parameters of controlled motion, loads and postures (all influenced by motor control) and the many presentations of back pain.

A classification scheme based on provocative motions, postures and loads forms an interesting clustering of patients which lends itself to different skill levels of the clinician. The more skilled clinicians would presumably form more clusters and have more clinical 'tools' to effectively deal with the more subtle presentations of faulty motor control. The less skilled would be able to be as effective as possible within the clusters they themselves determined.

6. Muscles of the torso are fundamentally different from those of the limbs

Muscles of the torso are fundamentally different from those of the limbs from a motor control perspective. Limb muscles create motion, torso muscles more often stop motion or control motion. The simple act of walking requires stiffness and stability of the spine and pelvis simply to lift one leg for swing while supporting body weight on the other. Without quadratus lumborum to assist in the lateral support of the swing-side of the pelvis, walking is not possible (Parry (1984) noted walking was not possible in those with quadratus lumborum paralysis). It neither shortens nor lengthens, but simply is activated to stiffen and stop motion. Consider opening a door where the hips and legs create a root to the ground, the arm reaches and pulls. If the spine then twists while transferring the torques up through the torso, many tissues become strained including the discs, ligaments, facets, etc. If the twisting torque is transferred through a torso sufficiently stiffened and controlled not to twist, relegating the motion to occur in the limbs, these potentially painful spine tissues are spared. This is a component of 'spine sparing movement strategy'. In spinal joints where small aberrant motions are present and cause pain, there really are no agonists or antagonists in the torso as all muscles are required to stabilize/stiffen and control motion generated elsewhere. This is an example using a lower demand task of daily living. In contrast, study of athletic performance (McGill (2009) contains many examples from a variety of sports) often shows that function is optimized when power is generated at the hips and transmitted through a stiffened 'core', or torso, with no 'energy leaks' (eccentric spine motion absorbing kinetic energy). This has a large impact on the approach to training torso muscles both for purposes of rehabilitation and pain control, and for performance enhancement. Examination of the architecture and mechanics of the abdominal wall, for example, shows that the wall uses the three layers as a structural composite to enhance stiffness and the production of hoop stresses (Brown and McGill 2008a, 2009). The rectus abdominis assists the production and transmission of these hoop stresses, developed by the obliques and transverse abdominis, around the torso via the lateral tendons that interrupt the series-arranged contractile portions within rectus (McGill 2007). Thus training the rectus with this special structure through the range of motion, as with a sit up for example, would not address one of the primary functions (actually the associated spine flexion with the sit up would mimic the disc herniation mechanism (Callaghan and McGill 2001)). In contrast, exercises designed to resist impending torso motion such as 'stir the pot' would enhance this function (McGill 2009). The practical implication is that some of the motor control principles to guide progressive exercise of the limbs may not hold true for muscles and movement of the torso.

7. Many injury mechanisms of the spine are controlled, or created, by the chosen motor control strategy

This opinion insinuates that back pain of 'insidious onset' may not be, and that it is actually caused by the movement patterns 'chosen' by the patient. The way a task is executed determines the posture of the spinal joints and the subsequent load placed on them. The loads determine the nature of the tissue damage. The various types of disc damage, for example, have been shown to be a function of posture, load and morphology (McGill et al. 2009c). Specifically, disc herniation is a function of repeated bending (Tampier et al. 2007), while annular delamination a function of repeated twisting (Marshall and McGill 2010), and endplate fracture a function of repeated or excessive compression (the textbook of Adams et al. (2002) forms an excellent base of evidence). In summary, the habitual patterns of movement and muscle activation in an individual determine the stress concentrations, which lead to the specific type of damage which influence the pain. In this way the motor control strategy modulates both the injury risk and the nature of the resulting tissue damage.

The obvious implication is that clinicians use therapeutic exercise to modulate pain by changing posture, movement and motor patterns in patients. Logically, injury and pain could be prevented the same way. But then there are counter arguments presented using examples of some athletes who seem to defy this logic, as they move in ways that create enormous stresses, and appear to avoid injury. A comment after working with many world-class athletes is that they are highly selected, gifted and adapted, and simply fall outside of what is 'normal'. While they are wonderful specimens to study, revealing mechanisms of exceptional function, sometimes they reveal their 'gifts' that simply are not helpful for a pained person.

8. Clinical technique during corrective exercise matters (corollary of previous section)

If the previous opinion has merit then the issue changes from 'it is not a matter of doing a corrective exercise', to a matter of 'doing the corrective exercise optimally'. Therapy can be easily modified to increase pain or take it away (McGill and Karpowicz 2009). The injury mechanism or the 'pain-inducing' mechanism is modulated by subtle postural changes and loads. Observation of some clinicians has convinced this author that they are oblivious to the role of the variables of motor control to determine the outcome of the patient. They do not recognize that poor movement represents a missed opportunity for success. But it is a joy to observe other clinicians who are vigilant to the movement flaws of the patient, correct them, and reduce their pain.

9. Important aspects of motor control have been obscured in the literature because functional variables are interrelated

A summary of the performance and injury literature would reveal that high power generation in the spine is problematical (McGill 2009). Power is the product of velocity and force. If the spine is moving segmentally (high velocity) then the force it is bearing must be low to control risk of damage. If the force it is bearing is high, the velocity of movement must be low to control risk. Thus the combination of spine bending while under load, i.e. their relationship to one another, determines the risk of the situation. Studying only one of the variables in isolation would obscure the risk potency. Consider another topic and example involving patient assessment. During testing of back extensor strength the torso, hips, shoulders and possibly limbs would need to be stiffened and stabilized to obtain a valid score. In contrast, the hips are designed to generate power with low risk. Valid hip strength and performance testing would need mobility and no doubt spine stiffening/stability, depending on the test device. Poor spine stability would obscure true hip function. Likewise, poor hip function and control compromises back/torso function. In fact asymmetrical hip motion and stiffness is a predictor of those at risk of developing back disorders (e.g. Ashmen et al. 1996) as is asymmetrical strength (Nadler et al. 2001). Disorders elsewhere in the anatomical linkage are suspected by various clinicians to be linked to back pain, but as of yet remain obscured in the scientific literature because of the multifactorial modulators. The point is that involvement of one variable is influenced by the performance and involvement of another. Barriers to understanding have affected both ends of the patient population – from the very disabled back pain sufferer to the elite performance athlete who only experiences pain when challenging the world record. Athletes are interesting to study as they have so much to reveal about mechanisms of spine and segment linkage function. Admittedly many are puzzled that the variables that characterize superior performance in athletes remains quite obscure. Why are the best athletes not the ones who have the strongest back strength scores? Consider some of the outstanding athletes who have dominated sports that obviously require strength, such as ice hockey or basketball, yet when tested are not the 'strongest'. Several of our recent studies have revealed variables that help define athletic success but they tend to be more neural or motor control in nature than strength. But it would be fair to state that many athletes train strength as a primary objective. For example, our recent study of elite mixed martial arts fighters (McGill et al. 2010), who need to punch and kick with speed and force, revealed that the fast and hard punch is initiated with a muscular pulse to stiffen the body to begin the propulsion of the arm. Then the speed of limb movement is enhanced with a subsequent phase of muscle relaxation. A second pulse is then created to stiffen the body to create a large 'effective mass' behind the impacting fist or foot. Thus the ability to strike very quickly and with high force not only requires rapid muscle contraction, but also rapid muscle relaxation. Without rapid relaxation the limb is slowed by the residual stiffness and viscosity causing poor performance. This is not routinely measured nor trained. This may be relevant to the back pained athlete who must react quickly. It also highlights the 'athleticism' needed for optimal function in non-athletes when a rapid response is needed in activities of daily living such as when arresting a slip, or when playing with children.

In summary, because many variables are interrelated the important variables of motor control have been obscured. Simply measuring the 'external end effect', such as a force on a transducer, or an 'internal trait variable', such as an EMG peak, from a muscle maintains the veil over motor control mechanisms. Post processing and modelling of the many variables is one approach to help enhance understanding, but this is much rarer in the 'motor control' literature when contrasted with other disciplines such as biomechanics.

10. Are clinicians training the critical variables or features to avoid the cause of back disorders and to enhance function and performance?

In many cases it is suggested that the answer is no. For example, consider the many 'strength' exercises for the back. Many clinics and training facilities are dominated by sagittal plane challenges and lifts and holds. Now consider the mechanics of walking and carrying a load that will eventually be needed by any patient. For example, the jet-lagged, fatigued traveller carrying a suitcase in one hand following 21 hours sitting on aeroplane seats that have no lumbar support and a bolster at shoulder level, further slumping their torso. Have they been prepared by a rehabilitation or training programme to meet the challenge? Our recent report of the spine mechanics utilized by strongman event athletes showed how they depended on the quadratus lumborum and abdominal obliques to accomplish one-armed carrying without failing (McGill et al. 2008). The task revealed the critical role of stabilizers such as quadratus lumborum and latissimus dorsi. It would be rare to have these anatomically lateral and frontal plane muscles as a focus in the clinic. A literature search will reveal that they have not received much scientific attention, but they are essential for walking and carrying. This opinion suggests a balanced treatment of the variables by scientists that are linked to back disorders will eventually lead to enhanced clinical practice.

11. Too many rehabilitation approaches are polluted by body building principles

While it is difficult to obtain the typical sets and repetitions of exercises used in clinics around the world, observation suggests that some try and isolate muscles, perhaps employing three sets of ten repetitions, training three times per week etc. The question is: are these approaches consistent with the principles of enhancing control of movement and muscles? Consider another situation of having a back pained patient perform a bench-press. In a standing posture one can only 'press' half of one's body weight without falling over. In contrast, a standing one-armed cable press would train the bench press mechanism in a standing posture, but studies show that it is the torso or core musculature that acts as the limiter (an analysis of these mechanics, and motor patterns are in Santana et al. (2007)). This may be considered an extreme example by some until a patient is thwarted or exacerbated from the action of pushing open a steel door at the entrance of the clinic. Thus a body building exercise was utilized (bench press) when it was the cable press ability that was needed by the patient to function. This example does show how important torso training is for back health and function, and that successful back function depends on the motor control proficiency of the entire linkage.

12. The transverse abdominis – the disconnect between evidence and clinical practice

Perhaps this is the most contentious issue for many. My colleague Professor Hodges approaches the transverse abdominis (TvA) issue from a neuroscience perspective while I approach it from a clinical/biomechanical perspective. The following discourse lays out a position.

There are three (and possibly four) postulates surrounding the clinical focus on TvA:

1. That people with low back pain have a delayed TvA.
2. That onset delay is unique to the TvA making it a select and specific marker of pathology.
3. That correcting the delay will treat pain (in other words it will have substantial impact on the mechanisms associated with function and pain).
4. And if 1–3 are true: that 'abdominal hollowing' at low levels of muscle activation in a supine posture is a valid way of training the TvA.

The neuroscience approach tries to detect the pathology, and then write movement engrams to correct the dysfunction. Hence, the approach of Professor Hodges' group of having a patient lie on their back to quiet the TvA muscle and then conduct low level contractions in isolation. Other clinical groups also attempt to isolate muscles to address other syndromes although they tend to use the same mental imagery to contract muscles but with much higher levels of contraction. For example, Professor Janda incorporated the gluteal muscles into the hip extensor pattern engram to correct the crossed pelvis syndrome (common in back pain individuals) with quite demanding contractions (Janda et al. 2007). Dr Hewett's group has been very successful in reducing knee ligament injury rates in female collegiate basketball players by creating new hip dominant movement engrams (Hewett et al. 2005). Again the exercises require demanding contraction levels. Dr Kolar's group in Prague use much more intense exercises for TvA contraction than the well known 'hollowing' approach (Kolar 2007). He also addresses the concerns regarding depressing the ribcage (to prevent rib flaring) to enhance breathing mechanics. He does this by having the patient lie on their backs but with the hips and knees flexed to 90 degrees. Holding this posture causes substantial abdominal wall contraction. Then the breath is exhaled to the normal full exhalation level and then forceful effort continues for complete expulsion of air from the lungs. This greatly enhances TvA activation to substantial levels. This paragraph has two implications: successfully changing muscle activation engrams are usually performed with exercises that create substantial muscle challenge; and engrams can be changed by isolating single muscles and by re-training with groups of muscles. There are several clinical tools to establish 'normal' muscle activation engrams but no single approach has proved to be superior with patients with back pain.

The biomechanical approach is used to assess the mechanics of the TvA and test the feasibility of claims about function. The TvA is the smallest of the abdominal wall muscles. The forces from the TvA are small and its contributions to moment production and spine stability are dwarfed by muscles such as the obliques, quadratus lumborum, latissimus dorsi and the entire erector spinae group (Kavcic et al. 2004). The TvA shares its tendon and fascial connections with the much larger and thicker internal oblique such that if it were delayed in activation, the internal oblique would dominate the shared tendon/fascia tension easily making up for any TvA deficit. There is no question that TvA is involved in building intra-abdominal pressure which is used by patients and athletes alike to stabilize their spine and bear more load (Cholewicki et al. 1999). The TvA has not been shown to not contract during these high load situations. But even if TvA were not active, the much larger internal oblique would still stiffen the abdominal wall creating the pressure vessel which carries some of the spine load. Intra-abdominal pressure (IAP) is an important mechanism when the spine loads are high but not so important when the loads are low (McGill and Norman 1987; McGill and Sharratt 1990). Further, the composite structure of the abdominal wall creates a 'super-stiffness' where the three layers bind forming enhanced strength and stiffness (higher than the individual muscles would suggest) which reduces the reliance on a much thinner and weaker TvA when creating wall stiffness (Brown and McGill 2008a). The internal oblique muscle dominates the mechanics in this regard. The biomechanical approach suggests that the mechanical consequence of a delayed contraction onset TvA is rather small. Nor does a hypothesis of TvA pathology fit the many mechanisms of mechanical back pain. For example, consider the common back pain exacerbator of prolonged sitting. It appears that the major contributor is the flexed posture of the intervertebral disc. Many mechanisms dominate spine curvature suggesting that intervention directed towards them would be far more productive than changing an activation onset engram of TvA.

Finding patients with a delayed TvA is very difficult – certainly not all back pain patients have a delay while some normal people have a delay. It is hard to obtain an impression of the percentage of subjects within the experimental groups with a delay because only average scores were reported and the studies had 15 or fewer subjects. A recent study of 48 chronic back pain patients did not find a feedforward delay unique to TvA in either the pained or the control group (Gubler et al. 2010). Further complicating the search for unique activation patterns of TvA is that delays may be modulated by fatigue (Allison and Henry 2002). One would suspect that fatigue would be an issue in those who respond to pain with constant guarding and bracing. The selection of the method to quantify the delay also affects the results. The choice of task affects the number of muscles that show delays (e.g. Cholewicki et al. (2002) who used a sudden load experiment rather than the more popular arm raise task). Finding delays in tasks more common to daily living would be helpful in understanding the motor control and biomechanical importance. For example, other variables of motor control disturbances are very blatant and easily measured in patients (these include strength, the flexion-relation phenomenon, both gross and segmental spine range of motion, muscle fatiguability, position sense, uncoordination, endurance, balance ability, and structural characteristics of muscles together with cognitive behavioural components linked to motor control, to name a few). However, some in the clinical community do not seem to collectively appreciate that many muscles display delays in back pain populations and that the patterns of delay among different muscles are helpful in classifying the nature of the link between motor control and pain. Instead they focus on TvA to the exclusion of other variables. Silfies and colleages (2009) reported delays in the arm raise experiment in several muscles. When grouping the entire back pain group as one there were delays in external oblique, lumbar multifidus and erector spinae compared with the non-pained control group. However, further subclassifying the patients into two clinical painful groups (not stable and stable) a different impression was formed as only the 'not stable' group demonstrated delays on average. Again, not all back pain patients showed a delay. Hubley-Kozey and Vezina (2002) demonstrated that populations of back pain subjects have many different responses in the motor control patterns during a task that challenged stability. Thus, many muscles show activation onset delays, and differences throughout the entire contraction pattern. There is no rationale that an onset delay in one muscle is enormously more critical than a delay in another. Furthermore, it would be more intriguing if delays were detectable in tasks of daily living and subsequently assessed with a kinetic analysis to determine the mechanical consequence of the delay. Delays are one minor variable, as one would be swayed if the entire time history of the muscle contraction pattern was distinguishable of a particular back pain group. Our collective work on athletic tasks suggests that even though muscles have different onsets their rate of force development is different such that the force peaks appear to coincide together (McGill et al. 2009a, 2009b both have several examples). Further, electromechanical delay appears to be substantially longer than most reported TvA delays such that the modulation of the actual force output of the muscle may be less affected than the magnitude of an onset delay would suggest. The final issue is one of muscle mechanics. Muscle onset/offset is the lowest form of EMG evidence. Modelling the activation profiles of muscles and the consequence of these forces on a three-dimensional skeleton, and understanding the forces, torques, stiffness and joint loads that result from onset delays, suggests these delays would not matter except for quite ballistic tasks. For example, tasks of holding loads while breathing heavily would be unaffected by a 70 ms delay of a single muscle (Wang and McGill 2008) although the timing for ballistic contractions could be slightly influenced (Vera-Garcia et al. 2007). However, most back pain sufferers are exacerbated by activities, such as prolonged sitting, standing and even repeated industrial tasks that would be unaffected by changes in muscle force occurring in less than 70 ms (i.e. reported delays). It is possible that some patients benefit from specific TvA training. If TvA were missing from a contraction pattern then training to encode it in the pattern engram is justifiable (although this has not been documented thus far). TvA training may enhance a patient's awareness of the existence of the abdominal wall and I have seen this in a qualitative sense (in patients who would be referred to as the motor awareness challenged) and appreciate the research. But experience suggests this is quite rare. In contrast, having followed every patient ever attending our clinic, this author is convinced that superior clinical results are achieved with a wide variety of abdominal activation techniques. In fact, encouraging muscle patterns including all muscles and combinations of muscles of the hips and torso can, in many patients, immediately reduce their pain. Consider the heel drop test that induces pain in a patient. Often repeating this test with an abdominal brace eliminates the pain. In contrast, hollowing the abdominals to isolate the TvA, or even the subtle visualization required to only activate the TvA at very low levels, rarely reduce pain. It is appreciated that this is usually done in a supine lying posture otherwise the TvA cannot be made inactive, but not all clinicians realize this. More often than not a brace (simply lightly stiffening the entire abdominal wall) will cause less pain. Yet occasionally a brace in some patients will increase their pain with this test. Alternatively, in such a patient, less abdominal contraction but more activation of the latissimus dorsi (and by biomechanical default pectoralis major) sometimes produces immediate relief. Obviously the contractions are 'tuned' to optimize stability/stiffness/control, reduce spine load, reduce aberrant joint micromotion, and effectively reduce pain. In summary, there are two issues. The first is that different patterns of co-contraction can reduce or eliminate pain during provocative tests and it is helpful for patients to understand which pattern is most helpful for a particular situation. TvA really does not help here. The second issue is training TvA to be included in the movement engram should it be missing in some patients. There is evidence of what would be considered relatively minor disruptions in TvA in an arm raise task but no evidence to suggest it is substantially perturbed in daily activities.

There is no issue with clinicians directing clinical effort towards TvA in these situations. I have a major concern when clinical focus is directed to TvA to the exclusion of all of the other easily documentable pathology of movement and muscle activation patterns. There are some clinicians who take all patients with back pain and begin isolation training of the TvA, even in patients who present with very recognizable disturbances in their motor patterns which are subsequently ignored with overzealous focus on TvA. For example, a patient may present with poor posture causing chronic muscle activity which loads the spine in compression. They may be bending painful discs because of their movement choices. Yet some clinicians fail to see these overt pain mechanisms and begin all back pain patients with isolated TvA training. Simple movement and posture training could have relieved their pain immediately. Perhaps even more disturbing is the number of high performance coaches from around the world who instruct their athletes to 'draw the navel towards the spine' to activate TvA, claiming this enhances stability while training or performing. Where they obtained this 'street level' impression is unknown, but it must be from lay colleagues propagating the myth as there is no evidence in the 'scientific' literature. A quick internet search will reveal a number who offer this instruction. Drawing the navel toward the spine reduces stability – increasing the distance between the abdominal wall and the spine enhances stability (Grenier and McGill 2007). The message is that back pain patients have many disturbances that require attention, and addressing them is justified with evidence for good clinical efficacy. The best initial approach is probably the one that has the largest potential to reduce pain and restore functional ability. Good clinicians have a wide array of clinical tools, and wisdom to use them.

The final issue deals with the patient trials where TvA was the focus of the intervention. Most studies involve the subtle 'drawing in' manoeuvre to re-train TvA but also include various abdominal exercises. It is suspect that it is the exercises that produce the reported clinical benefit. Koumantakis et al. (2005) studied two groups (one started with TvA-focused training and then progressed to full abdominal training, the other just initiated with abdominal wall training). This study suggested that in the average painful back, specific TvA training delayed recovery until full abdominal wall work was undertaken. The implication is to simply begin with stabilization training with exercises for the entire torso rather than any focused on TvA. A study by Cairns et al. (2006) also compared two groups: one with specific focus on TvA and multifidus added to active exercise typical in physical therapy; and the other with active exercise and manual therapy (their terms and definitions). This was not as clean a study as the Koumantakis study in that 'manual therapy' could have played a role. Nonetheless, there was no difference in the patient group outcome after a 12-month period.

Some clinical groups go though 'eras'. Not too long ago many physical therapists were taught to teach 'pelvic tilts' to their back pained patients (without critical discussion of whether they needed it or not). Eras, to such groups, come and go. In my opinion, the practice of some therapists to give TvA exercises to every patient with back pain is another era. This will be replaced by another in the future. However, it must be clarified given what I feel has been a misinterpretation by some. If pathology is found in a muscle or in any component of the spine, I am in full support of addressing it including TvA and multifidus training.

In summary, the answers to the postulates remain not fully understood and will direct future work. However, for those looking for a position on these issues now, I believe the evidence suggests that:

1. *People with low back pain have a delayed TvA.* Some people with back pain have a delayed TvA and some without pain have a delay. Larger studies suggest TvA delays are not a distinguishing feature of all back pain groups.
2. *Delays are unique to the TvA making it a select and specific marker of pathology.* Delays can occur in many muscles and appear to depend on the back pain classification group to which they belong. The delays also appear to depend on the task. But there are many other features of back pain that appear to be far more important than an activation delay. The full time history of the activation and force production of a muscle is more important.
3. *Correcting the delay will treat pain (in other words it will have substantial impact on the mechanisms associated with function and pain).* There is no evidence to support that correcting a delay is a superior way to reduce pain and enhance function. In contrast, several forms of exercise have been conclusively shown to be effective.

13. All muscles are important – the most important one at any particular time depends on many variables

When stated this opinion seems so obvious. Yet some clinicians appear to focus on muscles that they read about most often and ignore those that do not get attention in the journals that they read. I believe this is the case with TvA and multifidus. In the formative stage of developing the strategy to removing the cause of the pain in an individual (by changing their patterns of movement, muscle activation and frequency/repetition of these) some muscles may be extremely important. For example, encoding the gluteal muscles in the hip extension movement engram would be critical for those with the pain-induced extensor syndrome known as crossed pelvis syndrome (Janda et al. 2007). Changing sitting posture to make sitting tolerable may focus on hip flexors to flex the hips, tilting the pelvis forward and aligning the lumbar spine with less lumbar extensor contraction. Correction of the standing posture to minimize activation of the back extensors in those suffering with muscle cramps and spasms would be a very appropriate first step. The point is that all muscles will be required to execute optimal movement and joint loading. Many clinicians will not have read much about quadratus lumborum, yet the first functional loss from a paralyzed quadratus lumborum is the inability to walk (Parry 1984). It is a critical muscle for a compromised patient when walking up stairs or for a person to carry a suitcase (McGill et al. 2008). While the task context will change, it is a critical muscle for function and will be needed by every single back pain patient. Yet many clinicians will neglect it for the simple reason that is has not had the same number of research studies as TvA, for example. It is hoped that the eventual goal of rehabilitation programs should be to build capabilities in tasks requiring movement patterns to push, pull, lift, squat, lunge, carry asymmetrical loads and buttress torsional loads without twisting. The issue is about developing effective movement repertoires that spare joints. All muscles will be challenged as they contribute to the motor control schema and need to be activated properly.

14. Can the mechanics of TvA be documented with ultrasound?

The link between TvA muscle thickening, and activation (EMG) is obscured by the composite structure of the three layers of the abdominal wall. Fascial connections between TvA and internal oblique cause force crosstalk between them (Brown and McGill 2009) such that the force developed in one muscle is transferred to its adjacent layer. Further, we have not been able to find a link between muscle thickness and activation level, questioning whether the ultrasound measurement tool reveals biomechanical force production and function (Brown and McGill 2008c). For example, because of the composite wall architecture, a relaxed external oblique will thicken upon activation of internal oblique, falsely creating the illusion that it has been activated. Further, the relationship between activation, force production and stiffness is highly non-linear (Brown and McGill 2008b). In such a system every single variable would have to be controlled to evaluate and interpret the activation state of a muscle and then the measurements of 'muscle thickness' would need to be 'reprocessed' to appreciate the non-linearities. In summary, in most cases ultrasound is not equivalent to EMG for obtaining impressions of activation and subsequent interpretation of mechanics.

15. Are there patients who have developed the motor control wisdom to isolate and activate multifidus separately from other extensors?

I have only found one. Interestingly the motor strategy to isolate multifidus is a pattern that would be used to cause disc herniation. It is not the intention to downplay the role of multifidus, or the need for training it, as it is an important muscle like any other. It is emphasized that general erector spinae training includes multifidus along with other components of the erector spinae in a safer way and in a way that patients are able to perform. There is no evidence of an exercise that challenges just multifidus separately from the adjacent erector spinae muscles or that any patient could produce just multifidus activation. Perhaps it is just a distortion of nomenclature where some people refer to the erector spinae as 'multifidus'. In other words, there does not appear to be a 'multifidus' exercise.

16. No surgeon should be allowed to operate unless the cause of the tissue damage has been pointed out to the patient

First, surgery performed in cases of trauma, birth defects, real metastatic disease, etc. is necessary and not linked to issues of motor control. However, many surgical candidates with back pain have a history of slow or insidious onset. These are the ones who generally present with flawed motion and motor control patterns. For example, a patient who presents with a posterolateral disc bulge on the left side at L4/L5 has probably caused it by their own choice of movement patterns (McGill et al. 2009c). The specific cause is flexion bending with a bias to the right (Aultman et al. 2005). If the surgeon successfully repairs this but the patient continues with the flawed movement pattern, the patient has a high risk of either compromised healing or presenting in the future with the same condition at another spinal level, or both. This is a movement-based or 'motor control' back pain issue.

17. Motor control issues are probably the most important determinant of who will develop back disorders, and maintain the disorders

Recall that movement, resulting from muscle activation patterns, is included in any discussion of 'motor control' within this chapter. This opinion has been gained from the combination of working as a consultant to athletic teams and programmes together with conducting experimental studies. For example, having consulted with a number of Olympic programmes and sports organizations, both professional and amateur, watching the movement patterns of specific individuals early in the season motivated me to predict who would become injured and in what way. For example, in one team I predicted two players would sustain back complaints to the point of affecting their play (they showed the tendency to initiate movement with their spine rather than with their hips like their other teammates). Two would sustain ankle injuries because of the heavy pounding of poorly directed forces down their legs. One would sustain a knee injury as they used their knees to break motion rather than their hips. I correctly predicted four out of five (the knee case did not materialize that season). Movement patterns seen with the eye predicted who would become injured. In past years, I would have had the opportunity to spend time with clinicians like Vladamir Janda or Shirley Sarhmann and discuss with them how they 'saw' pathology when people moved and how they would diagnose it to a specific hip or knee, for example. Sure enough upon subsequent examination the knee or hip would reveal itself as faulty. Thus I am convinced skilled clinicians and coaches see the motor disturbances. The corollary is that this knowledge could be used to intervene and reduce the risk. Just a few studies have managed to do this in athletic populations (e.g. Hewett et al. 2005) but it needs to be done in non-athletic populations at risk. There are several studies ongoing where movement and motor patterns have been documented in occupational groups using a longitudinal study design, and so for now we must wait to see who develops painful disorders.

Using a more scientifically rigorous example, and a slightly different experimental paradigm, we conducted a study (McGill et al. 2003) on 76 workers all performing the same two physical jobs. In this group 26 had recurrent back episodes lasting on average a couple of weeks per year, but all were at work and functioning well on the testing day. Those workers who had recurrent painful back attacks differed from their healthy colleagues. When bending to pick up a coin from the floor they did so with more spine flexion and less hip flexion than their healthy colleagues. They had more back strength when tested. It was assumed that this was because they 'overused' their backs when working. Interestingly they had less back extensor muscle endurance. It became clear that while they were stronger, their lack of endurance caused them to 'break good form' when lifting, imposing stresses to their back which lead to tissue irritation. They had stiffer hips, particularly in flexion and internal rotation. Interestingly, their psychosocial markers were present on average, but were less important than those variables considered biomechanical and motor control in nature. Whether these were cause or consequence of their back disorders is open for debate, but it is suggested that they would hinder recovery.

It is now appreciated how important a hip examination is for back pain patients.

18. Every back pain patient should have a movement assessment together with provocative testing as part of an examination

The combination of biomechanics and motor control variables in provocative tests and movement assessment screens are perhaps the most powerful components of an examination to direct treatment of a back pained patient.

Just because a patient has the ability to move a certain way does not mean that they will move in a joint sparing way performing tasks of daily living. We screened 180 students to quantify their squat and lunge mechanics together with their hip and back range of motion (publication pending). Interestingly, there appeared to be little relationship between whether they could move in a joint sparing way versus whether they chose to move in a joint sparing way. Motor control patterns, or patterns of movement that spare joints, appear to be natural in some people and not in others. The implication is that training could be considered to correct the patterns in certain individuals. The clinical questions are: which method would be best to change patterns, and was the assumption correct that changing the patterns would be clinically effective?

Nonetheless, provocative testing as part of an assessment identifies the motions, postures and loads that exacerbate the pain experienced in that individual. It then becomes clear what a patient must avoid to reduce immediate further pain and reduction in the sensitivity to pain over time. The provocative tests also guide the starting level and choice of corrective exercise as that being below the threshold that initiates pain. Finally, some tests have shown to have prognostic value. Chorti et al. (2009) demonstrated that some provocative tests of spine instability (e.g. Hicks et al. 2005), which involve the application of load in specific postures and with different levels of muscle activation, had predictive value for which patient would have a better outcome with a specific approach (in this case stabilization exercise). In contrast, Parks et al. (2003) showed that spine range of motion had little ability to predict who would return to work in an occupational rehabilitation clinic setting. It is hoped that more evaluation of the clinical tests in the future will be conducted as this effort will be well rewarded.

CONCLUSIONS

Back pain patients present with many different patterns. Some are very simple to recognize and the treatment to modify the faulty movement is straightforward to design. Other patients present complex patterns where very thorough assessment and analysis is needed to form hypotheses to guide a course of treatment. With these patients the treatment is continually fine-tuned and forms an experiment in progress. The clinician will be humbled but will have better results as the treatment is progressed with every positive sign of progress. Understanding and manipulating motor control variables that govern movement patterns, and the way the movement is created with muscles, is paramount to success. Big picture thinking is important as is considering the details. Finally, I hope that the scientific/clinical community can work to achieve success in conquering suffering from back pain. The misery of patients who cannot enjoy life because of pain hits me daily. On the other hand, if the problems and issues are solved it will deny others the joy I have had with my colleagues in studying such a fascinating system.

REFERENCES

Adams, M., Bogduk, N., Burton, K., Dolan, P., 2002. The Biomechanics of Back Pain. Churchill Livingston, Edinburgh.

Allison, G.T., Henry, S.M., 2002. The influence of fatigue on trunk muscle responses to sudden arm movements, a pilot study. Clin Biomech 17, 414–417.

Ashmen, K.J., Swanik, C.B., Lephart, S.M., 1996. Strength and flexibility characteristics of athletes with chronic low back pain. J Sport Rehabil 5, 275–286.

Aultman, C.D., Scannell, J., McGill, S.M., 2005. Predicting the direction of nucleus tracking in bovine spine motion segments subjected to repetitive flexion and simultaneous lateral bend. Clin Biomech 20, 126–129.

Brown, S., McGill, S.M., 2008a. How the inherent stiffness of the in-vivo human trunk varies with changing magnitude of muscular activation. Clin Biomech 23, 15–22.

Brown, S., McGill, S.M., 2008b. Co-activation alters the linear versus non-linear impression of the EMG – torque relationship of trunk muscles. J Biomech 41, 491–497.

Brown, S., McGill, S.M., 2008c. An ultrasound investigation into the morphology of the human abdominal wall uncovers complex deformation patterns during contraction. Eur J Appl Physiol 104, 1021–1030.

Brown, S., McGill, S.M., 2009. Transmission of muscularly generated force and stiffness between layers of the rat abdominal wall. Spine 34, E70–E75.

Cairns, M.C., Foster, N.E., Wright, C., 2006. Randomized controlled trial of specific spinal stabilization exercises and controlled physiotherapy for recurrent low back pain. Spine 31, E670–E681.

Callaghan, J.P., McGill, S.M., 2001. Intervertebral disc herniation: studies on a porcine model exposed to highly repetitive flexion/extension motion with compressive force. Clin Biomech 16, 28–37.

Cholewicki, J., Juluru, K., McGill, S.M., 1999. The intra-abdominal pressure mechanism for stabilizing the lumbar spine. J Biomech 32, 13–17.

Cholewicki, J., Greene, H.S., Polzhofer, G.R., Galloway, M.T., Shah, R.A., Radebold, A., 2002. Neuromuscular function in athletes following recovery from a recent acute low back injury. J Orthop Sports Phys Ther 32, 568–575.

Chorti, A.G., Chortis, A.G., Strimpakos, N., McCarthy, C.J., Lamb, S.E., 2009. The prognostic value of symptom responses in the conservative management of spinal pain. Spine 34, 2686–2699.

Fritz, J., Whitman, J.M., Childs, J., 2005. Lumbar spine segmental mobility assessment: an examination of validity for determining intervention strategies in patients with low back pain. Arch Phys Med Rehabil 86, 1745–1752.

Grenier, S.G., McGill, S.M., 2007. Quantification of lumbar stability using two different abdominal activation strategies. Arch Phys Med Rehab 88, 54–62.

Gubler, D., Mannion, A.F., Pulkovski, N., Schenk, P., Gorelick, M., Helbling, D., et al., 2010. Ultrasound tissue Doppler imaging reveals no delay in abdominal muscle feedforward activity during rapid arm movements in patients with chronic low back pain. Spine 35, 1506–1513.

Hewett, T.E., Myer, G.D., Ford, K.R., 2005. Reducing knee and anterior cruciate ligament injuries among female athletes: a systematic review of neuromuscular training interventions. J Knee Surg 18, 82–88

Hicks, G.E., Fritz, J.M., Delitto, A., McGill, S.M., 2005. Preliminary development of a clinical prediction rule for determining which patients with low back pain will respond to a stabilization exercise program. Arch Phys Med Rehab 86, 1753–1762.

Hubley-Kozey, C.L., Vezina, M.J., 2002. Differentiating temporal electromyographic waveforms between those with chronic low back pain and healthy controls. Clin Biomech 17, 621–629.

Janda, V., Frank, C., Liebenson, C., 2007. Evaluation of muscular imbalance. In: Liebenson, C. (Ed.), Rehabilitation of the Spine. Lippincott Williams and Wilkins, Philadelphia.

Kavcic, N., Grenier, S., McGill, S., 2004. Determining the stabilizing role of individual torso muscles during rehabilitation exercises. Spine 29, 1254–1265.

Kolar, P., 2007. Facilitation of agonist-antagonist co-activation by reflex stimulation methods. In: Liebenson, C. (Ed.), Rehabilitation of the Spine. Lippincott Williams and Wilkins, Philadelphia.

Koumantakis, G.A., Watson, P.J., Oldham, J.A., 2005. Trunk muscle stabilization training plus general exercise versus general exercise only: randomized controlled trial of patients with recurrent low back pain. Phys Ther 85, 209–225.

Marshall, L., McGill, S.M., 2010. The role of axial torque/twist in disc herniation. Clin Biomech 25, 6–9.

McGill, S.M., 2007. Low Back Disorders: evidence based prevention and rehabilitation. Human Kinetics Publishers, Champaign Urbana.

McGill, S.M., 2009. Ultimate Back Fitness and Performance, fourth ed. Backfitpro Inc, Waterloo, Canada.

McGill, S.M., Karpowicz, A., 2009. Exercises for spine stabilization: motion/motor patterns, stability progressions and clinical technique. Arch Phys Med Rehab 90, 118–126.

McGill, S.M., Norman, R.W., 1987. An assessment of intra-abdominal pressure as a viable mechanism to reduce spinal compression. Ergonomics 30, 1565–1588.

McGill, S.M., Sharratt, M.T., 1990. The relationship between intra-abdominal pressure and trunk EMG. Clin Biomech 5, 59–67.

McGill, S.M., Grenier, S., Bluhm, M., Preuss, R., Brown, S., Russell, C., 2003. Previous history of LBP with work loss is related to lingering effects in biomechanical physiological, personal, and psychosocial characteristics. Ergonomics 46, 731–746.

McGill, S.M., McDermott, A., Fenwick, C., 2008. Comparison of different strongman events: trunk muscle activation and lumbar spine motion, load and stiffness. J Strength Cond Res 23, 1148–1161

McGill, S.M., Karpowicz, A., Fenwick, C., 2009a. Ballistic abdominal exercises: muscle activation patterns during a punch, baseball throw, and a torso stiffening manoeuvre. J Strength Cond Res 23, 898–905.

McGill, S.M., Karpowicz, A., Fenwick, C., 2009b. Exercises for the torso performed in a standing posture: motion and motor patterns. J Strength Cond Res 23, 455–464.

McGill, S.M., Tampier, C., Yates, J., Marshall, L., 2009c. Motion and load determines the pattern of annulus disruption. In: International Society for Study of the Lumbar Spine Annual Meeting. May, Miami, pp. 4–8.

McGill, S.M., Chaimberg, J.D., Frost, D., Fenwick, C., 2010. The double peak: how elite MMA fighters develop speed and strike force. J Strength Cond Res 24, 348–357.

Nadler, S.F., Malanga, G.A., Feinberg, J.H., Pryicien, M., Stitik, T.P., DePrince, M., 2001. Relationship between hip muscle imbalance and occurence of low back pain in collegiate athletes: a prospective study. Am J Phys Med Rehab 80, 572–577.

Parks, K.A., Crichton, K.S., Goldford, R.J., McGill, S.M., 2003. On the validity of ratings of impairment for low back disorders. Spine 28, 380–384.

Parry, C.B.W., 1984. Vicarious motions. In: Basmajian, J. (Ed.), Therapeutic Exercise, fourth ed. Williams and Wilkins, Baltimore.

Santana, J.C., Vera-Garcia, F.J., McGill, S.M., 2007. A kinetic and electro-myographic comparison of standing cable press and bench press. J Strength Cond Res 21, 1271–1279.

Silfies, S.P., Mehta, R., Smith, S.S., Kerduna, A.R., 2009. Differences in feedforward trunk muscle activity in subgroups of patients with mechanical low back pain, Arch Phys Med Rehab 90, 1159–1169.

Tampier, C., Drake, J., Callaghan, J., McGill, S.M., 2007. Progressive disc herniation: an investigation of the mechanism using radiologic, histochemical and microscopic dissection techniques. Spine 32, 2869–2874.

Vera-Garcia, F., Elvira, J.L.L., Brown, S.H.M., McGill, S.M., 2007. Effects of abdominal stabilization manoeuvres on the control of spine motion and stability against sudden trunk loading perturbations. J EMG Kines 17, 556–567.

Wang, S., McGill, S.M., 2008. Links between the mechanics of ventilation and spine stability. J Appl Biomech 24, 166–174.

| 8 |

The kinesiopathological model and mechanical low back pain

Linda R. Van Dillen*, Shirley A. Sahrmann† and Barbara J. Norton‡
*Program in Physical Therapy and Department of Orthopaedic Surgery, †Program in Physical Therapy, Department of Cell Biology and Physiology, Department of Neurology and Neurophysiology and ‡Program in Physical Therapy and Department of Neurology, Washington University School of Medicine at Washington University Medical Center, St Louis, Missouri, USA

Characteristic patterns of movements and alignments can be recognized in many musculoskeletal pain conditions, including mechanical low back pain (LBP). In some instances the patterns displayed by patients can be linked to a specific pathology, disease or injury. There are, however, several musculoskeletal pain conditions in which a specific causal link cannot be identified. A key question in all instances is whether the movements and alignments displayed by the person with musculoskeletal pain are a consequence of the condition or contribute to the development of the condition. One potential answer to this question may be found in the kinesiopathological model (Sahrmann 2002). A basic premise of the kinesiopathological model is that continual repetition of specific movements and alignments which are requisite to performing daily activities can lead to the development of musculoskeletal pain conditions (Fig. 8.1). The purposes of this chapter are to: (i) describe the kinesiopathological model; (ii) describe the application of the model to LBP; and (iii) review the findings from studies that have been conducted to test assumptions of the model in patients with LBP.

THE KINESIOPATHOLOGICAL MODEL

The kinesiopathological model, hereinafter referred to as the Model, describes a process that is proposed to contribute to the development, as well as the course, of many musculoskeletal pain conditions, including mechanical LBP. The process begins with repetition of a daily activity associated with specific movements or specific alignments. The repetitions are proposed to lead to adaptations in the musculoskeletal and neural systems, for example, changes in muscle strength, flexibility, stiffness, timing and level of muscle activity, to name just a few. Although such adaptations often may be beneficial, continual repetition of specific movements and alignments may be increasingly detrimental because the associated adaptations contribute to imbalances about the joint(s). For example, repeated trunk rotation to the right to reach for the phone (a trunk rotation activity) could cause the muscles that contribute to right trunk rotation to become shorter and stronger while the muscles that contribute to left trunk rotation to become longer and weaker. With continued repetition, the adaptations would result in alterations in the joint motions (accessory and physiological) and in joint alignments. The alterations due to repeated performance of trunk rotation to the right, in turn, lead to alterations in the motions and alignments associated with many other daily activities, i.e. patterns of altered movements and alignments. The repetition of altered patterns of movements and alignments are proposed to result in localized regions of tissue stress, symptoms and, eventually, tissue injury (Adams 2004). According to the Model, the deleterious process can be

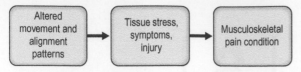

Figure 8.1 Sequence of events proposed for movements and alignments to contribute to development of musculoskeletal pain conditions according to the kinesiopathological model (Sahrmann 2002).

slowed by maintaining optimal joint mechanics. Optimal joint mechanics can be maintained by minimizing the repetition of the same movements and alignments with daily activities, moving joints throughout the ranges of all available motions, and assuming a variety of positions throughout the day.

THE KINESIOPATHOLOGICAL MODEL AND LOW BACK PAIN

The specific alteration proposed to contribute to LBP is the tendency for one or more lumbar joints to move *more readily* than adjacent joints, for example, other lumbar joints, the hip joints or thoracic joints. The tendency to move more readily occurs each time the person performs his or her daily activities. In this context, the definition of 'more readily' is movement that occurs sooner or proceeds farther than is ideal. As the daily activities are performed repeatedly throughout the day and some joints are moving more readily than others, some or all of the lumbar joints become *relatively more flexible* than other joints. Typically, the lumbar joints become more flexible in a *specific direction(s)*, for example, flexion, extension, rotation or some combination thereof. In such cases, the lumbar joint(s) are said to display a directional tendency (DT). Although the DT is presumed to develop over time primarily as the result of adaptations in the musculoskeletal and neural systems related to repeated movements and sustained postures, personal characteristics, such as, sex, activity level, anthropometrics and genetics, are considered to modify the rate and nature of the adaptations. The DT a person adopts is evidenced in specific patterns of altered movement and alignment used across multiple daily activities. The use of a specific pattern results in decreased variability in the types of lumbar joint movements and alignments used across the day. The reduction in variability then is considered to predispose a person to the development, or persistence and recurrence of LBP. Specifically, the exposure of spinal tissue to repeated low magnitude loading in the *same direction across a day* is proposed to contribute to the accumulation of tissue stress. Stresses on the tissue can contribute to symptoms, microtrauma and, potentially, macrotrauma. This set of events is considered

likely because repeated use of the patterns may allow minimal time for normal tissue adaptation to the stresses to occur. The Model further maintains that until the variables contributing to the use of the movement and alignment patterns are modified, the LBP has the potential to persist or recur. Figure 8.2 is a representation of the processes proposed to contribute to the development and course of LBP based on the Model.

Low back pain subgroups

The assumption that people with LBP display direction-specific movement and alignment patterns that contribute to their LBP suggests that there are different subgroups of people with LBP. The subgroups would differ based on the DT they display with activities. A standardized examination to identify the movement and alignment patterns associated with a DT, as well as related symptoms, has been developed; various measurement properties of the examination have been tested (Van Dillen et al. 1998; Luomajoki et al. 2007). The LBP subgroup labels are based on the lumbar region DT that is: (i) identified most consistently across items in the examination; and (ii) associated with the person's symptoms. The proposed subgroups are lumbar: (i) flexion; (ii) extension; (iii) rotation; (iv) rotation with flexion; and (v) rotation with extension. Identification of subgroups based on the DT and related symptoms has been pursued in an effort to identify more homogeneous groups of people with LBP to examine in studies of mechanisms contributing to LBP conditions and for the development of treatment programmes.

STUDIES OF SELECT ASPECTS OF THE KINESIOPATHOLOGICAL MODEL

Various studies have been conducted to examine aspects of the Model in people with LBP. One group of studies has used standardized clinical tests (Van Dillen et al. 1998; Luomajoki et al. 2007), designed to identify the pattern of movement, alignment (Henry et al. 2012) and symptoms that characterizes a person's relevant lumbar directional tendency. These studies have focused on whether there are subgroups of people with LBP based on symptoms and the DT identified with clinical tests (Van Dillen et al. 2003b; Trudelle-Jackson et al. 2008; Harris-Hayes et al. 2009), if the subgroups differ from people without LBP (Luomajoki et al. 2008), and the relationship of select test findings to symptom report (Van Dillen et al. 2001, 2009), sex (Scholtes and Van Dillen 2007), activity type (Van Dillen et al. 2003a, 2006), severity of the LBP condition (De Vito et al. 2007) and injury risk (Roussel et al. 2009). A second group of studies has used laboratory instrumentation to quantify the patterns of movement and alignment with clinical tests to examine

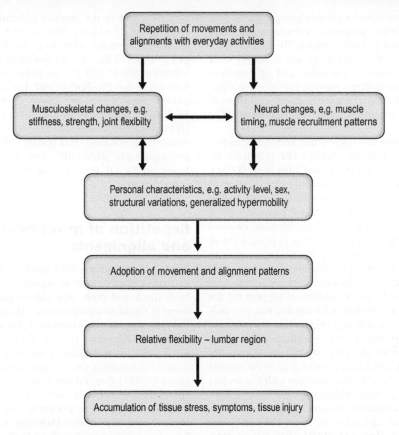

Figure 8.2 Details of the processes proposed for the development and course of low back pain based on the kinesiopathological model.

differences among LBP subgroups (Gombatto et al. 2007; Van Dillen et al. 2007), differences between people with LBP and people without LBP (Norton et al. 2004; Porter et al. 2009; Scholtes et al. 2009), sex differences (Gombatto et al. 2006) and mechanisms underlying clinical test findings (Gombatto et al. 2008b, 2009). In the following sections we describe findings from a subset of these studies that examine some of the major assumptions of the Model as applied to LBP. The studies examine whether: (i) people with LBP can be subgrouped based on movement and alignment patterns that reflect a specific DT; (ii) the DT identified with clinical tests is related to the types of repetitive movements that a person participates in regularly; and (iii) the DT a person displays is related to musculoskeletal, neural or personal factors or some interaction of these factors.

Movement and alignment patterns

One assumption of the Model is that people with LBP display movement and alignment patterns that reflect their DT and the patterns are used across a variety of activities.

In addition, it is assumed that there are different subgroups of people with LBP who differ based on the specific DT that characterizes their LBP condition. We tested this assumption by examining 188 people with LBP (72% chronic (Spitzer et al. 1987)) using a standardized examination that included clinical tests of movement and alignment performed in different positions (Van Dillen et al. 1998, 2003a). Each test is proposed to assess one of the following directional tendencies: flexion, extension, rotation, or a combination of rotation with flexion or rotation with extension. We predicted that a person would demonstrate positive findings across tests that assess a specific DT, for example, lumbar flexion. We also predicted that a person would demonstrate negative findings across tests that assess other directional tendencies. Thus, there would be groupings of tests that would represent different DTs that characterize different LBP subgroups. To test the prediction, a statistical technique referred to as factor analysis (Nunally and Bernstein 1994) was applied to two different random samples from the examination data. Factor analysis provides groupings of inter-correlated tests referred to as factors. We predicted that the factors retained from the two separate analyses would represent groups of tests consistent with the different proposed LBP subgroups. Three factors were identified in both samples. The factors represented groups of tests that were proposed to capture a DT for lumbar (i) extension, (ii) rotation and (iii) rotation with extension. These findings provide evidence that clinical test findings correlate in ways consistent with three of the proposed LBP subgroups, and the subgroups differ based on their DT.

To examine whether the clinical test findings from this data set were relevant to the person's LBP condition we conducted a secondary analysis (Van Dillen et al. 2003a). Typically, each clinical test that results in an increase in symptoms is immediately followed by a second test in which symptoms are monitored while the person's DT is systematically modified. The typical modification involves either (i) positioning the lumbar region in neutral (or as close as possible) or (ii) restricting the timing or amount of lumbar joint(s) movement while movement in other joints is encouraged. An improvement in symptoms with the second test would provide additional support for the importance of the DT observed with the first test. For each clinical test in which people reported an increase in symptoms, we analyzed symptom responses during the second test. We found that for the majority of tests (86%), the majority of people (76%±15%) reported an improvement in symptoms when their DT was modified with the second test. Similar findings with additional clinical tests have been reported in a sample that included larger proportions of people with acute and subacute LBP (42%) than our original study (Van Dillen et al. 2009). These data suggest that the DT displayed during clinical tests is related to a person's LBP symptoms and systematically changing the DT with performance of the tests improves symptoms.

We also tested the assumption that people with LBP display movement and alignment patterns that reflect their DT by comparing people in different LBP subgroups ($N=100$; 72% chronic) to each other, and to people without LBP (NoLBP; $N=60$) (Norton et al. 2004). The people with LBP were assigned to a subgroup based on their DT identified across clinical tests (Van Dillen et al. 2003b; Trudelle-Jackson et al. 2008). The subgroups examined were rotation with extension (RotExt; $N=62$), rotation with flexion (RotFlex; $N=18$) and extension (Ext; $N=20$). Because a person's DT can be reflected in his or her alignment we measured lumbar region alignment in standing. We predicted that: (i) the RotExt subgroup would stand in more lumbar extension than the NoLBP group and the RotFlex subgroup; and (ii) the RotExt and Ext subgroup would stand in the same amount of lumbar extension. To test these predictions we used a non-invasive, electromechanical digitizer and trigonometric method (Youdas et al. 1995) to quantify the lumbar curvature angle in the sagittal plane. All people were measured while maintaining a comfortable standing position. When the NoLBP group was compared to all LBP subjects there were

no differences in the amount of lumbar curvature angle (NoLBP: $40.2°±14.8°$; LBP: $42.5°±15.2°$). The RotExt subgroup, however, displayed more lumbar extension ($46.7°±14.7°$) than the (i) NoLBP group and (ii) RotFlex subgroup ($38.2°±14.1°$). In addition, the lumbar curvature angle for the RotExt and Ext ($43.4°±16.2°$) subgroups were the same. These data demonstrate that predictable differences in alignment could be identified: (i) between people with and people without LBP when the comparison was made to a specific LBP subgroup; and (ii) among people with LBP when they were subgrouped based on the DT with clinical tests from a standardized examination.

Repetition of movements and alignments

A second assumption of the Model is that a specific DT is, in part, a consequence of repetition of: (i) movements, both trunk and limb, that induce lumbar region movement in the same direction and (ii) sustained positions in the same direction. We examined this assumption by comparing an LBP group ($N=50$; chronic or recurrent (Von Korff 1994)) that regularly participated in sports that put rotational demands on the trunk and hips and a NoLBP group ($N=41$) that did not participate in rotation-related sports. Kinematics were captured during two active lower limb movement tests performed in prone, hip lateral rotation and knee flexion (Scholtes et al. 2009). We have found in prior work that these limb movement tests are often symptom-provoking in people with LBP (Van Dillen et al. 2001). The limb movements were also thought to be those that were frequently used during the sports activities and, thus, might impact the lumbopelvic region. Because people with LBP are thought to move the lumbar region more readily than people without LBP we predicted that the LBP group would display earlier lumbopelvic motion with each limb movement test than the NoLBP group. We indexed the person's DT by calculating the difference in time between the start of limb movement and the start of lumbopelvic rotation normalized to the limb movement time. We also measured subject characteristics, LBP history, sports participation and activity levels (Baecke et al. 1982). We found that the two groups were the same except for three of the kinematic variables. The groups displayed equal hip rotation (LBP: $44.28°±6.38°$; NoLBP: $41.59°±6.62°$), however, the LBP group had slightly less knee flexion ($114.28°±8.60°$) than the NoLBP group ($119.95°±9.31°$). As predicted, for both tests the LBP group rotated the lumbopelvic region earlier during the limb movement than the NoLBP group (Fig. 8.3A). Interestingly, the LBP group also had a greater magnitude of end-range lumbopelvic rotation than the NoLBP group with both limb movement tests (Fig. 8.3B). In addition, when the early lumbopelvic rotation was modified during

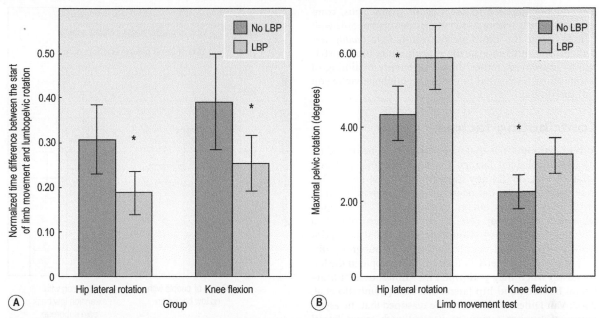

Figure 8.3 (A) Mean and 95% confidence intervals of ratios of the difference in time between the start of lumbopelvic rotation and the start of the limb movement normalized to the limb movement time for people with LBP and people without LBP. The ratios are provided for both groups for lumbopelvic rotation during two tests performed in prone, hip lateral rotation and knee flexion. The smaller the ratio the sooner the lumbopelvic region begins to move during the limb movement. The asterisk indicates a significant difference between the two groups. People with LBP rotate the lumbopelvic region earlier with both lower limb tests. (B) Mean and 95% confidence intervals of the maximal lumbopelvic rotation for people with LBP and people without LBP with two limb movement tests performed in prone, hip lateral rotation and knee flexion. The asterisk indicates a significant difference between the two groups. *(A) and (B) adapted from Scholtes, S.A., Gombatto, S.P., Van Dillen, L.R., 2009. Differences in lumbopelvic motion between people with and people without low back pain during two lower limb movement tests.* Clinical Biomechanics 24, 7, with permission from Elsevier.

the symptom-provoking limb movement tests, the majority of people reported an improvement in their symptoms with the tests (hip rotation: 93%; knee flexion: 88%). These findings support the idea that the DT displayed by a person with LBP is related to the types of trunk and limb movements the person performs on a regular basis and to the person's LBP symptoms. We identified a similar relationship between types of repetitive movements people participated in and the DT displayed with trunk and limb clinical tests in people with LBP who regularly performed two different types of leisure time activities; symmetrical activities and asymmetrical activities (Van Dillen et al. 2006).

An additional comparison was made between two groups who both participated in rotation-related sports; an LBP group (N=50) and a NoLBP group (N=25) (Porter et al. 2013). The same two normalized movement variables were measured as in the previously described study. We found that the kinematic variable to index a person's DT, the time between the start of the limb movement and the start of lumbopelvic rotation, was the same for both groups (hip rotation: LBP: 0.21±0.18, NoLBP: 0.20±0.13;

knee flexion: LBP: 0.25±0.21, NoLBP: 0.29±0.18). The two groups were also the same with regard to all other variables except their activity levels. Sport activity levels from the Baecke Habitual Activity Questionnaire (Baecke et al. 1982) were the same between the two groups (LBP: 3.68±0.55; NoLBP: 3.55±0.61). However, people with LBP reported a lower daily activity level (average work + leisure scores; 2.33±0.30) than people without LBP (2.65±0.54). These findings suggest two ideas. First, the activity a person participates in regularly appears to contribute to movement patterns related to the activity. Second, the imbalance between routine daily activities and higher intensity activities may be an important factor that interacts with a person's DT to contribute to an LBP condition. Interestingly, in the same cohort of subjects a preliminary analysis of a different clinical movement test, rocking backward from a quadruped position, demonstrated that the LBP group and the NoLBP group do not display the exact same lumbar region movement pattern across the test movement (Meroni et al. 2009). In the preliminary analysis, the LBP group displayed a greater magnitude of lumbopelvic movement *late* in the test movement compared to the NoLBP group. Thus, compared to people without LBP, the tendency of people with LBP to move the lumbopelvic region *more readily* was evident as a difference in the magnitude of lumbopelvic region movement rather than a difference in timing of initiation of movement between the lumbopelvic region and the limbs.

Contributing factors

A third assumption is that a person's DT can be related to: (i) musculoskeletal factors; (ii) neural factors; (iii) personal factors; or (iv) any interaction of these factors. We examined the potential relationship of a musculoskeletal factor, passive elastic energy, to a person's DT by comparing a RotExt subgroup (*N*=22; chronic or recurrent) to a NoLBP group (*N*=19) (Gombatto et al. 2008b). In prior work we found that people in the RotExt subgroup displayed more asymmetry in their DT than people in the Rot subgroup when they performed the clinical tests of trunk lateral bending and hip lateral rotation (Gombatto et al. 2007; Van Dillen et al. 2007). We reasoned that the asymmetry of lumbar region movement with trunk lateral bending could be, in part, a reflection of the passive resistance of structures in the trunk encountered across the trunk movement. Based on our prior study findings, we predicted that with trunk lateral bending the RotExt subgroup would be more asymmetrical in passive elastic energy of the trunk than a NoLBP group. A passive movement device, a motion capture system and surface electromyography (Gombatto et al. 2008a) were used to capture data to examine our prediction about lumbar region passive elastic energy. The instrumentation provided position and force data during passive trunk lateral bending on a friction-free surface. Trunk muscle activity was monitored during the trunk movement to assure that the movement was passive (Scannell and McGill 2003). The groups were the same with regard to subject characteristics, activity levels and end range of trunk lateral bending motion. The two groups were also no different in their total passive elastic energy (NoLBP: 103.55±10.46 Nmdeg; RotExt: 103.91±9.73 Nmdeg). The RotExt subgroup, however, displayed a greater difference in passive elastic energy between sides than the NoLBP group (Fig. 8.4). These data suggest that the LBP and NoLBP groups maintain the same overall level of passive tissue characteristics of the trunk in the frontal plane but, as predicted, the RotExt subgroup displays more asymmetry in these characteristics than the NoLBP group.

We also have examined the potential relationship between sex and a person's DT. Because men differ from women structurally and physiologically (Chow et al. 2000; Toft et al. 2003), it would follow that men may differ from women in their movement patterns. We have tested this relationship with select clinical movement tests (Scholtes and Van Dillen 2007; Van Dillen et al. 2007) as

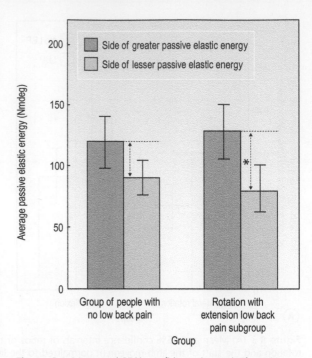

Figure 8.4 Mean and 95% confidence interval of passive elastic energy with each direction of trunk lateral bending for people in the Rotation with Extension LBP subgroup compared to people with no LBP. The side of greater elastic energy was compared to the side of lesser passive elastic energy for each group. The total passive elastic energy was the same between groups. The asterisk indicates a greater difference in passive elastic energy between sides, i.e. more asymmetry, in the Rotation with Extension subgroup when compared to the people with no LBP. *Reproduced from Gombatto, S.P., Norton, B.J., Scholtes, S.A., Van Dillen, L.R., 2008. Differences in symmetry of lumbar region passive tissue characteristics between people with and people without low back pain.* Clinical Biomechanics *23, 986, with permission from Elsevier.*

well as with instrumented measures of alignment (Norton et al. 2004). We first examined this relationship by comparing men (*N*=27) and women (*N*=19) with LBP in our cohort of people who participated in rotation-related sports (Gombatto et al. 2006). Kinematic data and LBP symptoms were recorded during the clinical test of active hip lateral rotation. We examined hip lateral rotation because there are data to suggest that men display more active and passive stiffness of the lower limbs than women (Gajdosik et al. 1990; Granata et al. 2002; Blackburn et al. 2004; Staron et al. 2000). We reasoned that if men have more lower limb stiffness than women, men may move the lumbar region more readily than women. To index the DT with hip lateral rotation we quantified the range of available lumbopelvic rotation used across the

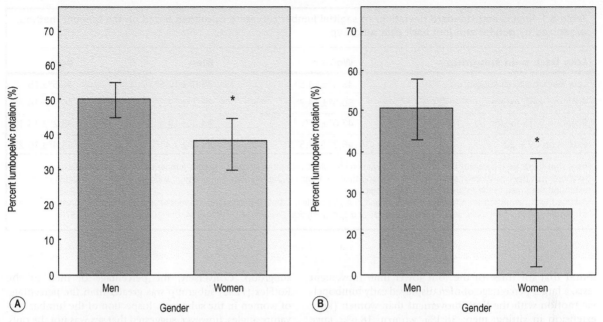

Figure 8.5 (A) Mean and standard deviation for the percent of lumbopelvic rotation motion attained at 60% of the maximum hip lateral rotation motion for men and women with LBP. The asterisk indicates that the men used more of their available lumbopelvic rotation than women at the 60% point of the hip lateral rotation motion. (B) Mean and standard deviation for the percent of lumbopelvic rotation motion attained at 60% of the maximum hip lateral rotation motion for men and women who reported an increase in LBP symptoms with the test movement. The asterisk indicates that the men used more of their available lumbopelvic rotation than women at the 60% point of the hip lateral rotation motion. *(A) and (B) reproduced from Gombatto, S.P., Collins, D.R., Sahrmann, S.A., Engsberg, J.R., Van Dillen, L.R., 2006. Gender differences in pattern of hip and lumbopelvic rotation in people with low back pain. Clinical Biomechanics 21, 263, with permission from Elsevier.*

range of the hip movement. Specifically, we calculated the percentage of maximum lumbopelvic rotation attained at increments of maximum hip lateral rotation. We predicted that the men with LBP would use a greater percentage of their total lumbopelvic motion in the *early* part of the limb movement than the women with LBP. Men and women were equal with regard to all subject characteristics except weight and LBP history. Compared to women, men were heavier (difference: 18.8±3.0 kg) and had a longer history of LBP (men: 8.1±6.2 years; women: 3.5±3.0 years). Men and women displayed the same amount of active hip lateral rotation (men: 44.7°±7.1°; women: 42.7°±5.2°) and lumbopelvic rotation (men: 6.1°±3.2°; women: 4.6°±2.0°). Men, however, completed more of their available lumbopelvic rotation in the *early* part of the hip rotation motion than women (Fig. 8.5A). When we examined only the people who specifically reported an increase in symptoms with the hip rotation test, the sex differences were even greater (Fig. 8.5B). Finally, a greater percentage of men (70.4%) reported an increase in symptoms with the hip rotation test than women (36.8%). This was the case even though baseline LBP symptom ratings between men and women were the same (verbal numeric pain

rating scale (0–10) (Jensen et al. 1986): men: 2.9°±1.4°; women: 3.9°±1.7°). These data suggest that men with LBP may have more of a tendency to move the lumbopelvic region early in a limb movement than women with LBP, and the lumbopelvic movement with the hip movement may be more likely to be associated with symptoms in men with LBP than women with LBP.

A second examination of the relationship between sex and a person's DT was based on a secondary analysis of a subset of clinical test responses obtained from the people with LBP in our factor analysis study described previously (Van Dillen et al. 2003b; Scholtes and Van Dillen 2007). The goal was to examine if the sex differences in kinematics we identified with the hip lateral rotation test would be generalized to other lower limb movement tests in a larger, more heterogeneous sample of people with LBP. The sample included 170 people with LBP (84 men, 86 women) who had participated in our standardized examination. Based on our prior study (Gombatto et al. 2006) we predicted that with each of the tests more men would display early lumbopelvic movement during the lower limb movement test than women. Men and women were the same with regard to all subject characteristics. We

Table 8.1 Means and standard deviations of sagittal lumbar curvature calculated based on the tangent method, organized by gender and low back pain subgroup.

Low back pain subgroup	Women	Men	Both
Low back pain (all subgroups)	48.8°±14.5°	35.0°±12.5°	42.5°±15.2°
Rotation with extension (N = 62)	50.5°±14.7°	39.7°±12.3°	46.7°±14.7°
Rotation with flexion (N = 18)	47.0°±9.7°	34.9°±14.4°	38.2°±14.1°
Extension (N = 20)	46.2°±17.5°	35.0°±7.4°	43.4°±16.2°

Note that there are differences between men and women consistent with other studies of sagittal lumbar curvature using surface measurement devices. Women stand in more extension than men. Men in the rotation with extension subgroup, however, stand in more extension than men in the rotation with flexion subgroup.
Adapted with permission from Norton, B.J., Sahrmann, S.A., Van Dillen, L.R., 2004. Differences in measurements of lumbar curvature related to gender and low back pain, *Journal of Orthopaedic and Sports Physical Therapy* 34 (9), 524–534. doi: 10.2519/jospt.2004.1570.

found that for three of the four lower limb movement tests, a larger percentage of men displayed early lumbopelvic motion with the limb movement than women (knee extension in sitting: men: 38.1%, women: 18.6%; knee flexion in prone: men: 45.2%, women: 19.8%; hip lateral rotation in prone: men: 66.3%, women: 32.6%). To examine the effect of symptoms on responses during a test we also analyzed the data from the subset of people who reported an increase in symptoms with a test. The findings were the same as for the group as a whole (knee extension in sitting: men: 58.1%, women: 26.9%; knee flexion in prone: men: 63.2%, women: 32.0%; hip lateral rotation in prone: men: 76.2%, women: 43.2%). These data provide additional support for the idea that sex may be a factor that contributes to lumbopelvic movement patterns, and that men may be more likely than women to display early lumbopelvic movement with lower limb movements. In addition, these data suggest that the early lumbopelvic movement during a test movement is present even when symptoms are reproduced during the test.

The relationship between sex and a person's DT was also examined in our previously described study using the electromechanical device to measure lumbar alignment in standing (Norton et al. 2004). Earlier studies based on non-invasive measures of sagittal plane spinal alignment have documented that women stand in more lumbar extension than men (Bergenudd et al. 1989; Youdas et al. 2000). Given these prior findings we wanted to know whether the differences in lumbar region alignment we identified among the different LBP subgroups were solely the result of differences in the distribution of men and women in the various subgroups. We predicted that differences in lumbar curvature angle among LBP subgroups would be related to sex. Overall, we found that there was a relationship between sex and LBP subgroup. The percentage of women in the RotExt (65%) and Ext (75%) subgroups was greater than the percentage of men in each

subgroup. Conversely, the percentage of men in the RotFlex (72%) subgroup was greater than the percentage of women in the subgroup. Inspection of the lumbar curvature angles, however, suggested that sex was not the only determinant of LBP subgroup (Table 8.1). We found that men and women in the RotExt subgroup were more extended than their counterparts in the RotFlex subgroup, but that men were not as extended as the women in either subgroup. On the other hand, women in the RotFlex subgroup were not as extended as women in the RotExt subgroup, but were more extended than men in either subgroup. These findings suggest that sex is not the sole determinant of a person's DT as reflected in lumbar region alignment. Sex along with other variables, for example, activity level or occupation, may modify the DT a person displays and, thus, the type of LBP condition he or she presents with.

SUMMARY

The processes described in the kinesiopathological model provide a potential explanation for the role of repetition of movements and alignments during everyday activities in the development and course of an LBP condition. Based on the Model a primary control issue considered to contribute to LBP is the tendency for one or more of the lumbar joints to move *more readily* than other joints. This tendency to move more readily is typically associated with a specific direction(s) such as flexion, extension, rotation or some combination, i.e. a directional tendency. The directional tendency is evidenced by an altered timing or magnitude of movement of one or more lumbar joints with performance of trunk or limb movements or when assuming positions. Recent studies provide initial support for three of the major assumptions of the Model. First, people with LBP display a tendency to move one or more of the lumbar joints more readily than other joints across a variety of movements and positions, and the directional tendency displayed assists in identifying subgroups of people with LBP. Second, the types of repetitive movements a person participates in regularly appear to be related to a person's directional tendency. Third, a person's directional tendency is related to select musculoskeletal and personal factors and the interaction of these factors. Additionally, the findings across studies suggest that the directional tendency a person displays is related to a person's LBP symptoms. Finally, the Model is intended to provide a framework for the role of potential physical and personal factors to a LBP condition. The Model does not account for other factors, for example, psychosocial variables, known to influence the presentation and course of an LBP condition.

ACKNOWLEDGEMENTS

The authors wish to thank Sara P. Gombatto PT, PhD and Sara S. Scholtes, DPT, PhD for their contributions to many of the studies described, and to Kate Baxter for assistance with adapting figures and tables for the text.

REFERENCES

Adams, M.A., 2004. Biomechanics of back pain. Acupuncture Med 22, 178–188.

Baecke, J.A., Burema, J., Frijters, J.E., 1982. A short questionnaire for the measurement of habitual physical activity in epidemiological studies. Am J Clin Nutr 36, 936–942.

Bergenudd, H., Nilsson, B., Uden, A., Willner, S., 1989. Bone mineral content, gender, body posture, and build in relation to back pain in middle age. Spine 14, 577–579.

Blackburn, J.T., Riemann, B.L., Padua, D.A., Guskiewicz, K.M., 2004. Sex comparison of extensibility, passive, and active stiffness of the knee flexors. Clin Biomech 19, 36–43.

Chow, R.S., Medri, M.K., Martin, D.C., Leekam, R.N., Agur, A.M., McKee, N.H., 2000. Sonographic studies of human soleus and gastrocnemius muscle architecture: Gender variability. Eur J Appl Physiol 82, 236–244.

De Vito, G., Meroni, R., Lanzarini, C., Barindelli, G., Della Morte, G.C., Valagussa, G., 2007. Pelvic rotation and low back pain. In: 6th Interdisciplinary World Congress on Low Back and Pelvic Pain. Barcelona, Spain, pp. 294.

Gajdosik, R.L., Giuliani, C.A., Bohannon, R.W., 1990. Passive compliance and length of the hamstring muscles of healthy men and women. Clin Biomech 5, 23–29.

Gombatto, S.P., Collins, D.R., Sahrmann, S.A., Engsberg, J.R., Van Dillen, L.R., 2006. Gender differences in pattern of hip and lumbopelvic rotation in people with low back pain. Clin Biomech 21, 263–271.

Gombatto, S.P., Collins, D.R., Engsberg, J.R., Sahrmann, S.A., Van Dillen, L.R., 2007. Patterns of lumbar region movement during trunk lateral bending in two different subgroups of people with low back pain. Phys Ther 87, 441–454.

Gombatto, S.P., Klaesner, J.W., Norton, B.J., Minor, S.D., Van Dillen, L.R., 2008a. Validity and reliability of a system to measure passive tissue characteristics of the lumbar region during trunk lateral bending in people with and people without low back pain. J Rehabil Res Dev 45, 1415–1429.

Gombatto, S.P., Norton, B.J., Scholtes, S.A., Van Dillen, L.R., 2008b. Differences in symmetry of lumbar region passive tissue characteristics between people with and people without low back pain. Clin Biomech 23, 986–995.

Gombatto, S.P., Norton, B.J., Sahrman, S.A., Strube, M.J., Van Dillen, L.R., 2009. Factors predicting lumbar region passive elastic energy in people with and people without low back pain. J Orthop Sports Phys Ther 39, A92.

Granata, K.P., Wilson, S.E., Padua, D.A., 2002. Gender differences in active musculoskeletal stiffness. Part I. Quantification in controlled measurements of knee joint dynamics. J Electromyogr Kinesiol 12, 119–126.

Harris-Hayes, M., Van Dillen, L.R., 2009. Inter-tester reliability of physical therapists classifying low back pain problems based on the movement system impairment classification system. Phys Med Rehabil 1, 117–126.

Henry, S.M., Van Dillen, L.R.., Trombley, A.L.., Dee, J.M., Bunn, J.Y., 2012. Reliability of novice raters in using the movement system impairment approach to classify people with low back pain. Manual Therapy http://dx.doi.org/10.1016/j.math.2012.06.008.

Jensen, M.P., Karoly, P., Braver, S., 1986. The measurement of clinical pain intensity: a comparison of six methods. Pain 27, 117–126.

Luomajoki, H., Kool, J., de Bruin, E., Airaksinen, O., 2007. Reliability of movement control tests in the lumbar spine. BMC Muscoskel Disord 8, 90–101.

Luomajoki, H., Kool, J., de Bruin, E.D., Airaksinen, O., 2008. Movement control tests of the low back; evaluation of the difference between patients with low back pain and healthy controls. BMC Muscoskel Disord 9, 170–181.

Meroni, R., DeVito, G., Sahrman, S.A., Van Dillen, L.R., 2009. Lumbopelvic motion with rocking back in quadriped: a comparison of three different populations. J Orthop Sports Phys Ther 39, A83.

Norton, B.J., Sahrmann, S.A., Van Dillen, L.R., 2004. Differences in measurements of lumbar curvature related to gender and low back pain. J Orthop Sports Phys Ther 34, 524–534.

Nunally, J.C., Bernstein, I.H., 1994. Factor analysis I: The general model and variance condensation. In: Vaicunas, J., Bslser, J.R. (Ed.), Psychometric Theory, third ed. McGraw-Hill, New York, pp. 447–490.

Porter, R.L., Scholtes, S.A., Van Dillen, L.R., 2013. Activity level and movement patterns in people with and people without chronic or recurrent low back pain who participate in rotation-related sports. Journal of Sport Rehabilitation in press.

Roussel, N., Nijs, J., Truijen, S., Mottram, S., Van Moorsel, A., Stassijns, G., 2009. Altered lumbo-pelvic movement control but not generalized joint hypermobility is associated with increased injury in dancers: a prospective study. Man Ther 14, 630–635.

Sahrmann, S.A., 2002. Diagnosis and Treatment of Movement Impairment Syndromes, first ed. Mosby, St Louis, MO.

Scannell, J.P., McGill, S.M., 2003. Lumbar posture – should it, and can it, be modified? A study of passive tissue stiffness and lumbar position during activities of daily living. Phys Ther 83, 907–917.

Scholtes, S.A., Van Dillen, L.R., 2007. Gender-related differences in prevalence of lumbopelvic region movement impairments in people with low back pain. J Orthop Sports Phys Ther 37, 744–753.

Scholtes, S.A., Gombatto, S.P., Van Dillen, L.R., 2009. Differences between people with and people without low back pain in lumbopelvic motion during two lower limb movement tests. Clin Biomech 24, 7–12.

Spitzer, W.O., LeBlanc, F.E., Dupuis, M., 1987. Scientific approach to the assessment and management of activity related spinal disorders: a monograph for clinicians. Report of the Quebec Task Force on Spinal Disorders. Spine 12, S1–S59.

Staron, R.S., Hagerman, F.C., Hikida, R.S., Murray, T.F., Hostler, D.P., Crill, M.T., 2000. Fiber type composition of the vastus lateralis muscle of young men and women. J Histochem Cytochem 48, 623–629.

Toft, I., Lindal, S., Bonaa, K.H., Jenssen, T., 2003. Quantitative measurement of muscle fiber composition in a normal population. Muscle Nerve 28, 101–108.

Trudelle-Jackson, E., Sarvaiya-Shah, S.A., Wang, S.S., 2008. Interrater reliability of a movement impairment-based classification system for lumbar spine syndromes in patients with chronic low back pain 1. J Orthop Sports Phys Ther 38, 371–376.

Van Dillen, L.R., Sahrmann, S.A., Norton, B.J., Caldwell, C.A., Fleming, D., McDonnell, M.K., et al., 1998. Reliability of physical examination items used for classification of patients with low back pain. Phys Ther 78, 979–988.

Van Dillen, L.R., Sahrmann, S.A., Norton, B.J., McDonnell, M.K., Caldwell, C.A., Bloom, N.J., et al., 2001. Effect of active limb movements on symptoms in patients with low back pain. J Orthop Sports Phys Ther 31, 402–413.

Van Dillen, L.R., Sahrmann, S.A., Norton, B.J., Caldwell, C.A., McDonnell, M.K., Bloom, N., 2003a. The effect of modifying patient-preferred spinal movement and alignment during symptom testing in patients with low back pain: a preliminary report. Arch Phys Med Rehabil 84, 313–322.

Van Dillen, L.R., Sahrmann, S.A., Norton, B.J., Caldwell, C.A., McDonnell, M.K., Bloom, N.J., 2003b. Movement system impairment-based categories for low back pain: stage 1 validation. J Orthop Sports Phys Ther 33, 126–142.

Van Dillen, L.R., Sahrmann, S.A., Caldwell, C.A., McDonnell, M.K., Bloom, N.J., Norton, B.J., 2006. Trunk rotation-related impairments in people with low back pain who participated in two different types of leisure activities: a secondary analysis. J Orthop Sports Phys Ther 36, 58–71.

Van Dillen, L.R., Gombatto, S.P., Collins, D.R., Engsberg, J.R., Sahrmann, S.A., 2007. Symmetry of timing of hip and lumbopelvic rotation motion in 2 different subgroups of people with low back pain. Arch Phys Med Rehabil 88, 351–360.

Van Dillen, L.R., Maluf, K.S., Sahrmann, S.A., 2009. Further examination of modifying patient-preferred movement and alignment strategies in patients with low back pain during symptomatic tests. Man Ther 14, 52–60.

Von Korff, M., 1994. Studying the natural history of back pain. Spine 19, 2041S–2046S.

Youdas, J.W., Suman, V.J., Garrett, T.R., 1995. Reliability of measurements of lumbar spine sagittal mobility obtained with the flexible curve. J Orthop Sports Phys Ther 21, 13–20.

Youdas, J.W., Garrett, T.R., Egan, K.S., Therneau, T.M., 2000. Lumbar lordosis and pelvic inclination in adults with chronic low back pain. Phys Ther. 80, 261–75.

The relationship between control of the spine and low back pain: a clinical researcher's perspective

Julie A. Hides
School of Physiotherapy, Australian Catholic University, McAuley Campus, Banyo, Queensland, Australia

CHAPTER CONTENTS

WHAT IS MOTOR CONTROL TRAINING FOR LOW BACK PAIN?

As research physiotherapists involved in the area of therapeutic exercise for low back pain (LBP), the approach of my colleagues and myself, as outlined in two textbooks, is often quoted as 'motor control training' (Richardson et al. 1999, 2004b). The first edition of our textbook addressed motor control training of muscles such as the transversus abdominis (TrA), multifidus, pelvic floor and diaphragm. This initial work was derived from clinical observations of people with LBP and development of novel research approaches, which allowed the morphology of the deep muscles to be investigated scientifically. The roles of these muscles in protecting the joints from injury and evidence of their dysfunction in LBP led to a new paradigm of exercise therapy to address motor control problems in these muscles. We also described clinical tests for the TrA and multifidus muscles, and described the use of imaging techniques for providing feedback of muscle contraction. In the second edition (Richardson et al. 2004b), we described integration of the rehabilitation of the muscles listed above with one joint and multi-joint muscles. In this chapter, I would like to discuss how our original research has continued to evolve and give some examples of contemporary management focussing on retraining motor control for people with LBP.

MOTOR CONTROL EXERCISE

A recent systematic review by Macedo et al. (2009) examined motor control training for persistent (subacute, chronic and recurrent) LBP. Of the 14 randomized controlled trials (RCTs) included, the results of 7 trials showed that motor control exercise was better than minimal intervention or as supplement to another intervention in reducing pain at short-term (<3 months), intermediate (3–12 months) and long-term (>1 year) follow-up and in reducing disability at long-term follow-up. Four trials found that motor control exercise was better than manual therapy for pain, disability and quality of life at intermediate follow-up, but the effects were small. Five trials found that motor control exercise was better than other forms of exercise in reducing disability at short-term follow-up. Macedo et al. (2009) concluded that in patients with chronic LBP, motor control exercise is more effective than minimal intervention and beneficial when added to another therapy for pain at all time points and for disability at long-term follow-up. It is still unclear which patients respond best to which type of exercise. Identifying subgroups of patients that benefit more from one intervention than another would seem to be one of the biggest challenges in LBP research. RCTs using motor control training as an intervention have been performed on specific defined subgroups of people with spondylolisthesis (O'Sullivan et al. 1997), acute LBP (Hides et al. , 1996, 2001), chronic LBP (Goldby et al. 2006) and pregnancy-related pelvic girdle pain (Stuge et al. 2004).

We have recently performed a series of studies of various designs on specific subgroups including elite cricketers (Hides et al. 2006, 2008b, 2010b), elite Australian Football League (AFL) players (Hides et al. 2010a, 2010b, 2011b, 2012; Stewart et al. 2010; Hides and Stanton 2012; Hyde et al. 2012), Olympians, elite weightlifters (Bonacci et al. 2011; Sitilertpisan et al. 2012), Australian ballet dancers (Gildea et al. 2009) and prolonged bed rest subjects (Hides 2007; Belavý et al. 2008, 2010a, 2011; Hides et al. 2011c). This chapter will discuss some of these studies to highlight some relevant points concerning motor control training from a clinical researcher's perspective. Also included is a detailed description of the motor control approach used, and then some clinical discussion points and key clinical points associated with the results of the studies we have performed.

RETRAINING MOTOR CONTROL IN ELITE AUSTRALIAN CRICKETERS

We studied motor control training in elite cricketers, as although these athletes have high levels of fitness and undergo intensive strength training programmes, they still suffer LBP. In a recent injury report conducted among Australian cricketers, it was shown that the incidence of LBP was 8%, and as high as 14% among fast bowlers (Orchard et al. 2002; Orchard and James 2003). In addition, the injury prevalence (games missed due to injury) was similar for fast bowlers and full contact football players (Orchard et al. 2002). Bowling workload (Dennis et al. 2003) and biomechanical analysis of bowling action (Portus et al. 2004) have been identified as two key issues in prevention of LBP in fast bowlers. However, the role of physical preparation in terms of specific muscle re-education had not been investigated prior to our series of studies. We studied elite cricketers attending a national training camp (Hides et al. 2006, 2008b, 2008c, 2010c). This presented a unique opportunity to study elite athletes over a defined assessment period, where participant training activities were standardized and monitored. The aims of the studies were to determine the effect of a staged motor control training program on: (i) the size and symmetry of the multifidus muscle; (ii) the motor control of the anterolateral abdominal muscles; and (iii) self-reported pain levels, in elite cricketers with and without

LBP. As part of the study, all of the cricketers underwent a full musculoskeletal assessment. Based on this assessment, cricketers were eligible for either the LBP group or the asymptomatic group. In all cases of those with current LBP, the subjects reported previous episodes of LBP and the location of the pain was unilateral in distribution. Participants in the study were undertaking a 13-week cricket training programme that consisted of 2×6 week blocks separated by a 1-week break.

Assessing muscle function of multifidus and the abdominal muscles

Cross-sectional areas (CSAs) of the multifidus muscle were measured from L2 to L5 vertebral levels using ultrasound imaging. Clinical muscle testing of the TrA muscle was conducted using a 'draw in' manoeuvre, viewed using magnetic resonance imaging (MRI) (Richardson et al. 2004a; Hides et al. 2006, 2008b, 2010a, 2011b, 2012). The CSA of the trunk (excluding subcutaneous tissue) was obtained by measuring around the perimeter of the trunk, in rested and contracted states. MRI has been used previously to demonstrate differences in ability to perform the drawing in manoeuvre in subjects with LBP (Richardson et al. 2004a; Hides et al. 2008b, 2010a, 2011b). Subjects with LBP were shown to be less able to decrease the CSA of their trunk (Richardson et al. 2004b; Hides et al. 2008b, 2010a, 2011b) (Figs 9.1 and 9.2). Decreasing the CSA of the trunk is achieved by a concentric shortening of the TrA muscle, with minimal contraction of the oblique abdominal muscles. While there is an increase in intra-abdominal pressure (IAP) associated with this (Cresswell et al. 1992), contraction of all of the abdominal muscles, in association with contraction of the diaphragm (Hodges et al. 2005) and pelvic floor muscles (Neumann and Gill 2002), may result in large increases in IAP (Morris et al. 1961; Agostini and Campbell 1970), such as experienced with coughing

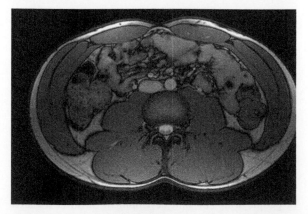

Figure 9.1 MRI of the trunk at the level of the L3–L4 disc before drawing in the abdominal wall.

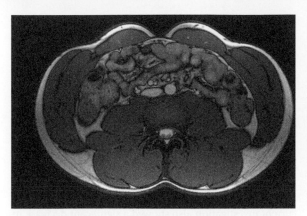

Figure 9.2 MRI of the trunk at the level of the L3–L4 disc while attempting to draw in the abdominal wall. In this case, the abdominal wall has bulged, in response to a global contraction of the rectus abdominis, oblique abdominal and transversus abdominis muscles.

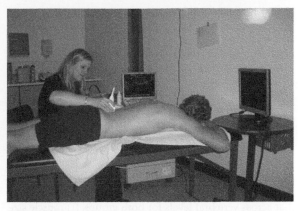

Figure 9.3 The athlete is learning to contract the multifidus muscle in prone lying whilst visually receiving feedback of muscle contraction by watching the ultrasound monitor.

(Neumann and Gill 2002). On MRI, a contraction of all of the abdominal muscles while attempting to draw in the abdominal wall may result in less decrease or even an increase in CSA of the trunk (Neumann and Gill 2002).

Motor control training

Subjects in the LBP group were provided with a 6-week motor control training programme (Richardson et al. 2004b). Instead of lifting weights in the gym, they initially undertook a programme of motor control training using ultrasound imaging to provide feedback of contraction of muscles including the multifidus and the TrA. They were taught to contract the TrA muscle (draw in the abdominal wall), isometrically contract the multifidus muscle with a focus on each vertebral level and draw up the deep pelvic floor (Hides et al. 1996, 2004). Subjects were asked if they could 'feel' the multifidus contacting, as perception of voluntary contraction of the segmental multifidus muscle may be indicative of the proprioceptive role of the multifidus muscle (Hides et al. 2004). Subjects were taught to co-contract the TrA, anterior pelvic floor and multifidus muscles. Subjects were encouraged to hold their contractions, while breathing normally, for at least 10 seconds and to repeat at least 10 times. Time was allocated for practice on a daily basis (15–30 minutes per day). All exercises were performed in a pain-free position and manner.

The cricketers were first taught to activate the muscles in lying positions (Fig. 9.3), and as performance improved, they were progressed to more functional upright (sitting and standing) positions. They were encouraged to maintain a lumbar lordosis and thoracic kyphosis when in upright positions, and were taught to perform voluntary contractions of the multifidus, TrA and pelvic floor muscles using ultrasound imaging to provide feedback in these

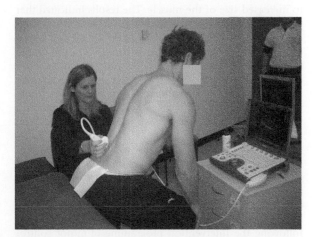

Figure 9.4 The athlete was taught to dissociate hip movements from lumbopelvic movements. This involved checking the ability to hold a lumbar lordosis and thoracic kyphosis while leaning forward from the hips. Ultrasound imaging was used to provide feedback of multifidus muscle contraction and maintenance of spinal position.

positions. They were also taught to dissociate hip movements from lumbopelvic movements. This involved checking the ability to hold a lumbar lordosis and thoracic kyphosis while leaning forward in sitting and standing positions, whilst breathing using the diaphragm (Fig. 9.4). Subjects were asked to lean forwards from the hips and substitution strategies were observed for. The most common substitution strategy observed was flexion of the lumbar spine, but some subjects extended at the thoracolumbar junction.

There was also an emphasis placed on gaining endurance of the multifidus muscle. This was trained by being able to lean forward from the hips and hold this position while maintaining a lumbar lordosis, thoracic kyphosis and while maintaining normal respiration. Ultrasound imaging was also used to provide feedback of multifidus contraction during this phase of training. Techniques of squatting and lunging were examined, and subjects were instructed to maintain their lumbar lordosis and thoracic kyphosis throughout the movement. After the 6-week motor control training programme, subjects in the LBP group were allowed to resume graduated weight training with the rest of the squad. Close monitoring of technique and maintenance of the spinal curves was continually monitored in the weights room.

The pattern of results for the multifidus muscle indicated that across vertebral levels for both groups; (i) muscle size increased during the course of the training camp; (ii) there was significant amount of muscle size asymmetry among these cricketers; and (iii) there was a significant decrease in asymmetry during the course of the training camp. At the L5 vertebral level, there was an additional effect related to increased size of the muscle. The results indicated that the increase in muscle size during the course of the training camp was not the same for both groups. At L5, multifidus muscle size was smaller in the cricketers with LBP at the start of the training camp, but this was not evident at the end of the training camp. At the L5 vertebral level, there was also a decrease in asymmetry during the course of the training camp, which was greater for the LBP group. There was also a 50% decrease in the mean reported pain level among the cricketers with LBP (Hides et al. 2008).

Results for the abdominal muscles showed that the contraction size for the CSA of the abdominal wall (expressed as a percentage change from the rest condition) for the asymptomatic group was similar at pre-camp and post-camp whereas the LBP group demonstrated a relative increase in contraction size from pre-camp to post-camp following the intervention programme of motor control exercises. The increase in thickness of the internal oblique (IO) muscle due to contraction (expressed as a percentage change from the rest condition) for the asymptomatic group was similar at pre-camp and post-camp, whereas the LBP group demonstrated a relative decrease in the amount of contraction of the IO muscle from pre-camp to post-camp following the intervention programme of motor control training exercises. In the case of the TrA muscle thickness, the increase in TrA thickness due to contraction for the asymptomatic group increased from pre-camp to post-camp, whereas the LBP group demonstrated a relative decrease in the amount of contraction of the TrA muscle from pre-camp to post-camp following the intervention programme of motor control exercises.

Clinical discussion points

The motor control training exercises used in these studies were low load in nature and did not induce pain. The cricketers in the LBP group stopped high resistance exercise while they learned to 'switch on' the multifidus, TrA and pelvic floor muscles prior to resuming higher load exercises. Ultrasound imaging was used to provide feedback of voluntary isometric contraction of the multifidus muscle to the subjects. The use of ultrasound imaging to provide feedback has been shown previously to enhance the ability to isometrically contract the multifidus muscle in normal subjects (Van et al. 2006). Using a rehabilitation protocol that involved progression from motor control training to high load exercise has been shown in a prior study to lead to hypertrophy of the multifidus muscle with a concomitant decrease in pain in subjects with chronic LBP (Danneels et al. 2001). Results of the current investigation also showed a significant decrease in reported pain levels for the subjects in the LBP group who underwent motor control training. This difference in pain scores (measured using a visual analogue scale or VAS) was statistically significant and exceeded the minimum clinically significant difference in VAS pain scores reported in clinical studies (Todd et al. 1996; Kelly 1998).

Results of studies performed on asymptomatic subjects without a history of LBP have previously shown that the multifidus muscle is symmetrical between sides (Hides et al. 1992, 1994, 1995, 2008a; Stokes et al. 2005). Hides et al. (1994) documented multifidus asymmetry in subjects with acute unilateral first episode LBP, and similar results were found in subjects with chronic LBP with unilateral pain presentations of greater than 12 weeks duration (Barker et al. 2004; Hides et al. 2008a). In all these cases, the smaller muscle was found ipsilateral to symptoms. In the elite cricketers studied, the asymmetry resolved (the smaller side increased in CSA) in subjects who underwent specific rehabilitation.

The effect of motor control training on an athlete's performance was not investigated in this study, although it is also used as a sport training method (Mills et al. 2005) and two RCTs have shown improvements in lower extremity power and agility (Mills et al. 2005) and increased vertical takeoff velocity (Butcher et al. 2007) in subjects who underwent trunk stability training (Butcher et al. 2007). Proposed explanations for this include optimization of the ability of the lower extremity muscles to provide force by providing a stable base from which the muscles could contract, enhancing the neural drive to the lower extremity muscles and increasing the overall awareness and control of trunk and pelvic position. Anecdotal reports from the current study may lend support to the latter explanation, as subjects with LBP who received the intervention commented that their ability to squat with weights was improved after intervention, as they could 'feel' where their backs were in space as they added load. This would be an advantage, as biomechanical models have suggested that the lumbar spine is best able to cope with compressive forces when it is positioned in a lordosis (Kiefer et al. 1997).

Differences between cricketers with and without LBP were also evident in their contraction of the TrA and IO muscles, measured by muscle thickness. At the start of the training camp, cricketers with LBP contracted both the IO and the TrA muscles *more* than the asymptomatic cricketers when they drew in their abdominal walls. Similar results have been presented in studies which compared automatic recruitment of the abdominal muscles among subjects with and without LBP in response to a simulated weight-bearing task (Hides et al. 2009a; Hyde et al. 2012). It has been proposed that a more general strategy of 'bracing' the abdominal muscles may lead to an increase in intra-abdominal pressure (Hides et al. 2009a). Therefore, despite the increased thickness of the IO and TrA muscles in the cricketers with LBP (contracting against the resistance of the increased intra-abdominal pressure), the TrA muscle could not concentrically shorten (slide) to the same extent as seen in those without LBP. By the end of the camp, the cricketers with LBP who received motor control training decreased the amount of contraction of both the IO and the TrA muscles when they drew in their abdominal walls. This finding makes sense if interpreted in the context of over-contraction of these muscles at the start of the training camp. Associated with this decrease in the amount of contraction of the TrA and IO muscles was an improvement in the ability to draw in the abdominal wall (reflected by the trunk CSA measure) and perform the muscle test for the TrA muscle. Overactivity of lumbopelvic muscles has been commonly observed among people with LBP (Lariviere et al. 2000; Ng et al. 2002; van Dieen et al. 2003; Hodges et al. 2003; Geisser et al. 2005). This may represent an attempt to confer generalized stiffness (Gardner-Morse and Stokes 1998) to the vertebral column or to increase intra-abdominal pressure, which can also confer generalized stiffening of the spine (Hodges and Moseley 2003; Hodges et al. 2005).

This result may hold important implications for exercise therapy. There is evidence that the TrA muscle is controlled independently of the other abdominal muscles (Hodges and Richardson 1996, 1998). Results from this study, where cricketers with LBP contracted the TrA (and IO) muscle more than the healthy subjects, would suggest that increasing the amount of contraction of the TrA muscle when performing motor control exercises may not be as important as improving the ability to contract the TrA muscle independently of the other abdominal muscles before progressing to higher load activities, where the abdominal muscles are more likely to contract together.

A further consideration in the implementation of the motor control training was the use of ultrasound imaging to provide feedback of the independent contraction of the TrA muscle. Ultrasound imaging has been successfully used to provide feedback to enhance motor re-learning in subjects with chronic LBP (Goldby et al. 2006) and has been shown to be superior to clinical instruction alone in normal subjects (Henry and Westervelt 2005). Furthermore, the use of ultrasound imaging in the specific motor control retraining of the TrA muscle (independently of the other abdominal muscles) has been shown to facilitate the development of changes in the timing of muscle activation that were evident not only immediately after training (Tsao and Hodges 2007) but also after 6 months (Tsao and Hodges 2008). By the end of the 13-week programme, which included progression to closed-chain exercises, cricketers with LBP were able to draw in the abdominal wall and significantly decrease the CSA of the trunk. Similar programmes of therapeutic exercise aimed at improving the motor control of the TrA muscle have previously reported a concomitant reduction in the severity (and recurrence) of LBP symptoms in non-athletic subjects with chronic LBP (O'Sullivan et al. 1997; Stuge et al. 2004; Goldby et al. 2006). While bowler workloads (Dennis et al. 2003, 2005) and technique (Elliot 2000) must also be considered, re-education of the ability to contract the TrA muscle independently of the other abdominal muscles in fast bowlers may help to stabilize the spine against the large forces induced on the spine when bowling (Elliot 2000), and may reduce the incidence and severity of LBP in this population.

Key clinical points from this research

- Atrophy of the multifidus muscle can present in elite athletes who are still able to perform their sports and train, including high loaded weight training.
- As the athletes were undergoing weight training prior to the studies described above, weight training alone may not be enough to induce hypertrophy of the multifidus muscle in athletes with LBP and associated atrophy of the multifidus muscle (if present).
- It would appear that retraining motor control prior to loaded activity is a sensible approach for hypertrophying the multifidus muscle.
- Endurance of the multifidus muscle and adequate proprioception of lumbopelvic and thoracic position may be important factors to consider in weight-bearing exercise.
- Adequate mobility of the thoracic spine, hips, and adequate dissociation of hips/lumbar spine motion (especially flexion/extension) and thoracic motion (rotation) would seem important factors to consider.
- Cricketers with LBP tended to overcontract their abdominal muscles, and did not exhibit independent control of their TrA muscle. An essential component of treatment was learning to decrease overactivity of the IO muscle, and to re-learn a diaphragmatic breathing pattern.
- Ultrasound imaging was deemed a useful tool in these studies, as a means of providing feedback of

appropriate patterns of contraction for the TrA and multifidus muscles. This was found to be of benefit in upright functional positions as well as during performance of exercises in the weights room.

EFFECTS OF DELOADING

Alterations in physical activity experienced during space-flight or prolonged bed rest have direct effects on the musculoskeletal system. Exposure to microgravity has been shown to lead to an increased incidence of LBP associated with abnormal lengthening of the spine (Wing et al. 1991), atrophy of spinal musculature (Leblanc et al. 1995), increased intervertebral disc (IVD) height and area (Leblanc et al. 1994, 1995) and altered IVD composition. Greater than 50% of astronauts complain of LBP during space missions (Wing et al. 1991), and astronauts have an increased incidence of disc protrusion when compared to a general or an army aviation population (Johnston et al. 1998). Astronauts undergo specific training programmes before and after spaceflight, to try to minimize the effects of loss of functional weight bearing and to help to prevent conditions such as LBP developing. LBP is also known to be a huge problem on Earth (Hicks et al. 2002), but it is difficult to perform longitudinal studies before and after the onset of LBP as development of insidious LBP may take a long time. This process is accelerated in spaceflight and prolonged bed rest, and these studies therefore offer a unique opportunity to study people before and after the onset of LBP. Bed rest studies are also useful as they allow testing of countermeasures and rehabilitation procedures both during and after periods of reduced functional weight bearing.

Countermeasures and rehabilitation procedures have traditionally aimed at reversing muscle atrophy and weakness which are assumed to be the result of LBP, spaceflight and prolonged bed rest, however this is not always the case. While some muscles do atrophy, other muscles increase in size under these conditions. For example laboratory studies have demonstrated the effects of induced pain (Hodges et al. 2003; Kiesel et al. 2008) or anticipation of pain (Neumann and Gill 2002) on muscle function in normal subjects, and demonstrated that while some muscles become inhibited (and atrophy), other muscles increase their activation in response to induced pain (Hodges et al. 2003).

This situation of differential atrophy between muscles also occurs in bed rest. Studies using MRI have demonstrated greater atrophy in the spinal extensor muscles than in the flexor muscles (Lee et al. 2003; Cao et al. 2005). The psoas muscle, a spinal flexor, has been shown not to change significantly in size during spaceflight (LeBlanc et al. 1995, 2000) and bed rest (Leblanc et al. 1992; Cao et al. 2005), with other more recent studies showing increases in psoas size during bed rest (Hides et al. 2007, 2009b; Belavý et al. 2008). In addition, recent works in prolonged bed rest have shown differential atrophy in the paraspinal (extensor) muscles with the multifidus muscle showing greater atrophy than the lumbar erector spinae at the lower lumbar levels (Hides et al. 2007, Belavý et al. 2011). In comparison, the abdominal flexor muscle group has been shown to increase in size during bed rest (Hides et al. 2007).

Some of the changes in bed rest have been observed to be long-lasting in nature. It took 28 days for the psoas muscle to return to its pre bed-rest size following re-ambulation (Hides et al. 2007) and changes in the multifidus muscle were still evident at 90 days after re-ambulation and return to normal activities (Belavý et al. 2008). Electromyographic studies have also shown the persistence of motor control changes in the lumbopelvic musculature up to 1 year after bed rest (Belavý et al. 2007a, 2007b, 2010b). Similar changes in muscle size have been reported for people with LBP for the multifidus (Leblanc et al. 1992, 1995; Hides et al. 1996, 1998; Danneels et al. 2000; Wallwork et al. 2009) and psoas muscles (Leblanc et al. 1995; Danneels et al. 2000; Stewart et al. 2010). This differential atrophy of the muscles during bed rest has also been linked to the development of LBP afterwards (Holguin et al. 2009; Belavý et al. 2011).

Motor control training

In a recent study, we trialled two intervention programmes after prolonged bed rest (Hides et al. 2011c). Subjects underwent 60 days of head-down tilt bed rest as part of the 2nd Berlin BedRest Study (BBR2–2). After bed rest they underwent one of two exercise programmes, trunk flexor and general strength training or specific motor control training. MRI of the lumbopelvic region was conducted at the start and end of bed rest and during the recovery period (14 and 90 days after re-ambulation). CSAs of the multifidus, psoas, lumbar erector spinae and quadratus lumborum (QL) muscles were measured from L1 to L5. Morphological changes including disc volume, spinal length, lordosis angle and disc height were also measured. Both exercise programmes restored the multifidus muscle to pre-bed rest size, but further increases in psoas muscle size were seen in the trunk flexor and general exercise group up to 14 days after bed rest. The trunk flexor and general strengthening programme resulted in greater decreases in disc volume and anterior disc height. The motor control training programme may be preferable to trunk flexor and general strength training after bed rest (when musculoskeletal structures are deconditioned) as it restored the CSA of the multifidus muscle without generating potentially harmful compressive forces through the spine.

MUSCLE IMBALANCE, MUSCLE ASYMMETRY AND MOTOR CONTROL TRAINING

Bed rest studies provide a good example of development of muscle imbalances. Sports which involve very specific training and loading patterns also have the potential to induce muscle imbalances, and muscle asymmetries. A recent longitudinal study was conducted to determine if muscle imbalance of trunk muscles exists in elite AFL players (Hides and Stanton 2012). AFL players were assessed at four time points over three playing seasons, and MRI was used to determine the CSAs of the multi-fidus (vertebral levels L2 to L5) and lumbar erector spinae muscles (L3), as well as the thickness of the TrA and IO muscles at L3. By the end of the playing season, results showed 11.1% atrophy for multifidus CSA and 21% atrophy for TrA thickness at rest. In comparison, the CSA of the lumbar erector spinae muscles increased by 3.6% and the thickness of the IO muscle increased by 11.8% compared with the start of the pre-season. Overall, the results of this study indicated that trunk muscles with a proposed role in torque production such as IO and lumbar erector spinae, increased in size over the playing season and reduced in size again by the start of the next season. The increase in size during the season could be expected as a result of higher loads associated with training and playing football. However, the results also indicated that local muscles such as the multifidus and TrA decreased in size over the playing season. This muscle imbalance was associated with playing football rather than with LBP.

In a longitudinal observational study, we examined the relationship between severity of pre-season hip, thigh and groin (HTG) muscle injuries, and lumbopelvic muscle size, asymmetry and function at the start and end of the pre-season (Hides et al. 2011a). In AFL, HTG muscle injuries have the highest prevalence and incidence rate. Deficits within the lumbopelvic region, such as impaired muscle function and muscle asymmetry, could contribute to injuries in the pre-season, and injury could in turn affect muscle size and function. MRI examinations were performed on 47 male elite AFL players at the start and at the end of the football pre-season. CSAs of multifidus, psoas major and QL muscles were measured, as well as change in trunk CSA due to voluntarily contracting the TrA muscle. Injuries occurring during pre-season training were routinely recorded by the club's performance staff at each training session. Results showed that players with more severe pre-season HTG injuries (more training sessions missed) had significantly smaller multifidus muscle CSA compared with players with no HTG injury. No relationship was found for size or asymmetry of the QL or psoas

major muscles, or ability to contract the TrA muscle through 'drawing in' of the abdominal wall. Small multi-fidus muscle size at L5 predicted five of six cases that incurred a more severe HTG injury. We have recently completed a study looking at players from six AFL clubs to replicate this finding.

Given that the small size of the multifidus muscle at the lumbo-sacral junction predicted HTG injuries in AFL players, a logical next step was to intervene using motor control training to see if this could affect injury rates. Other prospective studies have also shown that deficits in the control of the trunk can predict lower limb injuries (Zazulak et al. 2007a, 2007b). Zazulak et al. (2007b) showed that increased trunk displacement in response to sudden trunk force release (factors related to lumbopelvic stability) was predictive of knee and anterior cruciate ligament injuries in athletes. The rationale for this was that decreased neuromuscular control of the trunk, coupled with high ground reaction forces directed toward the body's centre of mass, compromised the dynamic stability of the knee joint and increased knee injury risk. LBP is also common amongst AFL players. We conducted a panel randomized intervention trial to examine the effect of a motor control training programme for elite AFL players with and without LBP (Hides et al., 2012). The outcome measures included CSA and symmetry of multifidus, QL and psoas muscles, and change in CSA of the trunk in response to an abdominal drawing in task. These measures of muscle size and function were performed using MRI. Availability of players for competition games was used to assess the effect of the intervention on the occurrence of injuries. The motor control programme involved performance of voluntary contractions of the multifidus and TrA muscles while receiving feedback from ultrasound imaging. As all players were to receive the intervention, the trial was delivered as a stepped-wedge design with three treatment arms (15 weeks intervention, 8 weeks intervention and a 'wait-list' control who received 7 weeks intervention toward the end of the playing season). Players participated in a pilates programme when they were not receiving the intervention. Results showed that the intervention programme was associated with an increase in multifidus muscle size relative to results for the control group. The programme was also associated with an improved ability to draw in the abdominal wall. Intervention was commensurate with an increase in availability for games and a high level of perceived benefit. Motor control training was also commensurate with decreased LBP in AFL players. In this study, footballers who received the intervention early in the season missed fewer games due to injury than those who received it late in the playing season.

Many sports are asymmetrical in nature, and asymmetry has been thought to possibly be related to injuries. Due to the proposed undesirable consequences of asymmetry, several coaching and training sources encourage players in sports involving kicking such as Australian Rules football (Parkin et al. 1987a, 1987b) and soccer (Mozes et al. 1985; McLean and Tumilty 1993) to practice using both legs during training. The rationale for this practice is to minimize potential asymmetrical forces acting on joints, reduce muscle imbalances and decrease the workload of the dominant leg which may eventually lead to overuse injuries (Anderson et al. 2001).

One trunk muscle that has been studied in cricketers is the QL muscle. Researchers have used imaging studies to reveal hypertrophy of the QL muscle ipsilateral to the bowling arm in fast bowlers (Wallace et al. 1997; Engstrom et al. 2007; Hides et al. 2008a; Ranson et al. 2008). Engstrom et al. (1999, 2007) and Walker et al. (1999) hypothesized that increased muscle development created an increased mechanical load on the neural arch resulting in contralateral bone stress injuries. However, care must be exercised when extrapolating from morphological studies. A mathematical model was developed to test this theory by De Visser et al. (2007). The model was used to estimate forces and moments delivered by the QL muscle on the L3 and L4 vertebrae during the bowling action. In contrast to the earlier studies which had predicted a relationship between hypertrophy of the QL muscle and development of injuries (Engstrom et al. 1999, 2007; Walker et al. 1999), the model predicted that asymmetry of the QL muscle may help to reduce bone stresses (De Visser et al. 2007).While it has not been shown that development of muscle asymmetry relates to injury, it is nevertheless important to determine if such asymmetries actually do exist in relation to specific sports.

As cricket is an asymmetrical sport, it is likely that asymmetries will develop in many trunk muscles. This may occur in all cricketers, not just the fast bowlers who are exposed to very high asymmetrical forces when they bowl. A recent MRI study (Hides et al. 2008b) showed that asymmetry of the QL muscle was present in cricketers of all positions. Among fast bowlers, it was found that asymmetry was related to the presence of LBP. Fast bowlers with LBP had the greatest asymmetry, whereas fast bowlers without LBP had no greater evidence of asymmetry of the QL muscle than other cricketers (not fast bowlers) in the squad. For the psoas muscle, it has been reported that asymmetry in fast bowlers is significantly greater than asymmetry in control subjects (Hides et al. 2008b) (Fig. 9.5). While increased loading and hypertrophy of muscles may be associated with sporting activities, results must be interpreted carefully as pain and muscle inhibition can lead to atrophy of muscles. Asymmetry of the psoas muscle has also been observed in subjects presenting with unilateral LBP with decreased CSA on the affected side (Barker et al. 2004). Thus athletes with LBP may present with competing influences of muscle hypertrophy due to increased activity levels and muscle atrophy due to pain and muscle inhibition.

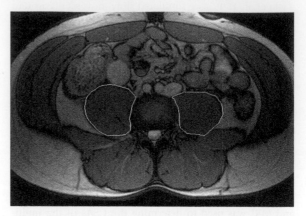

Figure 9.5 MRI of the trunk at the level of the L3–L4 disc in an elite cricketer. Asymmetry of the psoas muscle is evident, with the psoas on the right side (left of image) larger (outlined). There is also asymmetry between sides in the quadratus lumborum muscle (bigger on the left side) and oblique abdominal muscles (bigger on the right side).

Asymmetry of trunk muscles has also been investigated in AFL players in relation to their preferred kicking leg. Kicking is an asymmetrical and ballistic task which involves trunk rotation and hip flexion (Mozes et al. 1985; Anderson et al. 2001) and it has been proposed that kicking may contribute to muscle imbalances and induce torsion on the spine (Orchard et al. 1999; James 2002). The effect of kicking on muscles of the lower limb has been investigated (Orchard et al. 1999; Orchard 2001; Baczkowski et al. 2006). Researchers have identified the roles of specific muscles relative to the kicking and stance leg, and a link between muscle injuries and leg preference has been determined. However, muscles of the hip and lumbopelvic region have received less attention.

To determine if asymmetry relative to the preferred kicking leg exists for the psoas and QL muscles among elite AFL players, 54 players were assessed at three time points from 2005 to 2007 (start of pre-season, end of season and end of pre-season training) (Hides et al. 2010b). Number of injuries was also included as a risk factor. Results showed that at all three time points, the CSA of the psoas muscle was significantly greater ipsilateral to the kicking leg, while the CSA of the QL muscle was significantly greater on the side contralateral to the kicking leg (stance leg). While the primary aim of this study was focussed on asymmetry of the psoas and QL muscles, information about current lumbopelvic and/or lower limb injuries was collected at each time point. This kind of information is important, as in AFL players, it is unknown whether asymmetry of trunk muscles is a normal finding related to function for this group or is potentially problematical. Interestingly, increased psoas muscle size has been documented in athletes with LBP when compared with athletes without LBP (McGregor et al. 2002; Stewart et al. 2010). Results of the study indicated no overall effect for number of injuries on muscle size or asymmetry. However, this aspect could be further examined, as the relationship may be far more complex than can be explained by relating asymmetries to number of injuries. While it is quite possible that asymmetries of key lumbo-pelvic muscles may induce deleterious forces on the spine, it may be that the presence of an operational stability system (provided by other deep abdominal and paraspinal muscles such as the multifidus and lumbar erector spinae) may counter these forces and protect the spine from injury (Hides et al. 2010b). A possibility is that injuries ensue when the stability system is inadequate to negate the forces induced on the spine by the torque producing muscles. Future studies could investigate this aspect further.

The size of the psoas muscle has been examined in athletic and non-athletic populations. Assessments have been conducted in age-matched athletic and non-athletic adolescent girls (Peltonen et al. 1998). The sports undertaken by the athletic subjects included gymnastics, ballet and figure skating. The athletes assessed had greater absolute psoas muscle CSA and trunk flexion force than the control subjects, which was explained by their regular physical training. It would seem from these studies that it is important to examine muscle size and symmetry in different sports, as athletes may show prominent development in muscle groups used in their competitive activities and/or training regimes (Kanehisa et al. 2001, 2003). Muscle imbalances have the potential to exist between sides and between muscle groups. Hypertrophy of the psoas muscle in AFL players is most likely related to its role as a primary hip flexor (Bogduk et al. 1992; Penning 2000) (Fig. 9.6) as was seen in gymnasts, ballet dancers,

figure skaters (Peltonen et al. 1998) and cricketers (Ranson et al. 2008).

Key clinical points from these studies

- Asymmetry of trunk muscles may occur in athletes who participate in asymmetrical sports. It is unclear if the resultant asymmetry is a necessary response to the demands of the individual sport or if it is potentially harmful.
- Imbalance between the trunk flexor and extensor muscles may occur in various sports. In the presence of hypertrophy of muscles such as the psoas, exercises should be selected which do not over-recruit the already hypertrophied muscles. This may include factors such as position adopted for exercises and open versus closed chain exercise selection.
- Athletes may have muscles which are receiving competing influences of hypertrophy (due to demands of the sport) and atrophy (due to factors such as pain inhibition). A thorough individual muscle assessment will be required to determine the most appropriate exercise therapy approach.
- Studies on athletes have supported studies conducted on non-athletic populations in that motor control training is commensurate with a reduction in LBP.
- Assessment of muscle imbalance may be a useful screening tool which could be used by sporting teams.
- Although there are many factors to consider in association with decreasing rates of injuries in elite athletes, motor control training represents one approach which may be beneficial.

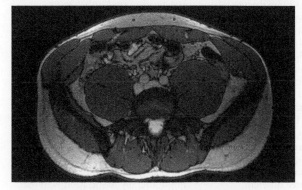

Figure 9.6 MRI of the trunk at the level of the L4–L5 disc in an elite AFL player, showing hypertrophy of the posas muscles bilaterally. The psoas muscles are also asymmetrical between sides, with a bigger muscle on the player's left side (to right of the image).

ACKNOWLEDGEMENTS

I would like to acknowledge the many researchers I have worked with in the projects discussed in this chapter, including: Professor Carolyn Richardson, Professor Warren Stanton, Associate Professor Stephen Wilson, Gunda Lambrecht, Dr Daniel Belavý, Professor Dieter Felsenberg, Jan Gildea, Dilani Mendis, Margot Sexton, Dr Kevin Sims, Dr Shaun McMahon, Lachlan Penfold, Nathan Carloss, Peter Stanton, Helen Littleworth, Mark Hollands, Dr Katie McMahon, Dr Mark Strudwick. BBR2 was funded by the European Space Agency, The University of Queensland, grant number FE 468/5–1 from the German Research Foundation (DFG). The Cricket project was funded by a grant from the Cricket Australia Sports Science Medicine Advisory Group (CASSMAG), and the AFL project was funded by a grant from the Lions AFC.

REFERENCES

Agostini, E., Campbell, E.J.M., 1970. The abdominal muscles. In: Campbell, E.J.M., Agostini, E., Newsom-Dvis, J. (Eds.), The Respiratory Muscles: mechanisms and neural control. Lloyd Luke, London, pp. 175–180.

Anderson, K., Strickland, S.M., Warren, R., 2001. Hip and groin injuries in athletes. Am J Sports Med 29, 521–533.

Baczkowski, K., Marks, P., Silberstein, M., Schneider-Kolsky, M.E., 2006. A new look into kicking a football: an investigation of muscle activity using MRI. Australasian Radiol 50, 324–329.

Barker, K.L., Shamley, D.R., Jackson, D., 2004. Changes in the cross-sectional area of multifidus and psoas in patients with unilateral back pain – the relationship to pain and disability. Spine 29, E515–E519.

Belavý, D.L., Richardson, C.A., Wilson, S.J., Felsenberg, D., Rittweger, J., 2007a. Tonic-to-phasic shift of lumbo-pelvic muscle activity during 8 weeks of bed rest and 6-months follow up. J Appl Physiol 103, 48–54.

Belavý, D.L., Richardson, C.A., Wilson, S.J., Rittweger, J., Felsenberg, D., 2007b. Superficial lumbopelvic muscle overactivity and decreased cocontraction after 8 weeks of bed rest. Spine 32, E23–E29.

Belavý, D.L., Hides, J.A., Wilson, S.J., Stanton, W., Dimeo, F.C., Rittweger, J., et al., 2008. Resistive simulated weightbearing exercise with whole body vibration reduces lumbar spine deconditioning in bed-rest. Spine 33, E121–E31.

Belavý, D.L., Armbrecht, G., Gast, U., Richardson, C.A., Hides, J.A., Felsenberg, D., 2010a. Countermeasures against lumbar spine deconditioning in prolonged bed rest: resistive exercise with and without whole body vibration. J Appl Physiol 109, 1801–1811.

Belavý, D.L., Ng, J.K.F., Wilson, S.J., Armbrecht, G., Stegeman, D.F., Rittweger, J., et al., 2010b. Influence of prolonged bed-rest on spectral and temporal electromyographic motor control characteristics of the superficial lumbo-pelvic musculature. J Electromyogr Kinesiol 20, 170–179.

Belavý, D.L., Armbrecht, G.P., Richardson, C.A., Felsenberg, D., Hides, J.A., 2011. Muscle atrophy and changes in spinal morphology: Is the lumbar spine vulnerable after prolonged bed-rest? Spine 36, 137–145.

Bogduk, N., Pearcy, M., Hadfield, G., 1992. Anatomy and biomechanics of psoas major. Clin Biomech 7, 109–119.

Bonacci, J., Green, D., Saunders, P.U., Franettovich, M., Blanch, P., Vicenzino, B., 2011. Plyometric training as an intervention to correct altered neuromotor control during running after cycling in triathletes: a preliminary randomised controlled trial. Phys Ther Sport 12, 15–21.

Butcher, S.J., Craven, B.R., Chilibeck, P.D., Spink, K.S., Sprigings, E.J., 2007. The effect of trunk stability training on vertical takeoff velocity. J Orthop Sports Phys Ther 37, 223–231.

Cao, P.H., Kimura, S., Macias, B.R., Ueno, T., Watenpaugh, D.E., Hargens, A.R., 2005. Exercise within lower body negative pressure partially counteracts lumbar spine deconditioning associated with 28-day bed rest. J Appl Physiol 99, 39–44.

Cresswell, A.G., Grundstrom, H., Thorstensson, A., 1992. Observations on intra-abdominal pressure and patterns of abdominal intramuscular activity in man. Acta Physiol Scand 144, 409–418.

Danneels, L.A., Vanderstraeten, G.G., Cambier, D.C., Witrouw, E.E., De Cuyper, H.J., 2000. CT imaging of trunk muscles in chronic low back pain patients and healthy control subjects. Eur Spine J 9, 266–272.

Danneels, L.A., Vanderstraeten, G.G., Cambier, D.C., Witrouw, E.E., Bourgois, J., Dankaerts, W., et al., 2001. Effects of three different training modalities on the cross sectional area of the lumbar multifidus muscle in patients with chronic low back pain. Br J Sports Med 35, 186–191.

de Visser, H., Adam, C.J., Crozier, S., Pearcy, M.J., 2007. The role of quadratus lumborum asymmetry in the occurrence of lesions in the lumbar vertebrae of cricket fast bowlers. Med Engineering Physics 29, 877–885.

Dennis, R., Farhart, R., Goumas, C., Orchard, J., 2003. Bowling workload and the risk of injury in elite cricket fast bowlers. J Sci Med Sport 6, 359–367.

Dennis, R.J., Finch, C.F., Farhart, P.J., 2005. Is bowling workload a risk factor for injury to Australian junior cricket fast bowlers? Br J Sports Med 39, 843–846.

Elliot, B., 2000. Back injuries and the fast bowler in cricket. J Sports Sci 18, 983–991.

Engstrom, C., Walker, D., Kippers, V., Hunter, J., Hanna, A.J., Buckley, R., 1999. A prospective study on back injury and muscle morphometry in junior cricket fast bowlers. In: Abstracts of the 5th IOC World Congress on Sport Sciences. Canberra, ACT, Sports Medicine Australia.

Engstrom, C.M., Walker, D.G., Kippers, V., Mehnert, A.J., 2007. Quadratus lumborum asymmetry and L4 pars injury in fast bowlers: A prospective MR study. Med Sci Sports Exercise 39, 910–917.

Gardner-Morse, M.G., Stokes, I.A., 1998. The effects of abdominal muscle coactivation on lumbar spine stability. Spine 23, 86–91.

Geisser, M.E., Ranavaya, M., Haig, A.J., Roth, R.S., Zucker, R., Ambroz, C., et al., 2005. A meta-analytic review of surface electromyography among persons with low back pain and normal, healthy controls. J Pain 6, 711–726.

Gildea, J., Hides, J., Stanton, W., Hodges, P., 2009. Low back pain is associated with changes in multifidus muscle size in ballet dancers, paper presented to Australian Physiotherapy Association National Conference Week, Sydney, Australia, October 2009.

Goldby, L.J., Moore, A., Doust, J., Trew, M.E., 2006. A randomized controlled trial investigating the efficiency of musculoskeletal physiotherapy on chronic low back disorder. Spine 31, 1083–1093.

Henry, S.M., Westervelt, K.C., 2005. The use of real-time ultrasound feedback in teaching abdominal hollowing exercises to healthy subjects. J Orthop Sports Phys Ther 35, 338–345.

Hicks, G.S., Duddleston, D.N., Russell, L.D., Holman, H.E., Shepherd, J.M., Brown, C.A., 2002. Low back pain. Am J Med Sci 324, 207–211.

Hides, J., Stanton, W., 2012. Muscle imbalance and elite australian rules football players: a longitudinal study of changes in trunk muscle size. J Athletic Training 47, 153–157.

Hides, J.A., Cooper, D.H., Stokes, M.J., 1992. Diagnostic ultrasound imaging for measurement of the lumbar multifidus muscle in normal young adults. Physiother Theory Pract 8, 19–26.

Hides, J.A., Stokes, M.J., Saide, M., Jull, G.A., Cooper, D.H., 1994. Evidence of lumbar multifidus muscle wasting ipsilateral to symptoms in patients with acute/subacute low back pain. Spine 19, 165–172.

Hides, J.A., Richardson, C.A., Jull, G.A., 1995. Magnetic resonance imaging and ultrasonography of the lumbar multifidus muscle: comparison of two different modalities. Spine 20, 54–58.

Hides, J.A., Richardson, C.A., Jull, G.A., 1996. Multifidus muscle recovery is not automatic after resolution of acute, first-episode low back pain. Spine 21, 2763–2769.

Hides, J.A., Richardson, C.A., Jull, G., 1998. Use of real-time ultrasound imaging for feedback in rehabilitation. Manual Ther 3, 125–131.

Hides, J.A., Jull, G.A., Richardson, C.A., 2001. Long-term effects of specific stabilizing exercises for first-episode low back pain. Spine 26, E243–248.

Hides, J.A., Richardson, C.A., Hodges, P.W., 2004. Local segmental control. In: Richardson, C.A., Hodges, P.W., Hides, J.A. (Eds.), Therapeutic Exercise for Lumbo-pelvic Stabilization: a motor control approach for the treatment and prevention of low back pain, 2nd edn. Churchill Livingstone, Edinburgh, pp. 185–219.

Hides, J., Wilson, S., Stanton, W., McMahon, S., Keto, H., McMahon, K., et al., 2006. An MRI investigation into the function of the transversus abdominis muscle during 'drawing-in' of the abdominal wall. Spine 31, E175–E8.

Hides, J.A., Belavý, D.L., Stanton, W., Wilson, S.J., Rittweger, J., Felsenberg, D., et al., 2007. Magnetic resonance imaging assessment of trunk muscles during prolonged bed rest. Spine 32, 1687–1692.

Hides, J., Gilmore, C., Stanton, W., Bohlscheid, E., 2008a. Multifidus size and symmetry among chronic LBP and healthy asymptomatic subjects. Manual Therapy 13, 43–49.

Hides, J., Stanton, W., Freke, M., Wilson, S., McMahon, S., Richardson, C., 2008b. MRI study of the size, symmetry and function of the trunk muscles among elite cricketers with and without low back pain. Br J Sports Med 42, 509–513.

Hides, J., Stanton, W., McMahon, S., Sims, K., Richardson, C.A., 2008c. Effect of stabilization training on multifidus muscle cross-sectional area among young elite cricketers with low back pain. J Orthop Sports Phys Ther 38, 101–108.

Hides, J.A., Belavý, D.L., Cassar, L., Williams, M., Wilson, S.J., Richardson, C.A., 2009a. Altered response of the anterolateral abdominal muscles to simulated weight-bearing in subjects with low back pain. Eur Spine J 18, 410–418.

Hides, J., Lambrecht, G., Richardson, C., Damann, V., Armbrecht, G., Pruett, C., et al., 2009b. Effect of motor control re-training and general trunk strengthening on trunk muscle size after 60 days bed-rest, paper presented to Australian Physiotherapy Association National Conference Week, Sydney, Australia, October 2009.

Hides, J.A., Boughen, C.L., Stanton, W.R., Strudwick, M.W., Wilson, S.J., 2010a. A magnetic resonance imaging investigation of the transversus abdominis muscle during drawing-in of the abdominal wall in elite Australian Football League players with and without low back pain. J Orthop Sports Phys Ther 40, 4–10.

Hides, J., Fan, T., Stanton, W., Stanton, P., McMahon, K., Wilson, S., 2010b. Psoas and quadratus lumborum muscle asymmetry among elite Australian Football League players. Br J Sports Med 44, 563–567.

Hides, J.A., Stanton, W.R., Wilson, S.J., Freke, M., McMahon, S., Sims, K., 2010c. Retraining motor control of abdominal muscles among elite cricketers with low back pain. Scand J Med Sci Sports 20, 834–842.

Hides, J.A., Brown, C.T., Penfold, L., et al., 2011a. Screening the lumbopelvic muscles for a relationship to injury of the quadriceps, hamstrings, and adductor muscles among elite Australian football league players. J Orthop Sports Phys Ther 41, 767–775.

Hides, J., Hughes, B., Stanton, W., 2011b. Magnetic resonance imaging assessment of regional abdominal muscle function in elite AFL players with and without low back pain. Manual Ther 16, 279–284.

Hides, J.A., Lambrecht, G., Richardson, C.A., Stanton, W.R., Armbrecht, G., Pruett, C., et al., 2011c. The effects of rehabilitation on the muscles of the trunk following prolonged bed rest. Eur Spine J 20, 808–818.

Hides, J.A., Stanton, W.R., Mendis, M.D., Gildea, J., Sexton, M.J., 2012. Effect of motor control training on muscle size and football games missed from injury. Med Sci Sports Exercise 44, 1141–1149.

Hodges, P.W., Moseley, G.L., 2003. Pain and motor control of the lumbopelvic region: effect and possible mechanisms. J Electromyogr Kinesiol 13, 361–370.

Hodges, P.W., Richardson, C.A., 1996. Inefficient muscular stabilization of the lumbar spine associated with low back pain. A motor control evaluation of transversus abdominis. Spine 21, 2640–2650.

Hodges, P.W., Richardson, C.A., 1998. Delayed postural contraction of transversus abdominis in low back pain associated with movement of the lower limb. J Spinal Disorders 11, 46–56.

Hodges, P.W., Moseley, G.L., Gabrielsson, A., Gandevia, S.C., 2003. Acute experimental pain changes postural recruitment of the trunk muscles in pain-free humans. Exp Brain Res 151, 262–271.

Hodges, P.W., Eriksson, A.E., Shirley, D., Gandevia, S.C., 2005. Intra-abdominal pressure increases stiffness of the lumbar spine. J Biomech 38, 1873–1880.

Holguin, N., Muir, J., Rubin, C., Judex, S., 2009. Short applications of very low-magnitude vibrations attenuate expansion of the intervertebral disc during extended bed rest. Spine J 9, 470–477.

Hyde, J., Stanton, W.R., Hides, J.A., 2012. Abdominal muscle response to a simulated weight-bearing task by elite Australian Rules football players. Human Movement Sci 31, 129–138.

James, T., 2002. Hypertonicity of the iliopsoas muscle. J Myo 1, 1–6.

Johnston, S.L., Wear, M.L., Hamm, P.B., 1998. Increased incidence of herniated nucleus pulposus among astronauts and other selected populations (abstract). Aviation Space Environ Med 69, 220.

Kanehisa, H., Nemoto, T., Fukunaga, T., 2001. Strength capabilities of knee extensor muscles in junior speed skaters. J Sports Med Phys Fitness 41, 46–53.

Kanehisa, H., Funato, K., Kuno, S., Fukunaga, T., Katsuta, S., 2003. Growth trend of the quadriceps femoris muscle in junior Olympic weight lifters: an 18-month follow-up survey. Eur J Appl Physiol 89, 238–242.

Kelly, A.M., 1998. Does the clinically significant difference in visual analog scale pain scores vary with gender, age, or cause of pain? Acad Emergency Med 5, 1086–1090.

Kiefer, A., Shirazi-Adl, A., Parnianpour, M., 1997. Stability of the human spine in neutral postures. Eur Spine J 6, 45–53.

Kiesel, K.B., Uhl, T., Underwood, F.B., Nitz, A.J., 2008. Rehabilitative ultrasound measurement of select trunk muscle activation during induced pain. Man Ther 13, 132–138.

Lariviere, C., Gagnon, D., Loisel, P., 2000. The comparison of trunk muscles EMG activation between subjects with and without chronic low back pain during flexion-extension and lateral bending tasks. J Electromyogr Kinesiol 10, 79–91.

Leblanc, A.D., Schneider, V.S., Evans, H.J., Pientok, C., Rowe, R., Spector, E., 1992. Regional changes in muscle mass following 17 weeks of bed rest. J Appl Physiol 73, 2172–2178.

Leblanc, A.D., Evans, H.J., Schneider, V.S., Wendt, R.E. 3rd, Hedrick, T.D., 1994. Changes in intervertebral disc cross-sectional area with bed rest and space-flight. Spine 19, 812–817.

Leblanc, A., Rowe, R., Schneider, V., Evans, H., Hedrick, T., 1995. Regional muscle loss after short-duration spaceflight. Aviation Space Environ Med 66, 1151–1154.

Leblanc, A., Lin, C., Shackelford, L., Sinitsyn, V., Evans, H., Belichenko, O., et al., 2000. Muscle volume, MRI relaxation times (T2), and body composition after spaceflight. J Appl Physiol 89, 2158–2164.

Lee, S.U., Hargens, A.R., Fredericson, M., Lang, P.K., 2003. Lumbar spine disc heights and curvature: upright posture vs. supine compression harness. Aviation Space Environ Med 74, 512–516.

Macedo, L.G., Maher, C.G., Latimer, J., McAuley, J.H., 2009. Motor control exercise for persistent, nonspecific low back pain: a systematic review. Phys Ther 89, 9–25.

McGregor, A.H., Anderton, L., Gedroyc, W.M., 2002. The trunk muscles of elite oarsmen. Br J Sports Med 36, 214–217.

McLean, B.D., Tumilty, D.M., 1993. Left-right asymmetry in 2 types of soccer kick. Br J Sports Med 27, 260–262.

Mills, J.D., Taunton, J.E., Mills, W.A., 2005. The effect of a 10-week training regimen on lumbo-pelvic stability and athletic performance in female athletes: a randomized-controlled trial. Phys Ther Sport 6, 60–66.

Morris, J.M., Lucas, D.B., Bresler, B., 1961. Role of the trunk in stability of the spine. J Bone Joint Surg 43A, 327–351.

Mozes, M., Papa, M.Z., Zweig, A., Horoszowski, H., Adar, R., 1985. Iliopsoas injury in soccer players. Br J Sports Med 19, 168–170.

Neumann, P., Gill, V., 2002. Pelvic floor and abdominal muscle interaction: EMG activity and intra-abdominal pressure. Int Urogynecol J Pelvic Floor Dysfunc 13, 125–132.

Ng, J.K.F., Richardson, C.A., Parnian-pour, M., Kippers, V., 2002. EMG activity of trunk muscles and torque output during isometric axial rotation exertion: a comparison between back pain patients and matched controls. J Orthop Res 20, 112–121.

Orchard, J., 2001. Intrinsic and extrinsic risk factors for muscle strains in Australian football. Am J Sports Med 29, 300–303.

Orchard, J., James, T., 2003. Cricket Australia injury report 2003, Official report version 3.2. Cricket Australia 1, 1–28.

Orchard, J., Walt, S., Mcintosh, A., Garlick, D., 1999. Muscle activity during the drop punt kick. J Sports Sci 17, 837–838.

Orchard, J., James, T., Alcott, E., Carter, S., Parhart, P., 2002. Injuries in Australian cricket at first class level 1995/1996 to 2000/2001. Br J Sports Med 36, 270–274.

O'Sullivan, P.B., Twomey, L.T., Allison, G.T., 1997. Evaluation of specific stabilizing exercise in the treatment of chronic low back pain with radiologic diagnosis of spondylolysis or spondylolisthesis. Spine 22, 2959–2967.

Parkin, D., Smith, R., Schokman, P., 1987a. Questions – facts, fads and fallacies. In: Parkin, D., Smith, R., Schokman, P. (Eds.), Premiership Football: how to train, play and coach Australian Football, second ed. Hargreen, Melbourne, Australia, p. 204.

Parkin, D., Smith, R., Schokman, P., 1987b. Skill development. In: Parkin, D., Smith, R., Schokman, P. (Eds.), Premiership Football: how to train, play and coach Australian Football, second ed. Hargreen, Melbourne, Australia, p. 19.

Peltonen, J.E., Taimela, S., Erkintalo, M., Salminen, J.J., Oksanen, A., Kujala, U.M., 1998. Back extensor and psoas muscle cross-sectional area, prior physical training, and trunk muscle strength – a longitudinal study in adolescent girls. Eur J Appl Physiol Occup Physiol 77, 66–71.

Penning, L., 2000. Psoas muscle and lumbar spine stability: a concept uniting existing controversies – Critical review and hypothesis. Eur Spine J 9, 577–585.

Portus, M., Mason, B.R., Elliott, B.C., Pfitzner, M.C., Done, R.P., 2004. Technique factors related to ball release speed and trunk injuries in high performance cricket fast bowlers. Sports Biomech 3, 263–284.

Ranson, C., Burnett, A., O'Sullivan, P., Batt, M., Kerslake, R., 2008. The lumbar paraspinal muscle morphometry of fast bowlers in cricket. Clin J Sport Med 18, 31–37.

Richardson, C.A., Jull, G.A., Hodges, P.W., Hides, J., 1999. Therapeutic Exercise for Spinal Segmental Stabilization in Low Back Pain. Churchill Livingstone, Edinburgh.

Richardson, C.A., Hides, J.A., Wilson, S., Stanton, W., Snijders, C.J., 2004a. Lumbo-pelvic joint protection against antigravity forces: motor control and segmental stiffness assessed with magnetic resonance imaging. J Gravitat Physiol 11, P119–122.

Richardson, C.A., Hodges, P.W., Hides, J.A., 2004b. Therapeutic Exercise for Lumbo-Pelvic Stabilization: a motor control approach for the treatment and prevention of low back pain. Churchill Livingstone, Edinburgh.

Sitilertpisan, P., Hides, J., Stanton, W., Paungmali, A., Pirusan, U., 2012. Multifidus muscle size and symmetry among elite weightlifters. Phys Ther Sport 13, 11–15.

Stewart, S., Stanton, W., Wilson, S., Hides, J., 2010. Consistency in size and asymmetry of the psoas major muscle among elite footballers. Br J Sports Med 44, 1173–1177.

Stokes, M., Rankin, G., Newham, D.J., 2005. Ultrasound imaging of lumbar multifidus muscle: normal reference ranges for measurements and practical guidance on the technique. Man Ther 10, 116–126.

Stuge, B., Veierod, M.B., Laerum, E., Vøllestad, N., 2004. The efficacy of a treatment program focusing on specific stabilizing exercises for pelvic girdle pain after pregnancy – a two-year follow-up of a randomized clinical trial. Spine 29, E197–E203.

Todd, K.H., Funk, K.G., Funk, J.P., Bonacci, R., 1996. Clinical significance of reported changes in pain severity. Ann Emerg Med 27, 485–489.

Tsao, H., Hodges, P.W., 2007. Immediate changes in feedforward postural adjustments following voluntary motor training. Exp Brain Res 181, 537–546.

Tsao, H., Hodges, P.W., 2008. Persistence of improvements in postural strategies following motor control training in people with recurrent low back pain. J Electromyogr Kinesiol 18, 559–567.

Van, K., Hides, J.A., Richardson, C.A., 2006. The use of real-time ultrasound imaging for biofeedback of lumbar multifidus muscle contraction in healthy subjects. J Orthop Sports Phys Ther 36, 920–925.

Van Dieen, J.H., Cholewicki, J., Radebold, A., 2003. Trunk muscle recruitment patterns in patients with low back pain enhance the stability of the lumbar spine. Spine 28, 834–841.

Walker, D., Engstrom, C., Buckley, R. 1999. Evaluating lumbar spine injuries in young athletes with magnetic resonance imaging. In: Abstracts of the 5th IOC World Congress on Sport Science. Canberra, ACT, Sports Medicine Australia.

Wallace, R., Neal, R., Engstrom, C., Hunter, J., Walker, D., Hanna, A., et al., 1997. A sticky wicket: the continuing problem of lumbar spine injuries in cricket fast bowlers. Sport Health 15, 6–9.

Wallwork, T.L., Stanton, W.R., Freke, M., Hides, J.A., 2009. The effect of chronic low back pain on size and contraction of the lumbar multifidus muscle. Man Ther 14, 496–500.

Wing, P.C., Tsang, I.K.Y., Susak, L., Gagnon, F., Gagnon, R., Potts, J.E., 1991. Back pain and spinal changes in microgravity. Orthop Clin North Am 22, 255–262.

Zazulak, B.T., Hewett, T.E., Reeves, N.P., Goldberg, B., Cholewicki, J., 2007a. Deficits in neuromuscular control of the trunk predict knee injury risk: a prospective biomechanical-epidemiologic study. Am J Sports Med 35, 1123–1130.

Zazulak, B.T., Hewett, T.E., Reeves, N.P., Goldberg, B., Cholewicki, J., 2007b. The effects of core proprioception on knee injury: a prospective biomechanical-epidemiological study. Am J Sports Med 35, 368–373.

Chapter |10|

Existing muscle synergies and low back pain: a case for preventative intervention

Jack P. Callaghan* and Erika Nelson-Wong[†]
*Faculty of Applied Health Sciences, University of Waterloo, Waterloo, Ontario, Canada, and [†]Rueckert–Hartman College of Health Professions,
School of Physical Therapy, Regis University, Denver, Colorado, USA

INTRODUCTION

Recruitment strategies, endurance and strength of torso musculature have all been examined for a potential link with low back pain (LBP) with mixed levels of success. One of the primary barriers has been the isolation of whether the inherent muscle responses were pre-existing to low back pain development or developed post-pain presentation. A second issue has been the examination of individual muscle responses in isolation from other agonist and antagonist muscle groups. This chapter examines the need for more integrative muscle control assessments examining the timing and co-activation of muscle groups. A case is made that low back pain may be linked to pre-existing muscle control strategies in asymptomatic individuals through the use of a subacute transient pain model induced by 2 hours of prolonged standing.

BACKGROUND

Many risk factors have been identified for the development of low back injury, including anthropometric characteristics, lumbar hypomobility, reduced lumbar lordosis, psychological distress and previous low back injury (Adams et al. 1999), as well as specific mechanical loading factors (Norman et al. 1998). However, LBP is a complex, multifactorial process with pathoanatomical, neurophysiological, physical and psychosocial components (Linton 2000; Kumar 2001; Waddell 2004) potentially contributing to low back dysfunction. Therefore, the effective prediction of who will develop LBP remains problematic (Leboeuf-Yde et al. 1997).

Prolonged standing as a risk factor for low back pain

Epidemiological studies have shown that standing occupations have a strong association with LBP (Andersen et al. 2007; Roelen et al. 2008). Checkout clerks and individuals in other occupations often have long periods of standing and are known to develop LBP as the length of time on their feet increases (Kim et al. 1994). In a 2-year prospective study of Danish workers across 30 different industries,

Andersen and colleagues (2007) found that requiring prolonged periods of occupational standing (>30 minutes out of each hour) was one of the strongest predictors of LBP with a hazard ratio of 2:1 (95% CI 1.3–3.3). Another study in Dutch workers reported that prolonged standing was related to increased pain reporting in the low back and thoracic region (Roelen et al. 2008). Prolonged standing has been strongly associated with LBP incidence, but not all workers exposed to prolonged standing will become LBP developers.

Altered muscle activation in the presence of low back pain

Differences in muscle activation patterns between people with LBP and healthy controls have been very well documented, although the interpretation of these differences remains a matter of debate (van Dieën et al. 2003b). Results vary depending upon whether participants were sub-classified or treated as a homogeneous LBP group. Findings also appear to be task-dependent. A common finding has been the presence of generally increased trunk muscle activation in individuals with LBP (Lariviere et al. 2000; van Dieën et al. 2003a; Burnett et al. 2004; Silfies et al. 2005; Dankaerts et al. 2006; Pirouzi et al. 2006). There is evidence that LBP also impacts coordination of trunk and hip musculature as differences in muscle onsets, offsets and durations have been found between those with LBP and healthy controls during different tasks, including single leg standing, and trunk flexion/extension cycles (Leinonen et al. 2000; Hungerford et al. 2003; Ferguson et al. 2004). Studies of fatigability in LBP patients versus control subjects have produced conflicting findings. Kankaanpaa and colleagues (1998) reported increased fatigability of the gluteus maximus and lumbar paraspinal muscles in LBP groups during an isometric back extension task. In contrast, da Silva et al. (2005) found no differences in lumbar paraspinal muscle fatigue or strength between LBP and control groups during three different assessment protocols.

The Flexion Relaxation Phenomenon (FRP) is a period of myoelectrical silence of the lumbar extensor muscles when an individual stands in full flexion, and has been confirmed in multiple studies of asymptomatic individuals (Paquet et al. 1994). It has been proposed that the FRP is an indication of loads being shifted to the passive structures (ligaments), or being taken over by deeper muscles not accessible by surface EMG recording (Callaghan and Dunk 2002). FRP can be quantified through a ratio of trunk extensor muscle activation in the upright position to muscle activation in the flexed position, or the Flexion Relaxation Ratio (FRR) (Dankaerts et al. 2006). FRP has been shown to be absent or diminished in LBP patients, although this effect appears to be achieved through a different muscle activation pattern (failure to relax the

extensors versus increased activation of the extensors) depending upon the patient's clinical sub-classification (Paquet et al. 1994; Dankaerts et al. 2006).

Agonist/antagonist co-activation has also been reported in LBP patients (van Dieën et al. 2003a; Dankaerts et al. 2006; Pirouzi et al. 2006), although not all studies have found this to be the case (Silfies et al. 2005). The presence of increased agonist/antagonist co-activation appears to be highly task-dependent.

Motor control patterns and low back pain: predisposing versus adaptive factors?

It is well known that motor control impairments occur with non-specific LBP. These are commonly considered to be secondary to pain (van Dieën et al. 2003b), and are proposed to be adaptive and protective in nature (van Dieën et al. 2003a). Because of this premise, it has been suggested that no attempt should be made to normalize or correct these 'adaptive' motor patterns (van Dieën et al. 2003a, 2003b; O'Sullivan 2005). Several research groups have suggested that there is also a 'maladaptive' motor control impairment where the alteration in motor pattern is not protective, but instead results in provocation of pain and abnormal tissue loading (Burnett et al. 2004; McGill 2004; O'Sullivan 2005). In these cases, it is suggested that correction of the maladaptive motor pattern may be beneficial.

It should be noted, however, that regardless of the terminology used ('adaptive' vs. 'maladaptive'), the motor pattern in question has previously been considered to be in response to some initial LBP or injury, and therefore both should essentially be considered to be adaptations of the motor control system to LBP. Since most prior research has utilized intact subject groups (those who already have a clinical presentation of LBP vs. healthy controls), it is impossible to answer the question of whether alterations in motor control are predisposing or adaptive in nature. The presence of a dysfunctional motor control pattern in a healthy individual may in fact predispose them to develop a non-specific LBP disorder for the same reasons that O'Sullivan's 'maladaptive' subgroup is thought to perpetuate and worsen their disorder through faulty movement and control (O'Sullivan, 2005).

The existing published studies that have investigated the pain–spasm–pain and pain adaptation models are largely based on animal studies, and artificially induced episodes of acute pain in humans through injection of noxious substances (van Dieen et al. 2003b). Both of these models suggest that altered motor control patterns are adaptive in nature, while one (pain–spasm–pain) can be considered to be 'maladaptive' and have the effect of perpetuating the painful disorder, and the other is appropriately adaptive and serves to protect the system (pain adaptation). Neither model allows for the possibility that altered motor control might actually be a contributing factor for the initial development of LBP, and might in some cases be considered to be causal.

Stabilization-based exercise as an intervention for low back pain

It is becoming widely accepted that patients who receive treatments that are matched to a sub-classification category have better outcomes than those receiving unmatched treatments (Fritz et al. 2007). Most clinical guidelines for the treatment of LBP include some form of supervised exercise as an intervention (Airaksinen et al. 2006); the appropriate prescription, optimal level of supervision and dosing, however, have been less well established. Exercise intervention for patients with LBP is an accepted part of physical therapy practice and is included as a stand-alone first-line treatment or as an adjunct to manual therapy in most practice patterns (Hayden et al. 2005; Ferreira et al. 2007). In a systematic review, Hayden and colleagues (2005) found that the most effective exercise intervention strategy was to individually tailor a programme to the patient, deliver it in a supervised format with regular follow-up with the therapist, and encourage patient adherence to the programme in order to achieve high dosage. These authors also reported that exercise programmes with an emphasis on muscle strengthening appeared to be most effective. Other research has investigated the response to

stabilization-based exercise intervention in patients with low back pain, with a primary focus on identification of predictive factors for positive outcomes (Hicks et al. 2005).

TRANSIENT LBP MODEL

A functionally induced LBP model was used as a prospective design to study factors linked to LBP development during prolonged standing exposures (Gregory and Callaghan 2008; Gregory et al. 2008; Nelson-Wong et al. 2008). The rationale for this protocol is that a percentage of individuals who have no prior history of LBP develop considerable levels of LBP during the common, functional task of prolonged standing. This allows for a standardized laboratory approach for the evaluation of biological responses and their relationship to pain development. This protocol has proven effective for inducing LBP in 40–65% of asymptomatic individuals with no lifetime history of LBP (Gregory and Callaghan 2008; Gregory et al. 2008; Nelson-Wong et al. 2008). This allows for separation of pain developers (PD) and non-pain developers (NPD) during the prolonged standing exposure. Using the pain grouping also allowed for investigation of an exercise-based intervention on factors deemed to be important in low back pain development (Fig. 10.1).

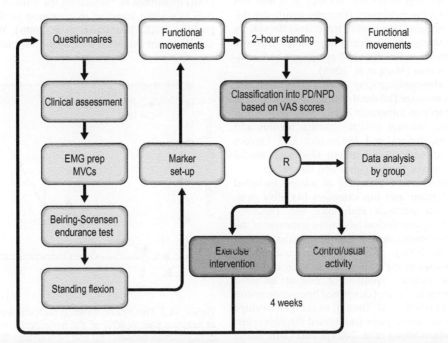

Figure 10.1 Flowchart of the experimental protocol for the two data collection days separated by a 4-week period.

The prolonged standing protocol involved standing at a workstation for a 2-hour period while completing simulated occupational tasks. Participants were constrained within a 1.12 m² area to be in contact with two force platforms but were otherwise allowed to shift their weight and move around within the limits of the force platforms.

To assess the pain developed, a 100 mm visual analogue scale (VAS) with end-point anchors of 'no pain' and 'worst pain imaginable' for the low back were completed at baseline and every 15 minutes. Additional clinically relevant measures were assessed including physical activity history (Minnesota Leisure Time Physical Activity Questionnaire, MPAQ (Folsom et al. 1986)), and a questionnaire to assess attitudes towards pain, injury and disability was completed (compilation of questions from the Cognitive Risk Profile for Pain, CRPP (Cook and DeGood 2006), Survey of Pain Attitudes-b, SOPA-b (Tait and Chibnall 1997) and the Fear Avoidance Beliefs Questionnaire, FABQ (Waddell et al. 1993)). Standardized physiotherapy assessments included active and passive hip and lumbar range of motion, assessment of core stability as demonstrated by active straight leg raise (ASLR) (Mens et al. 1999) and active side-lying hip abduction (AHAbd) (Nelson-Wong et al. 2009), time to fatigue in side support (McGill et al. 1999; Hicks et al. 2005), assessment of lumbar segmental mobility (Hicks et al. 2003) and prone instability testing (Hicks et al. 2003; Hicks et al. 2005).

Participants were considered to be PD if a change in VAS score greater than 10 mm from baseline was recorded. The 10 mm threshold VAS value was chosen, as 9 mm has been found to be the minimum clinically significant difference in VAS, representing a small treatment effect (Kelly 1998) and the Minimally Clinically Important Difference (MCID) for patients to feel their LBP symptoms had worsened was only 8 mm (Hagg et al. 2003).

Continuous electromyography (EMG) data were collected from 16 muscles (bilateral thoracic erector spinae, lumbar erector spinae, latissimus dorsi, rectus abdominis, external oblique, internal oblique, gluteus medius and maximus). Three-dimensional kinematics and kinetics were determined with an 8-segment rigid link model (bilateral feet, shanks, thighs, pelvis and thorax).

Primary biomechanical measures of interest included fatigability of lumbar and hip extensors (da Silva et al. 2005) during an extensor endurance test (Beiring–Sorenson position) and flexion relaxation response of the trunk and hip extensors during standing lumbar flexion (Dankaerts et al. 2006), as well as the acute muscle activation responses to the prolonged standing exposure. The muscle activation responses of interest included co-activation of muscle pairs (quantified by co-contraction coefficient, CCI (Lewek et al. 2004)), phase relationships of onsets between muscle pairs (quantified through cross-correlation (Nelson-Wong et al. 2009)), and Gaps analyses (Veiersted et al. 1990)).

RESPONSE TO INDUCED LBP

Baseline responses

The 43 participants clearly separated into two distinct groups, with 17 of the 43 (40%) participants being classified as PDs. The time developing pain (Fig. 10.2) resulted in averaged maximum VAS scores of 22.7 ± 2.91 mm for PD and 1.37 ± 0.45 mm for NPD. Both groups exhibited similar anthropometric characteristics, baseline VAS scores, physical activity levels, attitudes towards pain and disability, scores on the majority of the clinical assessment measures and extensor fatigability.

There were only two measures taken prior to pain development that related to the pain group classification. Individuals in the PD group demonstrated greater difficulty in maintaining the frontal plane position of the pelvis during active hip abduction in side-lying (AHAbd test) (Nelson-Wong et al. 2009). The AHAbd test was designed to challenge the trunk musculature during active lower limb movement in a destabilized position of side-lying with extended lower extremities. The finding that pain developers had greater difficulty controlling this movement and maintaining the trunk in a neutral position during a relatively low demand challenge supports the concept of decreased trunk control during an upright posture, and perhaps is an indicator of a pre-existing motor control deficiency in this group. The second measure that identified the PDs *a priori* was a flexion–relaxation response (FRR) quantified by calculating the ratio of muscle activation in upright standing to activation in the fully flexed position (FRR) (Dankaerts et al. 2006). While no back muscle group exhibited a different response between the

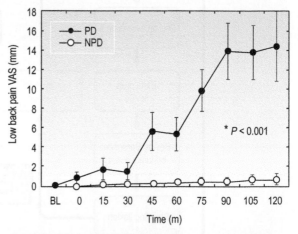

Figure 10.2 The 2-hour standing protocol was successful at inducing pain in 40% of the participants, with a clear differentiation between PD and NPD groups (time by group interaction significant at $P<0.001$).

pain groups, gluteus maximus was found to have an increased relaxation response (3.4 ± 6.8) in PDs compared with NPDs (0.91 ± 1.0), with a larger FRR value indicating higher muscle activation in upright standing than in the flexed position. The finding of increased FRR for the gluteus maximus in PD individuals is consistent with earlier reports of gluteal hypoactivity in patients with LBP (Leinonen et al. 2000).

Prolonged standing responses

There were very minor postural changes observed over the 2-hour standing exposure, with no differences detected between PD/NPD groups. Similarly, there were no substantial changes in low back joint kinetics that identified different responses between the PD and NPD groups.

Typical measures of muscle activation state, such as mean activation level, did not separate the PD and NPD groups for any back muscle. The only single muscle data analysis that reveled a PD/NPD difference was a measure of total Gap time (time the muscle spent at < 0.05% maximum voluntary contraction (MVC) over 15-minute blocks) for both right and left gluteus medius muscles. The NPD group consistently had longer total Gap times than the PD group for the bilateral gluteus medius muscles. The NPD group responded as the standing duration progressed by decreasing their total Gap time, where the PD group remained at a relatively constant Gap time throughout the entire standing exposure (Fig. 10.3).

Due to minimal difference in posture, low back joint kinetics and isolated muscle activation responses, analyses incorporating antagonistic and synergistic muscle activation patterns were undertaken to assess the involvement of motor control strategies on the development of LBP.

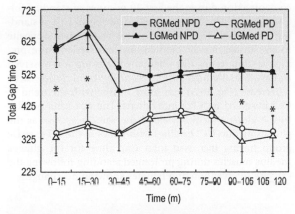

Figure 10.3 The total Gap time for bilateral gluteus medius muscles decreased over time for the NPD group, while it stayed relatively constant for the PD group during the standing exposure. NPD individuals had longer total Gap times than PDs for these muscles at the beginning and end of the standing protocol (* designates $P<0.05$).

First, trunk muscle activation profiles were cross-correlated against the right gluteus medius (RGMd) and the relative recruitment relationship was determined. The right gluteus medius muscle was chosen as a reference as it was at a distal endpoint of the kinetic chain for muscles being monitored, and enabled the discussion of muscle onsets within the context of 'top-down' versus 'bottom-up' control. A 'top-down' control strategy has been shown previously for the trunk muscles during walking and during perturbations in standing (Prince et al. 1994). There was a consistent pattern across both PD and NPD groups to activate the trunk muscles following the RGMd, indicating a predominantly 'bottom-up' control strategy. A second approach to assess muscle control as an explanatory factor in the LBP responses involved examining the co-contraction index (CCI) for all 120 possible muscle pair combinations. This approach successfully identified differences between the PD/NPD groups. All trunk flexor/extensor CCI combinations revealed higher levels of muscle co-activation for the PD group at the beginning and end of the 2-hour standing period. Average CCI values over 12 combinations of bilateral lumbar extensor muscles and six flexor groups revealed the PD group had higher levels of co-contraction and that the control strategy varied differently compared to the NPD group over the two hours (Fig. 10.4). A similar finding was also present for the bilateral gluteus medius muscles, with PDs having significantly higher levels of bilateral gluteus medius co-activation during the first and final 30 minutes of standing (Fig. 10.4).

When the CCI are linked with the pain scores, the PD group exhibited increased co-activation muscle patterns as a precursor to the increase in their subjective reports of pain development. During the time period from 30 to 90 minutes, the NPD group had an increase in trunk muscle co-activation without any commensurate increase in pain rating levels (Fig. 10.4a). The PD group showed the reverse pattern with a general decrease in muscle co-activation, although this was the time period where VAS rating was increasing the most (Fig. 10.4b). During this period of increased pain development, there was a strong negative correlation between VAS score and co-contraction index for the bilateral gluteus medius and trunk flexor-extensor groups ($r = -0.73$ and $r = -0.92$, respectively). The co-contraction indices for these muscle groups were negatively correlated ($r = -0.39$ for gluteus medius, and $r = -0.18$ for trunk flexor-extensors) for the PD and NPD groups, showing a clearly different muscle control strategy between the two groups.

IMPACT OF PREVENTATIVE INTERVENTION

The presence of pre-existing motor control strategies that may predispose an individual to developing LBP

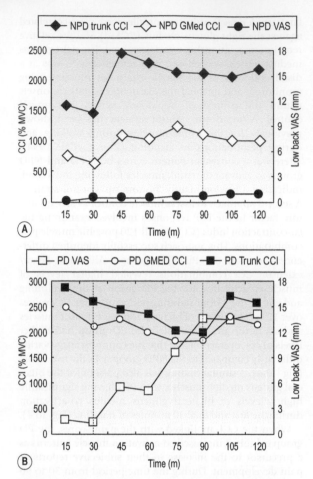

Figure 10.4 (A) Over the 2-hour prolonged standing period, the NPD group showed an average increase in co-activation of both the trunk flexor-extensor and bilateral gluteus medius muscles. (B) Corresponding to the steepest slope of VAS, the PD group had a decrease in co-activation of trunk flexor-extensors and bilateral gluteus medius muscles.

raises the question of whether these responses can be altered. A four-week exercise intervention was undertaken to determine if the muscle control strategies present in the PD group could be altered, and all 43 participants were re-tested with the 2-hour standing protocol after 4 weeks. Half of each of the PD/NPD groups was randomly assigned to exercise intervention or control/usual activity groups. The exercise programme was monitored and progressed on a weekly basis by a licensed physiotherapist, with participants completing exercises independently at home 3–5 times per week. The exercises were from stabilization-based programmes for clinical LBP patients (Hicks et al. 2005) and included: abdominal bracing with heel slides and straight leg raises; arm and leg extensions in quadruped; bridging in supine; standing rows with resistance band; side-bridge support; 'clamshells' in side-lying; and single leg wall-slide squat with abdominal bracing.

A subjective improvement in LBP during prolonged standing was found for the PD group assigned to exercise intervention with no change in either of the NPD groups' VAS scores or the PD control group.

The control groups (both PD and NPD) and the NPD exercise intervention group had no change in gluteus medius co-contraction during the second prolonged standing session after 4 weeks. A consistent pattern of trunk flexor/extensor CCI was present on the second test, however the control PD group and both NPD groups had lower CCI scores. The PD control group followed the same modulation of trunk CCI as was seen on the initial testing day, with a marked decrease in trunk CCI during the middle stages of standing (from 30 to 60 minutes) when LBP was increasing most rapidly. There were also no changes between the two test days in the muscle rest (Gaps analyses) for the bilateral gluteus medius for these three groups.

Pain developers' response to exercise intervention

The PD group responded in a positive fashion to the exercise intervention. There were alterations in the muscle control strategies that followed the reduction in LBP scores. There were gender-specific responses that were not present in the other three groups or present in the PD group during the initial testing session.

PD males responded to the exercise intervention with an overall decrease in the CCI of the gluteus medius muscles whereas females exhibited no change in this motor control strategy. Both genders demonstrated a change in the trunk flexor/extensor CCI with decreased co-contraction during the first 30 minutes of standing followed by an increase in trunk flexor/extensor CCI as standing progressed. This motor control pattern was opposite to the trunk muscle modulation observed on the pre-intervention testing day where the PD group was observed to have initially high CCI levels at the trunk followed by a decrease (Fig. 10.5) and more in line with the trend of CCI observed in NPD individuals. The rest time profiles in the gluteus medius yielded the same response as the gluteus medius CCI findings with males in the PD exercise group having increased total Gap time for the gluteus medius muscles during prolonged standing following the exercise intervention and females showing no change.

DISCUSSION AND IMPLICATIONS

Individuals with no present or historical indications of LBP have clear motor control strategies that predispose them to developing functionally induced LBP. The motor

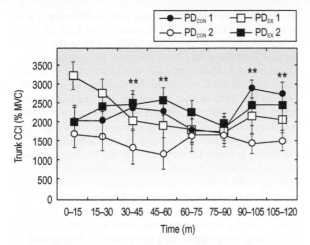

Figure 10.5 PD$_{EX}$ had an initial decrease, followed by increased trunk co-contraction. PD$_{CON}$ demonstrated decreased trunk co-contraction on day 2 throughout the 2-hour standing period.

control strategies were assessed using muscle co-contraction and the exhibited pain-inducing control strategies demonstrated positive pain mitigating responses to an exercise intervention.

Specific responses to a transient functionally induced LBP model revealed pre-existing low back and hip motor control strategies. Co-contraction of the bilateral gluteus medius muscles and trunk flexor/extensor muscles was a consistent finding in LBP developers. There was a consistent indication that NPD and PD individuals have very different muscle activation patterns, particularly at the hip, that manifest in the early stages of a prolonged standing task. Modulation of these patterns as standing exposure time increases also differs between the two groups. PD individuals demonstrated higher levels of muscle co-activation than NPD individuals immediately upon the initiation of the standing protocol, prior to any subjective reports of LBP. This supports the contention that this muscle co-activation pattern is not an adaptive response to LBP, and appears to be an important factor in the predisposition of individuals who experience LBP during standing. While PDs had higher initial levels of co-contraction, the muscle co-contraction control strategy for the PD group exhibited a decreasing trend in CCI over time whereas the NPDs increased their co-contraction levels. Increased trunk muscle co-activation during a prolonged posture may be an appropriate motor control strategy to maintain a relatively static posture in a pain-free state. The major difference in the muscle co-contraction strategy employed by the PD group was a reduction in CCI corresponding to the period of greatest pain development. During the final 30 minutes of standing the PD group increased their gluteus medius muscle co-activation levels

once more, and this was the time period where their VAS scores levelled off, or stabilized. The question remains as to whether this was an adaptive response to their increasing discomfort that resulted in a motor pattern change, or whether LBP was stabilizing for some other reason which allowed the participants to revert to their 'usual' muscle co-activation pattern.

There were additional muscle activation differences that are consistent with the findings of increased co-contraction at the hip in the PD group. Most notable are the total rest time (total Gap time) for the muscle groups at the hip that was less for the PD group than that of the NPD group. This suggests that there may be a fatigue component that ties into the development of LBP in these individuals. The different muscle activation patterns demonstrated by the PD group during the initial stages of standing may predispose them to fatigue as the task duration progresses. Van Dieën and colleagues (2009) found evidence of fatigue, as demonstrated by negative mean power frequency (MPF) slopes, in the lumbar extensors with sustained contractions at as low as 2% and 5% MVC with greater fatigue in muscles that had lower variability in activation level during a 30-minute exertion. The PDs in this study had a shorter total Gap duration in the hip musculature during prolonged standing, indicating that they had less variability in their muscle activation patterns than the NPDs. These findings suggest that the PD group might be more susceptible to fatigue during the prolonged standing task and this may be one potential mechanism for their LBP development.

Because the LBP developers in this study had difficulty with maintaining postural control when asked to perform a low-level challenge directed at the core trunk stabilizers during the AHAbd test, there is some support for the hypothesis that co-activation at the hip during prolonged standing is a compensatory motor control pattern that has been adopted by these individuals. This appears to be a dysfunctional muscle activation pattern in that it does not protect these individuals from developing pain during a common, low-level activity. Several studies have shown altered postural and trunk control in response to perturbations in individuals with LBP (Henry et al. 2006; Brumagne et al. 2008; Silfies et al. 2009). Therefore, impairments in trunk and pelvis control during a self-initiated perturbation (AHAbd) may be indicative that a similar deficiency to perturbation reported for LBP individuals exists in the PD group. Co-activation at the hip during standing may serve as an attempt to compensate for an inability to adequately utilize core trunk muscles for postural stability during prolonged standing.

With the implementation of an exercise intervention it was expected that if PDs were going to benefit by having decreased LBP, they would also have decreased co-contraction of these muscle groups. Male PDs in the exercise group had a general decrease in co-contraction of the gluteus medius muscles, however females in the same group did not demonstrate similar responses. A different response was observed for trunk flexor/extensor co-contraction with both genders having an initial decrease in trunk CCI, followed by increased co-contraction, where on the first day they initially had elevated CCI of the trunk, followed by a decrease as standing duration progressed. A response to training was also present in the total rest in the right gluteus medius. Males in the PD exercise group demonstrated longer total Gap lengths during the standing exposure, indicating they were increasing the amount of time the muscle was spending in the resting state following the exercise intervention. The presented theory that low-level muscle fatigue may be one of the mechanisms underlying the LBP development is supported by this increased rest time in the initial stages of standing, combined with decreased VAS scores. This is consistent with the finding of decreased CCI for this group. These changes and the decreased LBP VAS scores support the idea that co-contraction of the trunk flexor/extensor musculature may be beneficial for preventing LBP development during a static, prolonged posture. The PD exercise group may have been attempting to 'brace' the trunk musculature during standing since this bracing manoeuvre was emphasized during the exercise intervention. There was no change in the NPD exercise group, indicating no negative consequences associated with the exercise intervention as they did not have a pain experience on either collection day and therefore may not have altered any abdominal bracing or co-contraction control strategies. In contrast, it could be that gluteus medius co-contraction is a maladaptive response manifested as an inability to provide adequate postural control at the trunk, and is therefore a predisposing factor for LBP development.

Findings from the first year of a longitudinal follow-up of the test group indicate that low back pain development during a 2-hour standing exposure may predict an increased risk for future development of clinical LBP. In the initial 12 months after taking part in the study, 3 participants required medical intervention for LBP. Of these 3 individuals, 2 had been identified as PD in the experimental study and had been assigned to control groups. The other individual (also assigned to the control group) had been classified as NPD in this study using the threshold criteria of >10 mm change in VAS during the first standing exposure day. However, on the second testing day, this individual reported a change in VAS of 20 mm, a score that would have resulted in a classification of PD. Of further interest, the intervention that these individuals received consisted mainly of core stabilization exercises (similar to those described in this study) and all responded well to these. These preliminary findings indicate that, although these studies were conducted in an asymptomatic sample, early identification of subclinical control issues may be possible and early intervention aimed at preventing future LBP development may be appropriate and effective.

This chapter presents a case that many of the commonly accepted 'adaptations' to LBP may actually be present as predisposing factors prior to the manifestation of a clinical LBP problem, specifically identifying the association of hip abductor muscle co-activation prior to the development of LBP during standing. While the exact mechanisms of LBP development during standing remain elusive, it is clear from this study that exercise intervention directed at the trunk and hip does have some effect on the muscle activation patterns of those muscle groups during the functionally induced LBP. There was a significant decrease in subjective VAS scores in the exercise group; however, it is difficult to say unequivocally that this was entirely due to the exercise intervention. Accompanying changes in muscle activation patterns after training do indicate that there is a potential to intervene in individuals who have pre-existing motor control patterns that may predispose them to developing LBP.

REFERENCES

Adams, M.A., Mannion, A.F., Dolan, P., 1999. Personal risk factors for first-time low back pain. Spine 24, 2497–2505.

Airaksinen, O., Brox, J.I., Cedraschi, C., Hildebrandt, J., Klaber-Moffett, J., Kovacs, F.M., 2006. European guidelines for the management of chronic non-specific low back pain. Eur Spine J 15, S192–S300.

Andersen, J.H., Haahr, J.P., Frost, P., 2007. Risk factors for more severe regional musculoskeletal symptoms. Arthritis Rheum 56, 1355–1364.

Brumagne, S., Janssens, L., Knapen, S., Claeys, K., Suuden-Johanson, E.,

2008. Persons with recurrent low back pain exhibit a rigid postural control strategy. Eur Spine J 17, 1177–1184.

Burnett, A.F., Cornelius, M.W., Dankaerts, W., O'Sullivan, P.B., 2004. Spinal kinematics and trunk muscle activity in cyclists: a comparison between healthy controls and non-specific chronic low back pain subjects-a pilot investigation. Man Ther 9, 211–219.

Callaghan, J.P., Dunk, N.M., 2002. Examination of the flexion relaxation phenomenon in erector spinae muscles during short duration

slumped sitting. Clin Biomech. 17, 353–360.

Cook, A.J., Degood, D.E., 2006. The cognitive risk profile for pain: development of a self-report inventory for identifying beliefs and attitudes that interfere with pain management. Clin J Pain 22, 332–345.

Da Silva, R.A., Arsenault, A.B., Gravel, D., Lariviere, C., De Oliveira, E., 2005. Back muscle strength and fatigue in healthy and chronic low back pain subjects: a comparative study of 3 assessment protocols. Arch Phys Med Rehabil 86, 722–729.

Dankaerts, W., O'sullivan, P., Burnett, A., Straker, L., 2006. Altered patterns of superficial trunk muscle activation during sitting in nonspecific chronic low back pain patients: importance of subclassification. Spine 31, 2017–2023.

Ferguson, S.A., Marras, W.S., Burr, D.L., Davis, K.G., Gupta, P., 2004. Differences in motor recruitment and resulting kinematics between low back pain patients and asymptomatic participants during lifting exertions. Clin Biomech 19, 992–999.

Ferreira, M.L., Ferreira, P.H., Latimer, J., Herbert, R.D., Hodges, P.W., Jennings, M.D., et al., 2007. Comparison of general exercise, motor control exercise and spinal manipulative therapy for chronic low back pain: a randomized trial. Pain 131, 31–37.

Folsom, A.R., Jacobs, D.R., Caspersen, C.J., Gomez-Marin, O., Knudsen, J., 1986. Test–retest reliability of the Minnesota Leisure Time Physical Activity Questionnaire. J Chron Dis 39, 505–511.

Fritz, J., Cleland, J.A., Childs, J.D., 2007. Subgrouping patients with low back pain: evolution of a classification approach to physical therapy. J Orthop Sports Phys Ther. 37, 290–302.

Gregory, D.E., Brown, S.H.M., Callaghan, J.P., 2008. Trunk muscle responses to suddenly applied loads: do individuals who develop discomfort during prolonged standing respond differently? J Electromyogr Kinesiol 18, 495–502.

Gregory, D.E., Callaghan, J.P., 2008. Prolonged standing as a precursor for the development of low back discomfort: An investigation of possible mechanisms. Gait Posture 28, 86–92.

Hagg, O., Fritzell, P., Nordwall, A., 2003. The clinical importance of changes in outcome scores after treatment for low back pain. Eur Spine J 12, 12–20.

Hayden, J.A., Van Tulder, M., Tomlinson, G., 2005. Systematic Review: Strategies for using exercise therapy to improve outcomes in chronic low back pain. Ann Intern Med 142, 776–785.

Henry, S.M., Hitt, J.R., Jones, S.L., Bunn, J.Y., 2006. Decreased limits of stability in response to postural perturbations in subjects with low back pain. Clin Biomech 21, 881–892.

Hicks, G.E., Fritz, J.M., Delitto, A., McGill, S.M., 2005. Preliminary development of a clinical prediction rule for determining which patients with low back pain will respond to a stabilization exercise program. Arch Phys Med Rehabil 86, 1753–1762.

Hicks, G.E., Fritz, J.M., Delitto, A., Mishock, J., 2003. Interrater reliability of clinical examination measures for identification of lumbar segmental instability. Arch Phys Med Rehabil 84, 1858–1864.

Hungerford, B., Gilleard, W., Hodges, P., 2003. Evidence of altered lumbopelvic muscle recruitment in the presence of sacroiliac joint pain. Spine 28, 1593–1600.

Kankaanpaa, M., Taimela, S., Laaksonen, D., Hanninen, O., Airaksinen, O., 1998. Back and hip extensor fatigability in chronic low back pain patients and controls. Arch Phys Med Rehabil 79, 412–417.

Kelly, A.-M., 1998. Does the clinically significant difference in visual analog scale pain scores vary with gender, age, or cause of pain? Acad Emerg Med 5, 1086–1090.

Kim, J.Y., Stuart-Buttle, C., Marras, W.S., 1994. The effects of mats on back and leg fatigue. Appl Ergon 25, 29–34.

Kumar, S., 2001. Theories of musculoskeletal injury causation. Ergonomics 44, 17–47.

Lariviere, C., Gagnon, D., Loisel, P., 2000. The comparison of trunk muscles EMG activation between subjects with and without chronic low back pain during flexion-extension and lateral bending tasks. J Electromyogr Kinesiol 10, 79–91.

Leboeuf-Yde, C., Lauritsen, J.M., Lauritzen, T., 1997. Why has the search for causes of low back pain largely been nonconclusive? Spine 22, 877–881.

Leinonen, V., Kankaanpaa, M., Airaksinen, O., Hanninen, O., 2000. Back and hip extensor activities during flexion/extension: effects of low back pain and rehabilitation. Arch Phys Med Rehabil 81, 32–37.

Lewek, M.D., Rudolph, K.S., Snyder-Mackler, L., 2004. Control of frontal plane knee laxity during gait in patients with medial compartment knee osteoarthritis. Osteoarthritis Cartilage 12, 745–751.

Linton, S.J., 2000. A review of psychological risk factors in back and neck pain. Spine 25, 1148–1156.

McGill, S.M., 2004. Linking latest knowledge of injury mechanisms and spine function to the prevention of low back disorders. J Electromyogr Kinesiol 14, 43–47.

McGill, S.M., Childs, A., Liebenson, C., 1999. Endurance times for low back stabilization exercises: clinical targets for testing and training from a normal database. Arch Phys Med Rehabil 80, 941–944.

Mens, J.M., Vleeming, A., Snijders, C.J., Stam, H.J., Ginai, A.Z., 1999. The active straight leg raising test and mobility of the pelvic joints. Eur Spine J 8, 468–473.

Nelson-Wong, E., Flynn, T.W., Callaghan, J.P., 2009. Development of active hip abduction as a screening test for identifying occupational low back pain. J Orthop Sports Phys Ther 39, 649–657.

Nelson-Wong, E., Gregory, D.E., Winter, D.A., Callaghan, J.P., 2008. Gluteus medius muscle activation patterns as a predictor of low back pain during standing. Clin Biomech 23, 545–553.

Nelson-Wong, E., Howarth, S.J., Winter, D.A., Callaghan, J.P., 2009. Application of auto and cross-correlation analysis in human movement and rehabilitation research. J Orthop Sports Phys Ther 39, 287–295.

Norman, R., Wells, R., Neumann, P., Frank, J., Shannon, H., Kerr, M., 1998. A comparison of peak vs. cumulative physical work exposure risk factors for the reporting of low back pain in the automotive industry. Clin Biomech. 13, 561–573.

O'Sullivan, P., 2005. Diagnosis and classification of chronic low back pain disorders: maladaptive movement and motor control impairments as underlying mechanism. Man Ther 10, 242–255.

Paquet, N., Malouin, F., Richards, C.L., 1994. Hip–spine movement interaction and muscle activation patterns during sagittal trunk movements in low back pain patients. Spine 19, 596–603.

Pirouzi, S., Hides, J., Richardson, C., Darnell, R., Toppenberg, R., 2006. Low back pain patients demonstrate increased hip extensor muscle activity during standardized submaximal rotation efforts. Spine 31, E999–E1005.

Prince, F., Winter, D.A., Stergiou, P., Walt, S.E., 1994. Anticipatory control of upper body balance during human locomotion. Gait Posture 2, 19–25.

Roelen, C.A.M., Schreuder, K.J., Koopmans, P.C., Groothoff, J.W., 2008. Perceived job demands relate to self-reported health complaints. Occup Med (Lond) 58, 58–63.

Silfies, S.P., Bhattacharya, A., Biely, S., Smith, S.S., Giszter, S., 2009. Trunk control during standing reach: a dynamical system analysis of movement strategies in patients with mechanical low back pain. Gait Posture 29, 370–376.

Silfies, S.P., Squillante, D., Maurer, P., Westcott, S., Karduna, A.R., 2005. Trunk muscle recruitment patterns in specific chronic low back pain populations. Clin Biomech 20, 465–473.

Tait, R.C., Chibnall, J.T., 1997. Development of a brief version of the Survey of Pain Attitudes. Pain 70, 229–235.

Van Dieën, J.H., Cholewicki, J., Radebold, A., 2003a. Trunk muscle recruitment patterns in patients with low back pain enhance the stability of the lumbar spine. Spine 28, 834–841.

Van Dieën, J.H., Selen, L.P.J., Cholewicki, J., 2003b. Trunk muscle activation in low-back pain patients, an analysis of the literature. J Electromyogr Kinesiol 13, 333–351.

Van Dieën, J.H., Westebring-Van Der Putten, E.P., Kingma, I., De Looze, M.P., 2009. Low-level activity of the trunk extensor muscles causes electromyographic manifestations of fatigue in absence of decreased oxygenation. J Electromyogr Kinesiol 19, 398–406.

Veiersted, K.B., Westgaard, R.H., Andersen, P., 1990. Pattern of muscle activity during sterotyped work and its relation to muscle pain. Int Arch Occup Environ Health 62, 31–41.

Waddell, G., 2004. The back pain revolution. Churchill Livingstone, Edinburgh: New York.

Waddell, G., Newton, M., Henderson, I., Somerville, D., Main, C.J., 1993. A Fear-Avoidance Beliefs Questionnaire (FABQ) and the role of fear-avoidance beliefs in chronic low back pain and disability. Pain 52, 157–168.

Chapter |11|

Trunk muscle control and back pain: chicken, egg, neither or both?

G. Lorimer Moseley
Sansom Institute for Health Research, University of South Australia, Adelaide, and Neuroscience Research Australia, Sydney, Australia

INTRODUCTION

When one treads on a drawing pin, such that the flesh of one's toe is penetrated, blood vessels are broken open, wide and small diameter neurones are stimulated, inflammatory mediators are released, short loop reflexes are engaged, spinal neurones are upregulated, cytokines are recruited, adrenaline is liberated, blood is redistributed, heart rate is increased, and spatial attention is shifted. This bombardment of responses occurs without our knowledge – all we know is that it hurts! Once it hurts, we radically alter the way we move so as not to put our toe down, to get to somewhere safe so we can visually inspect the damage, to alert a sympathetic member of our community to our plight so that they can assist us in this goal, or to transport our toe to an appropriately trained member of the community so that they can assess and remove the danger.

The terrific complexity of this multi-systemic protective response, about nearly all of which *we are unaware*, reminds me of my old high-school teacher who, when she was obviously out of her depth on some issue of biology, would look whimsically out the window, hands raised to the heavens, and say 'Indeed, we are fearfully and wonderfully made ...' That pain is just one part of the protective response, the only one that is conscious – the only one that plunges *me* into an unpleasant sensory and emotional experience from which *I* would like to escape – reminds me of the fundamental principle of pain science that nociception is neither sufficient nor necessary for pain. Nociception does not make us visit the hospital, but pain does. Nociception does not make us bandage up our toe, but pain does. Nociception does not make us walk on our heel, foot turned out like a sand wedge, but pain does. The idea that pain and nociception are distinct is not new, but it has been swamped perhaps by the vigour with which we pursue easy solutions to difficult problems. In fact, over twenty years ago, Patrick Wall, perhaps the parent of modern pain science, stated on the basis of many experiments in animals and humans, that 'the mislabelling of nociceptors as pain fibres was not an elegant simplification but a most unfortunate trivialization' (Wall and McMahon 1986). Despite the substantial progress that has been made since then in our understanding of nociception and pain, his assertion remains as pertinent as ever – 75% of clinicians consider the statement 'pain receptors carry pain messages to the brain' to be true, which it is not (Moseley, Oltholf, Venema, Don and Wijers, unpublished data).

How then does one define the relationship between control of the trunk muscles and back pain? To take on what appears to me to be a gargantuan task, I will first describe how I think pain works. This is a conceptualization of pain rather than an account of the biological mechanisms that underpin it – to do the latter is beyond the scope of this chapter and the expertise of this author (and probably that of any single human!). I will then propose that pain and motor control are homeostatic responses that serve to maintain the condition of our tissues and to thus promote our longevity. In this sense, I consider them to be more epiphenomenal. That is, I think that activation of the trunk muscles is modulated by myriad factors *including* the implicit perception of the threat to which the back is exposed. I think that back pain emerges according to the implicit perception of threat to which the back is exposed and the biological advantage that is offered by making it hurt. I will also contend that back pain and trunk muscle activity are in some sense interrelated – that control of the trunk muscles can affect pain via nociceptive and non-nociceptive sensory input and that pain can affect motor control of the trunk muscles via concerted protective behaviours. Moreover, I will contend that motor commands can evoke pain after a period of associative learning. In keeping with this first rather contention-filled paragraph, in what follows I will take an hypothesis-generating approach rather than simply review the literature.

WHY DO THINGS HURT?

Pain emerges into consciousness from a pattern of activity in several brain areas. *Exactly* how this occurs is not known – we must first conquer the holy grail of how the brain produces consciousness if we are to understand how the brain produces pain. However, there is an immense and rapidly growing literature about why things hurt, why some things hurt more than others and how we can help things to hurt less. The bulk of the research concerns the contribution of nociception to pain. We now have a very detailed understanding of the peripheral nociceptor and a reasonably detailed understanding of the spinal nociceptor (see Fields et al. 2006; Meyer et al. 2006 for reviews). Nociceptors, or A-α (thin myelinated peripheral neurones) and C-fibres (thinner, unmyelinated peripheral neurones), respond to changes in their chemical, thermal or mechanical environment. Some nociceptors have very low thresholds for activation such that they respond to very small changes in tissue pH, or gentle mechanical stimulation (for example sensual touch – see Craig 2002 for a review), or subtle shifts in temperature. Many have high thresholds and it is this sub-group of A-α and C fibres that are more suitably called nociceptors because, in a normal state, they don't respond until the intensity of the stimulus is dangerous, or potentially so.

In highly controlled experiments, the more dangerous a stimulus, the more it hurts. For example, the nociceptive barrage, brain activation and pain evoked by a 56 °C rod touching the skin are greater than those evoked by an otherwise identical 42 °C rod touching the skin (Bushnell et al. 2002). However, modulating nociception is not the only way to modulate pain. For example: touching the skin with a −20 °C rod normally hurts, but simultaneously touching the skin with the same rod hurts more (about 3 more points on a 10-point scale) if one simultaneously sees a red light than if one simultaneously sees a blue light, even though the noxious input is identical. This effect is attributable to the inherent meaning of 'red' (hot), which is more dangerous than the inherent meaning we attach to 'blue' (cold) (Moseley and Arntz 2007). We also gain information from the appearance of a body part – when patients with chronic arm pain view their limb through a magnifying lens (that is, making it look bigger or more swollen), it hurts more, and becomes more swollen, than when they view it through clear glass or a minimizing lens (Moseley et al. 2008a). In fact, noxious input is not even necessary for pain: in an elegant series of experiments, supposedly normal volunteers (there is an argument that the 'normality' of people who volunteer for experimental pain studies is questionable – see Moseley et al. 2008b) placed their head inside what they thought was a head stimulator but was in fact a sham and did nothing whatsoever to the head. However, when the investigators turned up the stimulator's 'intensity knob', the volunteers began to report pain, the intensity of which was positively related to the setting on the intensity knob (Bayer et al. 1991; Bayer et al. 1998).

There are many contextual, sensory and cognitive factors that modulate pain (see Jones and Moseley 2007; Butler and Moseley 2003; Moseley 2007 for reviews), such that the notion that pain is a measure of the state of the tissues of the body is no longer biologically or phenomenologically defensible. Arguably more defensible is the notion that pain is a measure of the brain's judgement of the need to protect a body part. This is not a trivial shift in thinking because it requires us to accept that anything that affects the brain's judgement of threat to body tissues can affect pain. This model of pain accommodates the myriad experiments that show nociception modulates pain, but also accommodates the growing body of data that show factors other than nociception also modulate pain. Moreover, this model of pain accommodates the variability and diversity of the results of brain imaging studies into pain and lends itself to neurological mechanisms that are well established.

CONCEPTUALIZING THE NEUROLOGY OF PAIN

In an attempt to make sense of the growing body of literature showing that pain and nociception do not share an isomorphic relationship, Ron Melzack proposed the neuromatrix theory (Melzack 1990). It was not without critics, primarily because it did not postulate on the mechanisms involved (Keefe et al. 1996), but it has largely stood the test of time, its key tenets now embedded in the clinical and pain-related brain imaging literature (Giummarra et al. 2007; Tracey 2008; Seifert and Maihofner 2009). According to the neuromatrix theory, pain emerges into consciousness when a particular network of neurones, called a neurosignature (Melzack 1990) or neurotag (Butler and Moseley 2003), is activated. That is, pain is the output evoked by the pain neurotag. This conceptualization draws on the idea that the brain evokes responses across the systems of the body via the activation of neurotags. Everything the brain knows can be thought of as being held in neurotags, the output of which evokes a response, which may include the modulation of other neurotags. In this way, the pain neurotag can be modulated by myriad other neurotags, most notably neurotags that represent something relevant to danger to body tissues. If we return to the experiment in which a very cold stimulus evokes more pain if it is presented with a red light than if it is presented with a blue light, we have a method by which the neurotag that represents the meaning of 'red' upregulates the neurotag for hand pain, whereas the neurotag that represents the meaning of 'blue' downregulates it.

We can therefore define pain as an unpleasant sensory and emotional experience that is determined by the brain's judgement of threat to body tissue. Critically, this judgement occurs outside of consciousness. The fundamental distinction between this idea of pain and the previous model of pain put forward centuries ago is that pain does not provide a measure of the true threat to body tissue, but a measure of the brain's evaluation of that threat. In this way, pain is a potent homeostatic mechanism – it recruits consciousness and is therefore able to evoke targeted and intentional behavioural response of the entire organism.

PAIN AND MOTOR OUTPUTS AS A RESULT OF SOMETHING 'UPSTREAM'

Fundamental to Melzack's neuromatrix theory is the idea that pain and motor output are bifurcations of the same neurotag. This echoes previous ideas that we perceive things according to what we would do about them (see Noe 2005; and Wall 1994 for extension of this idea directly relevant to pain) and even though it is unlikely to be neuroanatomically accurate, motor outputs can certainly be thought of as being generated by activation of neurotags – pain and motor output that are consistent with protection of the body are likely to be activated together. Unlike pain, which emerges into consciousness, motor control is effected by muscles, which are accessed via

spinal and peripheral neurones and can be modulated by short and long latency sensory-motor arcs. However, cortical motor output depends on the brain's evaluation of the current state of the body and the perceived demands upon it, which means that the neurotags for motor control of the trunk muscles can be modulated by neurotags that represent anything that is relevant to the current state of the body or the perceived demands upon it.

As nociception provides the mechanism by which peripheral receptors inform the brain that danger exists, and therefore is a potent modulator of pain, so too proprioception provides the mechanism by which peripheral receptors inform the brain of the current state of the body, and the perceived demands upon it. Both nociception and proprioception are potent modulators of motor control. Moreover, as contextual and cognitive factors also modulate pain, so to do contextual and cognitive factors modulate motor control – one need only consider the deleterious effect that 'atmosphere' or 'performance anxiety' can have on motor performance.

With regards to trunk muscle control, cognitive variables have been related to back muscle activity during forward bending, lifting and voluntary arm movements (Watson et al. 1997; Marras et al. 2000; Moseley et al. 2004a, 2004b; Moseley and Hodges 2006). For example, experimentally induced back pain associated with voluntary arm movements augments postural activation of the upper abdominal muscles in advance of the movement (Moseley and Hodges 2005). When arm movements are no longer associated with back pain, postural activation of the upper abdominal muscles usually returns to normal. This effect of noxious stimulation is in itself evidence of modulation of motor control on the basis of a change in the perceived current state of the body – noxious input from the area implies that the back is injured or at risk of being injured and the augmentation of the upper abdominals is consistent with a more protective postural strategy (Moseley and Hodges 2006). Notably, postural activation of the upper abdominal muscles does not always return to normal. In fact, in one study by our group, three out of 16 (supposedly normal) healthy volunteers maintained the protective postural strategy even when arm movements were no longer associated with back pain (Moseley and Hodges 2006). Those three were characterized by beliefs that emphasized the vulnerability of one's back and an isomorphic relationship between pain and tissue damage.

MOTOR OUTPUT AND PAIN COULD BECOME LINKED VIA ASSOCIATIVE LEARNING

It has long been accepted that neurones that wire together fire together (Hebb 1949) – it seems reasonable that prolonged activation of neurotags for pain and for protective trunk muscle control strategies would be no exception. We have established in people with chronic arm pain that imagined movements of the arm increase pain and swelling even when there is no detectable muscle activity associated with the task (Moseley 2004; Moseley et al. 2008b). Preliminary data from 12 patients with chronic unremitting back pain corroborate that effect – prone patients rated their resting pain before and after imagining they were performing a series of trunk movements, or a series of neck movements, for 10 minutes. Pain was greater after the imagined trunk movements than it was before, but there was no change imparted by imagined neck movements (Chin et al. unpublished data). Further work is required to elucidate this effect, but it certainly seems possible that the command to move the back becomes sufficient to activate the back pain neurotag. If so, associative learning would seem the most likely explanation.

CONTROL OF THE TRUNK MUSCLES CONTRIBUTES TO PAIN

If control of the trunk muscles maintains the structural integrity of the spine, it follows that compromised control of the trunk muscles compromises the structural integrity of the spine. This situation should lead to activation of nociceptors in spinal structures, which will contribute to the brain's judgement that spinal tissues are under threat, thereby contributing to pain. This line of reasoning is intuitive and logically seductive. However, I contend that what exactly constitutes 'abnormal' or 'decreased' control of the trunk muscles is difficult to define, particularly when changes in motor control are appropriate if there is a change in the perceived status of, or perceived demands upon, the body. Current concepts in pain science, particularly as they relate to chronic pain, offer an alternative perspective: pain is protective as long as the tissues that are hurting need protecting. When the tissues do not need protecting, pain becomes the problem – it is considered maladaptive instead of adaptive, a disease in its own right (Cousins 2004). I contend that even in such states the problem lies upstream from pain – the problem lies with the brain's judgement of threat to body tissues. That is, the pain is an appropriate response to the judgement that tissue is in danger and needs protecting but the judgement itself is not appropriate because tissue is not in fact in danger. If we are to apply the same line of thinking to trunk muscle control – rather than considering persistent alterations in motor control as being the problem, perhaps the problem lies upstream from the motor output – perhaps the problem lies with the brain's judgement of the current state of, and perceived demands upon, the

back. Both aspects of this judgement can feasibly be disrupted in people with pain.

Inaccurate evaluation of the current state of the body

The brain holds representations, or maps, of the body and the space around it, which it uses to plan and modify motor commands (see Chapter 19). These cortical representations are thought to be in part innate and in part modified by ongoing input from proprioceptors and vision. They are also key in providing the sense that we have of our own body, that we own it and that it is always there, which are fundamental aspects of self-awareness (James 1890). The most studied cortical body maps lie in primary sensory cortex (S1) and primary motor cortex (M1) (Penfield and Boldrey 1937), however, the maps that are used to determine the current state and configuration of the body are probably held in posterior parietal cortex, where input from S1, M1, visual and association areas are integrated (Andersen et al. 1997; Das et al. 2001; Andersen and Buneo 2003). Unlike S1 and M1, the neural substrate of parietal body maps, sometimes called the working body maps because they are important for sensory-motor interaction, has not been elucidated. This means that we cannot detect alterations in the response profile of constituent neurones in the same way that we can for S1 and M1. In fact, S1 and M1 maps are relatively trivial: for S1, cutaneous stimulation evokes an electrical response that can be measured using electroencephalography (EEG) or a discrete change in blood oxygenation that can be measured using functional MRI (fMRI); for M1, transcranial magnetic stimulation (TMS) can be used to stimulate M1 and the electromyographical (EMG) response can be measured using recording electrodes placed over or in the target muscles. Notably, M1 is organized in a functional manner rather than an anatomical manner (Cheney and Fetz 1985; Grafton et al. 1991).

S1 and M1 body maps in people with recurrent or chronic back pain are different to those in healthy controls. For example, recording brain responses via magnetoencephalography (MEG) in response to cutaneous stimulation at the back and finger showed that while the location of the main response in S1 after finger stimulation was similar between patients and healthy controls, the peak response in S1 after back stimulation was about 3 cm (which constitutes many thousands of neurones) more medial, in people with chronic back pain (Flor et al. 1997). Changes in M1 representation of contraction of the deepest trunk muscle have also been reported in people with back pain (Tsao et al. 2008) – using TMS to evoke a contraction in transversus abdominis, the biggest EMG response was evoked by stimulation of M1 neurones that were situated posterior and lateral to the neurones that evoke the biggest EMG response in people without back pain. What is more, the shift in M1 representation was related to delayed contraction of transversus abdominis during voluntary arm movements.

How altered M1 maps of the trunk muscles relate to a change in trunk muscle control is not clear, nor is whether this shift in control contributes to pain. Training transversus abdominis both normalizes its M1 representation and its postural activation during arm movements (Tsao and Hodges 2008). It is not clear which aspect of training imparts the effect and there are many candidates, for example increased motor neurone excitability, correction of sensory maps or spatial coding of the body and altered cognitions about the perceived vulnerability of the back (see section below).

Although working body maps are more difficult to interrogate, there are correlational data that suggest they too may be disrupted in people with back pain. Both S1 representation and two-point discrimination (TPD) depend on inhibitory mechanisms within S1 (Taylor-Clarke et al. 2004), such that increased TPD threshold is considered a clear clinical signature of altered S1 representation (Flor et al. 1995; Maihofner et al. 2003). Accordingly, increased TPD threshold at the back is positively related with disrupted self-awareness of one's own back (Moseley 2008a) (as TPD threshold at the arm is positively related with disrupted self-awareness of one's arm in people with chronic arm pain (Maihofner et al. 2003; Moseley 2005)) and increased TPD threshold at the back in patients with chronic back pain is associated with a reduced capacity to voluntarily adopt specific lumbopelvic postures (Luomajoki and Moseley 2011). Taken together, these findings suggest that disrupted S1 body maps and the mechanisms that underpin those maps are associated with disruption of trunk muscle control.

How can we determine if this disruption actually involves the working body schema or simply reflects dysfunction of the output system itself? A pragmatic way to investigate the integrity of working body maps is via motor imagery (Coslett 1998; Schwoebel et al. 2001; Funk et al. 2005). For example, when we recognize a pictured limb as belonging to the left or the right side of the body, we make an initial judgement and then confirm or correct that judgement by mentally rotating our own limb to match the posture of that shown in the picture (Parsons and Fox 1998). That is, left/right judgements of pictured limbs require intact working body maps (Parsons 2001). This line of enquiry has been extended to interrogate working body maps of the trunk in people with back pain (Bray and Moseley 2011). In that study people with back pain and healthy controls performed a task in which they judged whether a pictured model had their trunk twisted to the left or to the right. Healthy controls were 80% accurate for the trunk task and the left/right hand judgement task. Remarkably, however, patients with back pain were 80% accurate on the hand task, but 50% accurate on

the trunk task – no better than chance. This finding is important because it suggests that the working body map of the trunk is so disrupted in people with back pain that they cannot use that map to differentiate left trunk rotation from right. We do not know whether performance on a left/right trunk rotation task relates to trunk muscle control but it seems a reasonable hypothesis to test.

These findings, taken together, would seem to strongly suggest that the brain's evaluation of the current state of the body might be fundamentally flawed in people with back pain. This has obvious implications for trunk muscle control because motor output to the trunk muscles will be inappropriate. This problem may also spark another one, because the central nervous system has in-built mechanisms to detect incongruence between the predicted and actual motor outcome of a command. The reafference principle (Von Holst 1950), whereby an exact copy of the command for movement (the 'efferent copy') is subtracted from sensory input about the actual movement ('reafference') to yield an error signal ('exafference'), and the corollary discharge model (Sperry 1950) sparked the idea, but an impressive amount of research has been undertaken since then (see Gandevia 1996 for review). One perspective on this error-detection system in people with chronic pain is that it increases pain because it alerts the brain to danger – that all is not as it should be (Harris 1999). This idea is intuitively sensible in light of the model of pain discussed earlier because anything that increases the implicitly perceived threat to body tissues should facilitate the pain neurotag. The detection of incongruence between the predicted and actual outcome of a movement would reasonably be considered as potentially dangerous. Although the idea is intuitively attractive, the several attempts to interrogate it have yielded contrasting results (McCabe et al. 2005; Moseley et al. 2006; McCormick et al. 2007). Another possibility that has recently emerged from experiments in people with chronic limb pain is that the problem lies with spatial representation, rather than somatotopic representation *per se*. People with chronic complex regional pain syndrome (CRPS) demonstrate a kind of spatial neglect that is confined to the area of space in which their affected limb normally resides (Moseley et al. 2009). This finding is consistent with the proposal that, in order to integrate body schematic information, stimuli on the body must be transformed from locations on the skin to locations in external space (Yamamoto and Kitazawa 2001; Kitazawa 2002; Haggard and Wolpert 2005; Gallace and Spence 2008) although this transformation depends to a certain extent on the specific nature of the task to be performed (Gallace et al. 2008). Therefore, it may be that a breakdown in the conversion to a spatial location underpins the problem with working body schema and the sensory-motor incongruence. Clearly, we are a long way from untangling this, but it is probably reasonable to conclude that incongruence between predicted and actual motor output does not cause pain in healthy controls, but it might in people with chronic pain in whom the protective neurotags are upregulated (see Moseley 2006; Lotze and Moseley 2007; McCabe et al. 2008 for reviews).

Inaccurate evaluation of the perceived demands upon the body

The second aspect of the brain's (unconscious) judgement that underpins motor control of the trunk muscles is that of the perceived demands upon the body. It is this judgement that is probably more open to modulation by non-proprioceptive sensory, cognitive and contextual factors. When healthy volunteers expect to experience back pain, postural activation of their trunk muscles associated with rapid arm movements mimics that observed in patients with back pain, and in healthy people with back pain induced by injection of hypertonic saline into their back muscles (Hodges and Richardson 1996; Hodges et al. 2003; Moseley et al. 2004a). Notably, changes in back muscle activation are not limited to the muscles that were injected and their coagonists. Thus, the anticipation of pain or injury to one's back is a cognitive factor that influences the perceived demands on the body, in which case it would alter trunk control. Further, most healthy participants who experience a short period of experimentally induced pain return to normal trunk muscle control when pain subsides. However, those who do not, give responses on the Pain Catastrophizing Scale (Sullivan et al. 1995), the Back Beliefs Questionnaire (Symonds et al. 1996) and the Survey of Pain Attitudes (Jensen and Karoly 1992) suggesting that they have beliefs and attitudes that emphasize the threat value of back pain and the vulnerability of the back. Notably, these participants are also characterized by a loss of the normal variability of the response once they have experienced back pain (Moseley and Hodges 2006).

Variability is critical for biological function and is thought to be important for motor learning, even when the motor output of interest is postural activation of the trunk muscles during limb movements. A large amount of research evaluates the variability of the motor constituents of a task (Latash et al. 2002). The finding of reduced variability in those who did not return to normal trunk muscle control during arm movements raised the possibility that cognitive factors can reduce variability of trunk muscle control strategies and therefore limit the capacity of the trunk control system to adapt to new demands. This idea is consistent with the notion that the robustness of motor tasks provides the freedom to generate exploratory variation in the task (McCollum and Leen 1989), persistent stimulation of perception–action systems, and motor learning and coordination (Riccio 1991). It seems reasonable to propose that, if exploratory variation is lost, then the perception–action system prevents adaptation to new

perceived demands. Such a cognitive control over motor output is particularly important for people with chronic back pain because they are characterized by beliefs that emphasize the vulnerability of their back and the catastrophic nature of back pain and back injury (Moseley et al. 2000; Sullivan et al. 2001).

There is a growing argument that protective motor strategies and a loss of variability is probably beneficial in the short term but may come at a cost if maintained long term. I have touched on this possibility elsewhere (Moseley et al. 2004a). It seems a sensible idea and is consistent with what we know of other protective strategies – protective activation of the sympathetic, immune or endocrine systems becomes problematic if maintained long term (see Butler and Moseley 2003; and Butler 2000 for reviews). It is an important consideration because it suggests that the way an individual conceptualizes pain and the vulnerability of their back could predispose them to recurrence or chronicity via a change in trunk muscle control. The final, somewhat speculative (but not outrageous) possibility is that this mechanism may predispose an individual to an initial episode of back pain. These issues evidently require further investigation, but they seem to emphasize a wide-ranging and multi-pronged approach to the elucidation of the relationship between trunk control and back pain. Notably, however, we should remember that, although it seems intuitively sensible and a seductive thesis, there are still no data that clearly show that the characteristic patterns of motor control of the trunk muscles that we see in people with back pain is causing their pain (see Chapter 18).

A MODEL OF THE RELATIONSHIP BETWEEN TRUNK CONTROL AND BACK PAIN

Figure 11.1 presents a schematic framework relating trunk control and back pain, although the relationship between trunk muscle control and back pain is far more complex than many clinicians and scientists would like to admit. I have tried to construct a perspective that draws on my research and clinical experience; it is thus, essentially, a limited model.

CONCLUSION

I consider pain and motor control to be outputs of the brain that reflect the brain's evaluation of the current state of the body and the perceived demands upon it. Importantly, I contend that this evaluation occurs outside of consciousness. This implies that back pain, and protective trunk muscle control strategies, that persist when the back

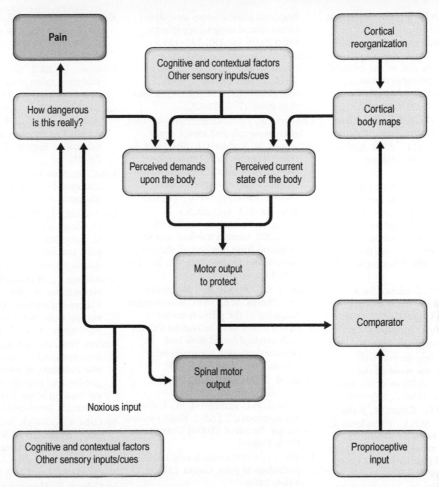

Figure 11.1 Proposed relationship between trunk muscle control and back pain.

is not in danger, reflect a problem with this evaluation and that they are, primarily, epiphenomenal, although they also affect one another indirectly. Changes in the brain's representation of the trunk, which occur as back pain persists, and cognitive and contextual factors that seem to become more common when back pain persists, probably contribute to problems with trunk control and may therefore contribute to pain. Data from other chronic pain states suggest that the command to move is sufficient to evoke pain, possibly via an associative learning process, and the same may also be true for back pain. Finally, cognitive and contextual factors may predispose an individual to recurrent episodes and, possibly (the speculative bit), be a cause of initial episodes of back pain.

REFERENCES

Andersen, R.A., Buneo, C.A., 2003. Sensorimotor integration in posterior parietal cortex. Adv Neurol 93, 159–177.

Andersen, R.A., Snyder, L.H., Bradley, D.C., Xing, J., 1997. Multimodal representation of space in the posterior parietal cortex and its use in planning movements. Ann Rev Neurosci 20, 303–330.

Bayer, T.L., Baer, P.E., Early, C., 1991. Situational and psychophysiological factors in psychologically induced pain. Pain 44, 45–50.

Bayer, T.L., Coverdale, J.H., Chiang, E., Bangs, M., 1998. The role of prior pain experience and expectancy in psychologically and physically induced pain. Pain 74, 327–331.

Bray, H., Moseley, G.L., 2011. Disrupted working body schema of the trunk in people with back pain. Br J Sports Med 45, 168–173.

Bushnell, M.C., Villemure, C., Strigo, I., Duncan, G.H., 2002. Imaging pain in the brain: The role of the cerebral cortex in pain perception and modulation. J Musculoskelet Pain 10, 59–72.

Butler, D., 2000. The sensitive nervous system. NOI Publications, Adelaide.

Butler, D., Moseley, G.L., 2003. Explain pain. NOI Group Publishing, Adelaide.

Cheney, P.D., Fetz, E.E., 1985. Comparable patterns of muscle facilitation evoked by individual corticomotoneuronal (CM) cells and by single intracortical microstimuli in primates: evidence for functional groups of CM cells. J Neurophysiol 53, 786–804.

Coslett, H.B., 1998. Evidence for a disturbance of the body schema in neglect. Brain Cogn 37, 527–544.

Cousins, M.C., 2004. Pain relief – a universal human right. Pain 112, 1–4.

Craig, A., 2002. How do you feel? Interoception: the sense of the physiological condition of the body. Nature Rev Neurosci 3, 655–666.

Das, A., Franca, J.G., Gattas, R., Kaas, J.H., Nicolelis, M.A.L., Timo-Iaria, C., et al., 2001. The brain decade in debate: VI. Sensory and motor maps: dynamics and plasticity. Braz J Med Biol Res 34, 1497–1508.

Fields, H., Basbaum, A., Heinricher, M., 2006. CNS mechanisms of pain modulation. In: McMahon, S.B., Koltzenburg, M. (eds), Textbook of Pain. Elsevier, London.

Flor, H., Braun, C., Elbert, T., Birbaumer, N., 1997. Extensive reorganization of primary somatosensory cortex in chronic back pain patients. Neurosci Lett 224, 5–8.

Flor, H., Elbert, T., Knecht, S., Wienbruch, C., Pantev, C., Birbaumer, N., et al., 1995. Phantom-limb pain as a perceptual correlate of cortical reorganization following arm amputation. Nature 375, 482–484.

Funk, M., Shiffrar, M., Brugger, P., 2005. Hand movement observation by individuals born without hands: phantom limb experience constrains visual limb perception. Exp Brain Res 164, 341–346.

Gallace, A., Soto-Faraco, S., Dalton, P., Kreukniet, B., Spence, C., 2008. Response requirements modulate tactile spatial congruency effects. Exper Brain Res 191, 171–186.

Gallace, A., Spence, C., 2008. The cognitive and neural correlates of 'tactile consciousness': a multisensory perspective. Consciousness and Cognition 17, 370–407.

Gandevia, S., 1996. Kinesthesia: roles for afferent signals and motor commands. In: Rothwell, L., Shepherd, J. (Eds.), Handbook of Physiology Section 12: Exercise: regulation and integration of multiple systems. Oxford University Press, New York.

Giummarra, M.J., Gibson, S.J., Georgiou-Karistianis, N., Bradshaw, J.L., 2007. Central mechanisms in phantom limb perception: the past, present and future. Brain Res Rev 54, 219–232.

Grafton, S.T., Woods, R.P., Mazziotta, J.C., Phelps, M.E., 1991. Somatotopic mapping of the primary motor cortex in humans: activation studies with cerebral blood flow and positron emission tomography. J Neurophysiol 66, 735–743.

Haggard, P., Wolpert, D.M., 2005. Disorders of body scheme. In: Freund, H.J., Jeannerod, M., Hallett, M., Leiguarda, I. (Eds.), Higher-order motor disorders. Oxford University Press, Oxford.

Harris, A.J., 1999. Cortical origin of pathological pain. Lancet 354, 1464–1466.

Hebb, D., 1949. The organization of behavior. Wiley, New York.

Hodges, P.W., Moseley, G.L., Gabrielsson, A., Gandevia, S.C., 2003. Experimental muscle pain changes feedforward postural responses of the trunk muscles. Exp Brain Res 151, 262–271.

Hodges, P.W., Richardson, C.A., 1996. Inefficient muscular stabilization of the lumbar spine associated with low back pain: a motor control evaluation of transversus abdominis. Spine 21, 2640–2650.

James, W., 1890. Principles of psychology. Henry Holt, New York.

Jensen, M.P., Karoly, P., 1992. Pain-specific beliefs, perceived symptoms severity and adjustment to chronic pain. Clin J Pain 8, 123–130.

Jones, L., Moseley, G.L., 2007. Pain. In: Porter, S. (Ed.), Tidy's Physiotherapy, 14th edn. Elsevier, Oxford.

Keefe, F.J., Lefebvre, J.C., Starr, K.R., 1996. From the gate control theory to the neuromatrix: revolution or evolution? Pain Forum 5, 143–146.

Kitazawa, S., 2002. Where conscious sensation takes place. Consciousness and Cognition 11, 475–477.

Latash, M.L., Scholz, J.P., Schoner, G., 2002. Motor control strategies revealed in the structure of motor variability. Exercise Sport Sci Rev 30, 26–31.

Lotze, M., Moseley, G.L., 2007. Role of distorted body image in pain. Curr Rheumatol Rep 9, 488–496.

Luomajoki, H., Moseley, G.L., 2011. Tactile acuity and lumbopelvic motor control in patients with back pain and healthy controls. Br J Sports Med 45, 437–440.

Maihofner, C., Handwerker, H.O., Neundorfer, B., Birklein, F., 2003. Patterns of cortical reorganization in complex regional pain syndrome. Neurology 61, 1707–1715.

Marras, W.S., Davis, K.G., Heaney, C.A., Maronitis, A.B., Allread, W.G., 2000. The influence of psychosocial stress, gender, and personality on mechanical loading of the lumbar spine. Spine 25, 3045–3054.

McCabe, C.S., Haigh, R.C., Blake, D.R., 2008. Mirror visual feedback for the treatment of complex regional pain syndrome (Type 1). Curr Pain Headache Rep 12, 103–107.

McCabe, C.S., Haigh, R.C., Halligan, P.W., Blake, D.R., 2005. Simulating sensory-motor incongruence in healthy volunteers: implications for a cortical model of pain. Rheumatology 44, 509–516.

McCollum, G., Leen, T., 1989. Form and exploration of mechanical stability limits in erect stance. J Motor Behav 21, 225–244.

McCormick, K., Zalucki, N., Hudson, M.L., Moseley, G.L., 2007. Faulty proprioceptive information disrupts motor imagery: an experimental study. Aust J Physiother 53, 41–45.

Melzack, R., 1990. Phantom limbs and the concept of a neuromatrix. Trends Neurosci 13, 88–92.

Meyer, R., Ringkamp, M., Campbell, J.N., Raja, S.N., 2006. Peripheral mechanisms of cutaneous nociception. In: McMahon, S.B., Koltzenburg, M. (Eds.), Textbook of Pain, fifth ed. Elsevier, London.

Moseley, G.L., 2004. Imagined movements cause pain and swelling in a patient with complex regional pain syndrome. Neurology 62, 1644.

Moseley, G.L., 2005. Distorted body image in complex regional pain syndrome. Neurology 65, 773–773.

Moseley, G.L., 2006. Making sense of S1 mania – are things really that simple? In: Gifford, L. (Ed.), Topical Issues in Pain Volume 5. CNS Press, Falmouth.

Moseley, G.L., 2007. Reconceptualising pain according to its underlying biology. Phys Ther Rev 12, 169–178.

Moseley, G.L., 2008a. I can't find it! Distorted body image and tactile dysfunction in patients with chronic back pain. Pain 140, 239–243.

Moseley, G.L., 2008b. Pain, brain imaging and physiotherapy – opportunity is knocking. Man Ther 13, 475–477.

Moseley, G.L., Arntz, A., 2007. The context of a noxious stimulus affects the pain it evokes. Pain 133, 64–71.

Moseley, G.L., Gallace, A., Spence, C., 2009. Space-based, but not arm-based, shift in tactile processing in complex regional pain syndrome and its relationship to cooling of the affected limb. Brain 132, 3142–3151.

Moseley, G.L., Hodges, P.W., 2005. Are the changes in postural control associated with low back pain caused by pain interference? Clin J Pain 21, 323–329.

Moseley, G.L., Hodges, P.W., 2006. Reduced variability of postural strategy prevents normalization of motor changes induced by back pain: a risk factor for chronic trouble? Behav Neurosci 120, 474–476.

Moseley, G.L., Hodges, P.W., Nicholas, M.K., 2000. The effect of neuroscience education on somatic perception and catastrophising in people with chronic low back pain – a randomised controlled trial. Annual Scientific Meeting of the Australian Pain Society. Melbourne.

Moseley, G.L., McCormick, K., Hudson, M., Zalucki, N., 2006. Disrupted cortical proprioceptive representation evokes symptoms of peculiarity, foreignness and swelling, but not pain. Rheumatology 45, 196–200.

Moseley, G.L., Nicholas, M.K., Hodges, P.W., 2004a. Does anticipation of back pain predispose to back trouble? Brain 127, 2339–2347.

Moseley, G.L., Nicholas, M.K., Hodges, P.W., 2004b. Pain differs from non-painful attention-demanding or stressful tasks in its effect on postural control patterns of trunk muscles. Exp Brain Res 156, 64–71.

Moseley, G.L., Parsons, T.J., Spence, C., 2008a. Visual distortion of a limb modulates the pain and swelling evoked by movement. Curr Biol 18, R1047–R1048.

Moseley, G.L., Zalucki, N., Birklein, F., Marinus, J., Hilten, J.J.V., Luomajoki, H., 2008b. Thinking about movement hurts: the effect of motor imagery on pain and swelling in people with chronic arm pain. Arthritis Care Res 59, 623–631.

Noe, A., 2005. Action in Perception (Representation and Mind). MIT Press, Boston, MA.

Parsons, L.M., 2001. Integrating cognitive psychology, neurology and neuroimaging. Acta Psychologica 107, 155–181.

Parsons, L.M., Fox, P.T., 1998. The neural basis of implicit movements used in recognising hand shape. Cogn Neuropsychol 15, 583–615.

Penfield, W., Boldrey, E., 1937. Somatic motor and sensory representation in the cerebral cortex of man studied by electrical stimulation. Brain 60, 389–443.

Riccio, G., 1991. Information in movement variability about the qualitative dynamics of posture and orientation. In: Newell, K., Corcos, D. (Eds.), Variability and Motor Control. Human Kinetics Publishers, Champaign, IL.

Schwoebel, J., Friedman, R., Duda, N., Coslett, H.B., 2001. Pain and the body schema: evidence for peripheral effects on mental representations of movement. Brain 124, 2098–2104.

Seifert, F., Maihofner, C., 2009. Central mechanisms of experimental and chronic neuropathic pain: findings from functional imaging studies. Cell Mol Life Sci 66, 375–390.

Sperry, R., 1950. Neural basis of the spontaneous optokinetic responses produced by visual neural inversion. J Comp Physiol Psychol 43, 482–489.

Sullivan, M.J.L., Bishop, S.R., Pivik, J., 1995. The Pain Catastrophizing Scale: development and validation. Psycholog Ass 7, 524–532.

Sullivan, M.J.L., Thorn, B., Haythornthwaite, J.A., Keefe, F., Martin, M., Bradley, L.A., et al., 2001. Theoretical perspectives on the relation between catastrophizing and pain. Clin J Pain 17, 52–64.

Symonds, T.L., Burton, A.K., Tillotson, K.M., Main, C.J., 1996. Do attitudes and beliefs influence work loss due to low back trouble? Occup Med (Lond) 46, 25–32.

Taylor-Clarke, M., Kennett, S., Haggard, P., 2004. Persistence of visual-tactile enhancement in humans. Neurosci Lett 354, 22–25.

Tracey, I., 2008. Imaging pain. Br J Anaesth 101, 32–39.

Tsao, H., Galea, M.P., Hodges, P.W., 2008. Reorganization of the motor cortex is associated with postural control deficits in recurrent low back pain. Brain 131, 2161–2171.

Tsao, H., Hodges, P.W., 2008. Persistence of improvements in postural strategies following motor control training in people with recurrent low back pain. Journal of Electromyography and Kinesiology 18, 559–567.

Von Holst, H., 1950. Relations between the central nervous system and the peripheral organs. Br J Anim Behav 2, 89–94.

Wall, P., 1994. Introduction to the edition after this one. Editorial. In: Wall, P., Melzack, R. (Eds.), The Textbook of Pain. Churchill-Livingstone, Edinburgh.

Wall, P., McMahon, S., 1986. The relationship of perceived pain to afferent nerve impulses. Trends Neurosci 9, 254–255.

Watson, P.J., Booker, C.K., Main, C.J., 1997. Evidence for the role of psychological factors in abnormal paraspinal activity in patients with chronic low back pain. J Musculo Pain 5, 41–56.

Yamamoto, S., Kitazawa, S., 2001. Reversal of subjective temporal order due to arm crossing. Nature Neurosci 4, 759–765.

Part | 3 |

Proprioceptive systems

Chapter |12|

Altered variability in proprioceptive postural strategy in people with recurrent low back pain

Simon Brumagne, Lotte Janssens, Kurt Claeys and Madelon Pijnenburg
Department of Rehabilitation Sciences, University of Leuven, Leuven, Belgium

INTRODUCTION

Patients with non-specific low back pain (LBP) have been observed to have altered motor and postural control (e.g. Hodges and Richardson 1996; Mientjes and Frank 1999; Brumagne, Cordo et al. 2004; Henry et al. 2006). Both an experimental finding and a clinical observation is the fact that some patients with LBP adopt two simple modes of postural control: a global trunk and body stiffening strategy (hyperactivity) and a passive postural strategy (hypoactivity), respectively (Hodges and Moseley 2003; van Dieën et al. 2003; Brumagne, Cordo et al. 2004; Henry et al. 2006; Brumagne et al. 2008a). In other words, in certain conditions these individuals activate all (global) trunk muscles in co-contraction. In other conditions these individuals do not activate trunk muscles and consequently, they will be hanging end of range in their spinal joints.

Depending on the time course, both positive and negative effects of co-contraction and passive control can be distinguished. Altered trunk muscle recruitment patterns might be functional in people with LBP (Lund et al. 1991), to prevent buckling of the spine during perturbations to which the patient could not adequately react (van Dieën et al. 2003). In contrast, increased activity of global trunk muscles in order to stabilize the spine may be at the cost of a loss of fine-tuning of intervertebral motion (Hodges and Moseley 2003). Furthermore, due to hyperactivity of the muscles, the muscles themselves could be painful (Johansson and Sojka 1991). Particularly, the presence of long-lasting static contractions (i.e. stabilizing co-contractions) might be a risk factor for chronic muscle pain (Sjøgaard et al. 2000). Moreover, increased co-contraction will lead to additional compressive forces acting on the spine (Granata and Marras 2000). In addition, these altered muscle activation patterns might hamper other bodily functions such as respiration (Hamaoui et al. 2002; Hodges et al. 2002), posture and movement (Dankaerts et al. 2009). Lastly, both hyperactivity of muscles (Djupsjöbacka et al. 1995; Thunberg et al. 2002) and hypoactivity/no muscle activity (Gandevia et al. 1992) might have a negative effect on proprioceptive acuity and consequently on proprioceptive control.

So, certain adopted postural strategies (e.g. stiffening) may be adequate in the short-term, but might be suboptimal and even a maladaption in the long run (Hodges and Moseley 2003).

Why do these people with LBP stiffen up to control their posture and movement? Currently, several mechanisms for trunk muscles co-contraction in people with acute and chronic LBP might explain these observations. Depending on the timeframe, pain itself, pain-adaptation (Lund et al. 1991; van Dieën et al. 2003), fear and fear of falling (Carpenter et al. 2001; Henry et al. 2006; Mok et al. 2007; Brumagne et al. 2008a), fear-avoidance beliefs

(Moseley and Hodges 2006) and muscle fatigue (Granata et al. 2004) have been described as possible underlying mechanisms.

Similar mechanisms are described for the observed passive control, including pain inhibition (Dickx et al. 2008), muscle fatigue (Caldwell et al. 2003) and psychological distress such as anxiety and depression (Verbunt et al. 2005).

An alternative but not mutually exclusive clarification may be *impaired proprioceptive control*. Altered proprioceptive control may induce similar changes in motor and postural control as described above (e.g. *pain-adaptation model*) and therefore may result in comparable possible consequences.

Low back pain is known to be a multi-factorial problem and the changes in motor and postural control will be task-dependent, related to the individual and hence highly variable between and probably within individuals. However, knowledge of all possible mechanisms may help to better identify subgroups of patients. Consequently, better and more specific interventions may be developed to prevent the high recurrence rate of LBP.

The 'impaired proprioceptive control' mechanisms will be further discussed below.

PROPRIOCEPTIVE CONTROL CHANGES OF THE LUMBOSACRAL REGION AS A POSSIBLE MECHANISM

Mechanical cumulative or repetitive stress (injury) might outwardly appear as a pure mechanical problem in origin. However, the underlying mechanism might describe a sensory processing problem. Due to a local or even a global proprioceptive impairment ('deafferentation') the central nervous system (CNS) may adopt a different postural strategy to overcome the loss of position and movement accuracy and precision (Ghez and Sainburg 1995; Gribble et al. 2003). This alternative strategy might be co-contraction or stiffening of the body or a body segment (e.g. trunk) to decrease the degrees of freedom to be controlled by the CNS. This might be a similar and less complex neural control mechanism as observed/ hypothesized in neurological conditions such as Parkinson's disease (Carpenter and Bloem 2011; Vaugoyeau and Azulay 2010; Wright et al. 2010), multiple sclerosis (Frzovic et al. 2000; Rougier et al. 2007) or dystonia (Byl et al. 1996; Torres-Russotto and Perlmutter 2008; Tamura et al. 2009). The pathological condition of (focal hand) dystonia particularly might be of interest for explaining similar observations. More specifically the *sensorimotor hypothesis of aberrant learning* might have analogous consequences in people with chronic LBP (Byl et al. 1996; Sanger and Merzenich 2000). If abnormal learning occurs due to repetition of abnormal or stereotypic

movements and postures, this could contribute to the maladaptive responsiveness and abnormal plasticity of the intracortical neurons in the sensory cortex (Byl et al. 2002; Tamura et al. 2009). This may in turn disturb motor function (Harbourne and Stergiou 2009; Tamura et al. 2009).

The importance of these aspects and the relation to LBP will be developed further later in this chapter.

Altered lumbosacral proprioception in people with LBP

Numerous studies have shown that individuals with LBP have altered (in most studies decreased) lumbosacral proprioception in different postures such as standing, sitting and four-point kneeling compared to healthy control subjects (e.g. Gill and Callaghan 1998; Brumagne et al. 2000; O'Sullivan et al. 2003). Although some studies did not show any differences in spine proprioception (Descarreaux et al. 2005; Asell et al. 2006) or only a direction-specific change in proprioception, indicating decreased acuity in the flexion direction but not in spinal extension (Newcomer et al. 2000). These changes in proprioceptive acuity have been seen in different populations such as young, middle-aged and elderly people, in highly active (e.g. professional ballet dancers) and sedentary people, in patients with mild and severe disability, in non-specific LBP and patients with spinal stenosis and disc herniation (e.g. Brumagne et al. 2000; Leinonen et al. 2002, 2003; O'Sullivan et al. 2003; Brumagne et al. 2004a; Brumagne et al. 2004b).

Several mechanisms have been described to influence lumbosacral proprioceptive acuity. Low back pain itself can have a direct negative effect on proprioceptive acuity, but cannot solely explain these changes taking into account the studies in patients with recurrent LBP (Brumagne et al. 2008b; Janssens et al. 2010). In these studies patients were tested when they were in a pain-free episode and they still showed altered proprioception. Moreover, acutely induced deep back pain did not show an effect on the stretch-reflex of the back muscles (Zedka et al. 1999). In addition to pain, back muscle fatigue and decreased blood supply might have a negative effect on lumbosacral position sense (Brumagne et al. 1999b; Taimela et al. 1999; Johanson et al. 2011; Janssens et al. 2012). Furthermore, proprioception may be impaired by the action exerted by the sympathetic nervous system on muscle spindle receptors. The sympathetic nervous system may have both an indirect effect on proprioception by decreasing the blood flow to skeletal muscles (Thomas and Segal 2004) and a direct effect on muscle spindles, generally characterized by a depression of the sensitivity to muscle length changes (Roatta et al. 2002). Moreover, sympathetic activation may also affect the basal discharge rate of the muscle spindles (Hellström et al. 2005). However, most of these results have to be confirmed in humans, since sympathetic modulation of muscle spindle afferent activity is mainly documented in animal studies and related to jaw and neck muscles (Passatore and Roatta 2006). Finally, older age has been described to have a negative effect on lumbosacral proprioceptive acuity, but this is more manifest in elderly individuals with LBP (Brumagne et al. 2004a).

As an important consideration, it should be pointed out that most studies on proprioceptive acuity in LBP are based on measures of position and movement sense. A possible limitation of this form of proprioception evaluation is the fact that position and movement sense assessments are based on a conscious control process and memory, while proprioceptive control is in general a subconscious process. Hence, this type of proprioception evaluation is an indirect measurement and may not grasp a comprehensive picture of proprioceptive control. In addition, most position and movement sense evaluations are performed in static postures such as standing or sitting. However, little is known about the proprioceptive control during more dynamic and complex tasks such as sit-to-stand in patients with LBP (Cordo and Gurfinkel 2004; Claeys et al. 2012).

The use of muscle vibration as an experimental probe can help in clarifying proprioceptive control in a more direct manner. Muscle vibration, often mistaken as a disturbance, is a powerful *stimulus* of muscle spindles and can induce kinesthetic illusions (Goodwin et al. 1972; Roll and Vedel 1982; Brumagne et al. 1999a; Cordo et al. 2005). Direction-specific responses can be expected if the CNS uses the afference of the stimulated muscles for postural control. Therefore, muscle vibration can be used both during experiments using the 'conscious' position sense paradigm (Brumagne et al. 2000) and during experimental setups where the 'subconscious' proprioceptive control is evaluated, such as in *postural balance* approach (see Fig. 12.1 and below).

Altered postural balance in people with LBP

The question arises whether the reports on altered lumbosacral proprioception are related to local dysfunction of proprioceptors (e.g. damaged/atrophied muscle spindles) thus affecting the quality of sensory reception used to track the spine, or to changes in central processing of these proprioceptive signals. Is it mainly a sensory impairment problem or an impaired sensory integration? Position and movement sense experiments are more inclined to target the receptor hypothesis. Based on recent studies, changes in central processing of proprioceptive signals (i.e. sensory integration) may play an important role in the observed altered proprioception in patients with LBP (Brumagne et al. 2004a; Brumagne et al. 2008b; della Volpe et al. 2006; Popa et al. 2007; Claeys et al. 2011).

For optimal postural control the CNS must identify and selectively focus on the sensory inputs (visual, vestibular and proprioceptive) that are providing the functionally most reliable input (Goodworth and Peterka 2009; Horlings et al. 2009). Through sensory re-weighting and gain control, the CNS must integrate the sensory signals adaptively to conflicting and complex postural conditions and to the task at hand. If some sensory signals are deemed unreliable, the CNS will increase the gain or upweigh another sensory system (e.g. vision over proprioception) or signals from a location within the proprioceptive system itself (e.g. ankle proprioceptive signals over back proprioceptive signals) and/or downweigh the unreliable sensory system or signals (Brumagne et al. 2004a; Carver et al. 2006; Claeys et al. 2011).

Additionally, proprioception plays an important role in the calibration of the internal representation of the body (Gurfinkel et al. 1995; Lackner and DiZio 2000). The same proprioceptive signals may be processed differently to information (interpretation) centrally, depending on which internal reference frame is chosen by the CNS. The process of selection of a reference frame and interpretation of proprioceptive signals are closely related to the mechanisms of a body scheme (Gurfinkel and Levik 1998). Plastic changes may occur in the brain that may alter the body image and body scheme due to chronic pain conditions (Moseley 2005) or tonic muscle activity as evoked by the Kohnstamm phenomenon or muscle vibration (Gilhodes et al. 1992; Brumagne, Smets et al. 2004; Ivanenko et al. 2006).

So, another approach (than 'conscious' position and movement sense evaluation) in assessing the role of proprioception is to evaluate postural balance, while keeping the signals from the visual (e.g. blindfolded) and vestibular systems (e.g. no head accelerations) relatively constant (Allum et al. 1998; Horlings et al. 2009).

No differences in postural sway between patients with LBP and healthy controls are seen during simple standing conditions. Even smaller sways are observed for the patient population (Brumagne, Cordo et al. 2004; Brumagne et al. 2008a, 2008b; Claeys et al. 2011). However, when the complexity of postural conditions increases (e.g. unstable support surface, translating platforms, unipedal stance, ballistic arm movements), postural sways increase significantly in patients with LBP compared to healthy individuals (Luoto et al. 1998; Mientjes and Frank 1999; Brumagne, Cordo et al. 2004; della Volpe et al. 2006; Henry et al. 2006; Mok et al. 2007; Popa et al. 2007; Brumagne et al. 2008a, 2008b; Claeys et al. 2011). Furthermore, during unstable sitting, larger sways are observed for the individuals with LBP compared to healthy controls, especially at the most difficult stability levels (Radebold et al. 2001; Van Daele et al. 2009).

Often, altered lumbosacral proprioception has been suggested as a possible mechanism for the observed decreased postural robustness and postural instability, although without a direct measurement of proprioception. Evaluating postural balance during complex postural

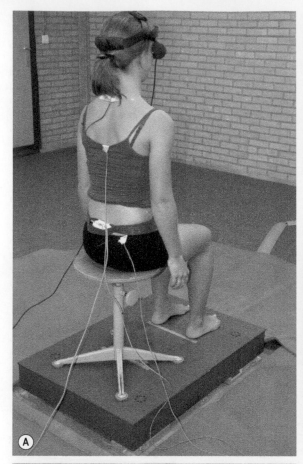

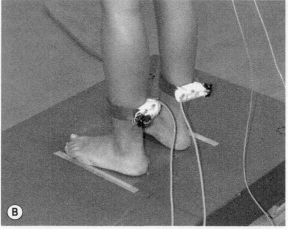

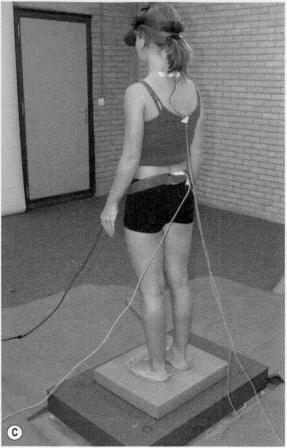

Figure 12.1 Experimental setup. (A) Sitting combined with back muscle vibration. (B) Ankle muscle vibration. (C) Standing on unstable support surface combined with back muscle vibration.

conditions combined with muscle vibration may lead to a more complete representation (Brumagne et al. 2008b).

As a final consideration, the observed changes in postural balance in people with LBP might be more related to altered sensory re-weighting (e.g. upweighting ankle proprioceptive signals and downweighting back muscle signals) (Brumagne, Cordo et al. 2004; della Volpe et al. 2006; Popa et al. 2007; Brumagne et al. 2008b; Claeys et al. 2011) and to changes in reference frames (e.g. offset in the subjective vertical) (Brumagne et al. 2008a) rather than a predominantly peripheral receptor and transmission problem. Accordingly, the individuals with LBP seem

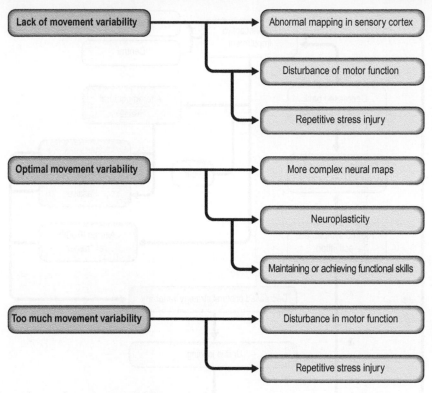

Figure 12.2 Different forms of movement variability.

to adopt a rigid postural control strategy instead of a multi-segmental postural control strategy, which seems suboptimal during more complex postural conditions and actually induces larger subsequent spinal motions (Mok et al. 2004, 2007; Henry et al. 2006; della Volpe et al. 2006; Popa et al. 2007; Brumagne et al. 2008a, 2008b; Van Daele et al. 2009).

DECREASED VARIABILITY IN PROPRIOCEPTIVE POSTURAL STRATEGIES AS A POSSIBLE MECHANISM

Variability is a fundamental property of biological systems and an optimal amount of variability in the motor constituents is important for postural and motor control and learning (Bernstein 1967; Fomin et al. 1976; Harbourne and Stergiou 2009). Lack of postural and movement variability describes biological systems that are overly rigid and unchanging, whereas too much movement variability portrays systems that are noisy and unstable. Both conditions characterize systems that are less compliant to perturbations which may cause or sustain a pathological

condition (Stergiou et al. 2006; Harbourne and Stergiou 2009) (see Fig. 12.2). The cause of decreased variability in postural coordination remains obscure.

A decrease in variability in anticipatory postural adjustments (APAs) has been observed when acute pain stimuli have been induced in the low back of healthy individuals. Moreover, in some subjects normal variability in postural strategy was not re-established even when the pain was stopped and these non-resolvers were characterized by more fear of movement that may induce LBP (Moseley and Hodges 2006). This decrease in variability in APAs has been confirmed in patients with chronic LBP (Jacobs et al. 2009). These authors found it unlikely that the decreased variability was neither due to biomechanical factors nor to reported pain and disability levels.

In addition, people with recurrent LBP seem to use the same proprioceptive postural strategy (i.e. strong reliance on ankle proprioceptive signals) even in postural conditions when this strategy is suboptimal, such as standing on an unstable support surface and sitting (Brumagne et al. 2006, 2008a, 2008b; Claeys et al. 2011). A similar rigid postural strategy can be evoked in healthy subjects when the inspiratory muscles and/or back muscles are experimentally fatigued (Janssens et al. 2010; Johanson et al. 2011).

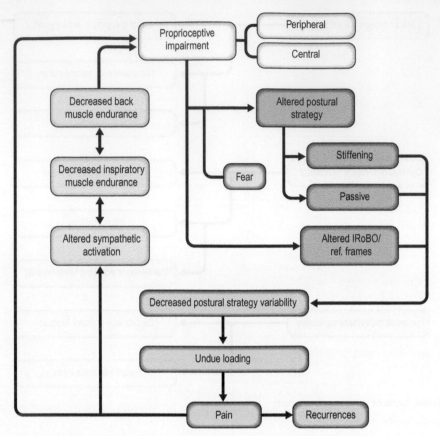

Figure 12.3 Proprioceptive impairment leading to decreased postural strategy variability and pain. IRoBO, internal representation of body orientation; ref., reference.

The dependence on other sensory systems (e.g. vision) and/or an increased reliance on proprioceptive signals from one location (i.e. ankle signals) observed in LBP may be an adaptive strategy to compensate for their proprioceptive deficits (e.g. at the low back). As the proprioceptive impairment progresses and during more complex postural conditions, the strategy consisting of re-weighting sensory inputs in favour of the visual sensory mode and single-joint control by stiffening (versus multi-segmental control) may no longer suffice. Moreover, the impaired adaptation and rigid postural strategy may even contribute to increased spinal loading due to poor or excessive stabilization of forces induced by movement (Mok et al. 2007). In addition, the lack of variability in posture and movement might lead to abnormal mapping of the sensory cortex, which in turn may lead to further altered postural and motor control (Merzenich and Jenkins 1993; Byl et al. 2002; Harbourne and Stergiou 2009).

Figure 12.3 summarizes how proprioception can be negatively influenced and how impaired proprioception may affect postural strategy and the internal representation of the body leading to decreased variability, undue loading and pain.

FUTURE DIRECTIONS

The proposed hypothesis of decreased variability in proprioceptive postural strategy as a possible mechanism of LBP may require further exploration in larger cohort studies in order to identify subgroups of patients. To elucidate the cause and effect relationship of LBP, prospective studies are necessary. Currently, we have undertaken a prospective study to underscore or refute this hypothesis. In the meantime, individuals with poor postural balance performance during standing have been shown to have an increased risk of LBP (Takala and Viikari-Juntura 2000). In addition, some aspects of proprioception such as decreased reflex control of trunk muscles during sitting, but not position sense, may be risk factors for causing and sustaining LBP in college athletes (Cholewicki et al. 2005; Silfies et al. 2007).

Refinement in methodology by creating better controlled postural conditions may assist in further revealing the underlying mechanisms (e.g. CAREN system, Barton et al. 2006). Moreover, if combined with functional (brain) imaging (e.g. functional magnetic resonance imaging (fMRI), diffusion tensor imaging, transcranial magnetic stimulation, functional near-infrared spectroscopy (fNIRS)) more direct insight into the central mechanisms may be provided. Recently, preliminary evidence of reorganization of trunk muscle representation at the *motor* cortex in individuals with recurrent LBP was provided and this reorganization seems to be associated with postural control impairments (Tsao et al. 2008). Functional near-infrared spectroscopy (fNIRS) may be a promising tool in postural control studies. As a non-invasive neuro-imaging method that measures changes in oxyhaemoglobin concentrations, it can be used in more functional postures and movements compared to fMRI (Shimada et al. 2005). Moreover, electromechanical devices (e.g. muscle vibrators) can be used in the experimental setting since NIRS measurements are not affected by electromagnetic noise.

To appraise variability in biological systems and thus in postural control, linear measures should be combined with non-linear measures such as approximate entropy and the Lyapunov exponent (Harbourne and Stergiou 2009).

Finally, preliminary results have shown that patients with recurrent LBP can change their proprioceptive control strategy by motor control exercises (combined with muscle vibration) (Brumagne et al. 2005). However, a more specific and direct proprioceptive training that is based on *sensing*, *localizing* and *discriminating* proprioceptive signals of specific trunk muscles during functional activities might be more effective in the long run. The emphasis is on how enhanced integration of sensory input can optimize the patient's capacity to change the stereotypical posture and movement patterns resulting in more flexible postural control strategies. Addressing variability in postural strategy might prove fruitful in the prevention of recurrence of LBP. The promotion of an optimal amount of movement variability in patients with LBP by incorporating a rich repertoire of postural and movement strategies allows the motor learning and the recovery of function not to be hard coded, but flexible to the individual needs (Harbourne and Stergiou 2009).

In summary, LBP may outwardly appear as a pure mechanical problem, however, the underlying mechanism may depict a sensory processing problem. People with LBP exhibiting a stiffening postural strategy may have an underlying proprioceptive control problem. This may lead to decreased variability in postural control strategies. If decreased variability in postural and motor control plays a role in sustaining LBP, rehabilitation of patients with recurrent LBP should include diversification of the postural and movement repertoire.

ACKNOWLEDGEMENTS

This work was supported by grants from the Research Foundation – Flanders (1.5.104.03 and G.0674.09). L.J. received a PhD fellowship of the Research Foundation – Flanders (FWO). M.P. is PhD fellow of the Agency for Innovation by Science and Technology – Flanders (IWT).

REFERENCES

Allum, J.H., Bloem, B.R., Carpenter, M.G., Hulliger, M., Hadders-Algra, M., 1998. Proprioceptive control of posture: a review of new concepts. Gait Posture 8, 214–242.

Asell, M., Sjölander, P., Kerschbaumer, H., Djupsjöbacka, M., 2006. Are lumbar repositioning errors larger among patients with chronic low back pain compared with asymptomatic subjects? Arch Phys Med Rehabil 87, 1170–1176.

Barton, G., Holmes, G., Hawken, M., Lees, A., Vanrenterghem, J., 2006. A virtual reality tool for training and testing core stability: a pilot study. Gait Posture 24, S101–S102.

Bernstein, N., 1967. Coordination of Movement. Pergamon Press, Oxford.

Brumagne, S., Lysens, R., Swinnen, S., Verschueren, S., 1999a. Effect of paraspinal muscle vibration on position sense of the lumbosacral spine. Spine 24, 1328–1331.

Brumagne, S., Lysens, R., Swinnen, S., Charlier, C., 1999b. Effect of exercise-induced fatigue on lumbosacral position sense. In: Proceedings of the 13th International Congress of the World Confederation for Physical Therapy, Yokohama, p. 171.

Brumagne, S., Cordo, P., Lysens, R., Swinnen, S., Verschueren, S., 2000. The role of paraspinal muscle spindles in lumbosacral position. Spine 25, 989–994.

Brumagne, S., Cordo, P., Verschueren, S., 2004a. Proprioceptive weighting changes in persons with low back pain and elderly persons during upright standing. Neurosci Lett 366, 63–66.

Brumagne, S., Smets, S., Staes, F., Van Deun, S., Stappaerts, K., 2004. Paraspinal muscle spasms as a mechanism for an altered internal representation in patients with low back pain. Abstract Book Spineweek 2004 SP8.

Brumagne, S., Valcke, R., Staes, F., Van Deun, S., Stappaerts, K., 2004b. Altered proprioceptive postural control in professional classic dancers with low back pain. Abstract Book Spineweek 2004 P145.

Brumagne, S., Devos, J., Maes, H., Roelants, M., Delecluse, C., Verschueren, S., 2005. Whole body and local spinal muscle vibration combined with segmental stabilization training improve trunk muscle control and back muscle endurance in persons with recurrent low back pain: a randomized controlled study. Eur Spine J 14, S31–S32.

Brumagne, S., Paulus, I., Van Deun, S., Bogaerts, A., Verschueren, S., Staes, F., 2006. A rigid proprioceptive postural control strategy in persons with recurrent low back pain during normal stance and standing on an unstable support surface. Society for Neuroscience Abstracts 347.1.

Brumagne, S., Janssens, L., Janssens, E., Goddyn, L., 2008a. Altered postural control in anticipation of postural instability in persons with recurrent low back pain. Gait and Posture 28, 657–662.

Brumagne, S., Janssens, L., Süüden-Johanson, E., Claeys, K., Knapen, S., 2008b. Persons with recurrent low back pain exhibit a rigid postural control strategy. Eur Spine J 17, 1177–1184.

Byl, N., Merzenich, M., Jenkins, W., 1996. A primate genesis model of focal dystonia and repetitive strain injury: I. Learning-induced dedifferentiation of the representation of the hand in the primary somatosensory cortex in adult monkeys. Neurology 47, 508–520.

Byl, N.N., Nagarajan, S.S., Merzenich, M.M., Roberts, T., McKenzie, A., 2002. Correlation of clinical neuromusculoskeletal and central somatosensory performance: variability in controls and patients with severe and mild focal hand dystonia. Neural Plast 9, 177–203.

Caldwell, J.S., McNair, P.J., Williams, M., 2003. The effects of repetitive motion on lumbar flexion and erector spinae muscle activity in rowers. Clin Biomech 18, 704–711.

Carpenter, M.G., Bloem, B.R., 2011. Postural control in Parkinson patients: a proprioceptive problem? Exp Neurol 227, 26–30.

Carpenter, M.G., Frank, J.S., Silcher, C.P., Peysar, G.W., 2001. The influence of postural threat on the control of upright stance. Exp Brain Res 138, 210–218.

Carver, S., Kiemel, T., Jeka, J.J., 2006. Modeling the dynamics of sensory reweighting. Biol Cybern 95, 123–134.

Cholewicki, J., Silfies, S.P., Shah, R.A., Greene, H.S., Reeves, N.P., Alvi, K., 2005. Delayed trunk muscle reflex responses increase the risk of low back injuries. Spine 30, 2614–2620.

Claeys, K., Brumagne, S., Dankaerts, W., Kiers, H., Janssens, L., 2011. Decreased variability in proprioceptive postural strategy during standing and sitting in people with recurrent low back pain. Eur J Appl Physiol 111, 115–123.

Claeys, K., Dankaerts, W., Janssens, L., Kiers, H., Brumagne, S., 2012. Altered preparatory pelvic control during the sit-to-stance-to-sit movement in people with non-specific low back pain. J Electromyogr Kinesiol (in press) PMID, 22595702.

Cordo, P.J., Gurfinkel, V.S., 2004. Motor coordination can be fully understood only by studying complex movements. Prog Brain Res 143, 29–38.

Cordo, P.J., Gurfinkel, V.S., Brumagne, S., Flores-Vieira, C., 2005. Effect of slow, small movement on the vibration-evoked kinesthetic illusion. Exp Brain Res 167, 324–334.

Dankaerts, W., O'Sullivan, P., Burnett, A., Straker, L., Davey, P., Gupta, R., 2009. Discriminating healthy controls and two clinical subgroups of nonspecific chronic low back pain patients using trunk muscle activation and lumbosacral kinematics of postures and movements: a statistical classification model. Spine 34, 1610–1618.

della Volpe, R., Popa, T., Ginanneschi, F., Spidalieri, R., Mazzocchio, R., Rossi, A., 2006. Changes in coordination of postural control during dynamic stance in chronic low back pain patients. Gait Posture 24, 349–355.

Descarreaux, M., Blouin, J.S., Teasdale, N., 2005. Repositioning accuracy and movement parameters in low back pain subjects and healthy control subjects. Eur Spine J 14, 185–191.

Dickx, N., Cagnie, B., Achten, E., Vandemaele, P., Parlevliet, T., Danneels, L., 2008. Changes in lumbar muscle activity because of induced muscle pain evaluated by muscle functional magnetic resonance imaging. Spine 33, E983–9.

Djupsjöbacka, M., Johansson, H., Bergenheim, M., Wenngren, B.I., 1995. Influences on the gamma-muscle spindle system from muscle afferents stimulated by increased intramuscular concentrations of bradykinin and 5-HT. Neurosci Res 22, 325–333.

Fomin, S.V., Gurfinkel, V.S., Feldman, A.G., Shtilkind, T.I., 1976. Moments in human leg joints during walking. Biofizika 21, 556–561.

Frzovic, D., Morris, M.E., Vowels, L., 2000. Clinical tests of standing balance: performance of persons with multiple sclerosis. Arch Phys Med Rehabil 81, 215–221.

Gandevia, S.C., McCloskey, D.I., Burke, D., 1992. Kinaesthetic signals and muscle contraction. Trends Neurosci 15, 62–65.

Ghez, C., Sainburg, R., 1995. Proprioceptive control of interjoint coordination. Can J Physiol Pharmacol 73, 273–284.

Gilhodes, J.C., Gurfinkel, V.S., Roll, J.P., 1992. Role of Ia muscle spindle afferents in post-contraction and post-vibration motor effect genesis. Neurosci Lett 135, 247–251.

Gill, K.P., Callaghan, M.J., 1998. The measurement of lumbar proprioception in individuals with and without low back pain. Spine 23, 371–377.

Goodwin, G.M., McCloskey, D.I., Matthews, P.B., 1972. Proprioceptive illusions induced by muscle vibration: contribution by muscle spindles to perception? Science 175, 1382–1384.

Goodworth, A.D., Peterka, R.J., 2009. Contribution of sensorimotor integration to spinal stabilization in humans. J Neurophysiol 102, 496–512.

Granata, K.P., Marras, W.S., 2000. Cost–benefit of muscle cocontraction in protecting against spinal instability. Spine 25, 1398–1404.

Granata, K.P., Slota, G.P., Wilson, S.E., 2004. Influence of fatigue in neuromuscular control of spinal stability. Hum Factors 46, 81–91.

Gribble, P.L., Mullin, L.I., Cothros, N., Mattar, A., 2003. Role of cocontraction in arm movement accuracy. J Neurophysiol 89, 2396–2405.

Gurfinkel, V.S., Ivanenko, YuP., Levik, YuS., Babakova, I.A., 1995. Kinesthetic reference for human orthograde posture. Neurosci 68, 229–243.

Gurfinkel, V.S., Levik, IuS., 1998. Reference systems and interpretation of proprioceptive signals. Fiziol Cheloveka 24, 53–63.

Hamaoui, A., Do, M., Poupard, L., Bouisset, S., 2002. Does respiration perturb body balance more in chronic low back pain subjects than in healthy subjects? Clin Biomech 17, 548–550.

Harbourne, R.T., Stergiou, N., 2009. Movement variability and the use of nonlinear tools. Phys Ther 89, 267–282.

Hellström, F., Roatta, S., Thunberg, J., Passatore, M., Djupsjöbacka, M., 2005. Responses of muscle spindles in feline dorsal neck muscles to electrical stimulation of the cervical sympathetic nerve. Exp Brain Res 165, 328–342.

Henry, S.M., Hitt, J.R., Jones, S.L., Bunn, J.Y., 2006. Decreased limits of stability in response to postural perturbations in subjects with low back pain. Clin Biomech 21, 881–892.

Hodges, P.W., Gurfinkel, V.S., Brumagne, S., Smith, T.C., Cordo, P.J., 2002. Coexistence of stability and mobility in postural control: evidence from postural compensation for respiration. Exp Brain Res 144, 293–302.

Hodges, P.W., Richardson, C.A., 1996. Inefficient muscular stabilization of the lumbar spine associated with low back pain. A motor control evaluation of transversus abdominis. Spine 21, 2640–2650.

Hodges, P.W., Moseley, G.L., 2003. Pain and motor control of the lumbopelvic region: effect and possible mechanisms. J Electromyogr Kinesiol 13, 361–370.

Horlings, C.G., Küng, U.M., Honegger, F., Van Engelen, B.G., Van Alfen, N., Bloem, B.R., et al., 2009. Vestibular and proprioceptive influences on trunk movements during quiet standing. Neuroscience 161, 904–914.

Ivanenko, Y.P., Wright, W.G., Gurfinkel, V.S., Horak, F., Cordo, P., 2006. Interaction of involuntary post-contraction activity with locomotor movements. Exp Brain Res 169, 255–260.

Jacobs, J.V., Henry, S.M., Nagle, K.J., 2009. People with chronic low back pain exhibit decreased variability in the timing of their anticipatory postural adjustments. Behav Neurosci 123, 455–458.

Janssens, L., Troosters, T., McConnell, A., Raymaekers, J., Goossens, N., Pijnenburg, M., et al., 2012. Suboptimal postural strategy and back muscle oxygenation during inspiratory resistive loading. Med Sci Sports Exerc, in press.

Janssens, L., Brumagne, S., Polspoel, K., Troosters, T., McConnell, A., 2010. The effect of inspiratory muscles fatigue on postural control in people with and without recurrent low back pain. Spine 35, 1088–1094.

Johansson, H., Sojka, P., 1991. Pathophysiological mechanisms involved in genesis and spread of muscular tension in occupational muscle pain and in chronic musculoskeletal pain syndromes: a hypothesis. Med Hypotheses 35, 196–203.

Johanson, E., Brumagne, S., Janssens, L., Pijnenburg, M., Claeys, K., Pääsuke, M., 2011. The effect of acute back muscles fatigue on postural control in individuals with and without recurrent low back pain. Eur Spine J 20, 2152–2159.

Lackner, J.R., DiZio, P.A., 2000. Aspects of body self-calibration. Trends Cogn Sci 4, 279–288.

Leinonen, V., Kankaanpää, M., Luukkonen, M., Kansanen, M., Hänninen, O., Airaksinen, O., et al., 2003. Lumbar paraspinal muscle function, perception of lumbar position, and postural control in disc herniation-related back pain. Spine 28, 842–848.

Leinonen, V., Määttä, S., Taimela, S., Herno, A., Kankaanpää, M., Partanen, J., et al., 2002. Impaired lumbar movement perception in association with postural stability and motor- and somatosensory-evoked potentials in lumbar spinal stenosis. Spine 27, 975–983.

Lund, J.P., Donga, R., Widmer, C.G., Stohler, C.S., 1991. The pain-adaptation model: a discussion of the relationship between chronic musculoskeletal pain and motor activity. Can J Physiol Pharmacol 69, 683–694.

Luoto, S., Aalto, H., Taimela, S., Hurri, H., Pyykkö, I., Alaranta, H., 1998. One-footed and externally disturbed two-footed postural control in patients with chronic low back pain and healthy control subjects. A controlled study with follow-up. Spine 23, 2081–2089.

Merzenich, M.M., Jenkins, W.M., 1993. Reorganization of cortical representations of the hand following alterations of skin inputs induced by nerve injury, skin island transfers, and experience. J Hand Ther 6, 89–104.

Mientjes, M.I., Frank, J.S., 1999. Balance in chronic low back pain patients compared to healthy people under various conditions in upright standing. Clin Biomech 14, 710–716.

Mok, N.W., Brauer, S.G., Hodges, P.W., 2004. Hip strategy for balance control in quiet standing is reduced in people with low back pain. Spine 29, E107–12.

Mok, N.W., Brauer, S.G., Hodges, P.W., 2007. Failure to use movement in postural strategies leads to increased spinal displacement in low back pain. Spine 32, E537–43.

Moseley, G.L., 2005. Distorted body image in complex regional pain syndrome. Neurology 65, 773.

Moseley, G.L., Hodges, P.W., 2006. Reduced variability of postural strategy prevents normalization of motor changes induced by back pain: a risk factor for chronic trouble? Behav Neurosci 120, 474–476.

Newcomer, K.L., Laskowski, E.R., Yu, B., Johnson, J.C., An, K.N., 2000. Differences in repositioning error among patients with low back pain compared with control subjects. Spine 25, 2488–2493.

O'Sullivan, P.B., Burnett, A., Floyd, A.N., Gadsdon, K., Logiudice, J., Miller, D., et al., 2003. Lumbar repositioning deficit in a specific low back pain population. Spine 28, 1074–1079.

Passatore, M., Roatta, S., 2006. Influence of sympathetic nervous system on sensorimotor function: whiplash associated disorders (WAD) as a model. Eur J Appl Physiol 98, 423–449.

Popa, T., Bonifazi, M., Della Volpe, R., Rossi, A., Mazzocchio, R., 2007. Adaptive changes in postural strategy selection in chronic low back pain. Exp Brain Res 177, 411–418.

Radebold, A., Cholewicki, J., Polzhofer, G.K., Greene, H.S., 2001. Impaired postural control of the lumbar spine is associated with delayed muscle response times in patients with chronic idiopathic low back pain. Spine 26, 724–730.

Roatta, S., Windhorst, U., Ljubisavljevic, M., Johansson, H., Passatore, M., 2002. Sympathetic modulation of muscle spindle afferent sensitivity to stretch in rabbit jaw closing muscles. J Physiol 540, 237–248.

Roll, J.P., Vedel, J.P., 1982. Kinaesthetic role of muscle afferents in man, studied by tendon vibration and microneurography. Exp Brain Res 47, 177–190.

Rougier, P., Faucher, M., Cantalloube, S., Lamotte, D., Vinti, M., Thoumie, P., 2007. How proprioceptive impairments affect quiet standing in patients with multiple sclerosis. Somatosens Mot Res 24, 41–51.

Sanger, T.D., Merzenich, M.M., 2000. Computational model of the role of sensory disorganization in focal task-specific dystonia. J Neurophysiol 84, 2458–2464.

Shimada, S., Hiraki, K., Oda, I., 2005. The parietal role in the sense of self-ownership with temporal discrepancy between visual and proprioceptive feedbacks. Neuroimage 24, 1225–1232.

Silfies, S.P., Cholewicki, J., Reeves, N.P., Greene, H.S., 2007. Lumbar position sense and the risk of low back injuries in college athletes: a prospective cohort study. BMC Musculoskelet Disord 8, 129.

Sjøgaard, G., Lundberg, U., Kadefors, R., 2000. The role of muscle activity and mental load in the development of pain and degenerative processes at the muscle cell level during computer work. Eur J Appl Physiol 83, 99–105.

Stergiou, N., Harbourne, R., Cavanaugh, J., 2006. Optimal movement variability: a new theoretical perspective for neurologic physical therapy. J Neurol Phys Ther 30, 120–129.

Taimela, S., Kankaanpää, M., Luoto, S., 1999. The effect of lumbar fatigue on the ability to sense a change in lumbar position: a controlled study. Spine 24, 1322–1327.

Takala, E.P., Viikari-Juntura, E., 2000. Do functional tests predict low back pain? Spine 25, 2126–2132.

Tamura, Y., Ueki, Y., Lin, P., Vorbach, S., Mima, T., Kakigi, R., et al., 2009. Disordered plasticity in the primary somatosensory cortex in focal hand dystonia. Brain 132, 749–755.

Thomas, G.D., Segal, S.S., 2004. Neural control of muscle blood flow during exercise. J Appl Physiol 97, 731–738.

Thunberg, J., Ljubisavljevic, M., Djupsjöbacka, M., Johansson, H., 2002. Effects on the fusimotor-muscle spindle system induced by intramuscular injections of hypertonic saline. Exp Brain Res 142, 319–326.

Torres-Russotto, D., Perlmutter, J.S., 2008. Task-specific dystonias: a review. Ann N Y Acad Sci 1142, 179–199.

Tsao, H., Galea, M.P., Hodges, P.W., 2008. Reorganization of the motor cortex is associated with postural control deficits in recurrent low back pain. Brain 131, 2161–2171.

Van Daele, U., Hagman, F., Truijen, S., Vorlat, P., Van Gheluwe, B., Vaes, P., 2009. Differences in balance strategies between nonspecific chronic low back pain patients and healthy control subjects during unstable sitting. Spine 34, 1233–1238.

van Dieën, J.P., Selen, L.P.J., Cholewicki, J., 2003. Trunk muscle activation in low-back pain patients, an analysis of the literature. J Electromyogr Kinesiol 13, 333–351.

Vaugoyeau, M., Azulay, J.P., 2010. Role of sensory information in the control of postural orientation in Parkinson's disease. J Neurol Sci 289, 66–68.

Verbunt, J.A., Seelen, H.A., Vlaeyen, J.W., Bousema, E.J., van der Heijden, G.J., Heuts, P.H., et al., 2005. Pain-related factors contributing to muscle inhibition in patients with chronic low back pain: an experimental investigation based on superimposed electrical stimulation. Clin J Pain 21, 232–240

Wright, W.G., Gurfinkel, V.S., King, L.A., Nutt, J.G., Cordo, P.J., Horak, F.B., 2010. Axial kinesthesia is impaired in Parkinson's disease: effects of levodopa. Exp Neurol 225, 202–209.

Zedka, M., Prochazka, A., Knight, B., Gillard, D., Gauthier, M., 1999. Voluntary and reflex control of human back muscles during induced pain. J Physiol 520, 591–604.

Chapter |13|

Proprioceptive contributions from paraspinal muscle spindles to the relationship between control of the trunk and back pain

Joel G. Pickar
Palmer Center for Chiropractic Research, Palmer College of Chiropractic, Davenport, Iowa, USA

INTRODUCTION

Relationships are two way streets. This is no less true for the relationship between control of the trunk and back pain. From the trunk's perspective, how could motor control of the trunk contribute to back pain? From the perspective of pain, how could pain affect motor control of the trunk? Our discussion will focus on the first half of this relationship, how control of the trunk could influence back pain. To address this relationship, we will first consider the endpoint by briefly summarizing our current understanding of pain mechanisms. These mechanisms provide the pathways by which motor control can relate to back pain.

PAIN

As a generalization, pain may be distinguished based upon the location of the stimulus that gives rise to it. This provides two broad categories of pain: psychological and somatic. Psychological pain is initiated by neurological processes within the brain. Reciprocally, somatic pain is initiated by stimuli outside of the brain. For the individual, the pain is equally real regardless of the source. Neural signals from both sources often converge to modify the sensations that one might have in response to input from either source alone. To wit, the same pain-producing stimuli, such as having a deep splinter removed under conditions in which one is focused on, versus distracted from, the process, can evoke different pain experiences (also see Moseley and Arntz 2007). We will focus on the sources and mechanisms that initiate somatic pain. The reader is referred to several excellent sources for the supporting literature (Treede et al. 1992; Cervero and Laird 1996; Wall et al. 2006; Sandkuhler 2009).

Nociceptive pain

Sherrington coined the termed 'nociception' in the early 1900s to describe the organism's ability to sense injurious stimuli. Nociception and the pain it produces require activation of specific peripheral receptive nerve endings in response to either impending tissue injury or to actual tissue injury. These nerve endings and their parent neurone are called nociceptors. Different classes of nociceptors respond directly to the physical energy contained in strong mechanical and extreme thermal stimuli. In addition, some classes respond indirectly to the injurious effects of these stimuli when cells in the traumatized tissues release inflammatory mediators. With back pain, mechanical and chemical stimuli are likely the two most relevant stimuli.

Nociceptive pain is considered normal or physiological because it notifies the organism that its well-being is being threatened and it elicits activity that removes or reduces the threat of injury. For example, mechanically sensitive nociceptors stimulated by creep deformation likely initiate positional adjustments during prolonged static postures. While there is a close correlation between the discharge rate of mechanically sensitive nociceptors and the subjective experience of pain, it is important to recognize that the mechanical threshold for discharge is below the pain threshold. Thus, activation of mechanically sensitive nociceptors does not necessarily evoke pain. In addition, the balance of input between mechanically sensitive nociceptors and non-nociceptors contributes to whether pain is experienced. Simultaneous mechanical input from low threshold receptors can gate the inflow of nociceptive signals (Van Hees and Gybels 1981).

Persistent nociceptive pain

This type of pain is on a continuum with nociceptive pain. It is considered normal and arises when the nociceptive stimulus is intense or prolonged. The consequence of such a nociceptive stimulus is a change in the response properties of the nociceptor and/or spinal cord neurons onto which the nociceptor synapses. The behavioral change in the nociceptor is termed 'peripheral sensitization' and 'central sensitization' for the spinal cord neuron. While it is clear from the literature that tissue damage sufficient to cause inflammation leads to sensitization, it is not clear whether mechanical stimulation sufficient in magnitude to stimulate nociceptors but not cause inflammation is also sufficient to produce sensitization.

Sensitization may manifest itself in two ways. First, the neurone's resting or spontaneous discharge may increase. While the mechanical stimulus may no longer be present, the nociceptor and/or first-order spinal cord neurone continue to transmit nociceptive signals upstream in the central nervous system. Second, a cell's excitation threshold may decrease, i.e. it becomes more excitable. Consequently, a noxious stimulus applied to the threatened or injured region may now evoke a greater discharge from the sensitized nociceptor, augmenting the sensation of pain (primary hyperalgesia). The sensitized nociceptor may also respond to non-noxious stimuli and evoke pain (allodynia). In addition, arising from central sensitization, noxious as well as non-noxious stimulation of the non-injured area may also induce pain (secondary hyperalgesia

and allodynia, respectively) as the spinal cord neurones discharge more or respond to formerly sub-threshold input, respectively.

Pathological pain

The predominant feature of pathological pain is that the individual experiences pain in the absence of either injury or threat of injury. Because the pain occurs in the absence of conditions that normally activate nociceptors, pathological pain has no adaptive or useful purpose. While injury may have occurred at one point in time, the pain persists despite completion of healing. Pathological pain most often arises from damage, not to the receptive endings of a peripheral nerve, but to the nerve itself or to the central nervous system. Structural changes lead to neural signalling that is independent of any noxious stimulus.

Proprioceptive pain

The axons of nociceptors involved in nociceptive and pathological pain are relatively small in diameter, and are either thinly myelinated or unmyelinated. Proprioceptive neurones, those with thickly myelinated, large diameter axons, appear also to contribute to at least one form of pain, namely delayed onset muscle soreness (Weerakkody et al. 2001, 2003). This pain arises from exercise in which a contracting muscle is forced to lengthen, i.e. contract eccentrically. Concentric contractions shorten muscle to induce movement; eccentric muscle contractions on the opposite side of the joint function as a brake to slow the movement. Control experimental protocols which (1) excluded sensitization of nociceptors, (2) selectively blocked large diameter afferents and (3) selectively stimulated low threshold mechanoreceptors were used to confirm that low threshold mechanoreceptors contributed to the soreness experienced after eccentric exercise (Weerakkody et al. 2001). The neuroanatomy and physiology that underlies the access these mechanoreceptors have to pain pathways is unknown. In the lumbar spine, a substantial amount of movement requires eccentric contraction of dorsal paraspinal muscles.

Sensory-motor-incongruity pain

Recognition of this type of pain is relatively new and the range of sensory incongruities that can give rise to it are not yet known (Harris 1999; Moseley and Gandevia 2005; McCabe et al. 2005, 2006). It appears to occur in the absence of tissue injury, being unrelated to the existence of any peripheral pathology. This seems particularly interesting relative to back pain because neither the occurrence nor severity of back pain corresponds with pathology seen with imaging studies (Hadler 2003; Jarvik et al. 2003).

The source of pain from sensory-motor incongruence is thought to arise in the brain but requires incongruous information from sensory pathways during body movement. Experimentally, individuals made to experience discordant sensory information *between* the visual and proprioceptive *systems* during movement of the extremities also experienced low level pain (McCabe et al. 2005). Sensory conflict in the brain was induced by having the individual move a limb hidden from view behind a mirror but having the individual view the mirror image of the unhidden, stationary limb which would be interpreted as a stationary, hidden limb. In contrast, individuals experiencing discordant sensory information incoherent *within* only the proprioceptive system, i.e. between muscle spindles and other forearm proprioceptors, only experienced peculiarity, foreignness and swelling but not pain (Moseley et al. 2006). Sensory conflict during movement was induced by stimulating muscle spindles using vibration to signal that the joint was extended more than it actually was. Common to these sensory conflict interventions was the development of an unusual sensory experience not apparently related to the nature of the actual stimulus.

That sensory conflicts can have physiological consequences is not new. Nausea arises when visual information regarding body movement is incongruent with sensory information from the proprioceptive and vestibular systems (Harrris 1999). It is known that feed-forward motor commands are constantly interacting with sensory feedback information for the construction of body maps and execution of movement (Prochazka 1996; Nielsen 2004; Knoblich et al. 2006). The simple act of reaching for a doorknob requires a body schema with which to identify in three dimensions where the limb is relative to the door knob (using proprioceptive visual information) in order to generate a motor command that at least begins to get the hand towards the door with accuracy and without injury. Conceptually, it seems reasonable to think that sensory conflicts regarding body position and movement could be interpreted by the brain as impending tissue injury. Pain from sensory-motor incongruence might be considered a form of pathological pain because tissue injury does not appear to be involved.

IMPORTANCE OF INTERSEGMENTAL MOTOR CONTROL

A number of considerations converge indicating the importance of motor control of both individual motion segments and the coordination between them for normal spine function and consequently for understanding back pain. Motor control of the trunk as a whole, and the lumbar spine in particular, must meet two biomechanical needs: (1) control of regional orientation and (2) control of individual motion segment translations and rotations while accomplishing regional orientation. While we know that 10–15% of low back pain arises from a well-defined

anatomical anomaly, such as infection (0.01%), inflammatory arthritis (0.3%), neoplasia (0.7%), visceral disease (2%), stenosis (3%), disc herniation, fracture, or degenerative changes (10%), which, in turn, produces nociceptive pain (see above), 85% of low back pain is considered idiopathic (Deyo and Weinstein 2001).

Mechanical abnormalities related to motion segment control were proposed as an aetiological factor in this higher occurring type of low back pain nearly 2 decades ago. At the 1988 workshop 'New Perspectives On Low Back Pain' sponsored by the National Institutes of Health and the American Academy of Orthopedic Surgeons (Schultz et al. 1989), the predominant hypothesis for explaining the aetiology of idiopathic low back pain was the presence of a mechanical derangement in a lumbar motion segment, a derangement caused by paraspinal muscle dysfunction, acute injury, degeneration and/or surgery. These, in turn, were thought to cause spinal instability and result in dysfunction and/or pain. The presence of an intervertebral motion abnormality that depended upon the magnitude and direction of the motion constituted a fundamental assumption underlying this hypothesis (Schultz et al. 1989). In addition, two interrelated systems were recognized as contributing to alterations in intervertebral motion and to spinal instability: passive elements of the spinal column and the neuromuscular control system (Schultz et al. 1989).

Since that time, many studies provide evidence for the importance of neuromuscular control of intersegmental kinematics for normal spinal function. Only a few are presented here to serve as background. It is well known that without active muscles, the osteoligamentous spine in the neutral erect position is unstable, buckling laterally in the coronal plane and progressively bending in the sagittal plane under a compressive axial load less than 100 N (Crisco et al. 1992). As the moving lumbar spine passes through a neutral erect position, lumbar paraspinal muscles are active (Cholewicki et al. 1997). Even small changes in the force from these lumbar muscles have large impacts on a motion segment's biomechanical behaviour. For example, *in vitro* experiments accompanied by a modelling approach that incorporated graded activity of one lumbar paraspinal muscle (Panjabi et al. 1989) show an increase in intersegmental stabilization with muscle inclusion. Graded increases in the muscle's modelled activity decreases both the neutral zone and the intersegmental range of motion: the intersegmental neutral zone decreases between 33% and 40% during flexion, extension and axial rotation but not lateral bending; the intersegmental range of motion decreases between 7% and 27% during extension and axial rotation but not flexion or lateral bending. The largest decrease in the neutral zone and range of motion during these manoeuvres occurs at low muscle forces (20 N compared with 40 N and 60 N). Similarly, very small increases in muscle activity (1–3% of maximal voluntary contraction) of lumbar multifidus, iliocostalis and thoracic longissimus muscles at L2–L4 are sufficient to restore segmental stability (defined by a potential energy minimum) of the lumbar spine even when loading moments are increased to 75% of body weight (Cholewicki and McGill 1996). Incorporating the force vectors of five paraspinal muscles into a modelling approach increases the stabilization of an individual lumbar motion segment: the intersegmental neutral zone decreases (range: 76–83%) during flexion, extension, axial rotation and lateral bending and intersegmental range of motion decreases (range: 55–93%) during flexion, extension, axial rotation and lateral bending (Wilke et al. 1995). Multifidus muscle accounts for 40–80% of the increased stability during sagittal flexion–extension, 45% during axial rotation, and 10–20% during lateral bending, suggesting that neuromuscular mechanisms controlling multifidus muscle activity alone could functionally impact the motion segment especially during flexion–extension and axial rotation. Abnormal control of multifidus muscle may contribute to the fact that mechanical injury to the intervertebral disc occurs most often during loading moments that combine flexion, lateral bending and axial rotation (Nordin and Balagué 1996). A videofluoroscopic study by Cholewicki and McGill has provided direct evidence that individual motion segment behavior is controlled by the motor control system, and in the extreme, that abnormal kinematics can occur when that control is inadequate.

MOTOR CONTROL IN GENERAL

Underlying posture and movement is the integration of feed-forward signals from the brain with feedback signals from peripheral proprioceptors (Nielsen 2004). The role of proprioceptive input is strikingly brought to light from the experiences of an individual with an unusual neuropathy wherein he lost all large diameter primary afferent fibres (Cole 1995). When a room was darkened, thus removing his visual input yet maintaining his vestibular input, this individual would nonetheless collapse to the floor. He would not know where he was in space, his central nervous system being uninformed of his ground contact and the relationships between his body segments. Even in the absence of conscious perception, proprioceptive signals provide the central nervous system with information about the body's location in space. These signals help shape the occurrence, timing and pattern of muscle recruitment, provide feedback with which to identify errors in executed movements (Prochazka 1996; Nielsen 2004), and contribute to neural representations (internal maps) of a body schema (Knoblich et al. 2006). While input from joint, skin and muscle receptors contributes to our proprioceptive sense, the input from muscles is thought to predominate (Prochazka 1996). The role of ligaments is not clear because their discharge is often

not graded with joint movement (Prochazka 1996; Grigg 2001).

The muscle spindle holds a particular fascination because it is anatomically and physiologically complex. It is the only sensory receptor whose sensitivity can be controlled by neural output from the CNS. While muscle spindles in particular have been studied extensively in appendicular muscles, until recently little was known about their position and movement sensitivities or their central synaptic organization in the lumbar spine (Pickar 1999; Pickar and Wheeler 2001; Akatani et al. 2004; Ge et al. 2005; Durbaba et al. 2006; Durbaba et al. 2007; Cao and Pickar 2009; Cao, Pickar et al. 2009).

MUSCLE SPINDLES, INTERSEGMENTAL MOTOR CONTROL AND PAIN

Our lab has been studying the physiology of lumbar paraspinal muscle spindles. Using the cat as an experimental preparation, we have recorded activity from individual muscle spindles in lumbar paraspinal muscles while imposing passive movements upon a vertebra to which the parent muscle attaches. This is accomplished in a relatively intact lumbar spine (Fig. 13.1). The preparation has been described previously (Pickar 1999; Ge et al. 2005). Briefly, an L5 laminectomy exposes the spinal cord where the L6 dorsal roots enter. Paraspinal tissues extending caudally from the L6 vertebra, including muscles innervated by the L6 dorsal root, are left intact. Muscle spindle afferents in the L6 dorsal root are identified and their activity recorded. Controlled actuations are applied to the L6 vertebra using its spinous process. The response of muscle spindle afferents to vertebral position and movement can be determined.

High sensitivity

We investigated the responsiveness of lumbar paraspinal muscle spindles to both a change in vertebral position (Cao, Pickar et al., 2009) and the velocity with which the change occurs (Cao, Khalsa et al. 2009). Our results indicate that spindles in the intersegmental multifidus and longissimus muscles have finer signalling resolution compared with spindles in extremity muscles. For the study of positional sensitivity, we used controlled actuations of the L6 vertebra (0.2, 0.4, 0.6, 0.8 and 1.2 mm) applying displacements in the horizontal plane in the cranial direction. Using geometry, we estimated the increase in muscle length for each actuation distance and determined the spindles' mean instantaneous discharge frequency at each length. Position sensitivity was determined as the slope of the relationship between the estimated change in muscle

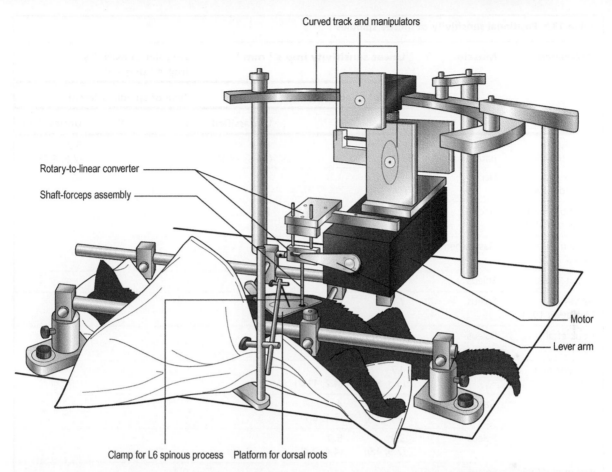

Curved track and manipulators

Rotary-to-linear converter

Shaft-forceps assembly

Motor

Lever arm

Clamp for L6 spinous process   Platform for dorsal roots

Figure 13.1 Set-up for recording from lumbar paraspinal muscle spindles and mechanically actuating the L6 lumbar vertebra.

length and mean instantaneous frequency. In addition, we recorded strain in the L6–L7 facet joint capsule. Based upon previously established relationships between intersegmental angles and facet joint capsule strains in the cat lumbar vertebral column during lumbar flexion, we related actuation distance to the intervertebral angle that could give rise to the joint capsule strain. Thus, positional sensitivity was quantified as discharge rate relative to muscle length and to joint angle. Table 13.1 compares the sensitivity of muscle spindles in the lumbar axial muscles with those in appendicular muscles. The estimates of mean position sensitivity (16.3 imp s^{-1} mm^{-1} ($10.6-22.1$, lower, upper 95% confidence interval)) and mean angular sensitivity (5.2 imp s^{-1} mm^{-1} ($2.6-8.0$, $P = 0.003$)) were more than 3.5 times greater compared with appendicular muscle spindles. The confidence intervals did not contain any of the estimates for static sensitivity of appendicular spindles previously reported in the literature.

Similarly, spindles in the lumbar paraspinal muscles were more sensitive to the velocity of vertebral movement in comparison to appendicular muscles (summarized in

Table 13.2). One millimetre actuations delivered at 0.5, 1.0 and 2.0 mm/s were applied at the L6 spinous process. Several response measures were used to make the comparisons. A 'slow velocity component' was measured as the slope of the relationship between displacement during the constant velocity ramp and instantaneous discharge frequency and a 'quick velocity component' was the slope's intercept at zero displacement. The sensitivities of these components to increasing velocity were at least 5–10 times greater compared to those reported for appendicular muscle spindles. A 'peak component' was determined as the highest discharge rates occurring near the end of the ramp compared with control. Its measure of velocity sensitivity was 2.9 imp s^{-1} mm^{-1} (0.2, 5.5 95% confidence interval) similar to that for cervical paraspinal muscles as well as appendicular muscles. The large dynamic sensitivity of lumbar paraspinal muscle spindles may help ensure control of intervertebral motion during changes in spinal orientation. Factors that adversely affect either proprioceptive input or its central integration may contribute to motor control errors that ultimately cause pain.

149

Table 13.1 Positional sensitivity of muscle spindles

Reference	Muscle	Linear sensitivity imp s⁻¹ mm⁻¹			Angular sensitivity imp s⁻¹ degree⁻¹		
		Type of spindle afferent			Type of spindle afferent		
		I	II	Unclassified	I	II	Unclassified
Cao, Pickar et al. 2009	Lumbar paraspinal			16.3 (10.6, 22.1)			5.2 (2.6, 8.0)
Bolton and Holland 1998	Neck						~2.3
Richmond and Abrahams 1979	Neck			1.4, −2.3			
Botterman and Eldred 1982	Gastrocnemius	2.1	3.2				
Granit 1958	Soleus	3.5					
Harvey and Matthews 1961	Soleus	7.7	6.0				
Houk et al. 1981	Soleus	3.1 (2.4, 3.8)	2.2 (1.9, 2.5)				
Lennerstrand 1968	TA + EDL	4.7 (3.3, 5.1)	7.7 (4.2, 11.2)				
	Gastrocnemius	2.6 (1.8, 3.4)	4.4 (2.1, 6.7)				
	Soleus	3.9 (2.9, 4.9)	5.9 (4.4, 7.4)				
Wei et al. 1986	Soleus				0.4		
	TA				0.6		
Windhorst et al. 1975	EDL	2.15					
Cheney and Preston 1976	Soleus	2.9	2.4		1.1	0.9	
Cordo et al. 2002	Finger extensors				0.4 (0.2, 0.6)		
Edin and Vallbo 1990	Finger extensors	1.7	2.8		0.23	0.33	
Vallbo 1974	Finger flexors				0.18	0.14	

TA, tibialis anterior; EDL, extensor digitorum longus.
Values in parentheses indicate lower and upper 95% confidence intervals.

Table 13.2 Dynamic sensitivity of muscle spindles

Reference	Muscle	Quick velocity		Slow velocity	
		Component imp s^{-1}	Sensitivity (imp/s)(mm/s) or (imp/s)/(degree/s)	Component imp s^{-1} mm^{-1} or imp s^{-1} degree^{-1}	Sensitivity (imp/s/mm)(mm/s) or (imp/s/degree)/(degree/s)
Cao, Khalsa et al. 2009	Lumbar paraspinal	Uncl: 28.4–35.8	Uncl: 4.80 (2.90, 6.7) *Uncl: 1.16 (−0.57, 2.89)*	Uncl: 20.5–23.9 *Uncl: 5.4–6.2*	Uncl: −2.10 (−0.45, −3.75) *Uncl: −0.16 (−0.04, −0.30)*
Lennerstrand 1968	Soleus and lateral gastrocnemius	I°: 0 II°: 0	I°: 0 II°: 0	I°: ~2.2 II°: 0	I°: 0 II°: 0
Grill and Hallett 1995	Finger extensors	Uncl: <5	*Uncl ~0.9*	*Uncl 0.027 (0.010, 0.042)*	

I°, primary muscle spindle afferent; II°, secondary muscle spindle afferent; Uncl, unclassified muscle spindle afferent.
Means or range of means: values in parentheses indicate lower and upper 95% confidence intervals.

History-dependent effects on muscle spindle responsiveness

One factor that may compromise the accuracy of proprioceptive signalling from lumbar paraspinal muscle spindles is thixotropy. Materials with this property are characterized by their capacity to change their behaviour from a liquid to a gel in the absence of a shear stress and then back to a liquid in the presence of a shear stress. In other words, the material's viscosity depends upon its previous history with shear stress. Intrafusal muscle fibres of the spindle apparatus behave thixotropically (Hill 1968; Hufschmidt and Schwaller 1987; Proske et al. 1993). They contain polymeric chains of actin and myosin between which actomyosin crossbridges spontaneously form within seconds of a muscle remaining at a fixed length, i.e. in the absence of a shearing force. These crossbridges are relatively stable, having a slower turnover rate compared with the recycling crossbridges that form during active muscle contraction. The tautness or stiffness of the intrafusal fibre contributes to the timing and fidelity with which muscle stretch is transmitted to the spindle's central region where the sensory terminal of the muscle spindle afferent is deformed (McMahon 1984; Mileusnic et al. 2006).

Our interest in this history-dependent property and its implications for motor control of the lumbar spine arose from previous studies revealing the adverse effects it produces on proprioceptive signalling in limb muscles of the human and cat (Gregory et al. 1986, 1987, 1988; Gregory et al. 1990; Wood et al. 1996). For example, in humans, foot repositioning errors can be evoked experimentally by passively holding the ankle in a position that either shortens or stretches the calf muscles. Upon asking an individual to reposition their foot to a reference position, the previous hold-short position causes an undershoot and hold-long causes an overshoot. Underlying these repositioning errors are altered responses in proprioceptive reflex pathways. The size of the Achilles tendon jerk reflex is larger after triceps surae contraction with the foot plantarflexed (i.e., calf muscles held short) than with the foot dorsiflexed. Conversely, the H reflex is smaller after hold-short than after hold-long.

These 'muscle-history' effects are related to changes in resting spindle discharge (Gregory et al. 1987, 1988; Gregory et al., 1990). When a muscle is held in a static position, either directly by isolating its tendon or indirectly by moving the joint, the intrafusal myofilaments crosslink and stiffen at the new position. Upon subsequent muscle shortening, the stiffened fibres become slack or kink and the sensory terminals are unloaded. Conceptually, this would be similar to pushing together the ends of a stiff piece of piano wire wherein it would either bend or kink. Conversely, subsequent lengthening generates more tension in the already stiffened fibres and augments deformation of the sensory terminals. When the ankle is returned to a reference position after being held-short compared with being held-long, the history-conditioned muscle spindle afferents have a higher discharge rate both at rest and in response to tapping the Achilles tendon. The larger afferent barrage to tapping evokes a larger reflex muscle contraction. The increased resting discharge provides a background of inhibition to the motoneuronal pool of the triceps surae muscles. Because the H reflex does not require activation of the spindles, its magnitude depends upon central mechanisms of excitability. Owing to inhibition of α-motoneurones occurring in response to increases in background spindle discharge (Granit 1950), the magnitude of the H reflex is diminished. The exact synaptic mechanism is not known but may be due to presynaptic inhibition (Gregory et al. 1990; but see Wood et al. 1996). Conversely, hold-long decreases resting discharge and removes the background inhibition. These changes in the magnitude of spindle discharge are also accompanied by delays in the onset of muscle spindle discharge after hold-long history (Morgan et al. 1984; Gregory et al. 1986).

These findings led us to wonder whether the biomechanical history of a spinal motion segment would alter the responsiveness of muscle spindles in lumbar paraspinal muscles attaching to that segment. From a biomechanical perspective, this appeared a sensible consideration for two reasons. First, a neutral zone has been described for intersegmental kinematics (Panjabi 1992). Experimentally, it is recognized by a region of movement trajectory where resistance to movement is low, i.e. intersegmental stiffness is minimal. This region is thought to underlie the experimental observation that spinal stability appears lowest in the neutral posture and that appropriate muscle activation appears critical to maintain stability in the neutral posture (Cholewicki and McGill 1996; Cholewicki et al. 1997). The presence of a neutral zone implies a range of movement wherein a motion segment's position is not uniquely determined and may not reflect the regional spinal posture. While this variation in intersegmental position despite identical regional orientation has not yet been shown directly, regional spinal postures can be quite different despite a sagittally balanced vertebral column with C7 over S1 (Claus et al. 2009). If thixotropic effects in muscle spindles were established within the neutral zone at a given intervertebral position and the zone's low stiffness then allowed a positional change to occur, spindles would not accurately report the new position. Secondly, lengthening or shortening histories could be established by intervertebral positions maintained longer than usual due to several conditions including sustained postures, sustained spinal loading, articular adhesions or asymmetrical alterations in passive muscle tone. The history established by these 'hold' situations would create an error signal from the spindle during a subsequent postural change.

We created biomechanical history using the experimental preparation shown in Figure 13.1. The biomechanical protocols held a lumbar vertebra in each of three positions that stretched, shortened or did not change the paraspinal muscles relative to an intermediate position (Fig. 13.2). Hold-long and hold-short were confirmed by the presence of increased and decreased spindle discharge, respectively, compared to hold-intermediate. Subsequent to establishing each positional history, the vertebra was returned to an identical position, the intermediate position (static test), and then moved in the direction that stretched the muscle (dynamic test). The effect of this biomechanical history on proprioceptive signalling was determined by comparing spindle discharge between hold-intermediate and hold-short or hold-long for each of the two tests. We have explored how the duration of spinal motion segment position as well as its magnitude and direction affect lumbar paraspinal muscle spindle responsiveness.

The responsiveness of multifidus and longissimus muscle spindles to identical vertebral positions or identical changes in position is decreased when the previous history has unloaded the spindle apparatus; it is increased when the previous history has loaded it (Ge et al. 2005). Hold-long decreases resting spindle discharge by more than 15 impulses per second. While hold-short does the converse by increasing resting discharge, it does so to a lesser absolute magnitude compared to hold-long (~5 impulses/s). These thixotropic effects in the paraspinal muscles are fully developed within 3–4 seconds of the hold history. Hold-long has a time constant of 2.6 s and hold-short 1.1 s (Ge et al. 2005). Very small vertebral displacements (0.05–0.11 mm) elicit these effects (Ge et al. 2006) and the magnitude of the altered responsiveness saturates between 0.32 and 0.53 mm of vertebral actuation in the posterior–anterior direction. Positional histories along all three cardinal axes will produce these proprioceptive errors (Pickar et al. 2008). Positional changes in the anatomical plane closest to that of the facet joint, i.e. the sagittal plane, produce the largest decrease in spindle responsiveness.

The apparent importance of proprioceptive input from lumbar paraspinal muscle spindles (indicated by their high position and dynamic sensitivities compared with appendicular muscles), their thixotropic property which alters their responsiveness, and anticipated reflex changes caused by these alterations suggest several ways that spinal motor control relates to back pain. Muscle spindle-induced alterations in the reflex timing or recruitment of paraspinal muscles could alter the instantaneous axis of intersegmental motion, abnormally loading spinal tissues and activating mechanonociceptors. Such nociceptive pain (see 'Pain' section above) would evoke protective behavior and/or serve as a warning of imminent injury. If the abnormal loading were sustained and sufficiently large, inflammatory mediators may be released from the loaded tissue. Persistent nociceptive pain (see 'Pain' section above) would continue until the proprioceptive, biomechanical and inflammatory conditions were ameliorated. In addition to these forms of pain, thixotropic-induced alterations in muscle spindle input could lead to sensory-motor-incongruity pain (see 'Pain' section above). Neural signals from non-thixotropic-dependent low threshold receptors located in the extracellular space of fascia, ligaments, intervertebral disc and either

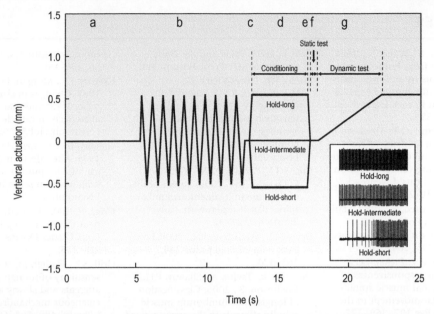

Figure 13.2 Schematic of the protocol to establish vertebral history. **a** Pre-deconditioning: vertebra maintained at intermediate position for 5 s. **b** Deconditioning: vertebra moved ventrally then dorsally 10 times between maximal displacements (10 mm/s) to create identical initial conditions across protocols. **c** Preconditioning: vertebra maintained at intermediate position for 0.5 s. **d** Conditioning: vertebra held at the intermediate, long, or short position for 4 s. Hold-long history loaded and hold-short history unloaded the muscle spindle relative to the effect of hold-intermediate as shown in the inset. **e** Return to the intermediate position. **f** Static test: vertebra maintained at intermediate position for 0.5 s. Mean instantaneous discharge frequency (MIF) following hold-intermediate was subtracted from that after hold-long and hold-short. **g** Dynamic test: vertebra slowly moved to the displacement of the hold-long direction. The mean spindle discharge frequency (MF) following hold-intermediate was subtracted from that after hold-long and hold-short. Inset shows discharge during the 2 tests. *Reproduced from Cao, D.Y., Pickar, J.G., 2009. Thoracolumbar fascia does not influence proprioceptive signalling from lumbar paraspinal muscle spindles in the cat. Journal of Anatomy 215, 417–424, with permission from John Wiley and Sons.*

intersegmental or global muscles would be discordant with the thixotropically derived error signals from the paraspinal muscle spindles. The central nervous system's expectation of a pattern of sensory input from its proprioceptive system would not match the motor pattern of the existing body schema and might be experienced as painful. Body-based therapeutic interventions and training may correct or override this discordance.

SUMMARY

The ideas expressed in this chapter regarding the relationship between motor control and pain are based upon several presumptions. First, appropriate motor control of intersegmental spinal kinematics during regional movements is crucial for normal biomechanics of the vertebral column. Because muscle spindles appear quite sensitive to changes in vertebral position and the rate of movement, we might expect that peripheral or central processes that adversely affect this proprioceptive input will significantly affect motor control of the spine. Secondly, motion segments have a neutral zone where there is low resistance to vertebral movement and therefore the positional relationship between vertebra of a motion segment is not uniquely determined by global position. Due to thixotropy, the responsiveness of the peripheral spindle apparatus is very sensitive to small and short-lasting changes in vertebral position along any of the cardinal axes of motion. Positional changes within the neutral zone may lead to proprioceptive errors from muscle spindles. Alterations in muscle spindle input may lead to strains that inflame spinal tissues and thereby exciting nociceptors, evoking nociceptive pain. In addition, muscle spindle signalling errors induced by thixotropy may produce incoherent proprioception and contribute to sensory-motor-incongruity pain.

REFERENCES

Akatani, J., Kanda, K., Wada, N., 2004. Synaptic input from homonymous group I afferents in m. longissimus lumborum motoneurons in the L4 spinal segment in cats. Exper Brain Res 156, 396–398.

Bolton, P.S., Holland, C.T., 1998. An *in vivo* method for studying afferent fibre activity from cervical paravertebral tissue during vertebral motion in anaesthetised cats. J Neurosci Methods 85, 211–218.

Botterman, B.R., Eldred, E., 1982. Static stretch sensitivity of Ia and II afferents in the cat's gastrocnemius. Pflugers Arch 395, 204–211.

Cao, D.Y., Khalsa, P.S., Pickar, J.G., 2009. Dynamic responsiveness of lumbar paraspinal muscle spindles during vertebral movement in the cat. Exp Brain Res 197, 369–377.

Cao, D.Y., Pickar, J.G., 2009. Thoracolumbar fascia does not influence proprioceptive signaling from lumbar paraspinal muscle spindles in the cat. J Anat 215, 417–424.

Cao, D.Y., Pickar, J.G., Ge, W., Ianuzzi, A., Khalsa, P.S., 2009. Position sensitivity of feline paraspinal muscle spindles to vertebral movement in the lumbar spine. J Neurophysiol 101, 1722–1729.

Cervero, F., Laird, J.M., 1996. From acute to chronic pain: mechanisms and hypotheses. Prog Brain Res 110, 3–15.

Cheney, P.D., Preston, J.B., 1976. Classification and response characteristics of muscle spindle afferents in the primate. J Neurophysiol 39, 1–8.

Cholewicki, J., McGill, S.M., 1996. Mechanical stability of the *in vivo* lumbar spine: implications for injury and chronic low back pain. Clinical Biomechanics 11, 1–15.

Cholewicki, J., Panjabi, M.M., Khachatryan, A., 1997. Stabilizing function of trunk flexor-extensor muscles around a neutral spine posture. Spine 22, 2207–2212.

Claus, A.P., Hides, J.A., Moseley, G.L., Hodges, P.W., 2009. Different ways to balance the spine: subtle changes in sagittal spinal curves affect regional muscle activity. Spine (Phila PA 1976) 34, E208–E214.

Cole, J., 1995. Pride and the Daily Marathon. MIT Press, Boston, MA.

Cordo, P.J., Flores-Vieira, C., Verschueren, S.M.P., Inglis, J.T., Gurfinkel, V., 2002. Position sensitivity of human muscle spindles: Single afferent and population representations. J Neurophysiol 87, 1186–1195.

Crisco, J.J., Panjabi, M.M., Yamamoto, I., Oxland, T.R., 1992. Euler stability of the human ligamentous lumbar spine: Part II experiment. Clin Biomech 7, 27–32.

Deyo, R.A., Weinstein, J.N., 2001. Low back pain. N Engl J Med 344, 363–370.

Durbaba, R., Taylor, A., Ellaway, P.H., Rawlinson, S., 2006. Classification of longissimus lumborum muscle spindle afferents in the anaesthetized cat. J Physiol 571, 489–498.

Durbaba, R., Taylor, A., Ellaway, P.H., Rawlinson, S.R., 2007. Spinal projection of spindle afferents of the longissimus lumborum muscles of the cat. J Physiol 580, 659–675.

Edin, B.B., Vallbo, A.B., 1990. Dynamic response of human muscle spindle afferents to stretch. J Neurophysiol 63, 1297–1306.

Ge, W., Cao, D., Pickar, J.G., 2006. Very small changes in vertebral position evoke muscle history dependent changes in paraspinal muscle spindle discharge. Soc Neurosci Abstr 650.2.

Ge, W., Long, C.R., Pickar, J.G., 2005. Vertebral position alters paraspinal muscle spindle responsiveness in the feline spine: effect of positioning duration. J Physiol 569, 655–665.

Granit, R., 1950. Reflex self-regulation of muscle contraction and autogenetic inhibition. J Physiol 13, 351–372.

Granit, R., 1958. Neuromuscular interaction in postural tone of the cat's isometric soleus muscle. J Physiol 143, 387–402.

Gregory, J.E., Mark, R.F., Morgan, D.L., Patak, A., Polus, B., Proske, U., 1990. Effects of muscle history on the stretch reflex in cat and man. J Physiol 424, 93–107.

Gregory, J.E., Morgan, D.L., Proske, U., 1986. Aftereffects in the responses of cat muscle spindles. J Neurophysiol 56, 451–461.

Gregory, J.E., Morgan, D.L., Proske, U., 1987. Changes in size of the stretch reflex of cat and man attributed to aftereffects in muscle spindles. J Neurophysiol 58, 628–640.

Gregory, J.E., Morgan, D.L., Proske, U., 1988. Aftereffects in the responses of cat muscle spindles and errors of limb position sense in man. J Neurophysiol 59, 1220–1230.

Grigg, P., 2001. Properties of sensory neurons innervating synovial joints. Cells Tissues Organs 169, 218–225.

Grill, S.E., Hallett, M., 1995. Velocity sensitivity of human muscle spindle afferents and slowly adapting type II cutaneous mechanoreceptors. J Physiol 489, 593–602.

Hadler, N.M., 2003. MRI for regional back pain: need for less imaging, better understanding. JAMA 289, 2863–2865.

Harris, A.J., 1999. Cortical origin of pain. Lancet 354, 1464–1466.

Harvey, R.J., Matthews, P.B., 1961. The response of de-efferented muscle spindle endings in the cat's soleus to slow extension of the muscle. J Physiol 157, 370–392.

Hill, D.K., 1968. Tension due to interaction between the sliding filaments in resting striated muscle – the effect of stimulation. J Physiol 199, 637–684.

Houk, J.C., Rymer, W.Z., Crago, P.E., 1981. Dependence of dynamic response of spindle receptors on muscle length and velocity. J Neurophysiol 46, 143–166.

Hufschmidt, A., Schwaller, I., 1987. Short-range elasticity and resting tension of relaxed human lower leg muscles. J Physiol 391, 451–465.

Jarvik, J.G., Hollingworth, W., Martin, B., Emerson, S.S., Gray, D.T., Overman, S., et al., 2003. Rapid magnetic resonance imaging vs. radiographs for patients with low back pain. JAMA 289, 2810–2818.

Knoblich, G., Thornton, I., Grosjean, M., Shiffrar, M., 2006. Human Body Perception from the Inside Out. Oxford University Press, Oxford.

Lennerstrand, G., 1968. Position and velocity sensitivity of muscle spindles in the cat. I. Primary and secondary endings deprived of fusimotor activation. Acta Physiol Scand 73, 281–299.

McCabe, C.S., Haigh, R.C., Halligan, P.W., Blake, D.R., 2005. Simulating sensory-motor incongruence in healthy volunteers: implications for a cortical model of pain. Rheumatology (Oxford) 44, 509–516.

McCabe, C.S., Haigh, R.C., Halligan, P.W., Blake, D.R., 2006. Re: Sensory-motor incongruence and reports of 'pain', by G. L. Moseley and S. C. Gandevia (Rheumatology 2005;44:1083-1085). Rheumatology (Oxford) 45, 644–645.

McMahon, T.A., 1984. Muscles, Reflexes, and Locomotion. Princeton University Press, Princeton, NJ.

Mileusnic, M.P., Brown, I.E., Lan, N., Loeb, G.E., 2006. Mathematical models of proprioceptors. I. Control and transduction in the muscle spindle. J Neurophysiol 96, 1772–1788.

Morgan, D.L., Prochazka, A., Proske, U., 1984. The after-effects of stretch and fusimotor stimulation on the responses of primary endings of cat muscle spindles. J Physiol 356, 465–477.

Moseley, G.L., Arntz, A., 2007. The context of a noxious stimulus affects the pain it evokes. Pain 133, 64–71.

Moseley, G.L., Gandevia, S.C., 2005. Sensory-motor incongruence and reports of 'pain'. Rheumatology (Oxford) 44, 1083–1085.

Moseley, G.L., McCormick, K., Hudson, M., Zalucki, N., 2006. Disrupted cortical proprioceptive representation evokes symptoms of peculiarity, foreignness and swelling, but not pain. Rheumatology (Oxford) 45, 196–200.

Nielsen, J.B., 2004. Sensorimotor integration at spinal level as a basis for muscle coordination during voluntary movement in humans. J Appl Physiol 96, 1961–1967.

Nordin, M., Balagué, F., 1996. Biomechanics and ergonomics in disk herniation accompanied by sciatica. In: Weinstein, J.N., Gordon, S.L. (eds), Low Back Pain. American Academy of Orthopedic Surgeons, Rosemont, IL, pp. 23–48.

Panjabi, M.M., 1992. The stabilizing system of the spine. Part II. Neutral zone and instability hypothesis. J Spinal Disord 5, 390–397.

Panjabi, M.M., Kuniyoshi, A., Duranceau, J., Oxland, T., 1989. Spinal stability and intersegmental muscle forces: a biomechanical model. Spine 14, 194–199.

Pickar, J.G., 1999. An in vivo preparation for investigating neural responses to controlled loading of a lumbar vertebra in the anesthetized cat. J Neurosci Methods 89, 87–96.

Pickar, J.G., Cao, D.Y., Ge, W., 2008. The responsiveness of lumbar paraspinal muscle spindles is affected by the history of vertebral position along 3 orthogonal axes of vertebral motion. Society for Neuroscience 180.10.

Pickar, J.G., Wheeler, J.D., 2001. Response of muscle proprioceptors to spinal manipulative-like loads in the anesthetized cat. J Manip Physiol Ther 24, 2–11.

Prochazka, A., 1996. Proprioceptive feedback and movement regulation. In: Rowell, L.B., Shepherd, J.T. (eds), Handbook of Physiology. American Physiological Society, Bethesda, MD, pp. 89–127.

Proske, U., Morgan, D.L., Gregory, J.E., 1993. Thixotropy in skeletal muscle and in muscle spindles: a review. Progr Neurobiol 41, 705–721.

Richmond, F.J.R., Abrahams, V.C., 1979. Physiological properties of muscle spindles in dorsal neck muscles of the cat. J Neurophysiol 42, 604–615.

Sandkuhler, J., 2009. Models and mechanisms of hyperalgesia and allodynia. Physiol Rev 89, 707–758.

Schultz, A., Carter, D., Grood, E., King, A., Panjabi, M., 1989. Posterior support structures – Part B: Basic science perspectives. In: Frymoyer, J.W., Gordon, S.L. (eds), New Perspectives on Low Back Pain. American Academy of Orthopedic Surgeons, Park Ridge, IL, pp. 249–275.

Treede, R.D., Meyer, R.A., Raja, S.N., Campbell, J.N., 1992. Peripheral and central mechanisms of cutaneous hyperalgesia. Progr Neurobiol 38, 397–421.

Vallbo, A.B., 1974. Afferent discharge from human muscle spindles in non-contracting muscles. Steady state impulse frequency as a function of joint angle. Acta Physiol Scand 90, 303–318.

Van Hees, J., Gybels, J., 1981. C nociceptor activity in human nerve during painful and non painful skin stimulation. J Neurol Neurosurg Psychiatry 44, 600–607.

Wall, P.D., McMahon, S.B., Koltzenburg, M., 2006. Wall and Melzack's Textbook of Pain. Elsevier/Churchill Livingstone, Philadelphia, PA.

Weerakkody, N.S., Percival, P., Hickey, M.W., Morgan, D.L., Gregory, J.E., Canny, B.J., et al., 2003. Effects of local pressure and vibration on muscle pain from eccentric exercise and hypertonic saline. Pain 105, 425–435.

Weerakkody, N.S., Whitehead, N.P., Canny, B.J., Gregory, J.E., Proske, U., 2001. Large-fiber mechanoreceptors contribute to muscle soreness after eccentric exercise. J Pain 2, 209–219.

Wei, J.Y., Simon, J., Randic, M., Burgess, P.R., 1986. Joint angle signaling by muscle spindle receptors. Brain Res 370, 108–118.

Wilke, H.J., Wolf, S., Claes, L.E., Arand, M., Weisand, A., 1995. Stability increase of the lumbar spine with different muscle groups: a biomechanical in vitro study. Spine 20, 192–198.

Windhorst, U., Meyer-Lohmann, J., Schmidt, J., 1975. Correlation of the dynamic behaviour of deefferented primary muscle spindle endings with their static behaviour. Pflugers Arch 357, 113–122.

Wood, S.A., Gregory, J.E., Proske, U., 1996. The influence of muscle spindle discharge on the human H reflex and the monosynaptic reflex in the cat. J Physiol 497, 279–290.

Chapter | 14 |

Time-dependent mechanisms that impair muscle protection of the spine

Patricia Dolan and Michael A. Adams
Centre for Comparative and Clinical Anatomy, University of Bristol, Bristol, UK

CHAPTER CONTENTS

INTRODUCTION

It is becoming clear that a failure of muscle control can lead to spinal injury and pain. The purpose of this chapter is to explain some of the underlying mechanisms in terms of muscle physiology and tissue biomechanics. The first section provides an updated account of the 'injury model' of back pain, which incorporates genetic inheritance and the human personality as well as mechanical loading. This is followed by a short description of muscle reflexes, and how they normally enable the back muscles to protect the spine from injury. Unfortunately, muscle protection can be impaired by a range of time-dependent mechanisms that involve soft tissue creep and muscle fatigue, and these are considered in detail. The final section provides some brief conclusions, and suggestions for future research.

THE 'INJURY MODEL' OF BACK PAIN

Severe injuries require little discussion: collisions and falls can obviously damage spinal tissues and cause pain. Fractured vertebrae are relatively easy to visualize and treat, and some soft tissue injuries can also be visualized using MRI. It is well established that human intervertebral discs can herniate (Adams and Hutton 1982) or suffer internal disruption (Adams et al. 2000) as a result of traumatic loading, and the underlying mechanisms have recently been explained by experiments on animal tissues (Tampier et al. 2007; Veres et al. 2008, 2010) and by finite-element mathematical models (Shirazi-Adl 1989; Schmidt et al. 2007).

More controversial is the potential for repetitive loading of physiological magnitude to cause fatigue failure of spinal tissues, leading to degenerative changes and pain. But even here the weight of evidence is now considerable. Early experiments on cadaver spines showed that repetitive flexion and compression of a motion segment can generate radial fissures, annular protrusion and in some cases nuclear extrusion (Fig. 14.1) (Adams and Hutton 1985; Gordon et al. 1991). More recent experiments on animal tissues have induced these lesions under more modest levels of compressive loading (Callaghan and McGill 2001). Not surprisingly, disc injuries become more frequent and more severe as the magnitude of compressive loading increases. It is now possible to quantify both bending and compressive loading of the human spine *in vivo* (Adams and Dolan 1991; Dolan and Adams 1993) and there can be little doubt that manual handling of weights as light as 10 kg can generate forces on the spine

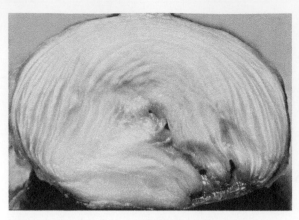

Figure 14.1 Posterolateral radial fissure typical of those found in cadaveric lumbar discs generated by repetitive loading in bending and compression. *Reproduced from Adams, M.A., Bogduk, N., Burton, K., Dolan, P., 2006. The Biomechanics of Back Pain, 2nd edn. Churchill Livingstone, with permission from Elsevier.*

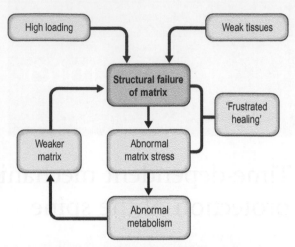

Figure 14.2 Modified injury model suggesting how mechanical factors may be involved in spinal degeneration and pain. Damage can be caused by high forces acting on normal tissue, or more moderate repetitive forces acting on tissue that has been weakened by factors such as an unfavourable genetic inheritance, age-related changes, or wear and tear ('fatigue') loading. Abnormal matrix stresses resulting from injury interfere with tissue metabolism, resulting in weakening and further structural damage. This 'vicious circle' can be characterized as 'frustrated healing' because of the inability of the relatively low cell population to repair the damaged matrix. *Adapted from Adams, M.A., Dolan, P., McNally, D.S., 2009. The internal mechanical functioning of intervetrebral discs and articular cartilage, and its relevance to matrix biology. Matrix Biology 28:384–389, with permission from Elsevier.*

sufficient to cause fatigue failure of spinal tissues (Dolan et al. 1994).

Physical disruption of intervertebral discs (and articular cartilage) alters the mechanical environment experienced by the tissue's cells (Adams et al. 2000, 2009): regions of particularly low and high stress are created, both of which inhibit disc cell metabolism (Ishihara et al. 1996) and precipitate progressive degenerative changes (Adams and Roughley 2006). Abundant proof of this comes from animal models of disc degeneration, which show that, regardless of the precise nature of the physical disruption, or the size of the animal, degeneration inevitably follows injury (Osti et al. 1990; Holm et al. 2004). Equivalent, though less controlled evidence is available for humans (Kerttulla et al. 2000). Attempts at repair are frustrated by the extremely low cellularity of intervertebral discs, and by the practical difficulty of unloading the human spine (Fig. 14.2). Inflammatory processes are evident in injured discs (Peng et al. 2005, 2009) and are amplified by repeated re-injury (Ulrich et al. 2007). Inflammation affects nociceptive nerve endings, leading to pain-sensitization phenomena in the peripheral annulus (Olmarker 2008) and nerve root (Goupille et al. 2007), which explain why fairly gentle mechanical probing can reproduce severe discogenic back pain (Kuslich et al. 1991). Injury to spinal ligaments can similarly lead to inflammation (Solomonow et al. 2003). Links between disc pathology and pain are notoriously variable, possibly because narrowed discs are stress-shielded by their neural arch (Pollintine et al. 2004) but it is nevertheless true that certain structural defects in intervertebral discs are strongly correlated to a history of severe back pain (Videman and Nurminen 2004).

This updated injury model of severe back pain is supported by many epidemiological surveys that implicate excessive mechanical loading in the aetiology of back pain. Particularly high risks of back pain are associated with rapid bending and twisting (Marras et al. 1993; Fathallah et al. 1998) and with incidents that involve sudden muscular efforts (Magora 1973), both of which lead to increased muscle activation (Magnusson et al. 1996; Wilder et al. 1996; van Dieën et al 1998) and increased compressive loading of the spine (Dolan et al. 1994; Mannion et al. 2000). Frequent and heavy lifting performed in flexed or twisted postures increases the risk of low back pain (Marras et al. 1993; Fathallah et al. 1998) and disc prolapse (Kelsey et al. 1984; Mundt et al. 1993), and extreme forward bending increases the risk of disc herniation (Seidler et al. 2003).

The injury model has been criticized in recent years because its early proponents supposed that mechanical loading provided a complete explanation of back pain. We now know that other factors are involved, including genetic inheritance (Hartvigsen et al. 2009) and the human personality (Adams et al. 1999), so that exposure to mechanical loading explains only a modest proportion of work-related back pain (Burton 1997; Ferguson and

Marras 1997; Macfarlane et al. 1997; Adams et al. 1999). Nevertheless, mechanical influences remain the best understood and most easily modified causes of back pain, and no other cause has been shown to be more important. Injury risk obviously depends on the strength of tissues as much as on the severity of loading, and tissue strength depends on genetic inheritance, metabolite transport, and age. Furthermore, all skeletal tissues are able to strengthen in response to repetitive non-damaging mechanical loading (Goodship et al. 1979; Porter et al. 1989) so that, in the words of Nietzsche, 'what does not kill him makes him stronger'. Mechanical loading is good for backs, unless it becomes excessive for any particular back. The importance of these considerations can be appreciated from recent twin studies: genetic inheritance explained over 70% of the variance in 'who gets disc degeneration' in a population of middle-aged women (Sambrook et al. 1999). But genetic influences on tissue degeneration are only half as great when specific spinal levels are considered, and when the study population is more diverse in age and occupation (Battie et al. 2008). Genetic influences on back pain are more modest again (Hartvigsen et al. 2009). Once back pain occurs, all aspects of the patient's behaviour, including responses to treatment, are influenced by psychosocial factors (Burton et al. 2005; Adams et al. 2012), and some of these are themselves influenced by pain (Mannion et al. 1996).

MUSCLES PROTECT THE SPINE FROM INJURY

Muscles of the trunk can do little to protect the spine during violent collisions or falls, especially if the external forces rise to damaging levels before the muscles have time to react. And during emergencies such as epileptic seizures, when neurological inhibition is over-ridden, the muscles themselves can generate forces high enough to injure the underlying spine (Vascancelos 1973). Under most circumstances, however, the trunk muscles ensure that spinal movements stay within safe limits, so that injuries are avoided. To do this effectively, the muscles must be able to contract with sufficient force, speed and endurance to prevent excessive movements, and to maintain stability during activities such as lifting (Fig. 14.3).

The central nervous system coordinates muscle activity using sensory information from a wide range of mechanoreceptor afferents found in muscle (Yamashita et al. 1993b; Roberts et al. 1995) and other tissues (Yahia et al. 1992; McLain and Pickar 1998). The most rapid reflexes are monosynaptic reflexes initiated by muscle spindles that lie within skeletal muscle, parallel to the extrafusal fibres. Muscle spindles are sensitive to changes in muscle length, and are innervated by primary (IA) and secondary (II) muscle afferents that synapse directly with alpha

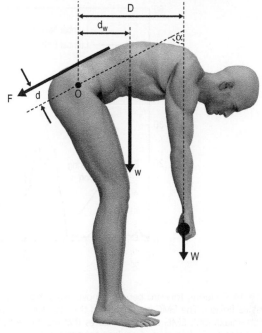

$$EM = F \times d = W \times D + w \times d_w$$
$$C = F + (W + w) \times \cos \alpha$$

Figure 14.3 During manual handling activities, back muscles must generate an extensor moment (EM) to counter the forward bending moment due to upper body weight (w) and the weight being lifted (W). The small lever arm of the back muscles requires high muscle forces to generate the required extensor moments. *Reproduced from Adams, M.A., Bogduk, N., Burton, K., Dolan, P., 2006. The Biomechanics of Back Pain, 2nd edn. Churchill Livingstone, with permission from Elsevier.*

motor neurones in the spinal cord. Primary afferents detect both strain and strain rate, and enable the muscle to contract rapidly (typically within 30–50 msec) in response to a sudden increase in muscle length (Dietz 1992; Sinkjaer et al. 1999). Secondary afferents, in contrast, are sensitive to static stretch and are slow-adapting. The small intervertebral muscles have a particularly high density of muscle spindles compared to the longer paraspinal muscles (Nitz and Peck 1986), suggesting that they play an important role in controlling relative motion between adjacent vertebrae. Afferents in these muscles can also initiate efferent activity in motor neurones at neighbouring levels, suggesting the presence of an intersegmental reflex (Kang et al. 2002) that allows for a coordinated reflex response at multiple spinal levels.

Muscle spindles are not the only afferents involved in these control pathways. Mechanoreceptors are found also in ligaments (Rhalmi et al. 1993), thoracolumbar fascia (Yahia et al. 1992), apophyseal joint capsules (McLain and

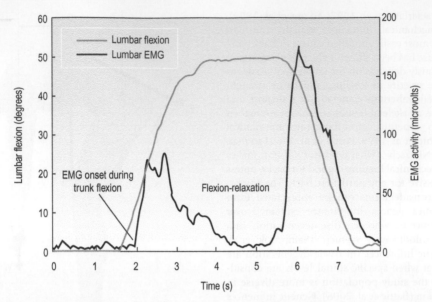

Figure 14.4 During forward bending movements, back muscles are activated in order to decelerate the trunk and prevent excessive flexion. The EMG graph shows the 'deceleration' peak from the lumbar erector spinae, followed by a period of 'flexion–relaxation'. EMG silence indicates that resistance to forward bending is now provided by the stretched passive tissues of the spine (including intramuscular connective tissue).

Pickar 1998) and intervertebral discs (Yamashita et al. 1993b; Roberts et al. 1995). In the disc (Yamashita et al. 1993b) and joint capsule (Cavanaugh et al. 1997), afferent activity is usually initiated only under severe loading conditions, suggesting that receptors in these tissues may be more important in nociception than proprioception. However, lower threshold afferents have been identified in spinal ligaments and in the apophyseal joint capsule, as well as in muscle and tendon (Yamashita et al. 1993a, 1993b), suggesting a proprioceptive function that contributes to the sensorimotor control of trunk movement. A specific ligamentomuscular reflex has been confirmed on anaesthetized patients and animals, in which stretching of the supraspinous ligament initiates reflex contractions of the multifidus muscle (Solomonow et al. 1998). Reflex activity in multifidus and longissimus can also be initiated by electrically stimulating afferents in the discs and capsules, with the size of this reflex response increasing if afferents in more than one tissue are stimulated simultaneously (Stubbs et al. 1998; Holm et al. 2002).

Evidently, trunk muscle activity is controlled by many reflex pathways as well as by voluntary activation. Feedback from such a wide variety of sensory afferents helps to ensure that trunk muscles are activated in such a way as to prevent excessive spinal movements (Fig. 14.4), but without generating inordinately high compressive forces on the spine. However, recent evidence suggests that several time-dependent effects can alter the sensitivity of mechanoreceptor afferents, and impair the sensorimotor

control of muscle activation. These mechanisms will be considered next.

TIME-DEPENDENT MECHANISMS THAT IMPAIR MUSCLE PROTECTION OF THE SPINE

Tensile creep in stretched tissues

Sensory feedback from mechanoreceptor afferents is based on their ability to detect altered loading in the surrounding tissue. Muscle spindles are believed to respond primarily to strain and strain rate, but other mechanoreceptors in muscle, skin and joint capsules appear to be capable of responding to a variety of stimuli, with stress being the dominant one (Khalsa et al. 1996; Ge and Khalsa 2002, 2003). In most engineering materials, stress (force per unit area) and strain (% change in length) are simply related so that changes in one automatically reflect changes in the other. However, several skeletal soft tissues exhibit viscoelastic and poroelastic mechanical properties where strain depends not only on stress but also on the duration or speed of loading. Generally, when a load is applied to a soft tissue, it expels water from that tissue, allowing strain to increase progressively as a function of time even if stress remains constant. This process is called 'creep'. Similarly, if such a tissue is subjected to a constant stretch, fluid expulsion allows the tension within it to fall over time, a phenomenon known as 'stress-relaxation'. In either case, the nature of the stress–strain relationship changes over time, with potentially serious biological consequences. For example, if a mechanoreceptor (like an engineer!) found it convenient to infer stress by measuring the strain it causes, and if the mechanoreceptor was accustomed to slow-acting mechanical forces that cause considerable creep, then it would underestimate tissue stress if the loading was applied so rapidly that little of the expected time-dependent strain had time to occur. Alternatively, if a mechanoreceptor was sensitive to stress then it would tend to underestimate tissue strain following prolonged or repetitive loading that caused substantial creep.

There is now direct evidence from animal models that the sensitivity of mechanoreceptors in spinal tissues can be altered by their recent loading history in the manner suggested above. Studies on anaesthetized cats have shown that cyclic (Solomonow et al. 1999) or sustained (Solomonow et al. 2002) loading of the supraspinous ligament can attenuate the reflex response initiated in the multifidus muscle. The fall in reflex activity occurs rapidly and the authors postulated that this was due to stress-relaxation in the ligament. They confirmed this by adding a pre-load to the ligament, which brought about an immediate recovery of the reflex response during subsequent stretches (Solomonow et al. 1999). If the ligament was left to recover naturally, then reflex activation remained impaired several hours after loading, suggesting that chronic stretching can have long-lasting effects on mechanoreceptor sensitivity (Gedalia et al. 1999; Claude et al. 2003).

Afferent activity in muscle spindles also appears to be influenced by their prior stretching (Morgan et al. 1984; Gregory et al. 1988, 1998; Avela et al. 1999). Lengthening of muscle reduces spindle sensitivity so that the muscle must then be stretched to a greater extent in order to initiate spindle firing. However, recent shortening of a muscle acts to increase spindle sensitivity so that a subsequent stretch applied to the muscle increases spindle firing at the same muscle length. These 'after effects' appear to be caused by mechanical changes in the muscle tissue rather than by muscle fatigue because they occur after just a few seconds (Hagbarth et al. 1985; Avela et al. 1999). Altered sensitivity of muscle spindles is thought to be due to thixotrophic effects caused by the formation of stable crossbridges within the intrafusal fibres (Ge and Pickar 2008). These crossbridges remain attached for longer periods than those that form during dynamic contractions, so that intrafusal fibres become slack (and hence less sensitive) if they have previously been lengthened. Conversely, they become taut (and hence more sensitive) if they have previously been shortened (Hufschmidt and Schwaller 1987; Proske et al. 1993).

The above findings have important implications concerning reflex protection of the spine under conditions

that lengthen the muscles and induce tensile creep in spinal tissues. Cadaver studies have shown that just 5 minutes of sustained full flexion applied to lumbar motion segments produces significant creep that reduces resistance to bending by 42% (Adams and Dolan 1996) while *in vivo* studies in cats suggest that small vertebral displacements of 1–2 mm held for just a few seconds are sufficient to reduce the sensitivity of spindles in the paraspinal muscles (Ge et al. 2005). In human volunteers, slumped postures that flex the lumbar spine increase range of flexion (McGill and Brown 1992) and impair spinal position sense (Dolan and Green 2006; Sanchez et al. 2006) (Fig. 14.5), suggesting that afferent feedback may be disturbed by tensile creep in soft tissues.

Compressive creep in intervertebral discs

Under conditions of chronic loading, the effects of creep in tensile structures are likely to be exacerbated by compressive creep in the discs. Disc creep is a slow process that takes hours to achieve equilibrium (McMillan et al. 1996). Over the course of a day, the loss of fluid arising from sustained compressive loading reduces the volume of human lumbar discs by approximately 20% (Botsford

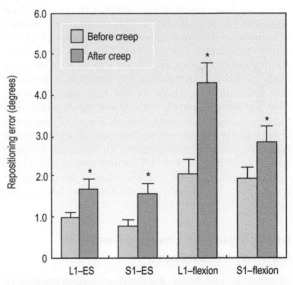

Figure 14.5 Sitting in a flexed posture for 1 hour increases spinal re-positioning errors. These were measured at the level of the first lumbar (L1) and the first sacral (S1) vertebrae using an electromagnetic motion analysis device, the 3-Space Fastrak (Polhemus, Vermont, USA). Differences in re-positioning errors were significant in both erect standing (ES) and flexed postures (*$P < 0.005$) and were greater in flexion than in standing ($P < 0.001$). Bars indicate the SEM.
Based on data from Sanchez et al. (2006).

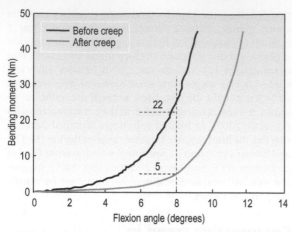

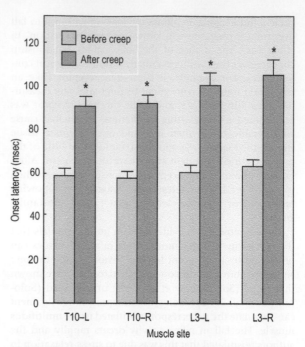

Figure 14.6 Bending stiffness curves obtained from a cadaveric lumbar motion segment, before and after 2 hours of compressive creep loading at 1.5 kN. At 8° of flexion, the bending moment resisted decreased by 77%, from 22 Nm to 5 Nm, as a result of increased slack in the disc and ligaments. *Reproduced from Adams, M.A., Bogduk, N., Burton, K., Dolan, P., 2006. The Biomechanics of Back Pain, 2nd edn. Churchill Livingstone, with permission from Elsevier.*

Figure 14.7 Onset latency of the erector spinae muscles, during a sudden perturbation of the trunk, increased significantly after sitting flexed for 1 hr (*$P < 0.001$), an activity known to cause creep in spinal tissues. Data shown are the mean values obtained from 15 healthy subjects, recorded from the right (R) and left (L) erector spinae at thoracic (T10) and lumbar (L3) levels. Bars indicate the SEM. *Based on data from Sanchez-Zuriaga et al. (2010).*

et al. 1994). The resulting fall in disc height brings the vertebrae closer together, and slackens the intervertebral ligaments (Zhao et al. 2005). This reduces the resistance to bending of the osteoligamentous spine (Fig. 14.6) in a similar manner to that observed following tensile ligamentous creep (Adams and Dolan 1996) and is therefore likely to reduce mechanoreceptor firing in response to spinal flexion. Conversely, in the early morning when discs are fully hydrated, the spine is much stiffer, and bending moments increase two- to three-fold compared to later in the day, suggesting that these changes in spinal stiffness are not fully compensated for by modified muscle activity (Adams et al. 1987). This may explain why advice to avoid bending in the first few hours of the day caused a significant fall in pain and disability in chronic back pain sufferers (Snook et al. 1998).

Investigating creep effects in human volunteers

In order to investigate the functional consequences of creep, we compared the amplitude and onset latency (i.e. delay) of back muscle activation in response to a sudden perturbation of the trunk, before and after a period of sustained flexion. Subjects sat for one hour in an easy chair so that their lumbar spine was flexed by at least 70% (Sanchez-Zuriaga et al. 2010), and during this time the back was fully supported in order to avoid muscle fatigue. A modest amount of creep in the soft tissues was

confirmed by a 4% increase in lumbar range of flexion. After the intervention, the amplitude of reflex muscle activity recorded from the erector spinae muscles was unchanged. However, onset latency increased by approximately 60% in both lumbar and thoracic muscles (Fig. 14.7). Onset latencies before creep were between 60 and 65 ms. These values are similar to those reported previously for the trunk muscles (Radebold et al. 2001; Herrmann et al. 2006; Vera-Garcia et al. 2006) suggesting that the initial muscle response was reflex in nature (Wilder et al. 1996; Dietz 1992) and was probably mediated by non-spindle afferents (Hasan and Stuart 1984; Matthews 1984; Lundberg et al. 1987). The lack of any change in the amplitude of the response shows that afferent activity was delayed but not diminished by creep, and this is consistent with a shift in the stress–strain relationship of the ligaments as suggested by earlier animal experiments (Solomonow et al. 1999). The increased latencies indicate that muscles were activated later in the flexion movement when tissue strains would be greater, suggesting that the mechanoreceptor afferents that initiated the reflex were sensitive to stress rather than strain.

These findings suggest a mechanism whereby sustained or repeated flexion of the trunk can impair protective reflexes. A delay in reflex activation during forward bending tasks would cause a slower deceleration of the trunk leading to increased levels of lumbar flexion that may increase the risk of tissue injury. Under dynamic loading conditions, there is also the potential for fatigue to develop in active muscles, and recent studies suggest that this also may impair sensorimotor function.

Muscle fatigue

Fatigue represents a normal physiological response to exercise which is due largely to local changes in the muscle but may also be influenced by central factors. It is often cited as a contributing factor to back injury, and there is some evidence that people with more fatigable muscles are at greater risk of developing first-time back pain (Biering-Sorensen 1984; Mannion et al. 1997).

Fatigue is characterized by contractile failure in individual muscle fibres (Bigland-Ritchie et al. 1986a), and at submaximal workloads this is initially compensated for by the recruitment of additional motor units to help maintain contraction force (Bigland-Ritchie et al. 1986a; Garland et al. 1994; Dolan et al. 1995). As exercise continues, central drive may fall (Bigland-Ritchie et al. 1986b; Gandevia et al. 1996) and this, together with the loss of contractility, contributes to a loss of force-generating capacity by the muscle.

Changes in muscle activation during fatigue may be influenced by altered input from muscle afferents as a result of metabolic changes within the muscle (Bigland-Ritchie et al. 1986b). Studies on human volunteers have reported reduced firing of IA spindle afferents during sustained contractions at moderate load (Macefield et al. 1991) and this may act to attenuate reflex activation of the fatigued muscle. However, reduced spindle firing may also affect cortical excitability and thereby influence higher levels of motor control (Stuart et al. 2002). Animal studies suggest that non-spindle (group II and group III) muscle afferents show increased firing during sustained contractions, especially when the muscle becomes ischaemic (Hayward et al. 1991). These findings suggest that different muscle afferents show different responses to fatigue that may be influenced by the loading conditions, and that increased activation of some muscle afferents may compensate for reduced activity in others in order to preserve sensorimotor function under adverse conditions.

Investigating muscle fatigue effects in human volunteers

The functional consequences of muscle fatigue on sensorimotor function have been investigated previously by examining changes in balance control, proprioception and reflex muscle activation. Numerous studies have shown that muscle fatigue increases postural sway (Davidson et al. 2004; Madigan et al. 2006; Pline et al. 2006; Vuillerme et al. 2002a, 2002b), impairs proprioception (Skinner et al. 1986; Taimela et al. 1999; Bjorklund et al. 2000; Pline et al. 2005; Ribeiro et al. 2007), and delays balance recovery following postural perturbations (Davidson et al. 2009). However, the effects of fatigue on reflex activation appear to be more variable. Reflex latency appears to be unaffected by fatigue (Hortobagyi et al. 1991; Herrmann et al. 2006), but reflex amplitude has been reported to increase (Hakkinen and Komi 1983; Hortobagyi et al. 1991; Herrmann et al. 2006), or decrease (Garland and McComas 1990; Balestra et al. 1992; Hagbarth et al. 1995). These contrasting findings may reflect differences in the extent of muscle fatigue induced by the experimental protocols, or they may be attributable to changes in muscle temperature or the variable responses of muscle spindles to different types of contraction.

In order to clarify matters, we further investigated back muscle reflexes following muscle fatigue (Sanchez-Zuriaga et al. 2010). Fatigue was induced using the Biering Sorensen test, which involves holding the unsupported upper body horizontal against the effects of gravity until the position can no longer be maintained. This test has two advantages: the isometric nature of the contraction induces marked fatigue of the back extensor muscles (Mannion and Dolan 1994), and the test position avoids any ligamentous creep or muscle lengthening, which, as mentioned previously, can have marked effects on reflex muscle activity. Results showed no change in the timing or amplitude of reflex activation, suggesting that any force decrement in fatigued muscle fibres was not compensated for by increased motor unit recruitment.

Another study has examined the effects of *dynamic* muscle fatigue on back muscle reflexes. Repeated flexion and extension movements were used to fatigue the muscles, and this increased the reflex EMG amplitude, even after EMG was normalized for load, suggesting that force generated by the reflex was increased (Hermann et al. 2006). The loading protocol used in this study may have caused creep as well as fatigue and may also have induced thixotrophic effects within the muscle spindles, which could explain the different response when compared to the effects of isometric fatigue.

Do these time-dependent mechanisms cause back pain?

Laboratory studies have shown that repetitive bending and lifting activities can lead to increased spinal flexion (Trafimow et al. 1993; van Dieën et al. 1998; Dolan and Adams 1998) and increased bending stresses on the osteoligamentous spine (Dolan and Adams 1998). Increased spinal flexion could be due to mechanical changes in the soft tissues, as discussed in the previous section.

However, it might also be due to muscle fatigue which leads to reduced force-generating capacity (Bigland-Ritchie et al. 1986b; Taylor et al. 2000), altered afferent input (Macefield et al. 1991; Taylor et al. 2000) and impaired proprioception (Lattanzio et al. 1997; Pedersen et al. 1998), all of which could contribute to impaired motor responses. Increased bending stresses on the spine during repetitive bending could lead to the accumulation of fatigue damage, increasing the risk of injury in the manner suggested by both experimental (Adams and Hutton 1985; Gordon et al. 1991; Callaghan and McGill 2001) and mathematical models (Schmidt et al. 2007).

Time-dependent changes in spinal tissues may also act to increase the risk of acute injury to the spine as a result of sudden overload. Sudden perturbations of the trunk normally lead to a strong and rapid activation of the back muscles (Marras et al. 1987; Mannion et al. 2000), which acts to protect the spine from excessive movement. The extent of muscle activation appears to be unaffected by the removal of audiovisual cues, suggesting that the response is largely reflex in nature (Mannion et al. 2000). A marked delay in reflex activation of the back muscles caused by creep in the soft tissues of the spine would lead to an impaired ability to respond rapidly to sudden perturbations (Sanchez-Zuriaga et al. 2010) and this may increase the risk of injury. Some evidence to support this is provided by a recent prospective study in college athletes which found that people who had longer trunk muscle latencies at baseline were more likely to sustain a back injury during the 2–3 year follow-up (Cholewicki et al. 2005). Delays in reflex activation, which can develop as a result of soft tissue creep, would therefore appear to be a risk factor for future back pain.

CONCLUSIONS

In vitro studies and mathematical models have explained how mechanical loading can induce injury in spinal tissues. In life, the trunk muscles normally act to control the movements of the trunk to ensure that spinal loading remains within safe limits. However, time-dependent changes in the soft tissues, as a result of creep and fatigue, can alter sensorimotor function and impair the ability of trunk muscles to protect the underlying spinal tissues from injury.

Once back injury occurs, pain (Radebold et al. 2001; Hodges 2001; Hodges et al. 2003) or even the anticipation of pain (Moseley et al. 2004) may further alter sensorimotor processing leading to greater impairments of muscle function that may leave the spinal tissues even more vulnerable to injury. The end result may be a vicious circle of repetitive injury, muscle dysfunction and chronic pain. Future prospective studies are required to identify those aspects of sensorimotor function such as delayed or reduced reflex activation, impaired proprioception and balance, and altered muscle recruitment patterns, that are most predictive of future back pain. Such information will enable more targeted interventions to be developed in order to minimize these functional impairments and reduce the risk of back pain.

REFERENCES

Adams, M.A., Bogduk, N., Burton, K., Dolan, P., 2012. The Biomechanics of Back Pain, 3rd edn. Edinburgh, Churchill Livingstone.

Adams, M.A., Dolan, P., 1991. A technique for quantifying the bending moment acting on the lumbar spine in vivo. J Biomech 24, 117–126.

Adams, M.A., Dolan, P., 1996. Time-dependent changes in the lumbar spine's resistance to bending. Clin Biomech 11, 194–200.

Adams, M.A., Dolan, P., Hutton, W.C., 1987. Diurnal variations in the stresses on the lumbar spine. Spine 12, 130–137.

Adams, M.A., Dolan, P., McNally, D.S., 2009. The internal mechanical functioning of intervertebral discs and articular cartilage, and its relevance to matrix biology. Matrix Biol 28, 384–389.

Adams, M.A., Freeman, B.J., Morrison, H.P., Nelson, I.W., Dolan, P., 2000. Mechanical initiation of intervertebral disc degeneration. Spine 25, 1625–1636.

Adams, M.A., Hutton, W.C., 1985. Gradual disc prolapse. Spine 10, 524–531.

Adams, M.A., Hutton, W.C., 1982. Prolapsed intervertebral disc. A hyperflexion injury. 1981 Volvo Award in Basic Science. Spine 7, 184–191.

Adams, M.A., Mannion, A.F., Dolan, P., 1999. Personal risk factors for first-time low back pain. Spine 24, 2497–2505.

Adams, M.A., Roughley, P.J., 2006. What is intervertebral disc degeneration, and what causes it? Spine 31, 2151–2161.

Avela, J., Kyrolainen, H., Komi, P.V., 1999. Altered reflex sensitivity after repeated and prolonged passive muscle stretching. J Appl Physiol 86, 1283–1291.

Balestra, C., Duchateau, J., Hainaut, K., 1992. Effects of fatigue on the stretch reflex in a human muscle. Electroencephalogr Clin Neurophysiol 85, 46–52.

Battie, M.C., Videman, T., Levalahti, E., Gill, K., Kaprio, J., 2008. Genetic and environmental effects on disc degeneration by phenotype and spinal level: a multivariate twin study. Spine 33, 2801–2808.

Biering-Sorensen, F., 1984. Physical measurements as risk indicators for low-back trouble over a one-year period. Spine 9, 106–119.

Bigland-Ritchie, B., Cafarelli, E., Vollestad, N.K., 1986a. Fatigue of submaximal static contractions. Acta Physiol Scand Suppl 556, 137–148.

Bigland-Ritchie, B.R., Dawson, N.J., Johansson, R.S., Lippold, O.C., 1986b. Reflex origin for the slowing of motoneurone firing rates in fatigue of human voluntary contractions. J Physiol 379, 451–459.

Bjorklund, M., Crenshaw, A.G., Djupsjobacka, M., Johansson, H., 2000. Position sense acuity is diminished following repetitive low-intensity work to fatigue in a simulated occupational setting. Eur J Appl Physiol 81, 361–367.

Botsford, D.J., Esses, S.I., Ogilvie-Harris, D.J., 1994. In vivo diurnal variation in intervertebral disc volume and morphology. Spine 19, 935–940.

Burton, A.K., 1997. Back injury and work loss. Biomechanical and psychosocial influences. Spine 22, 2575–2580.

Burton, A.K., Bartys, S., Wright, I.A., Main, C.J., 2005. Obstacles to recovery from musculoskeletal disorders in industry. (Research Report 323). HSE Books, London, (Available at www.hse.gov.uk/research/rrhtm.)

Callaghan, J.P., McGill, S.M., 2001. Intervertebral disc herniation: studies on a porcine model exposed to highly repetitive flexion/extension motion with compressive force. Clin Biomech 16, 28–37.

Cavanaugh, J.M., Ozaktay, A.C., Yamashita, T., Avramov, A., Getchell, T.V., King, A.I., 1997. Mechanisms of low back pain: a neurophysiologic and neuroanatomic study. Clin Orthop 335, 166–180.

Cholewicki, J., Silfies, S.P., Shah, R.A., Greene, H.S., Reeves, N.P., Alvi, K., et al., 2005. Delayed trunk muscle reflex responses increase the risk of low back injuries. Spine 30, 2614–2620.

Claude, L.N., Solomonow, M., Zhou, B.H., Baratta, R.V., Zhu, M.P., 2003. Neuromuscular dysfunction elicited by cyclic lumbar flexion. Muscle Nerve 27, 348–358.

Davidson, B.S., Madigan, M.L., Nussbaum, M.A., 2004. Effects of lumbar extensor fatigue and fatigue rate on postural sway. Eur J Appl Physiol 93, 183–189.

Davidson, B.S., Madigan, M.L., Nussbaum, M.A., Wojcik, L.A., 2009. Effects of localized muscle fatigue on recovery from a postural perturbation without stepping. Gait Posture 29, 552–557.

Dietz, V., 1992. Human neuronal control of automatic functional movements: interaction between central programs and afferent input. Physiol Rev 72, 33–69.

Dolan, K.J., Green, A., 2006. Lumbar spine reposition sense: the effect of a 'slouched' posture. Man Ther 11, 202–207.

Dolan, P., Adams, M.A., 1998. Repetitive lifting tasks fatigue the back muscles and increase the bending moment acting on the lumbar spine. J Biomech 31, 713–721.

Dolan, P., Adams, M.A., 1993. The relationship between EMG activity and extensor moment generation in the erector spinae muscles during bending and lifting activities. J Biomech 26, 513–522.

Dolan, P., Earley, M., Adams, M.A., 1994. Bending and compressive stresses acting on the lumbar spine during lifting activities. J Biomech 27, 1237–1248.

Dolan, P., Mannion, A.F., Adams, M.A., 1995. Fatigue of the erector spinae muscles. A quantitative assessment using 'frequency banding' of the surface electromyography signal. Spine 20, 149–159.

Fathallah, F.A., Marras, W.S., Parnianpour, M., 1998. The role of complex, simultaneous trunk motions in the risk of occupation-related low back disorders. Spine 23, 1035–1042.

Ferguson, S.A., Marras, W.S., 1997. A literature review of low back disorder surveillance measures and risk factors. Clin Biomech 12, 211–226.

Gandevia, S.C., Allen, G.M., Butler, J.E., Taylor, J.L., 1996. Supraspinal factors in human muscle fatigue: evidence for suboptimal output from the motor cortex. J Physiol 490, 529–536.

Garland, S.J., Enoka, R.M., Serrano, L.P., Robinson, G.A., 1994. Behavior of motor units in human biceps brachii during a submaximal fatiguing contraction. J Appl Physiol 76, 2411–2419.

Garland, S.J., McComas, A.J., 1990. Reflex inhibition of human soleus muscle during fatigue. J Physiol 429, 17–27.

Ge, W., Khalsa, P.S., 2002. Encoding of compressive stress during indentation by slowly adapting type I mechanoreceptors in rat hairy skin. J Neurophysiol 87, 1686–1693.

Ge, W., Khalsa, P.S., 2003. Encoding of compressive stress during indentation by group III and IV muscle mechano-nociceptors in rat gracilis muscle. J Neurophysiol 89, 785–792.

Ge, W., Long, C.R., Pickar, J.G., 2005. Vertebral position alters paraspinal muscle spindle responsiveness in the feline spine: effect of positioning duration. J Physiol 569, 655–665.

Ge, W., Pickar, J.G., 2008. Time course for the development of muscle history in lumbar paraspinal muscle spindles arising from changes in vertebral position. Spine J 8, 320–328.

Gedalia, U., Solomonow, M., Zhou, B.H., Baratta, R.V., Lu, Y., Harris, M., 1999. Biomechanics of increased exposure to lumbar injury caused by cyclic loading. Part 2. Recovery of reflexive muscular stability with rest. Spine 24, 2461–2467.

Goodship, A.E., Lanyon, L.E., McFie, H., 1979. Functional adaptation of bone to increased stress. An experimental study. J Bone Joint Surg 61A, 539–546.

Gordon, S.J., Yang, K.H., Mayer, P.J., Mace, A.H., Jr, Kish, V.L., Radin, E.L., 1991. Mechanism of disc rupture. A preliminary report. Spine 16, 450–456.

Goupille, P., Mulleman, D., Paintaud, G., Watier, H., Valat, J.P., 2007. Can sciatica induced by disc herniation be treated with tumor necrosis factor alpha blockade? Arthritis Rheum 56, 3887–3895.

Gregory, J.E., Morgan, D.L., Proske, U., 1988. Aftereffects in the responses of cat muscle spindles and errors of limb position sense in man. J Neurophysiol 59, 1220–1230.

Gregory, J.E., Wise, A.K., Wood, S.A., Prochazka, A., Proske, U., 1998. Muscle history, fusimotor activity and the human stretch reflex. J Physiol 513, 927–934.

Hagbarth, K.E., Bongiovanni, L.G., Nordin, M., 1995. Reduced servo-control of fatigued human finger extensor and flexor muscles. J Physiol 485, 865–872.

Hagbarth, K.E., Hagglund, J.V., Nordin, M., Wallin, E.U., 1985. Thixotropic behaviour of human finger flexor muscles with accompanying changes in spindle and reflex responses to stretch. J Physiol 368, 323–342.

Hakkinen, K., Komi, P.V., 1983. Electromyographic and mechanical characteristics of human skeletal muscle during fatigue under voluntary and reflex conditions. Electroencephalogr Clin Neurophysiol 55, 436–444.

Hartvigsen, J., Nielsen, J., Kyvik, K.O., Fejer, R., Vach, W., Iachine, I., et al., 2009. Heritability of spinal pain and consequences of spinal pain: a comprehensive genetic epidemiologic analysis using a population-based sample of 15,328 twins ages 20–71 years. Arthr Rheum 61, 1343–1351.

Hasan, Z., Stuart, D.G., 1984. Mammalian muscle receptors. In: Davidoff, R.A. (ed.) Handbook of the Spinal Cord. Dekker, New York, pp. 559–607.

Hayward, L., Wesselmann, U., Rymer, W.Z., 1991. Effects of muscle fatigue on mechanically sensitive afferents of slow conduction velocity in the cat triceps surae. J Neurophysiol 65, 360–370.

Herrmann, C.M., Madigan, M.L., Davidson, B.S., Granata, K.P., 2006. Effect of lumbar extensor fatigue on paraspinal muscle reflexes. J Electromyogr Kinesiol 16, 637–641.

Hodges, P., 2001. Changes in motor planning of feedforward postural responses of the trunk muscles in low back pain. Exp Brain Res 141, 261–266.

Hodges, P.W., Moseley, G.L., Gabrielsson, A., Gandevia, S.C., 2003. Experimental muscle pain changes feedforward postural responses of the trunk muscles. Exp Brain Res 151, 262–271.

Holm, S., Holm, A.K., Ekstrom, L., Karladani, A., Hansson, T., 2004. Experimental disc degeneration due to endplate injury. J Spinal Disord Tech 17, 64–71.

Holm, S., Indahl, A., Solomonow, M., 2002. Sensorimotor control of the spine. J Electromyogr Kinesiol 12, 219–234.

Hortobagyi, T., Lambert, N.J., Kroll, W.P., 1991. Voluntary and reflex responses to fatigue with stretch-shortening exercise. Can J Sport Sci 16, 142–150.

Hufschmidt, A., Schwaller, I., 1987. Short-range elasticity and resting tension of relaxed human lower leg muscles. J Physiol 391, 451–465.

Ishihara, H., McNally, D.S., Urban, J.P., Hall, A.C., 1996. Effects of hydrostatic pressure on matrix synthesis in different regions of the intervertebral disk. J Appl Physiol 80, 839–846.

Kang, Y.M., Choi, W.S., Pickar, J.G., 2002. Electrophysiologic evidence for an intersegmental reflex pathway between lumbar paraspinal tissues. Spine 27, E56–63.

Kelsey, J.L., Githens, P.B., White, A.A., Holford, T.R., Walter, S.D., O'Connor, T., et al., 1984. An epidemiologic study of lifting and twisting on the job and risk for acute prolapsed lumbar intervertebral disc. J Orthop Res 2, 61–66.

Kerttula, L.I., Serlo, W.S., Tervonen, O.A., Paakko, E.L., Vanharanta, H.V., 2000. Post-traumatic findings of the spine after earlier vertebral fracture in young patients: clinical and MRI study. Spine 25, 1104–1108.

Khalsa, P.S., Hoffman, A.H., Grigg, P., 1996. Mechanical states encoded by stretch-sensitive neurons in feline joint capsule. J Neurophysiol 76, 175–187.

Kuslich, S.D., Ulstrom, C.L., Michael, C.J., 1991. The tissue origin of low back pain and sciatica: a report of pain response to tissue stimulation during operations on the lumbar spine using local anesthesia. Orthop Clin North Am 22, 181–187.

Lattanzio, P.J., Petrella, R.J., Sproule, J.R., Fowler, P.J., 1997. Effects of fatigue on knee proprioception. Clin J Sport Med 7, 22–27.

Lundberg, A., Malmgren, K., Schomburg, E.D., 1987. Reflex pathways from group II muscle afferents. 3. Secondary spindle afferents and the FRA: a new hypothesis. Exp Brain Res 65, 294–306.

Macefield, G., Hagbarth, K.E., Gorman, R., Gandevia, S.C., Burke, D., 1991. Decline in spindle support to alpha-motoneurones during sustained voluntary contractions. J Physiol 440, 497–512.

Macfarlane, G.J., Thomas, E., Papageorgiou, A.C., Croft, P.R., Jayson, M.I., Silman, A.J., 1997. Employment and physical work activities as predictors of future low back pain. Spine 22, 1143–1149.

Madigan, M.L., Davidson, B.S., Nussbaum, M.A., 2006. Postural sway and joint kinematics during quiet standing are affected by lumbar extensor fatigue. Hum Mov Sci 25, 788–799.

Magnusson, M.L., Aleksiev, A., Wilder, D.G., Pope, M.H., Spratt, K., Lee, S.H., et al, 1996. Unexpected load and asymmetric posture as etiologic factors in low back pain. Eur Spine J 5, 23–35.

Magora, A., 1973. Investigation of the relation between low back pain and occupation. IV. Physical requirements: bending, rotation, reaching and sudden maximal effort. Scand J Rehabil Med 5, 186–190.

Mannion, A.F., Adams, M.A., Dolan, P., 2000. Sudden and unexpected loading generates high forces on the lumbar spine. Spine 25, 842–852.

Mannion, A.F., Connolly, B., Wood, K., Dolan, P., 1997. The use of surface EMG power spectral analysis in the evaluation of back muscle function. J Rehabil Res Dev 34, 427–439.

Mannion, A.F., Dolan, P., 1994. Electromyographic median frequency changes during isometric contraction of the back extensors to fatigue. Spine 19, 1223–1229.

Mannion, A.F., Dolan, P., Adams, M.A., 1996. Psychological questionnaires: do 'abnormal' scores precede or follow first-time low back pain? Spine 21, 2603–2611.

Marras, W.S., Lavender, S.A., Leurgans, S.E., Rajulu, S.L., Allread, W.G., Fathallah, F.A., et al., 1993. The role of dynamic three-dimensional trunk motion in occupationally- related low back disorders. The effects of workplace factors, trunk position, and trunk motion characteristics on risk of injury. Spine 18, 617–628.

Marras, W.S., Rangarajulu, S.L., Lavender, S.A., 1987. Trunk loading and expectation. Ergonomics 30, 551–562.

Matthews, P.B., 1984. Evidence from the use of vibration that the human long-latency stretch reflex depends upon spindle secondary afferents. J Physiol 348, 383–415.

McGill, S.M., Brown, S., 1992. Creep response of the lumbar spine to prolonged full flexion. Clin Biomech 7, 43–46.

McLain, R.F., Pickar, J.G., 1998. Mechanoreceptor endings in human thoracic and lumbar facet joints. Spine 23, 168–173.

McMillan, D.W., Garbutt, G., Adams, M.A., 1996. Effect of sustained loading on the water content of intervertebral discs: implications for disc metabolism. Ann Rheum Dis 55, 880–887.

Morgan, D.L., Prochazka, A., Proske, U., 1984. The after-effects of stretch and fusimotor stimulation on the responses of primary endings of cat muscle spindles. J Physiol 356, 465–477.

Moseley, G.L., Nicholas, M.K., Hodges, P.W., 2004. Does anticipation of back pain predispose to back trouble? Brain 127, 2339–2347.

Mundt, D.J., Kelsey, J.L., Golden, A.L., Pastides, H., Berg, A.T., Sklar, J., et al., 1993. An epidemiologic study of non-occupational lifting as a risk factor for herniated lumbar intervertebral disc. The Northeast Collaborative Group on Low Back Pain. Spine 18, 595–602.

Nitz, A.J., Peck, D., 1986. Comparison of muscle spindle concentrations in large and small human epaxial muscles acting in parallel combinations. Am Surg 52, 273–277.

Olmarker, K., 2008. Puncture of a lumbar intervertebral disc induces changes in spontaneous pain behavior: an experimental study in rats. Spine 33, 850–855.

Osti, O.L., Vernon-Roberts, B., Fraser, R.D., 1990. 1990 Volvo Award in experimental studies. Anulus tears and intervertebral disc degeneration. An experimental study using an animal model. Spine 15, 762–767.

Pedersen, J., Ljubisavljevic, M., Bergenheim, M., Johansson, H., 1998. Alterations in information transmission in ensembles of primary muscle spindle afferents

after muscle fatigue in heteronymous muscle. Neuroscience 84, 953–959.

Peng, B., Chen, J., Kuang, Z., Li, D., Pang, X., Zhang, X., 2009. Expression and role of connective tissue growth factor in painful disc fibrosis and degeneration. Spine 34, E178–182.

Peng, B., Wu, W., Hou, S., Li, P., Zhang, C., Yang, Y., 2005. The pathogenesis of discogenic low back pain. J Bone Joint Surg 87B, 62–67.

Pline, K.M., Madigan, M.L., Nussbaum, M.A., 2006. Influence of fatigue time and level on increases in postural sway. Ergonomics 49, 1639–1648.

Pline, K.M., Madigan, M.L., Nussbaum, M.A., Grange, R.W., 2005. Lumbar extensor fatigue and circumferential ankle pressure impair ankle joint motion sense. Neurosci Lett 390, 9–14.

Pollintine, P., Dolan, P., Tobias, J.H., Adams, M.A., 2004. Intervertebral disc degeneration can lead to 'stress-shielding' of the anterior vertebral body: a cause of osteoporotic vertebral fracture? Spine 29, 774–782.

Porter, R.W., Adams, M.A., Hutton, W.C., 1989. Physical activity and the strength of the lumbar spine. Spine 14, 201–203.

Proske, U., Morgan, D.L., Gregory, J.E., 1993. Thixotropy in skeletal muscle and in muscle spindles: a review. Progr Neurobiol 41, 705–721.

Radebold, A., Cholewicki, J., Polzhofer, G.K., Greene, H.S., 2001. Impaired postural control of the lumbar spine is associated with delayed muscle response times in patients with chronic idiopathic low back pain. Spine 26, 724–730.

Rhalmi, S., Yahia, L.H., Newman, N., Isler, M., 1993. Immunohistochemical study of nerves in lumbar spine ligaments. Spine 18, 264–267.

Ribeiro, F., Mota, J., Oliveira, J., 2007. Effect of exercise-induced fatigue on position sense of the knee in the elderly. Eur J Appl Physiol 99, 379–385.

Roberts, S., Eisenstein, S.M., Menage, J., Evans, E.H., Ashton, I.K., 1995. Mechanoreceptors in intervertebral discs. Morphology, distribution, and neuropeptides [see comments]. Spine 20, 2645–2651.

Sambrook, P.N., MacGregor, A.J., Spector, T.D., 1999. Genetic

influences on cervical and lumbar disc degeneration: a magnetic resonance imaging study in twins. Arth Rheum 42, 366–372.

Sanchez, D., Adams, M.A., Dolan, P., 2006. Spinal proprioception and back muscle activation are impaired by spinal 'creep' but not by fatigue. J Biomech 39, S33.

Sanchez-Zuriaga, D., Adams, M.A., Dolan, P., 2010. Is activation of the back muscles impaired by creep or muscle fatigue? Spine 35, 517–525.

Schmidt, H., Kettler, A., Heuer, F., Simon, U., Claes, L., Wilke, H.J., 2007. Intradiscal pressure, shear strain, and fiber strain in the intervertebral disc under combined loading. Spine 32, 748–755.

Seidler, A., Bolm-Audorff, U., Siol, T., Henkel, N., Fuchs, C., Schug, H., et al., 2003. Occupational risk factors for symptomatic lumbar disc herniation; a case-control study. Occup Environ Med 60, 821–830.

Shirazi-Adl, A., 1989. Strain in fibers of a lumbar disc. Analysis of the role of lifting in producing disc prolapse. Spine 14, 96–103.

Sinkjaer, T., Andersen, J.B., Nielsen, J.F., Hansen, H.J., 1999. Soleus long-latency stretch reflexes during walking in healthy and spastic humans. Clin Neurophysiol 110, 951–959.

Skinner, H.B., Wyatt, M.P., Hodgdon, J.A., Conard, D.W., Barrack, R.L., 1986. Effect of fatigue on joint position sense of the knee. J Orthop Res 4, 112–118.

Snook, S.H., Webster, B.S., McGorry, R.W., Fogleman, M.T., McCann, K.B., 1998. The reduction of chronic nonspecific low back pain through the control of early morning lumbar flexion. A randomized controlled trial. Spine 23, 2601–2607.

Solomonow, M., Baratta, R.V., Zhou, B.H., Burger, E., Zieske, A., Gedalia, A., 2003. Muscular dysfunction elicited by creep of lumbar viscoelastic tissue. J Electromyogr Kinesiol 13, 381–396.

Solomonow, M., Zhou, B.H., Baratta, R.V., Lu, Y., Harris, M., 1999. Biomechanics of increased exposure to lumbar injury caused by cyclic loading: Part 1. Loss of reflexive muscular stabilization. Spine 24, 2426–2434.

Solomonow, M., Zhou, B., Baratta, R.V., Zhu, M., Lu, Y., 2002. Neuromuscular disorders associated with static lumbar flexion: a feline model. J Electromyogr Kinesiol 12, 81–90.

Solomonow, M., Zhou, B.H., Harris, M., Lu, Y., Baratta, R.V., 1998. The ligamento-muscular stabilizing system of the spine. Spine 23, 2552–2562.

Stuart, M., Butler, J.E., Collins, D.F., Taylor, J.L., Gandevia, S.C., 2002. The history of contraction of the wrist flexors can change cortical excitability. J Physiol 545, 731–737.

Stubbs, M., Harris, M., Solomonow, M., Zhou, B., Lu, Y., Baratta, R.V., 1998. Ligamento-muscular protective reflex in the lumbar spine of the feline. J Electromyogr Kinesiol 8, 197–204.

Taimela, S., Kankaanpaa, M., Luoto, S., 1999. The effect of lumbar fatigue on the ability to sense a change in lumbar position. A controlled study. Spine 24, 1322–1327.

Tampier, C., Drake, J.D., Callaghan, J.P., McGill, S.M., 2007. Progressive disc herniation: an investigation of the mechanism using radiologic, histochemical, and microscopic dissection techniques on a porcine model. Spine 32, 2869–2874.

Taylor, J.L., Butler, J.E., Gandevia, S.C., 2000. Changes in muscle afferents, motoneurons and motor drive during muscle fatigue. Eur J Appl Physiol 83, 106–115.

Trafimow, J.H., Schipplein, O.D., Novak, G.J., Andersson, G.B., 1993. The effects of quadriceps fatigue on the technique of lifting. Spine 18, 364–367.

Ulrich, J.A., Liebenberg, E.C., Thuillier, D.U., Lotz, J.C., 2007. ISSLS prize winner: repeated disc injury causes persistent inflammation. Spine 32, 2812–2819.

van Dieën, J.H., van der Burg, P., Raaijmakers, T.A.J., Toussaint, H.M., 1998. Effects of repetitive lifting on kinematics: inadequate anticipatory control or adaptive changes? J Motor Behaviour 30, 20–32.

Vascancelos, D., 1973. Compression fractures of the vertebra during major epileptic seizures. Epilepsia 14, 323–328.

Vera-Garcia, F.J., Brown, S.H., Gray, J.R., McGill, S.M., 2006. Effects of different levels of torso coactivation on trunk muscular and kinematic responses to posteriorly applied sudden loads. Clin Biomech 21, 443–455.

Veres, S.P., Robertson, P.A., Broom, N.D., 2008. ISSLS prize winner: microstructure and mechanical disruption of the lumbar disc annulus: part II: how the annulus fails under hydrostatic pressure. Spine 33, 2711–2720.

Veres, S.P., Robertson, P.A., Broom, N.D., 2010. ISSLS prize winner: how loading rate influences disc failure mechanics: a microstructural assessment of internal disruption. Spine 35, 1897–1908.

Videman, T., Nurminen, M., 2004. The occurrence of anular tears and their relation to lifetime back pain history: a cadaveric study using barium sulfate discography. Spine 29, 2668–2676.

Vuillerme, N., Danion, F., Forestier, N., Nougier, V., 2002a. Postural sway under muscle vibration and muscle fatigue in humans. Neurosci Lett 333, 131–135.

Vuillerme, N., Forestier, N., Nougier, V., 2002b. Attentional demands and postural sway: the effect of the calf muscles fatigue. Med Sci Sports Exerc 34, 1907–1912.

Wilder, D.G., Aleksiev, A.R., Magnusson, M.L., Pope, M.H., Spratt, K.F., Goel, V.K., 1996. Muscular response to sudden load. A tool to evaluate fatigue and rehabilitation. Spine 21, 2628–2639.

Yahia, L., Rhalmi, S., Newman, N., Isler, M., 1992. Sensory innervation of human thoracolumbar fascia. An immunohistochemical study. Acta Orthop Scand 63, 195–197.

Yamashita, T., Cavanaugh, J.M., Ozaktay, A.C., Avramov, A.I., Getchell, T.V., King, A.I., 1993a. Effect of substance P on mechanosensitive units of tissues around and in the lumbar facet joint. J Orthop Res 11, 205–214.

Yamashita, T., Minaki, Y., Oota, I., Yokogushi, K., Ishii, S., 1993b. Mechanosensitive afferent units in the lumbar intervertebral disc and adjacent muscle. Spine 18, 2252–2256.

Zhao, F., Pollintine, P., Hole, B.D., Dolan, P., Adams, M.A., 2005. Discogenic origins of spinal instability. Spine 30, 2621–2630.

Part | 4 |

Clinical evidence of control approach

Chapter |15|

Effectiveness of exercise therapy for chronic non-specific low back pain

Marienke van Middelkoop*, Sidney M. Rubinstein†, Arianne Verhagen*, Raymond Ostelo†‡, Bart W. Koes* and Maurits van Tulder†‡
*Department of General Practice, Erasmus Medical Centre, Rotterdam, The Netherlands, †Department of Epidemiology and Biostatistics and EMGO Institute for Health and Care Research, VU University Medical Centre, Amsterdam, The Netherlands and ‡Department of Health Sciences and EMGO Institute for Health and Care Research, VU University, Amsterdam, The Netherlands

CHAPTER CONTENTS

BACKGROUND

Low back pain is usually defined as pain, muscle tension, or stiffness localized below the costal margin and above the inferior gluteal folds, with or without leg pain (sciatica). Low back pain is typically classified as being 'specific' or 'non-specific'. Specific low back pain refers to symptoms caused by a specific pathophysiologic mechanism, such as hernia nucleus pulposus (HNP), infection, inflammation, osteoporosis, rheumatoid arthritis, fracture or tumour. Specific underlying diseases can be identified only in about 10% of the patients (Deyo et al. 1992). The vast majority of patients (up to 90%) are labelled as having non-specific low back pain, which is defined as symptoms without clear specific cause, i.e. low back pain of unknown origin. Spinal abnormalities on radiographs and MRI are not strongly associated with non-specific low back pain, because many people without any symptoms also show these abnormalities (van Tulder et al. 1997).

Non-specific low back pain is usually classified according to duration as acute (less than 6 weeks), subacute (between 6 weeks and 3 months) or chronic (longer than 3 months) low back pain. In general, prognosis is good and most patients with an episode of non-specific low back pain will recover within a couple of weeks. However, back pain among primary care patients is often a recurrent problem with fluctuating symptoms. The majority of back pain patients will have experienced a previous episode and acute exacerbations of chronic low back pain are common. Low back pain (LBP) is not only a tremendous medical problem, but also a huge socioeconomic problem in Western countries due to high rates of disability and work absenteeism (Andersson 1999). It is important to provide effective and cost-effective interventions to improve patient outcomes and get maximum benefits within available health care budgets.

Evidence-based medicine has become increasingly more important over the past decade. The management of low back pain has been positively affected by the availability of more scientific research and better use of critical appraisal techniques to evaluate and apply research findings (Chou 2005). The randomized controlled trial remains the gold standard of evidence on effectiveness of therapeutic interventions, but, there are many other sources and types of evidence relevant to clinical practice. A large number of systematic reviews are available within and outside the framework of the Cochrane Back Review Group that have evaluated the therapeutic interventions for low back pain by critically appraising and summarizing randomized trials (Bombardier et al. 1997; Bouter et al. 2003). This large body of evidence has greatly improved our understanding of what does and does not work for low back pain. The evidence from trials and reviews have formed the basis for clinical practice guidelines on the management of low back pain that have been developed in various countries around the world.

Two recent papers summarized the quality and content of 25 international clinical guidelines on the management of low back pain (Koes et al. 2001; Bouwmeester et al. 2009). There seems to be consensus about the optimal management for acute low back pain. Recommendations for treatment of acute low back pain were rather consistent among the various international guidelines:

- Reassure patients on the favourable prognosis, if available provide printed patient information.
- Advise patients to stay active.
- Discourage bed rest.
- Prescribe medication if necessary (preferably time-contingent):
  - paracetamol/acetaminophen
  - non-steroidal anti-inflammatory drugs.
- If patients do not improve, spinal manipulation is an option for pain relief.

Exercise therapy was not recommended for acute low back pain in any of the guidelines. However, all guidelines recommended exercise therapy for patients with chronic non-specific low back pain.

Exercise therapy is probably the most widely used type of conservative treatment worldwide. A systematic Cochrane review published in 2005 found that exercise therapy significantly reduces pain and improves function in adults with chronic low back pain, particularly in patients visiting primary care providers because of back pain (Alexandre et al. 2001). Since the publication of the Cochrane review, new studies have been published investigating various types of exercise interventions for chronic low back pain. The present chapter provides an update of the evidence on exercise therapy compared to other interventions, but also on the comparison of different types of exercise in patients with chronic low back pain.

METHODS

Literature search, inclusion criteria and study selection

A literature search was performed using the following electronic databases: MEDLINE, EMBASE, CINAHL, CENTRAL and PEDro (up to 22 December 2008). References from the relevant studies were screened in order to identify any additional studies. The language was limited to English, Dutch and German. The search strategy outlined by the Cochrane Back Review Group (CBRG) was perused. Two reviewers working independently from each other conducted the electronic searches.

The inclusion criteria were as follows:

- Randomized controlled trials of two or more interventions.
- The study population should consist of adults, older than 18 years, with non-specific chronic low back pain that persisted for 12 weeks or more.
- RCTs studying any type of exercise therapy. *Exercise therapy* was defined as 'a series of specific movements with the aim of training or developing the body by a routine practice or physical training to promote good physical health' (Bendix et al. 1995). Additional treatments were allowed provided that the intervention of interest was the main contrast between the intervention groups included in the study.
- RCTs including subjects with specific low back pain caused by pathological entities, such as vertebral spinal stenosis, ankylosing spondylitis, scoliosis, coccydynia, were excluded. The diagnosis for these specific entities had to be confirmed by means of an MRI or another diagnostic tool. Trials on post-partum low back pain or pelvic pain due to pregnancy were also excluded as well as postoperative studies and prevention studies.
- The following self-reported outcome measures were assessed in this review: pain intensity (e.g. visual analogue scale (VAS), McGill pain questionnaire), back-specific disability (e.g. Roland Morris, Oswestry Disability Index), perceived recovery (e.g. overall improvement), return to work (e.g. return to work status, sick leave days) and side effects. The primary outcomes for this overview were pain and physical functional status. Studies with a follow-up less than one day were excluded.

Two authors independently screened the abstracts and titles retrieved by the search strategy and applied the inclusion criteria. The full text of the article was obtained if the abstract seemed to fulfil the inclusion criteria or if eligibility of the study was unclear. All full text articles were compiled and screened on inclusion criteria by the two authors, independently. Any disagreements between the authors were resolved by discussion and consensus. A third author was consulted if disagreements persisted.

Assessment of methodological quality and quality of evidence

Two reviewers conducted the risk of bias assessment, independently. Risk of bias of the individual studies was assessed using the criteria list advised by the CBRG, which consists of 11 items. Items were scored as positive if they did fulfil the criteria and negative when there was a clear risk of bias, and marked as inconclusive if there was insufficient information. Differences in assessment were discussed during a consensus meeting. A total score was computed, and high quality was defined as fulfilling six or more (more than 50%) of the internal validity criteria (range 0 to 11).

GRADE (Grades of Recommendation, Assessment, Development and Evaluation) was used to evaluate the overall quality of evidence and the strength of the recommendations (Chatzitheodorou et al. 2007). Quality of evidence of a specific outcome was based upon the following principal measures:

- Limitations (due to for example, study design)
- Consistency of results
- Indirectness (e.g. generalizability of the findings)
- Precision (e.g. sufficient data)
- Other considerations, such as reporting bias.

The overall quality was considered to be high when RCTs with a low risk of bias provided consistent, sufficient and precise results for a particular outcome; however, the quality of the evidence was downgraded by one level when one of the factors described above was not met. The following grades of evidence were applied:

High quality: Further research is very unlikely to change our confidence in the estimate of effect.
Moderate quality: Further research is likely to have an important impact on our confidence in the estimate of effect and may change the estimate.
Low quality: Further research is very likely to have an important impact on our confidence in the estimate of effect and is likely to change the estimate.
Very low quality: We are very uncertain about the estimate.

Data extraction and analysis

The same two review authors who performed the risk of bias assessment conducted the data extraction,

independently from one another. Data were extracted onto a standardized web-based form. Comparison therapies were combined into main clusters of presumed effectiveness (no treatment/waiting list controls, other interventions). Separate analyses were planned for each type of exercise therapy, each type of control, each main outcome measure, and time of follow-up (post-treatment: short-term = closest to 3 months, intermediate = closest to 6 months and long-term = closest to 12 months). If trials reported outcomes only as graphs, the means scores and standard deviations were estimated from these graphs.

For continuous data, results are presented as weighted mean differences (WMD). All scales were converted to 100-point scales. For dichotomous data, a relative risk (RR) was calculated, and the event was defined as the number of subjects recovered. A test for heterogeneity was calculated using the Q-test (Chi-square) and I^2. Confidence intervals (95% CI) were calculated for each effect. A random effects model was used and funnel plots were examined for publication bias.

If standard deviations were not reported, we calculated it using reported values of confidence intervals if possible. If the standard deviation of the baseline score was reported, this score was forwarded. Finally, if none of these data were reported, an estimation of the standard deviation was based on study data (population and score) of other studies.

In order to correct for bias introduced by 'double-counting' of subjects of trials that had two control groups in the same meta-analyses, the number of subjects of these trials was divided by two.

RESULTS OF THE REVIEW

Description of studies

Thirty-seven studies (3957 patients) were included (see Table 15.1). Multiple publications were found for Bendix et al. (1995, 1996, 1998), Gudavalli et al. (Cambron et al. 2006a, 2006b; Gudavalli et al. 2006), Niemistö et al. (2003, 2005), and Smeets et al. (2006, 2008). Information from all publications was used for assessment of risk of bias and data extraction, but only the first or most prominent publication was used for citation of these studies.

The results of the risk of bias assessment are shown in Table 15.1. All studies were described as randomized, however the method of randomization was only explicit in 75.7% ($N = 28$) of the studies. Only 15 studies (40.5%) met six or more of the criteria, which was our preset threshold for low risk of bias. Only the criteria regarding the baseline characteristics, timing of outcome measures and description of dropouts were met by 50% or more of the included randomized trials.

Table 15.1 Risk of bias of studies investigating exercise therapy for chronic low back pain

First-named author, year	Randomization adequate?	Allocation concealed?	Groups similar at baseline?	Patient blinded?	Care provider blinded?	Outcome assessor blinded?	Co-interventions avoided or similar?	Compliance acceptable?	Drop-out rate described and acceptable?	Timing outcome assessment similar?	Intention-to-treat analysis?	Total score
Alexandre et al. 2001	?	+	?	-	-	?	?	?	?	+	+	5
Bendix et al. 1995	+	-	+	-	-	+	+	+	+	+	-	7
Chatzitheodorou et al. 2007*	+	?	+	-	-	?	?	?	?	+	?	3
Chown et al. 2008	+	?	+	-	-	-	?	-	-	+	-	3
Critchley et al. 2007*	+	+	+	-	-	-	?	?	?	+	+	5
Deyo et al. 1990	+	+	+	-	-	+	+	+	+	+	-	8
Donzelli et al. 2006*	?	?	?	+	-	-	?	?	?	+	?	3
Elnaggar et al. 1991	+	+	+	-	-	+	+	-	-	+	+	6
Ferreira et al. 2007*	+	+	+	-	-	-	-	+	+	+	+	8
Frost et al. 1995 (1998)	+	+	+	-	-	+	+	+	+	+	+	8
Galantino et al. 2004	+	?	?	-	?	-	?	?	-	+	-	2
Gladwell et al. 2006*	?	?	-	-	-	+	?	+	-	-	-	3
Goldby et al. 2006*	+	?	+	-	-	+	?	-	+	+	?	4
Gudavalli et al. 2006*	+	+	+	-	-	+	?	?	-	+	+	6
Gur et al. 2003	?	?	+	-	-	-	?	?	+	+	+	4
Harts et al. 2008	+	+	+	-	-	-	?	+	-	+	+	6
Hildebrandt et al. 2000	+	+	+	-	-	-	+	-	-	+	+	6
Johannsen et al. 1995	-	?	?	-	-	-	-	-	-	-	-	1

Study	1	2	3	4	5	6	7	8	9	10	11	Total
Kankaanpaa et al. 1999	+	+	–	–	–	?	+	+	+	+	–	6
Koldas Doğan et al. 2008	?	+	–	–	–	?	?	+	+	+	?	3
Lewis et al. 2005*	?	–	–	–	+	+	+	+	+	+	+	7
Machado et al. 2007*	?	+	+	+	+	?	–	–	+	+	+	5
Mannion et al. 1999	+	+	+	+	+	+	+	+	+	+	+	11
Marshall et al. 2008*	?	+	–	–	?	?	?	+	+	+	–	3
Niemistö et al. 2003 (2005)	+	+	–	–	–	+	+	+	+	+	+	8
Risch et al. 1993	+	+	–	–	–	–	–	+	+	+	+	4
Rittweger et al. 2002	+	+	–	–	–	?	?	+	+	+	–	5
Roche et al. 2007*	?	+	?	–	?	?	?	+	+	+	?	4
Sherman et al. 2005*	+	+	–	–	+	+	+	+	+	+	+	8
Sjögren et al. 2005*	?	?	?	–	?	+	+	+	+	+	?	4
Smeets et al. 2006* (2008)	+	+	–	+	+	+	+	+	+	+	+	9
Tekur et al. 2008	+	+	–	–	–	?	?	+	?	?	?	4
Tritilanunt et al. 2001	?	+	–	–	–	?	–	+	+	+	–	4
Turner et al. 1990	+	+	–	–	–	–	–	–	+	+	–	4
Williams et al. 2005*	?	+	–	–	?	+	?	–	+	+	?	4
Yelland et al. 2004	+	+	–	–	–	+	+	+	+	+	+	8
Yozbatiran et al. 2004	?	+	–	–	–	?	+	+	+	+	+	5

+, Fulfils criteria; –, did not fulfil criteria; ?, unclear whether this item fulfils criteria.
*New studies (not included in Cochrane reviews).

Effectiveness of exercise therapy (Table 15.2)

Exercise therapy vs. waiting list controls/no treatment

Eight studies were identified as comparing some type of exercise therapy to waiting list controls or no treatment (Turner et al. 1990; Risch et al. 1993; Alexandre et al. 2001; Galantino et al. 2004; Sjögren et al. 2005; Gladwell et al. 2006; Smeets et al. 2006; Harts et al. 2008). Five studies reported post-treatment data only, because after the treatment period the waiting list controls also received the treatment. Only two studies (Alexandre et al. 2001; Smeets et al. 2006) had intermediate or long-term follow-up.

All studies reported data that could be used in the statistical pooling. The pooled mean difference of the five studies reporting post-treatment pain intensity was not statistically significant (−4.51 (95% CI −9.49, 0.47)). The WMD for post-treatment improvement in disability was −3.63 (95% CI −8.89, 1.63). The pooled mean WMD for pain intensity at intermediate follow-up was −16.46 (95% CI −44.48, 11.57). Only one study (102 people) reported intermediate outcomes for disability and long-term outcomes for pain intensity and disability. There were no differences between the group receiving exercise therapy and the waiting list control group (Smeets et al. 2006).

Therefore, there is low quality evidence (serious limitations, imprecision) that there is no statistically significant difference in pain reduction and improvement of disability between exercise therapy and no treatment/waiting list controls.

Exercise therapy vs. usual care/advice to stay active

A total of six studies (Hildebrandt et al. 2000; Niemistö et al. 2003; Frost et al. 2004; Yelland et al. 2004; Koldas Doğan et al. 2008; Tekur et al. 2008) investigated the effect of exercise therapy compared to usual care. Four of these studies had an intermediate or long-term follow-up. Statistical pooling of three studies (Frost et al. 2004; Koldas Doğan et al. 2008; Tekur et al. 2008) showed a significant decrease in pain intensity and disability in favour of the exercise group (WMD −9.23 (95% CI −16.02, −2.43)) and −12.35 (95% CI −23.00,−1.69), respectively. One study (Koldas Doğan et al. 2008) reported on pain and disability at short-term follow-up, and found no statistically significant differences between the exercise group and the control group receiving home exercises. Two studies (Niemistö et al. 2003; Frost et al. 2004) showed a statistically significant pooled WMD for disability at intermediate follow-up of −5.43 (95% CI −9.54, −1.32). One study (Niemistö et al. 2003) found a statistically significant difference at intermediate follow-up for pain relief for

the exercise group compared to the usual care group. Three studies (Frost et al. 2004; Yelland et al. 2004; Niemistö et al. 2005) reported on pain and/or disability at long-term follow-up. The pooled WMD for pain was not statistically significant (−4.94 (95% CI −10.45, 0.58)); the WMD for disability was statistically significant in favour of the exercise group (WMD −3.17 (95% CI −5.96, −0.38)).

One study (Hildebrandt et al. 2000) reported recovery at post-treatment and during intermediate and long-term follow-up. There was a statistically significant difference between the groups at 3 and 6 months follow-up in favour of the exercise group compared with usual care (P<0.001). Eighty percent of the patients in the exercise group regarded themselves recovered at 3 months follow-up versus 47% in the usual care group.

There is low quality evidence (serious limitations, imprecision) for the effectiveness of exercise therapy compared to usual care on pain intensity and disability.

Exercise therapy vs. back school/education

Three studies with a high risk of bias were identified (Williams et al. 2005; Donzelli et al. 2006; Goldby et al. 2006). Post-treatment results for disability were reported in two studies, with a significant pooled WMD of −11.20 (95% CI −16.78, −5.62). One study reported on pain post-treatment and found no statistically significant difference between both intervention groups (Williams et al. 2005). The pooled mean differences for pain and disability at 3 months follow-up were −7.63 (95% CI −17.20, 1.93) and −2.55 (95% CI −10.07, 4.97), respectively.

Two studies (Donzelli et al. 2006; Goldby et al. 2006) reported intermediate outcomes on pain, and three studies (Sherman et al. 2005; Donzelli et al. 2006; Goldby et al. 2006) reported on disability. The pooled WMDs showed no statistically significant differences between the groups: −5.58 (95% CI −16.65, 5.48) and −4.42 (95% CI −9.90, 1.05), respectively. Only one study (N = 346) reported long-term outcomes, and these were not statistically significantly different between the groups (Goldby et al. 2006).

The data provided very low quality evidence (serious limitations, imprecision and inconsistency) that there was no statistically significant difference in effect on pain and disability at short-term and intermediate follow-up for exercise therapy compared to back school/education.

Exercise therapy vs. behavioural treatment

Three studies, one with a low risk of bias, were identified comparing exercise therapy with a behavioural treatment (Elnaggar et al. 1991; Yozbatiran et al. 2004; Williams et al. 2005). Two studies reported post-treatment pain and disability and the pooled WMDs were 1.21 (95% CI −5.42, 7.84) and 0.34 (95% CI −2.64, 3.31), respectively.

Table 15.2 Summary effect estimates for exercise therapy in chronic low back pain patients

1. Exercise vs. no treatment/sham/placebo/waiting list controls

Outcome or subgroup	Studies	Participants	Statistical method	Effect estimate
1.1 Pain post-treatment	5	268	Mean difference (IV, random, 95% CI)	−4.51 (−9.49, 0.47)
1.2 Disability post-treatment	6	331	Mean difference (IV, random, 95% CI)	−3.63 (−8.89, 1.63)
1.3 Pain during intermediate follow-up	2	137	Mean difference (IV, random, 95% CI)	−16.46 (−44.48, 11.57)

2. Exercise therapy vs. usual care

Outcome or subgroup	Studies	Participants	Statistical method	Effect estimate
2.1 Pain post-treatment	2	108	Mean difference (IV, random, 95% CI)	−9.23 (−16.02, −2.43)
2.2 Disability post-treatment	3	188	Mean difference (IV, random, 95% CI)	−12.35 (−23.00, −1.69)
2.3 Disability during intermediate follow-up	2	267	Mean difference (IV, random, 95% CI)	−5.43 (−9.54, −1.32)
2.4 Pain at long-term (12 months) follow-up	2	301	Mean difference (IV, random, 95% CI)	−4.94 (−10.45, 0.58)
2.5 Disability at long-term (12 months) follow-up	3	377	Mean difference (IV, random, 95% CI)	−3.17 (−5.96, −0.38)

3. Exercise therapy vs. back school/education

Outcome or subgroup	Studies	Participants	Statistical method	Effect estimate
3.1 Disability post-treatment	2	139	Mean difference (IV, random, 95% CI)	−11.20 (−16.78, −5.62)
3.2 Pain at short-term (3 months) follow-up	3	200	Mean difference (IV, random, 95% CI)	−7.63 (−17.20, 1.93)
3.3 Disability after short-term (3 months) follow-up	3	200	Mean difference (IV, random, 95% CI)	−2.55 (−10.07, 4.97)
3.4 Pain at intermediate (6 months) follow-up	2	141	Mean difference (IV, random, 95% CI)	−5.58 (−16.65, 5.48)
3.5 Disability at intermediate (6 months) follow-up	3	241	Mean difference (IV, random, 95% CI)	−4.42 (−9.90, 1.05)

4. Exercise vs. behavioural treatment

Outcome or subgroup	Studies	Participants	Statistical method	Effect estimate
4.1 Pain post-treatment	2	146	Mean difference (IV, random, 95% CI)	1.21 (−5.42, 7.84)
4.2 Disability post-treatment	2	146	Mean difference (IV, random, 95% CI)	0.34 (−2.64, 3.31)
4.3 Pain during intermediate follow-up	3	258	Mean difference (IV, random, 95% CI)	−2.23 (−7.58, 3.12)
4.4 Disability during intermediate follow-up	3	258	Mean difference (IV, random, 95% CI)	1.97 (−3.55, 7.48)

Continued

Table 15.2 Summary effect estimates for exercise therapy in chronic low back pain patients—cont'd

4.5 Pain during long-term follow-up	3	247	Mean difference (IV, random, 95% CI)	−0.88 (−6.34, 4.58)
4.6 Disability during long-term follow-up	3	243	Mean difference (IV, random, 95% CI)	2.77 (−3.43, 8.96)
5. Exercise vs. TENS/laser/passive modalities				
Outcome or subgroup	**Studies**	**Participants**	**Statistical method**	**Effect estimate**
5.1 Pain post-treatment	5	286	Mean difference (IV, random, 95% CI)	−9.33 (−18.80, 0.13)
5.2 Disability post-treatment	5	286	Mean difference (IV, random, 95% CI)	−2.59 (−8.03, 2.85)
5.3 Pain during short-term follow-up	2	162	Mean difference (IV, random, 95% CI)	1.72 (−6.05, 9.50)
5.4 Disability during short-term follow-up	2	162	Mean difference (IV, random, 95% CI)	1.02 (−0.38, 2.42)
6. Exercise vs. manipulation/manual therapy				
Outcome or subgroup	**Studies**	**Participants**	**Statistical method**	**Effect estimate**
6.1 Pain post-treatment	3	395	Mean difference (IV, random, 95% CI)	5.67 (1.99, 9.35)
6.2 Disability post-treatment	3	398	Mean difference (IV, random, 95% CI)	2.16 (−0.96, 5.28)
6.3 Pain during short-term follow-up	2	326	Mean difference (IV, random, 95% CI)	−1.33 (−10.44, 7.79)
6.4 Disability during short-term follow-up	2	326	Mean difference (IV, random, 95% CI)	0.29 (−3.15, 3.72)
6.5 Pain during intermediate follow-up	3	461	Mean difference (IV, random, 95% CI)	−0.49 (−12.22, 11.23)
6.6 Disability during intermediate follow-up	3	461	Mean difference (IV, random, 95% CI)	2.38 (−5.16, 9.93)
6.7 Pain during long-term follow-up	4	515	Mean difference (IV, random, 95% CI)	2.09 (−2.94, 7.13)
6.8 Disability during long-term follow-up	5	553	Mean difference (IV, random, 95% CI)	−0.70 (−3.14, 1.74)

All three studies reported intermediate and long-term follow-up on pain intensity and disability. For intermediate follow-up the pooled WMDs for pain and disability were −2.23 (95% CI −7.58, 3.12) and 1.97 (95% CI −3.55, 7.48), respectively. Long-term results showed a pooled WMD for pain intensity of −0.88 (95% CI −6.34, 4.58) and a pooled WMD for disability of 2.77 (95% CI −3.43, 8.96).

There is low quality evidence (serious limitations, imprecision) that there are no statistically significant differences between exercise therapy and behavioural therapy on pain intensity and disability at short- and long-term follow-up.

Exercise therapy vs. TENS/laser therapy/ultrasound/massage

Five studies, two with a low risk of bias, were identified comparing exercise therapy with passive therapies such as TENS, low-level laser therapy, ultrasound and thermal therapy (Deyo et al. 1990; Kankaanpaa et al. 1999; Gur et al. 2003; Chatzitheodorou et al. 2007; Koldas Doğan et al. 2008). The pooled WMD for post-treatment pain intensity was −9.33 (95% CI −18.80, 0.13) and for post-treatment disability −2.59 (95% CI −8.03, 2.85). Two studies (Deyo et al. 1990; Koldas Doğan et al., 2008) reported on short-term pain intensity and disability and the pooled mean differences were 1.72 (95% CI −6.05, 9.50) and 1.02 (95% CI −0.38, 2.42), respectively. One study with a low risk of bias (Kankaanpaa et al. 1999) reported intermediate and long-term outcomes, and found a statistically significantly difference for pain intensity of 16.8 and 21.2 points, respectively, in favour of exercise therapy. Also a statistically significant difference was found for disability.

Low quality evidence (serious limitations, inconsistency, imprecision) was provided that there is no statistically significant difference in effect between exercise therapy compared to TENS/laser/ultrasound/massage on the outcomes pain and disability at short-term follow-up.

Exercise therapy vs. manual therapy/manipulation

Five studies, two with a low risk of bias, were identified comparing exercise treatment with spinal manipulation or manual therapy (Goldby et al. 2006; Gudavalli et al 2006; Ferreira et al. 2007; Chown et al. 2008; Marshall and Murphy 2008). Post-treatment data were available for three studies. The pooled WMDs for pain intensity and disability were 5.67 (95% CI 1.99, 9.35) and 2.16 (95% CI −0.96, 5.28), respectively. One study reported a statistically significant difference in global perceived effect post-treatment (Ferreira et al. 2007) in favour of spinal manipulation. Two studies reported short-term effects on pain intensity and disability and the pooled WMDs were −1.33 (95% CI −10.11, 7.79) and 0.29 (95% CI −3.15, 3.72), respectively (Goldby et al. 2006; Gudavalli et al. 2006). Intermediate results on pain and disability were reported by three studies (Ferreira et al. 2007; Goldby et al. 2006; Gudavalli et al. 2006) and the pooled WMDs were −0.49 (95% CI −12.22, 11.23) and 2.38 (95% CI −5.16, 9.93), respectively. All studies reported long-term results on disability and the pooled WMD was −0.70 (95% CI −3.14, 1.74). Four studies reported long-term results on pain intensity and the pooled WMD was 2.09 (95% CI −2.94, 7.13). Global perceived effect was reported by one study during intermediate and long-term follow-up. No statistically significant differences between groups were found in this study (Ferreira et al. 2007).

The data provided low quality evidence (inconsistency, imprecision) that there was no statistically significant difference in effect (pain intensity and disability) for exercise therapy compared to manual therapy/manipulation at short- and long-term follow-up.

Exercise therapy vs. psychotherapy

One study with a high risk of bias was identified (Machado et al. 2007). Post-treatment results showed a statistically significant difference in disability scores between both groups in advantage of the exercise group. No post-treatment differences between both groups were found for pain intensity. At 6 months follow-up, both disability and pain intensity scores were lower in the exercise group compared to the psychotherapy group, but not statistically significant.

Exercise therapy vs. other forms of exercise therapy

Eleven studies compared different exercise interventions with each other (Elnaggar et al. 1991; Johannsen et al. 1995; Tritilanunt and Wajanavisit 2001; Rittweger et al. 2002; Yozbatiran et al. 2004; Lewis et al. 2005; Sherman et al. 2005; Ferreira et al. 2007; Roche et al. 2007; Harts et al. 2008; Mannion et al. 1999). Data from these studies could not be pooled because of the heterogeneity of the types of interventions.

Two studies found statistically significant differences between different exercise interventions. One study (Tritilanunt and Wajanavisit 2001), with a high risk of bias, reported statistically significant difference in pain relief at 3 months follow-up of an aerobic exercise training programme compared with a lumbar flexion exercise programme of 3-months. One large trial (Ferreira et al. 2007) with a low risk of bias (N = 240) compared a general exercise programme (strengthening and stretching) with a motor control exercise programme (improving function of specific trunk muscles) of 12 weeks. The motor control exercise group had slightly better outcomes (mean adjusted between group difference function 2.9 and global perceived effect 1.7) than the general exercise group at 8 weeks. Similar group outcomes were found at 6 and 12 months follow-up.

A total of nine studies did not find any statistically significant differences between the various exercise interventions (Elnaggar et al. 1991). Sherman et al. (2005) compared a 12-week yoga (viniyoga) programme with a 12-week conventional exercise class programme. Back-related function in the yoga group was superior to the exercise group at 12 weeks.

Motor control exercise

In 2009 Macedo and colleagues published a systematic review on motor control exercise for persistent (subacute, chronic and recurrent) non-specific low back pain. Fourteen randomized controlled trials were included. The authors reported that seven trials found that motor control exercise was better than minimal intervention or as supplement to another intervention in reducing pain at short-term follow-up (WMD 14.3, 95% CI 20.4, 8.1), intermediate follow-up (WMD 13.6, 95% CI 22.4, 4.1), and long-term follow-up (WMD 14.4, 95% CI 23.1, 5.7) and in reducing disability at long-term follow-up (WMD 10.8, 95% CI 18.7, 2.8). There were no differences in disability at short-term and intermediate-term follow-up. Short-term follow-up was defined as less than 3 months, intermediate-term follow-up as between 3 and 12 months, and long-term follow-up as more than 12 months.

Four trials found that motor control exercise was better than manual therapy for pain (WMD 5.7, 95% CI 10.7, 0.8), disability (WMD 4.0, 95% CI 7.6, 0.4), and quality-of-life (WMD 6.0, 95% CI 11.2, 0.8) at intermediate follow-up, but the effects were small. There were no differences at short-term and long-term follow-up.

Five trials found that motor control exercise was better than other forms of exercise in reducing disability at short-term follow-up (WMD 5.1, 95% CI 8.7, 1.4).

Macedo et al. (2009) concluded that in patients with chronic low back pain, motor control exercise is more effective than minimal intervention and beneficial when added to another therapy for pain at all time points and for disability at long-term follow-up only. Motor control exercise is not more effective than manual therapy or other forms of exercise.

DISCUSSION OF RESULTS

The effectiveness of exercise therapy

No significant treatment effects of exercise therapy compared to no treatment/waiting list controls were found on pain intensity and disability. Compared to usual care, pain intensity and disability were significantly reduced by exercise therapy at short-term follow-up. Motor control exercise was more effective than minimal intervention and beneficial when added to another therapy for pain at all time points and for disability at long-term follow-up only. This overview included 11 studies comparing different types of exercise treatments with each other. Very small to no differences were found in these studies.

The Cochrane review published in 2005 on the effectiveness of exercise for low back pain found evidence for the effectiveness on pain and function in chronic patients (Hayden et al. 2005). We also found evidence for the effectiveness for exercise therapy compared to usual care. However, we applied strict inclusion criteria regarding chronic low back pain, so our meta-analyses excluded some of the studies included in the Cochrane review, but also included some new studies. Nevertheless, results are comparable despite the new studies that are conducted in the last years. It is therefore also striking that the quality of the included studies was still generally poor resulting in a potentially high risk of bias. Blinding of the patient and blinding of the care provider were not properly conducted in many studies. Blinding of patients is also difficult in many RCTs investigating the effectives of exercise therapy. The quality of future RCTs in the field of back pain should be improved to reduce bias in systematic reviews

and overviews, as it has been demonstrated that statistical pooling of trials with a high risk of bias may result in overestimation of treatment effects.

Of particular note is the heterogeneity among the studies. This heterogeneity could have been caused by differences in interventions, differences in control groups, duration of the intervention and the risk of bias of the different studies. Therefore, the results of the meta-analyses with heterogeneity should be interpreted with some caution.

Further research is very likely to have an important impact on our confidence in the estimate of effect and is likely to change the estimate. These studies should focus on specific populations and these should be well described. Further, more studies are needed to investigate the different forms of exercise interventions and finally, the description of these studies should include the compliance and co-interventions of the study groups.

The evidence on motor control exercise for chronic low back pain seems promising. Many types of exercises for low back pain are not strongly supported by pathophysiological or biomechanical studies. Aerobic exercises for low back pain, for example, were developed based on general principles of sports medicine. However, the underlying mechanisms of action of motor control exercise are supported by several studies (Hides et al. 1996; Hodges and Richardson 1996, 1998). Motor control exercise was developed based on the principle that individuals with low back pain have a lack of control of the trunk muscles, for example, the transversus abdominis and the multifidus muscles. The idea is to use a motor learning approach to retrain the optimal control and coordination of the spine. The intervention involves the training of pre-activation of the deep trunk muscles, with progression toward more complex static, dynamic and functional tasks integrating the activation of deep and global trunk muscles.

Although motor control exercise was more effective than minimal intervention for chronic low back pain, there were no differences when compared to other types of exercises. It is still unclear which patients respond best to which type of exercise. Whether individuals with reduced motor control benefit more from motor control exercise should be evaluated in future studies. Identifying subgroups of patients that benefit more from one intervention than another is one of the biggest challenges in low back pain research. Some promising initiatives have been published, such as the McKenzie method (McKenzie and May 2003), classification-based algorithm (Fritz et al. 2003), primary care back pain screening tool (Hill et al. 2008), and the Orebro Musculoskeletal Pain Screening Questionnaire (Linton and Hallden 1998).

Evidence-based practice

Opponents of evidence-based practice have criticized using the randomized controlled trial in a dogmatic way and refused to acknowledge that other study designs may also produce valid data about the outcome of interventions (Borgerson, 2009). The focus on randomized trials as the paradigm of study design to answer any clinical question is obviously wrong. Randomized trials are the gold standard for questions related to the effectiveness of preventive or therapeutic interventions, but not necessarily the best option for answering questions related to adverse effects, prognosis or diagnosis. Also, evidence on effectiveness from non-randomized observational studies may be utilized if little evidence from randomized trials is available. There are also situations in which effectiveness cannot be assessed by randomized trials because of practical or ethical reasons. Although rare, before–after experiments are sometimes valued in evidence-based medicine. If the treatment results in a dramatic effect and if the natural course of the condition is stable, bias can be ruled out as an explanation. Insulin for diabetes, suturing for repairing large wounds and defibrillation for ventricular fibrillation, for example, are interventions that were accepted without any evidence from randomized trials (Glasziou et al., 2007).

In general, however, randomized controlled trials are the preferred design to evaluate effectiveness of therapeutic interventions. There are examples where empirical evidence has resulted in better treatment in practice. Advising low back pain patients to stay active rather than lie in bed is one example (Deyo et al., 1986; Malmivaara et al., 1995). Bed rest had been the mainstay of treatment for low back pain for decades, until randomized controlled trials showed that staying active is more beneficial than staying in bed. Without these randomized trials, physicians may never have changed their practice and might still be advocating bed rest for low back pain.

Implications for practice

Exercise therapy is not effective for acute low back pain. Exercise therapy is effective for chronic low back pain, but there is no evidence that any type of exercise is clearly more effective than others. Subgroups of patients with low back pain may respond differently to various types of exercise therapy, but it is still unclear which patients benefit most from what type of exercises. Adherence to exercise prescription is usually poor, so supervision by a therapist is recommended. If home exercises are prescribed, strategies to improve adherence should be used. Patient's preferences and expectations should be considered when deciding which type of exercise to choose.

REFERENCES

Alexandre, N.M., de Moraes, M.A., Correa Filho, H.R., Jorge, S.A., 2001. Evaluation of a program to reduce back pain in nursing personnel. Rev Saude Publica 35, 356–361.

Andersson, G.B., 1999. Epidemiological features of chronic low-back pain. Lancet 354, 581–585.

Bendix, A.E., Bendix, T., Haestrup, C., Busch, E., 1998. A prospective, randomized 5-year follow-up study of functional restoration in chronic low back pain patients. Eur Spine J 7, 111–119.

Bendix, A.F., Bendix, T., Ostenfeld, S., Bush, E., Andersen, 1995. Active treatment programs for patients with chronic low back pain: a prospective, randomized, observer-blinded study. Eur Spine J 4, 148–152.

Bendix, A.F., Bendix, T., Vaegter, K., Lund, C., Frolund, L., Holm, L., 1996. Multidisciplinary intensive treatment for chronic low back pain: a randomized, prospective study. Cleve Clin J Med 63, 62–69.

Bombardier, C., Esmail, R., Nachemson, A.L., Back Review Group Editorial

Board, 1997. The Cochrane Collaboration Back Review Group for spinal disorders. Spine 22, 837–840.

Borgerson, K., 2009. Valuing evidence: bias and the evidence hierarchy of evidence-based medicine. Perspect Biol Med 52, 218–233.

Bouter, L.M., Pennick, V., Bombardier, C., The Editorial Board of the Back Review Group, 2003. Cochrane Back Review Group. Spine 28, 1215–1218.

Bouwmeester, W., van Enst, A., van Tulder, M., 2009. Quality of low back pain guidelines improved. Spine 34, 2562–2567.

Cambron, J.A., Gudavalli, M.R., Hedeker, D., McGregor, M., Jedlicka, J., Keenum, M., et al., 2006a. One-year follow-up of a randomized clinical trial comparing flexion distraction with an exercise program for chronic low-back pain. J Altern Complement Med 12, 659–668.

Cambron, J.A., Gudavalli, M.R., McGregor, M., Jedlicka, J., Keenum, M., Ghanayem, A.J., et al., 2006b. Amount of health care and self-care

following a randomized clinical trial comparing flexion-distraction with exercise program for chronic low back pain. Chiropr Osteopat 14, 19.

Chatzitheodorou, D., Kabitsis, C., Malliou, P., Mougios, V., 2007. A pilot study of the effects of high-intensity aerobic exercise versus passive interventions on pain, disability, psychological strain, and serum cortisol concentrations in people with chronic low back pain. Phys Ther 87, 304–312.

Chou, R., 2005. Evidence-based medicine and the challenge of low back pain: where are we now? Pain Practice 5, 153–178.

Chown, M., Whittamore, L., Rush, M., Allan, S., Stott, D., Archer, M., 2008. A prospective study of patients with chronic back pain randomised to group exercise, physiotherapy or osteopathy. Physiotherapy 94, 21–28.

Critchley, D.J., Ratcliffe, J., Noonan, S., Jones, R.H., Hurley, M.V., 2007. Effectiveness and cost-effectiveness of three types of physiotherapy used to reduce chronic low back pain disability: a pragmatic randomized trial with economic evaluation. Spine 32, 1474–1481.

Deyo, R.A., Diehl, A.K., Rosenthal, M., 1986. How many days of bed rest for acute low back pain? A randomized clinical trial. N Engl J Med 315, 1064–1070.

Deyo, R.A., Walsh, N.E., Martin, D.C., Schoenfeld, L.S., Ramamurthy, S., 1990. A controlled trial of transcutaneous electrical nerve stimulation (TENS) and exercise for chronic low back pain. N Engl J Med 322, 1627–1634.

Deyo, R.A., Rainville, J., Kent, D.L., 1992. What can the history and physical examination tell us about low back pain? JAMA 268, 760–765.

Donzelli, S., Di Domenica, E., Cova, A.M., Galletti, R., Giunta, N., 2006. Two different techniques in the rehabilitation treatment of low back pain: a randomized controlled trial. Eura Medicophys 42, 205–210.

Elnaggar, I.M., Nordin, M., Sheikhzadeh, A., Parnianpour, M., Kahanovitz, N., 1991. Effects of spinal flexion and extension exercises on low-back pain and spinal mobility in chronic mechanical low-back pain patients. Spine 16, 967–972.

Ferreira, M.L., Ferreira, P.H., Latimer, J., Herbert, R.D., Hodges, P.W., Jennings, M.D., et al., 2007. Comparison of general exercise, motor control exercise and spinal manipulative therapy for chronic low back pain: A randomized trial. Pain 131, 31–37.

Fritz, J.M., Delitto, A., Erhard, R.E., 2003. Comparison of classification-based physical therapy with therapy based on clinical practice guidelines for patients with acute low back pain: a randomized clinical trial. Spine 28, 1363–1371.

Frost, H., Klaber Moffett, J.A., Moser, J.S., Fairbank, J.C., 1995. Randomised controlled trial for evaluation of fitness programme for patients with chronic low back pain. BMJ 310, 151–154.

Frost, H., Lamb, S.E., Klaber Moffett, J.A., Fairbank, J.C., Moser, J.S., 1998. A fitness programme for patients with chronic low back pain: 2-year follow-up of a randomised controlled trial. Pain 75, 273–279.

Frost, H., Lamb, S.E., Doll, H.A., Carver, P.T., Stewart-Brown, S., 2004. Randomised controlled trial of physiotherapy compared with advice for low back pain. BMJ 329, 708.

Galantino, M.L., Bzdewka, T.M., Eissler-Russo, J.L., Holbrook, M.L., Mogck, E.P., Geigle, P., et al., 2004. The impact of modified Hatha yoga on chronic low back pain: a pilot study. Altern Ther Health Med 10, 56–59.

Gladwell, V., Head, S., Haggar, M., Beneke, R., 2006. Does a program of pilates improve chronic non-specific low back pain? J Sport Rehabil 15, 338–350.

Glasziou, P., Chalmers, I., Rawlins, M., McCulloch, P., 2007. When are randomised trials unnecessary? Picking signal from noise. BMJ 334, 349–351.

Goldby, L.J., Moore, A.P., Doust, J., Trew, M.E., 2006. A randomized controlled trial investigating the efficiency of musculoskeletal physiotherapy on chronic low back disorder. Spine 31, 1083–1093.

Gudavalli, M.R., Cambron, J.A., McGregor, M., Jedlicka, J., Keenum, M., Ghanayem, A.J., et al., 2006. A randomized clinical trial and subgroup analysis to compare flexion–distraction with active exercise for chronic low back pain. Eur Spine J 15, 1070–1082.

Gur, A., Karakoc, M., Cevik, R., Nas, K., Sarac, A.J., Karakoc, M., 2003. Efficacy of low power laser therapy and exercise on pain and functions in chronic low back pain. Lasers Surg Med 32, 233–238.

Harts, C.C., Helmhout, P.H., de Bie, R.A., Staal, J.B., 2008. A high-intensity lumbar extensor strengthening program is little better than a low-intensity program or a waiting list control group for chronic low back pain: a randomised clinical trial. Aust J Physiother 54, 23–31.

Hayden, J.A., van Tulder, M.W., Malmivaara, A., Koes, B.W., 2005. Exercise therapy for treatment of non-specific low back pain. Cochrane Database Syst Rev CD000335.

Hides, J.A., Richardson, C.A., Jull, G.A., 1996. Multifidus muscle recovery is not automatic after resolution of acute, first-episode low back pain. Spine 21, 2763–2769.

Hildebrandt, V.H., Proper, K.I., van den Berg, R., Douwes, M., van den Heuvel, S.G., van Buuren, S., 2000. [Cesar therapy is temporarily more effective in patients with chronic low back pain than the standard treatment by family practitioner: randomized, controlled and blinded clinical trial with 1 year follow-up]. Ned Tijdschr Geneeskd 144, 2258–2264.

Hill, J.C., Dunn, K.M., Lewis, M., Mullis, R., Main, C.J., Foster, N.E., et al., 2008. A primary care back pain screening tool: identifying patient subgroups for initial treatment. Arthritis Rheum 59, 632–641.

Hodges, P.W., Richardson, C.A., 1998. Delayed postural contraction of transversus abdominis in low back pain associated with movement of the lower limb. J Spinal Disord 11, 46–56.

Hodges, P.W., Richardson, C.A., 1996. Inefficient muscular stabilisation of the lumbar spine associated with low back pain: a motor control evaluation of transversus abdominis. Spine 21, 2640–2650.

Johannsen, F., Remvig, L., Kryger, P., Beck, P., Warming, S., Lybeck, K., et al., 1995. Exercises for chronic low back pain: a clinical trial. J Orthop Sports Phys Ther 22, 52–59.

Kankaanpaa, M., Taimela, S., Airaksinen, O., Hanninen, O., 1999. The efficacy of active rehabilitation in chronic low back pain. Effect on pain intensity, self-experienced disability, and lumbar fatigability. Spine 24, 1034–1042.

Koes, B.W., van Tulder, M.W., Ostelo, R., Kim Burton, A., Waddell, G., 2001. Clinical guidelines for the management of low back pain in primary care: an international comparison. Spine 26, 2504–2513.

Koldas Doğan, S., Sonel Tur, B., Kurtais, Y., Atay, M.B., 2008. Comparison of three different approaches in the treatment of chronic low back pain. Clin Rheumatol 27, 873–881.

Lewis, J.S., Hewitt, J.S., Billington, L., Cole, S., Byng, J., Karayiannis, S., 2005. A randomized clinical trial comparing two physiotherapy interventions for chronic low back pain. Spine 30, 711–721.

Linton, S.J., Hallden, K., 1998. Can we screen for problematic back pain? A screening questionnaire for predicting outcome in acute and subacute back pain. Clin J Pain 14, 209–215.

Macedo, L.G., Maher, C.G., Latimer, J., McAuley, J.H., 2009. Motor control exercise for persistent, nonspecific low back pain: a systematic review. Phys Ther 89, 9–25.

Machado, L.A., Azevedo, D.C., Capanema, M.B., Neto, T.N., Cerceau, D.M., 2007. Client-centered therapy vs exercise therapy for chronic low back pain: a pilot randomized controlled trial in Brazil. Pain Med 8, 251–258.

McKenzie, R., May, S., 2003. Mechanical Diagnosis and Therapy. Spinal Publications, Waikanae, New Zealand.

Malmivaara, A., Häkkinen, U., Aro, T., Heinrichs, M.L., Koskenniemi, L., Kuosma, E., et al., 1995. The treatment of acute low back pain – bed rest, exercises, or ordinary activity? N Engl J Med 332, 351–355.

Mannion, A.F., Muntener, M., Taimela, S., Dvorak, J., 1999. A randomized clinical trial of three active therapies for chronic low back pain. Spine 24, 2435–2448.

Marshall, P., Murphy, B., 2008. Self-report measures best explain changes in disability compared with physical measures after exercise rehabilitation for chronic low back pain. Spine 33, 326–338.

Niemistö, L., Lahtinen-Suopanki, T., Rissanen, P., Lindgren, K.A., Sarna, S., Hurri, H., 2003. A randomized trial of combined manipulation, stabilizing exercises, and physician consultation compared to physician consultation alone for chronic low back pain. Spine 28, 2185–2191.

Niemistö, L., Rissanen, P., Sarna, S., Lahtinen-Suopanki, T., Lindgren, K.A., Hurri, H., 2005. Cost-effectiveness of combined manipulation, stabilizing exercises, and physician consultation compared to physician consultation alone for chronic low back pain: a prospective randomized trial with 2-year follow-up. Spine 30, 1109–1115.

Risch, S.V., Norvell, N.K., Pollock, M.L., Risch, E.D., Langer, H., Fulton, M., et al., 1993. Lumbar strengthening in chronic low back pain patients. Physiologic and psychological benefits. Spine 18, 232–238.

Rittweger, J., Just, K., Kautzsch, K., Reeg, P., Felsenberg, D., 2002. Treatment of chronic lower back pain with lumbar extension and whole-body vibration exercise: a randomized controlled trial. Spine 27, 1829–1834.

Roche, G., Ponthieux, A., Parot-Shinkel, E., Jousset, N., Bontoux, L., Dubus, V., et al., 2007. Comparison of a functional restoration program with active individual physical therapy for patients with chronic low back pain: a randomized controlled trial. Arch Phys Med Rehabil 88, 1229–1235.

Sherman, K.J., Cherkin, D.C., Erro, J., Miglioretti, D.L., Deyo, R.A., 2005. Comparing yoga, exercise, and a self-care book for chronic low back pain: a randomized, controlled trial. Ann Intern Med 143, 849–856.

Sjögren, T., Nissinen, K.J., Jarvenpaa, S.K., Ojanen, M.T., Vanharanta, H., Malkia, E.A., 2005. Effects of a workplace physical exercise intervention on the intensity of headache and neck and shoulder symptoms and upper extremity muscular strength of office workers: a cluster randomized controlled cross-over trial. Pain 116, 119–128.

Smeets, R.J., Vlaeyen, J.W., Hidding, A., Kester, A.D., van der Heijden, G.J., Knottnerus, J.A., 2008. Chronic low back pain: physical training, graded activity with problem solving training, or both? The one-year post-treatment results of a randomized controlled trial. Pain 134, 263–276.

Smeets, R.J., Vlaeyen, J.W., Hidding, A., Kester, A.D., van der Heijden, G.J., van Geel, A.C., et al., 2006. Active rehabilitation for chronic low back pain: cognitive-behavioral, physical, or both? First direct post-treatment results from a randomized controlled trial [ISRCTN22714229]. BMC Musculoskelet Disord 7, 5.

Tekur, P., Singphow, C., Nagendra, H.R., Raghuram, N., 2008. Effect of short-term intensive yoga program on pain, functional disability, and spinal flexibility in chronic low back pain: a randomized control study. J Alt Complement Med 14, 637–644.

Tritilanunt, T., Wajanavisit, W., 2001. The efficacy of an aerobic exercise and health education program for treatment of chronic low back pain. J Med Assoc Thai 84, S528–S533.

Turner, J.A., Clancy, S., McQuade, K.J., Cardenas, D.D., 1990. Effectiveness of behavioral therapy for chronic low back pain: a component analysis. J Consult Clin Psychol 58, 573–579.

van Tulder, M.W., Assendelft, W.J., Koes, B.W., Bouter, L.M., et al., 1997. Spinal radiographic findings and nonspecific low back pain. A systematic review of observational studies. Spine 22, 427–434.

Williams, K.A., Petronis, J., Smith, D., Goodrich, D., Wu, J., Ravi, N., et al., 2005. Effect of Iyengar yoga therapy for chronic low back pain. Pain 115, 107–117.

Yelland, M.J., Glasziou, P.P., Bogduk, N., Schluter, P.J., McKernon, M., 2004. Prolotherapy injections, saline injections, and exercises for chronic low-back pain: a randomized trial. Spine 29, 9–16; discussion 16.

Yozbatiran, N., Yildirim, Y., Parlak, B., 2004. Effects of fitness and aquafitness exercises on physical fitness in patients with chronic low back pain. The Pain Clinic 16, 35–42.

Part | 5 |

State-of-the-art reviews

Chapter 16

How can models of motor control be useful for understanding low back pain?

N. Peter Reeves*, Jacek Cholewicki*, Mark Pearcy[†] and Mohamad Parnianpour[‡]
*Department of Osteopathic Surgical Specialties, College of Osteopathic Medicine, Michigan State University, East Lansing, Michigan, USA,
[†]Institute of Health and Biomedical Innovation, Queensland University of Technology, Brisbane, Queensland, Australia, and [‡]Department of Information and Industrial Engineering, Hanyang University, Ansan, Republic of Korea, and Department of Mechanical Engineering, Sharif University of Technology, Tehran, Iran

INTRODUCTION

There are several classes of models that have been used in the past for studying spinal loading, stability and risk of injury (see Reeves and Cholewicki (2003) for a review of past modelling approaches), but for the purpose of this chapter we will focus primarily on models used to assess motor control and its effect on spine behaviour.

This chapter comprises four sections. The first discusses why a shift in modelling approaches is needed to study motor control issues. We will argue that the current approach for studying the spine system is limited and not well suited for assessing motor control issues related to spine function and dysfunction. The second section will explore how models can be used to gain insight into how the central nervous system (CNS) controls the spine, linking with the next section, which will address how models of motor control can be used in the diagnosis and treatment of low back pain (LBP). The final section will deal with the issue of model verification and validity. This

issue is important since modelling accuracy is critical for obtaining useful insight into the behaviour of the system being studied.

A SHIFT IN MODELLING APPROACHES

First, it is important to note that all systems must be stable to perform their function. For the spine system, stable behaviour allows it to bear loads and permits controlled movement, while avoiding injury and pain. What does it mean, however, when we say that something is stable? There is a great deal of confusion about the term stability. Richard Bellman, an expert on stability, once wrote that 'stability is a heavily loaded term with an unstable definition' (Bellman 1953). This is particularly true when stability is applied to the spine (Reeves et al. 2007a, 2007b). In the past, researchers have argued that stability is a mechanical entity and should be treated as such (Pope and Panjabi 1985). Although stability applies to mechanical systems, it is not limited to just this class of systems. For example, we can study stability of electrical, biological, or social systems. Stability also applies to a system that is inherently unstable, but has control elements that give it stable behaviour. The human spine fits into this category: the osteoligamentous spine is mechanically unstable but the neuromuscular system stabilizes the spine under amazingly large mechanical compression loads.

The choice of definition for stability can have significant implications for how the system is studied. For instance, currently, the prevalent biomechanical definition of spine stability is based on the elastostatic approach first derived by Bergmark (1989). This mechanically based definition can be broken down into two components: 'elasto' referring to the elastic properties of the system, such as trunk muscle stiffness, and 'static' referring to the fact that the spine system is frozen in time, meaning it is not moving. Hypothetical perturbations are applied to the spine in this static configuration to determine if it is stable. The system is stable if the potential energy in the system increases when displaced, which indicates that the non-perturbed position is at an energy minimum – a necessary requirement for stability. Using this approach, it became apparent that muscles and the stiffness they provide are essential for maintaining spine stability (Bergmark 1989; Gardner-Morse et al. 1995; Cholewicki and McGill 1996; Cholewicki et al. 1997; Granata and Marras 2000). Not surprisingly, muscle stiffness became linked with stability.

There are a few limitations with the elastostatic approach, particularly if we are interested in applying them to study control (Reeves and Cholewicki 2009). In Chapter 2 a stick balancing example was used to describe how the CNS achieves stability for an inherently unstable system. Mechanically speaking, an upright stick in the palm of the hand is unstable. The stick when perfectly vertical is not at an energy minimum, but in fact at an energy maximum and will seek a lower energy configuration. If we apply the elastostatic approach to the stick balancing example, it would predict that the system is unstable. But we know if we apply forces to the base of the stick using the hand in the correct fashion, the stick can be stabilized. In instances when control is important, the elastostatic approach is not adequate as shown with our stick balancing system, and may lead to incorrect predictions of whether the system is stable or unstable. Therefore, for investigating issues related to motor control, this approach does not provide much insight. Moreover, this approach, which represents a static characterization of stability, places too much emphasis on stiffness, which represents displacement-related feedback, and ignores the damping property of the system, which represents velocity-related feedback. For dynamic systems such as the spine, both displacement and velocity-related feedback control are required (Reeves and Cholewicki 2009).

Have the static models of stability (e.g. Bergmark 1989; Cholewicki and McGill 1996; Granata and Marras 2000) outlived their usefulness? The work performed using elastostatic analyses of stability contributed a tremendous amount of knowledge and sprung new hypotheses. With some assumptions such analyses could be applied to the quasi-static tasks, such as lifting, that rely on a static and rigid trunk to transmit forces from the hands to the lower limbs and the floor. We have learned from these studies about the interplay between inter- and multi-segmental

muscles (muscles spanning one motion segment and muscles spanning multiple motion segments, respectively) and their contribution to the overall stability of the spine (Bergmark 1989; Crisco and Panjabi 1991). When the proper ratio between inter- and multi-segmental muscle recruitment is maintained, the general finding arose that more trunk muscle co-activation leads to a more robust spine (less likely to buckle) while under load. While true, such findings disregard the fact that the CNS has the ability to sense position and motion of the spine and change the activation level of the trunk muscles accordingly – feedback control. It is possible that in quasi-static tasks, muscle co-activation is the dominant mechanism assuring spine stability. However, the majority of common tasks, such as walking, running, skiing, riding a horse, or balancing on one leg, involve motion in the spine. In fact, the performance in these tasks would degrade and the task would break down if the spine was maintained stiff and rigid (Reeves et al. 2006). Instead, it has been shown that muscle activation is controlled through a combination of muscle co-activation and reflex responses (Moorhouse and Granata 2007), allowing the spine to maintain some level of suppleness. Reliance in part on reflex responses (CNS feedback control) has the advantage that it is a more efficient mechanism for stabilizing the spine than the metabolically costly muscle co-activation strategy. With reflex responses, timing of activation becomes an issue. At this point, static analysis of a system's stability is no longer applicable as it cannot account for timing of muscle activation.

So what type of modelling approach is better suited for studying motor control of the spine and its effect on back pain? Given that *control* is the issue, we would argue that an approach that is based on control theory would be useful. Control theory has been developed in a branch of science known as Systems Science. At the formal end of the systems approach is mathematical theory, which has been used to elucidate laws of control. These control laws have been applied to determine what control input is necessary, first to make the system stable and then to make it respond in some desirable way. These control laws are applicable to any system, and therefore, could be applied to the study of the spine to gain insight into spine function and dysfunction.

An additional benefit of the systems approach is the fact it can integrate knowledge. Systems Science is an interdisciplinary field of study. Therefore, researchers studying different parts of the spine system can integrate their knowledge into a comprehensive model of the system. We believe that the research community needs to shift away from the traditional reductionist approach, which does not appear well suited for studying LBP (Reeves and Cholewicki 2009). We argue that the application of a systems approach is better suited for studying back pain, given its multi-factorial nature and heterogeneity.

HOW CAN MODELS BE USED TO EXPLORE THEORIES OF MOTOR CONTROL?

It is a well-known theory that feedback control is used to provide stability. Briefly, information about the 'state' of the system (displacement and velocity of mass(es)) is used to apply control input to the system (Fig. 16.1). The conversion of spine displacement and velocity information to force, which acts on the spine, determines the overall behaviour of the system. For instance, a higher gain on displacement feedback control generates more force acting on the spine for a given displacement. Since the CNS can adjust feedback gains (control logic), there is considerable flexibility in how the CNS can stabilize the spine. (For more insight into feedback control and spine stability, see Reeves et al. 2007a, 2007b.)

Once stability is achieved, the interest shifts to other control issues, such as performance, robustness and efficiency. A system that performs well can stay close to the undisturbed position or movement trajectory after a perturbation. A system that is robust can maintain stable behaviour for both small and large perturbations. A robust system can also handle large changes in the system without affecting its performance significantly. For instance, a robust control system for the spine can handle changes to the spinal column (i.e. mechanical changes due to degenerative disc disease) without having the system's performance significantly affected by the change. When dealing with biological systems with limited power and energy, the issue of efficiency is also important. Ideally, we would like to control the spine in an efficient manner to avoid fatigue.

As mentioned, there are a number of strategies or muscle recruitment patterns that will ensure that the spine is stable. Strategies that keep the spine stable represent a set of 'stable solutions'. Within this stable set, some solutions are better for performance, robustness and efficiency. Most likely, the CNS chooses a particular solution out of the many to optimize the system. Optimization of the system will be based on some 'objective function'. For instance, the objective of the system may be to minimize energy demands required to maintain spine stability. In this instance, the CNS would reduce trunk muscle activation to the lowest possible levels, close to the point of instability. But it is likely that the CNS wants a margin of safety, so it may also have the objective to make the system robust. The point is, many concurrent and even competing objectives (maximize performance, robustness and/or efficiency) may be used to choose a particular control strategy. One of the more interesting areas of research is the application of optimal control theory. This theory can predict the optimal recruitment patterns that would satisfy some desired objective function of the system. Alternatively, it may be possible to determine what the CNS is optimizing based on the trunk muscle recruitment patterns (Xu et al. 2010). This type of analysis is extremely complex and the types of physical activities that we can model this way are limited at present, but the theoretical advances in computational methodology are forthcoming, which should facilitate modelling.

There is another type of modelling approach which treats the spine system as a 'black box' instead of the implicit representation of the system. Ideally, we would like to model the spine in a way that captures completely its complexity. However, this is not always possible: it is difficult to predict with accuracy the motion of all vertebrae in all planes of motion, although new methods now coming online will help (Anderst et al. 2008; Li et al. 2008; Wang et al. 2008); it is difficult to predict muscle activation of the deep trunk muscles; and it is very time-consuming to customize anatomy representation to an individual, which would ensure bio-fidelity. Instead of developing extremely detailed spine models, others have treated the system as a black box in which insight into a system can be achieved by looking at the response of the system during the execution of a task (Tanaka et al. 2009). For instance, this type of analysis can be used to determine how many state variables are needed to represent the system. Therefore, it is possible to adjust the complexity of the model based on dimensionality analysis. These models have also been used to predict the limits of stability for a given task. For example, using this type of analysis, it may be possible to locate the state space boundaries (limits on trunk displacement and velocity) for torso stability. Potentially, this type of approach can be used to assess the effects of factors affecting motor control on the region of stability. For instance, does fatigue decrease the region of stability, suggesting that stable behaviour is limited to smaller or slower trunk movements?

Learning and adaptation are other areas of motor control that continue to draw attention. For instance, how do we learn the dynamics of a task, or for that matter, the dynamics of the spine? There is growing evidence that

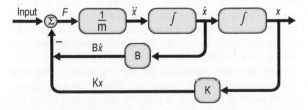

Figure 16.1 A feedback control system. Force (F) acts on a mass (m) and determines the acceleration ($\ddot{x}$), velocity ($\dot{x}$), and displacement (x) of the system. Gains B and K convert the velocity and displacement information to force and feed it back to affect the behaviour of the system.

people form internal models that characterize system dynamics (Conditt et al. 1997; Burdet et al. 2001). Therefore, execution of a task does not require rote learning of specific movements. Instead, with experience and the formation of internal models, the CNS can predict the necessary motor commands to accomplish the task. For example, when walking on a ship's deck in rough seas, it is possible for the CNS to send a feed-forward command to control the postural muscles to accommodate the rolling motion once the task is learned. By using feed-forward responses, the performance of the system is improved (less postural sway) while minimizing energy expenditure. Therefore, in situations in which disturbances can be predicted, the CNS can utilize internal models and feed-forward control instead of relying exclusively on feedback control.

Recently, a model of motor control learning was developed that explains how the CNS learns task dynamics and uses this information to adjust muscle recruitment patterns (Franklin et al. 2008). What makes this model unique is that it can account for learning in stable and unstable environments. For tasks that are stable, the model predicts that CNS will use reciprocal muscle activation to compensate for predictable disturbances. For instance, if the rolling seas are consistently periodic, then the CNS will tune postural control muscles to activate muscles that counteract the predictable disturbance. However, if the rolling seas are more variable and less predictable, then the CNS would tend to co-activate agonist and antagonist muscles to increase the trunk's mechanical impedance to counteract disturbances that can come from any direction. Therefore, depending on the task and the nature of disturbances, the CNS can shift from co-activation to reciprocal activation or vise versa. Therefore, the model predicts why co-activation is initially high when learning new tasks and then decreases with learning. It also explains why co-activation increases with fatigue, which increases noise in the neuromuscular system. Although the model of motor control learning was developed with upper extremity experiments, it represents a general scheme of motor control, which is applicable to the spine system as well.

WHAT IS THE USEFULNESS OF MODELS FOR DIAGNOSIS AND TREATMENT?

The clinical application of motor control models to the problem of LBP might not be far away. A general framework for the diagnosis and treatment has recently been presented (Xu et al. 2010). However, further research into a number of areas is required to test the validity and practicality of the approach.

In terms of diagnosis, it is important to know if people with LBP have a different objective function than healthy individuals. It appears that people with LBP have higher levels of co-activation (Lariviere et al. 2000; Marras et al. 2001; van Dieën et al. 2003). It is possible that people with LBP are weighting performance or robustness over efficiency. For example, people with LBP may want to minimize spine kinematic disturbances and are not concerned with the additional energy expenditure. Alternatively, it is possible that people with LBP have motor control impairments that increase the noise in the system, which would increase the level of co-activation to compensate for this random disturbance. The next important question to ask, if differences in objective functions exist, is whether rehabilitation should restore motor control to that of healthy individuals. It is possible that minimizing spine kinematic disturbances is important for protecting an injured spine. But it is also possible that this strategy has nothing to do with protecting the spine, but instead represents a dysfunctional coping strategy. In a recent study, the presentation of a painful stimulus resulted in altered muscle recruitment patterns, which persisted following the removal of the painful stimulus (Hodges et al. 2003; Moseley et al. 2004). Perhaps, following a painful episode, motor control strategies are confined to a non-optimal solution and need to be reset. In terms of rehabilitation, is it possible to reset motor control strategies? This is another important question that needs to be addressed. Others have shown that it is possible to modify motor control in the upper extremity using force fields generated a by robotic manipulandum (Burdet et al. 2001; Franklin et al. 2003, 2008). Perhaps, a similar approach can be used for back pain rehabilitation.

In addition to specific diagnosis and rehabilitation, models of motor control can be used to test current treatment paradigms. For example, there is a lot of interest in the importance of multifidus, which has been shown to atrophy in some individuals with LBP (Hides et al. 1994, 1996). Many back pain programmes stress retraining this so-called important spine stabilizer. But is it an important spine stabilizer, or more specifically, what happens to the spine behaviour when this muscle is affected by back pain? A multi-segmental, multi-muscle spine model can be developed to analyze the behaviour of the spine with and without multifidus atrophy. We may find that energy demands on the spine system increase as a result of shifting of muscle loading, which would support rehabilitation of this muscle. This same type of model could also be used to explore spine behaviour for muscle synergy patterns, which may be different between healthy and back pain groups. Recently, a method for finding muscle synergies has been developed using a triaxial dynamometer (Talebian et al. 2010). It is possible that people with LBP have fewer options (degrees of freedom) to control the spine than healthy individuals. If this is the case, it is also possible that less efficient control strategies are within the stable set of solutions for the back pain group. If this is the case, is it possible to decouple muscle activation in the back pain group?

Another important contribution that can be made with models of motor control is determining whether something that is statistically significant is clinically relevant. For instance, there are a number of studies that have shown that people with LBP have longer reflex responses than healthy individuals (Magnusson et al. 1996; Radebold et al. 2000, 2001; Reeves et al. 2005). Other studies have found that some people with LBP have impaired spine proprioception (Newcomer et al. 2000; Leinonen et al. 2002). But it is unclear if these documented differences affect the behaviour of the spine system significantly. By modelling the system, it is possible to run simulations with various impairments to determine how robust the system is to different types of impairment. Simulations can be run with a single impairment or combinations of impairments. With most chronic conditions, a widening array of biological processes or parts of the system are affected. Therefore, to properly study chronic LBP, it will be important to apply a systems approach (instead of a reductionist approach), which is possible with parametric models of motor control.

MODEL VERIFICATION AND VALIDITY

Mathematical models are written to simulate natural processes in order to predict behaviour that will give insight into how the processes occur and, clinically, to provide an aid to diagnosis and treatment. This reduces the requirement for expensive experiments and can take the place of experiments that would be difficult to justify ethically or would be too difficult actually to undertake. However, models are only as good as the underlying assumptions used to develop them, and the algorithms and data that are put into them. In order to give credence to the results of simulations undertaken with models, a process of model verification and validation must be undertaken.

Verification is the process of assessing that the algorithms and mathematical techniques used in the model are in themselves correct. This sounds relatively easy but in complex models requires particular attention to ensure errors are not inadvertently included. For example, in simulations, inappropriate choice of time steps can lead to accumulating numerical errors.

Validation can be achieved on one level by using the model to simulate a phenomenon that can also be solved analytically. The next level is to ensure that the model simulates the correct outcome for the concepts and boundary conditions used to set up the model in the first place.

The model can then be tested against more complex scenarios. If the model is then used to predict behaviour beyond the original boundary conditions it is necessary to clearly establish its sensitivity to changes in its parameters. This may set limits on which parameters in the model can be used to evaluate various scenarios whilst holding those that are very sensitive to within defined limits.

One method that may be applicable is the use of Monte Carlo simulations that allow large samples from the distribution of inputs (while considering their uncertainty) to be run by the model to result in outcome variables that would also be represented by a distribution (Hughes and An 1997; Rohlmann et al. 2009). Close analyses of the results often show which parameters are more important and require more precision to increase the resolution or sensitivity of the model. Computational power is increasing and will allow us to use these powerful stochastic approaches to model not only what we know but also the uncertainty with which we can presently estimate inputs.

By following these processes of verification and validation, the modeller is able to demonstrate clearly the efficacy and value of a model for simulating particular scenarios. This step of defining clearly what a model can and cannot do provides the user of the outcomes with evidence for confidence in the predictions of the simulations achieved by the model. These issues of verification, validation and sensitivity analysis are discussed comprehensively in the review literature and the reader is directed to the following articles: Viceconti et al. (2005), which discusses the requirements for publication of peer reviewed articles on models; Anderson et al. (2007), which discusses expectations for computational biomechanics; and Jones and Wilcox (2008) for expectations of models to analyze the spine.

For now we may still have to make certain clinical and professional judgements when asked about estimations of various biomechanical parameters predicted by present models during varying tasks (Sparto and Parnianpour 2001). Cross-validation may be one way to gain more confidence to navigate the uncertainty until we find accessible and less invasive gold standards to validate our models (McNally et al. 1996; Rohlmann et al. 2008; Arjmand et al. 2010).

ACKNOWLEDGEMENT

The authors wish to thank Associate Professor Clayton Adam from QUT for his advice in preparing the section on model validation.

REFERENCES

Anderson, A.E., Ellis, B.J., Weiss, J.A., 2007. Verification, validation and sensitivity studies in computational biomechanics. Comput Methods Biomech Biomed Eng 10, 171–184.

Anderst, W.J., Vaidya, R., Tashman, S., 2008. A technique to measure three-dimensional in vivo rotation of fused and adjacent lumbar vertebrae. Spine J 8, 991–997.

Arjmand, N., Gagnon, D., Plamondon, A., Shirazi-Adl, A., Lariviere, C., 2010. A comparative study of two trunk biomechanical models under symmetric and asymmetric loadings. J Biomech 43, 485–491.

Bellman, R.E., 1953. Stability Theory of Differential Equations. McGraw–Hill Book Co., New York.

Bergmark, A., 1989. Stability of the lumbar spine: a study in mechanical engineering. Acta Orthop Scand Suppl 230, 1–54.

Burdet, E., Osu, R., Franklin, D.W., Milner, T.E., Kawato, M., 2001. The central nervous system stabilizes unstable dynamics by learning optimal impedance. Nature 414, 446–449.

Cholewicki, J., McGill, S.M., 1996. Mechanical stability of the in vivo lumbar spine: implications for injury and chronic low back pain. Clin Biomech 11, 1–15.

Cholewicki, J., Panjabi, M.M., Khachatryan, A., 1997. Stabilizing function of trunk flexor–extensor muscles around a neutral spine posture. Spine 22, 2207–2212.

Conditt, M.A., Gandolfo, F., Mussa-Ivaldi, F.A., 1997. The motor system does not learn the dynamics of the arm by rote memorization of past experience. J Neurophysiol 78, 554–560.

Crisco 3rd, J.J., Panjabi, M.M., 1991. The intersegmental and multisegmental muscles of the lumbar spine. A biomechanical model comparing lateral stabilizing potential. Spine 16, 793–799.

Franklin, D.W., Burdet, E., Tee, K.P., Osu, R., Chew, C.M., Milner, T.E., et al., 2008. CNS learns stable, accurate, and efficient movements using a simple algorithm. J Neurosci 28, 11165–11173.

Franklin, D.W., Osu, R., Burdet, E., Kawato, M., Milner, T.E., 2003. Adaptation to stable and unstable dynamics achieved by combined impedance control and inverse dynamics model. J Neurophysiol 90, 3270–3282.

Gardner-Morse, M., Stokes, I.A., Laible, J.P., 1995. Role of muscles in lumbar spine stability in maximum extension efforts. J Orthop Res 13, 802–808.

Granata, K.P., Marras, W.S., 2000. Cost–benefit of muscle cocontraction in protecting against spinal instability. Spine 25, 1398–1404.

Hides, J.A., Richardson, C.A., Jull, G.A., 1996. Multifidus muscle recovery is not automatic after resolution of acute, first-episode low back pain. Spine 21, 2763–2769.

Hides, J.A., Stokes, M.J., Saide, M., Jull, G.A., Cooper, D.H., 1994. Evidence of lumbar multifidus muscle wasting ipsilateral to symptoms in patients with acute/subacute low back pain. Spine 19, 165–172.

Hodges, P.W., Moseley, G.L., Gabrielsson, A., Gandevia, S.C., 2003. Experimental muscle pain changes feedforward postural responses of the trunk muscles. Exp Brain Res 151, 262–271.

Hughes, R.E., An, K.N., 1997. Monte Carlo simulation of a planar shoulder model . Med Biol Eng Comput 35, 544–548.

Jones, A.C., Wilcox, R.K., 2008. Finite element analysis of the spine: towards a framework of verification, validation and sensitivity analysis. Med Eng Phys 30, 1287–1304.

Lariviere, C., Gagnon, D., Loisel, P., 2000. The comparison of trunk muscles EMG activation between subjects with and without chronic low back pain during flexion-extension and lateral bending tasks. J Electromyogr Kinesiol 10, 79–91.

Leinonen, V., Maatta, S., Taimela, S., Herno, A., Kankaanpaa, M., Partanen, J., et al., 2002. Impaired lumbar movement perception in association with postural stability and motor- and somatosensory-evoked potentials in lumbar spinal stenosis. Spine 27, 975–983.

Li, G., Van de Velde, S.K., Bingham, J.T., 2008. Validation of a non-invasive fluoroscopic imaging technique for the measurement of dynamic knee joint motion. J Biomech 41, 1616–1622.

Magnusson, M.L., Aleksiev, A., Wilder, D.G., Pope, M.H., Spratt, K., Lee, S.H., et al., 1996. European Spine Society – the AcroMed Prize for Spinal Research 1995. Unexpected load and asymmetric posture as etiologic factors in low back pain. Eur Spine J 5, 23–35.

Marras, W.S., Davis, K.G., Maronitis, A.B., 2001. A non-MVC EMG normalization technique for the trunk musculature: Part 2. Validation and use to predict spinal loads. J Electromyogr Kinesiol 11, 11–18.

McNally, D.S., Shackleford, I.M., Goodship, A.E., Mulholland, R.C., 1996. In vivo stress measurement can predict pain on discography. Spine 21, 2580–2587.

Moorhouse, K.M., Granata, K.P., 2007. Role of reflex dynamics in spinal stability: intrinsic muscle stiffness alone is insufficient for stability. J Biomech 40, 1058–1065.

Moseley, G.L., Nicholas, M.K., Hodges, P.W., 2004. Does anticipation of back pain predispose to back trouble? Brain 127, 2339–2347.

Newcomer, K.L., Laskowski, E.R., Yu, B., Johnson, J.C., An, K.N., 2000. Differences in repositioning error among patients with low back pain compared with control subjects. Spine 25, 2488–2493.

Pope, M.H., Panjabi, M., 1985. Biomechanical definitions of spinal instability. Spine 10, 255–256.

Radebold, A., Cholewicki, J., Panjabi, M.M., Patel, T.C., 2000. Muscle response pattern to sudden trunk loading in healthy individuals and in patients with chronic low back pain. Spine 25, 947–954.

Radebold, A., Cholewicki, J., Polzhofer, G.K., Greene, H.S., 2001. Impaired postural control of the lumbar spine is associated with delayed muscle response times in patients with chronic idiopathic low back pain. Spine 26, 724–730.

Reeves, N.P., Cholewicki, J., 2003. Modeling the human lumbar spine for assessing spinal loads, stability, and risk of injury. Crit Rev Biomed Eng 31, 73–139.

Reeves, N.P., Cholewicki, J., 2009. Expanding our view of the spine system. Eur Spine J 19, 331–332.

Reeves, N.P., Cholewicki, J., Milner, T.E., 2005. Muscle reflex classification of low-back pain. J Electromyogr Kinesiol 15, 53–60.

Reeves, N.P., Cholewicki, J., Narendra, K.S., 2007a. Re: Spine stability: the six blind men and the elephant. Clin Biomech 22, 487–488.

Reeves, N.P., Everding, V.Q., Cholewicki, J., Morrisette, D.C., 2006. The effects of trunk stiffness on postural control during unstable seated balance. Exp Brain Res 174, 694–700.

Reeves, N.P., Narendra, K.S., Cholewicki, J., 2007b. Spine stability: The six blind men and the elephant. Clin Biomech 22, 266–274.

Rohlmann, A., Graichen, F., Kayser, R., Bender, A., Bergmann, G., 2008. Loads on a telemeterized vertebral body replacement measured in two patients. Spine 33, 1170–1179.

Rohlmann, A., Mann, A., Zander, T., Bergmann, G., 2009. Effect of an artificial disc on lumbar spine biomechanics: a probabilistic finite element study. Eur Spine J 18, 89–97.

Sparto, P.J., Parnianpour, M., 2001. Generalizability of trunk muscle EMG and spinal forces. IEEE Eng Med Biol Mag 20, 72–81.

Talebian, S., Mousavi, S.J., Olyaei, G.R., Sanjari, M.A., Parnianpour, M., 2010. The effect of exertion level on activation patterns and variability of trunk muscles during multidirectional isometric activities in upright posture. Spine 35, E443–E451.

Tanaka, M.L., Nussbaum, M.A., Ross, S.D., 2009. Evaluation of the threshold of stability for the human spine. J Biomech 42, 1017–1022.

van Dieën, J.H., Cholewicki, J., Radebold, A., 2003. Trunk muscle recruitment patterns in patients with low back pain enhance the stability of the lumbar spine. Spine 28, 834–841.

Viceconti, M., Olsen, S., Nolte, L.P., Burton, K., 2005. Extracting clinically relevant data from finite element simulations. Clin Biomech 20, 451–454.

Wang, S., Passias, P., Li, G., Li, G., Wood, K., 2008. Measurement of vertebral kinematics using noninvasive image matching method-validation and application. Spine 33, E355–E361.

Xu, Y., Choi, J., Reeves, N.P., Cholewicki, J., 2010. Optimal control of the spine system. J Biomech Eng 132, 051004.

Chapter |17|

Targeting interventions to patients: development and evaluation

Linda R. Van Dillen* and Maurits van Tulder†
*Program in Physical Therapy and Department of Orthopaedic Surgery, Washington University School of Medicine at Washington University Medical Center, St Louis, Missouri, USA, and †Department of Epidemiology and Biostatistics, Department of Health Sciences and EMGO Institute for Health and Care Research, VU University Medical Centre, Amsterdam, The Netherlands

CHAPTER CONTENTS

STATUS OF RESEARCH REGARDING MANAGEMENT OF LOW BACK PAIN

Mechanical low back pain is usually classified into specific low back pain, non-specific low back pain and radicular syndrome. In 85–95% of the patients a specific diagnosis based on pathoanatomical causes is lacking, and these are diagnosed as having 'non specific' low back pain (Waddell 2005). The lack of a clear pathoanatomical basis to low back pain has led to a large variation in diagnoses, and an array of poorly studied interventions (Poitras et al. 2005). There was a promise that randomized controlled trials could provide answers on questions such as 'which intervention is most effective for which patient', but after the publication of more than 1,000 randomized controlled trials on low back pain there is still a lack of evidence regarding the most effective strategies for matching individual patients to particular interventions. The Cochrane Back Review Group acknowledged the limited role of randomized controlled trials in providing useful information on aspects of low back pain management other than efficacy and effectiveness, and stated that additional etiological, diagnostic and prognostic studies are needed to identify varieties, natural courses, or more homogeneous subgroups of patients with low back pain (Bouter et al. 2003). The identification of homogenous subgroups based on evidence-based classification algorithms was determined to be a priority for primary care research on low back pain as early as 1996 (Borkan and Cherkin 1996).

POTENTIAL NEED TO SUBGROUP PEOPLE WITH LOW BACK PAIN

Subgrouping of patients and targeting interventions to the patients' needs seems important in providing optimal care to low back pain patients. Recent research findings suggest the existence of low back pain subgroups (e.g. Fritz et al. 2007, Dankaerts et al. 2009; Silfies et al. 2009), but there is a lack of consensus as to how these subgroups should be identified and a continuous debate whether the identification of low back pain subgroups is necessary to improve treatment efficiency and reduce costs (Abraham and Killackey-Jones 2002; Wand and O'Connell 2008; Billis et al. 2007). Patients with chronic low back pain may be classified into two types: (1) 'persistent low back pain patients' who do not demonstrate significant psychological distress and (2) patients with a 'chronic low back pain syndrome' characterized by significant functional impairment and behavioural and psychological co-morbidities (Long et al. 2004). Several others have supported this classification description, but terms differ for the second group from 'failed back syndrome' (Turk 2002), 'medically incongruent pain group' (Reesor and Craig 1988) to 'problem backs' (Waddell et al. 1980). It has been advocated that these 'chronic low back pain syndrome' patients should be assessed and treated using a multi-factorial treatment approach, which addresses the complex psychosocial issues and focuses on restoring physical capacity (Gatchel 2001). Screening tools are needed to identify these patients.

SYSTEMS FOR SUBGROUPING

Over the years, many attempts have been made to classify patients with low back pain into more homogeneous subgroups with the goal of assisting in treatment direction. In 2007, Billis et al. identified 39 diagnostic and treatment-based classification systems. Most of the classification systems were based on biomedical features (pathoanatomic and/or clinical signs and symptoms) whereas fewer classification systems used psychosocial or biopsychosocial features. The majority of the classification systems were based on a judgemental approach, relying on clinical experience and intuition. A minority were derived using prospective study designs.

Four of the systems identified by Billis et al. have had a significant amount of research conducted examining the characteristics of the proposed system. The four systems vary in the degree of biomedical and psychosocial features used to identify the low back pain subgroups. All four systems, however, have the common purpose to assist in directing conservative treatment. The systems include the McKenzie Method classification system (McKenzie), the Treatment-based classification system (TBC), the Movement System Impairment classification system (MSI) and the O'Sullivan classification system (OS). We will review details of each, describe the general procedures for subgrouping and review the research related to reliability and validity of the system. Specifically, we will focus on research examining whether (1) clinicians can classify patients with low back pain reliably, (2) there are unique subgroups of people with low back pain and (3) matching treatment to a patient's classification results in better outcomes than an alternative treatment.

McKenzie Method classification system

The McKenzie system was originally described by McKenzie in 1981 and updated by McKenzie and May in 2003. The major low back pain subgroups proposed are postural, dysfunction and derangement. There is also an 'other' classification for patients who do not fit the criteria for classification. The derangement subgroup is further divided into four groups that differ based on location of symptoms. These include (1) central symmetrical without distal symptoms, (2) central symmetrical with distal symptoms, (3) unilateral asymmetrical symptoms to the knee and (4) unilateral asymmetrical symptoms below the knee. The major subgroups are those that are proposed to exist within the non-specific low back pain classification and who respond in a specific way when subjected to different mechanical forces. Mechanically based treatment is then prescribed based on the patient's responses. Mechanical treatment in the McKenzie system refers to treatment with repeated movements and sustained postures, as well as education to use patient-specific postures in functional activities. The names of the McKenzie subgroups describe the proposed tissue dysfunction that contributes to the person's clinical presentation. For example, internal displacement of the intervertebral disc is proposed to underlie the symptoms and signs of the derangement subgroup. The system is intended for use with patients who report symptoms in the back with or without radiating symptoms and with any stage of acuity (acute, subacute, chronic).

The McKenzie Method of classification uses findings from the clinical examination (history and physical). The findings that characterize each subgroup are based on a judgement by a clinical expert in mechanical therapy (McKenzie). The most important findings for subgrouping are the symptom responses with standardized tests of movements and positions in the examination. Tests include single and repeated trunk movements and sustained trunk postures. Assessments of trunk alignment and movement are also made. Tests are performed in loaded (gravity-affected) and unloaded (gravity-minimized) positions. In general, treatment includes repeated spine movements and postures or sustained postures that produce a consistent improvement in symptoms or mechanical function, as well as education.

Five studies have specifically examined the reliability of examiners classifying patients with low back pain using the McKenzie system. Patient samples included all stages of acuity. The earliest study by Kilby et al. (1990) involved two McKenzie-trained physical therapists who classified 41 patients with low back pain using a simultaneous examination design. Relatively low agreement was obtained for the overall classification into subgroups and classification into the derangement subgroups, i.e. 58.5% and 57%, respectively. In a much larger study Riddle et al. (1993) tested the reliability of 49 physical therapists to classify 363 patients. The therapists had an average of five years of clinical experience; 16 had postgraduate training in the McKenzie system. Therapists were given a written summary of the McKenzie Method of examination and classification. Reliability achieved was poor, with a kappa value of 0.26. Specific training did not affect the results. Razmjou et al. (2000) had two physical therapists trained in the McKenzie system conduct simultaneous examination on 45 patients. The kappa value for the overall classification into subgroups was good (0.70), and for classifying the derangement subgroups was excellent (0.96). In a study by Clare et al. (2004), 50 McKenzie-trained physical therapists reviewed 25 cases presented on McKenzie assessment forms. They obtained a fair kappa value (0.56) for assigning the overall classification. A kappa value of 0.68 was obtained for classifying the derangement subgroups. In another study using a simultaneous examination design two McKenzie-trained physical therapists classified 25 patients with low back pain (Clare et al. 2005). Reliability for the overall classification and for classifying the derangement subgroups was excellent, with kappa values of 1.0 and 0.84, respectively. Together these studies suggest that therapists trained in the McKenzie system can attain fair to excellent levels of reliability.

A small number of randomized controlled trials have specifically evaluated the efficacy of treatment matched to a patient's McKenzie classification compared to an alternative treatment. Stankovic and Johnell (1990) compared the effect of McKenzie-matched treatment to Mini-Back School in 100 patients with acute low back pain with and without radiating symptoms. At three weeks patients receiving McKenzie treatment displayed greater improvement than patients in the Mini-Back School treatment on five of seven measures of impairments and work-related function. At 52 weeks the McKenzie group was better than the Mini-Back School group in pain and movement, number of recurrences, medical care seeking and mean sick leave. A comparison of McKenzie-matched treatment, chiropractic manipulation and an educational booklet was made in 321 people with low back pain with varying stages of acuity and no nerve root compression (Cherkin et al. 1998). Short-term outcomes revealed no differences among the groups in symptom behaviour, function or disability. Long-term outcomes revealed greater costs for McKenzie and chiropractic treatment compared to education. Petersen et al. (2002) conducted a randomized controlled trial comparing McKenzie-matched treatment to a strengthening protocol in 260 patients with chronic low back pain and no nerve root compression. Outcomes of pain and disability were analyzed with an intention to treat analysis. There were no differences in outcomes between the two treatment groups at any time point (2, 4 and 12 months). Schenk et al. (2003) randomized 25 people with subacute lumbar radiculopathy to a McKenzie-matched treatment or spinal mobilization. After three treatments, the McKenzie-matched group displayed greater improvements in pain and disability compared to the mobilization group. Finally, 230 patients with low back pain of varying levels of acuity were classified based on the McKenzie system and then randomized to one of three treatments: McKenzie-matched treatment, treatment opposite the matched treatment and a non-directional treatment (Long et al. 2004). Outcomes were analyzed after two weeks of treatment. There was a greater improvement in all outcomes (pain, disability, use of medications, work and depression) in the McKenzie-matched treatment compared to the other two treatments. Finally, in a recent randomized controlled trial of 148 patients with acute low back pain, participants were assigned to receive a treatment programme based on the McKenzie method and first-line care (advice, reassurance and time-contingent acetaminophen) or first-line care alone, for 3 weeks. Results showed statistically significant but clinically non-relevant differences in short-term pain outcomes. There were no differences in function, disability and global perceived effect. Based on these studies, McKenzie-matched treatment does not appear to have a clear benefit above the other conservative treatments examined. However, the specific characteristics of the patients who best respond to McKenzie-matched treatment are still not fully understood and need further research.

Treatment-based classification system

The TBC system was originally proposed by Delitto et al. (1995). The system was developed in response to perceived limitations in some of the McKenzie classifications and to define additional subgroups. Recently Fritz et al. (2007) provided an update of the findings that characterize each proposed subgroup based on research conducted over the past 10 years. There are four low back pain subgroups proposed, each named for the treatment for which the patient is most likely to respond. The subgroups include (1) manipulation, (2) stabilization, (3) specific exercise (flexion, extension, lateral glide), and (4) traction. The specific exercise subgroup parallels the derangement subgroup in the McKenzie system. The TBC subgroups describe patients with acute low back pain with or without radiating symptoms. The subgroups proposed can exist within the specific and non-specific low back pain classifications.

Similar to the McKenzie system, the TBC system uses findings from the clinical examination to subgroup patients. The original description of the findings that characterized each of the four subgroups was based on judgement of a group of clinical experts (Delitto et al. 1989, 1995). Subsequent studies have used clinical prediction rule methods to refine the findings that characterize some of the subgroups (Fritz et al. 2007). Similar to the McKenzie examination, symptoms are monitored with tests of single and repeated trunk movements and sustained trunk postures. Additional tests include judgments of trunk alignment, quality and magnitude of trunk movement, symptom and mobility assessment with passive intervertebral movement, passive straight leg raising and neurological screening. A decision-making algorithm of self-report and clinical examination findings is used to assist in classification. The specifics of the treatments vary with classification as indicated by the name of each of the proposed subgroups.

The reliability of examiners to classify patients has been examined in four studies. Fritz and George (2000) investigated the inter-rater reliability of classifying patients into one of the four TBC subgroups using seven physical therapists familiar with the system and 43 patients with acute low back pain. They achieved a kappa value of 0.49. Kiesel et al. (2007) achieved a slightly higher kappa value (0.65) when eight physical therapists familiar with the classification system examined 30 patients who were in various stages of low back pain. In the study of Heiss et al. (2004) 45 patients with acute low back pain were classified by four physical therapists unfamiliar with the classification system. They found a low kappa value (0.15). Fritz et al. (2006) investigated inter-rater reliability of 30 physical therapists (novice = 10, experienced = 10, expert = 10) who classified 60 patient vignettes. They reported a kappa value of 0.60. In sum, these findings provide preliminary evidence that physical therapists who are familiar with the classification system can obtain a clinically acceptable level of inter-rater reliability.

Since the early 1990s several development and validation studies have been conducted on each of the four TBC interventions and the complete classification system (Delitto et al. 1993; Flynn et al. 2002; Fritz et al. 2003; McKenzie and May 2003; Schenk et al. 2003; Childs et al. 2004; Long et al. 2004; Hicks et al. 2005; Fritz, Childs et al. 2005; Fritz, Whitman et al. 2005; Brennan et al. 2006; Browder et al. 2007; Fritz, Cleland et al. 2007; Fritz, Lindsay et al. 2007a). Two studies have investigated the validity of the complete classification system. As the studies used different randomized controlled designs, they answered different research questions. Fritz et al. (2003) investigated the effectiveness of the overall treatment approach of the classification system (classification decision-making and treatment protocols) whereas Brennan et al. (2006) focused on the effectiveness of the classification decision-making. Fritz et al. (2003) compared treatment according to the classification system with clinical guidelines (low-stress aerobic exercises and advice to remain active) for 78 patients with acute, work-related low back pain in a randomized controlled trial. They found statistically significant better results for the outcomes of disability and return to work for patients receiving classification-based treatment at the four-week follow-up, but not at the one-year follow-up. Their results support the efficacy of the overall treatment approach of the classification system. However, the results may have been due to the treatment protocols that were used and not the classification decision-making process. Brennan et al. (2006) classified 123 patients with low back pain

less than 90 days (acute and subacute) based on the classification algorithm. All patients were randomized to receive specific exercises, manipulation or stabilization regardless of their classification. Outcomes were evaluated between patients who had received 'matched treatment' (according to the classification rules) and 'unmatched' (non-classification) treatment. The authors found a statistically significant reduction in disability favoring the matched treatment group after four and 52 weeks. Although intention-to-treat strategies were described to account for subjects lost to follow-up, subject attrition reduces the strength of the conclusions relating to the clinical prediction rules used to classify in the TBC system.

Movement System Impairment classification system

The MSI classification system was described in 2002 by Sahrmann. Five low back pain subgroups have been proposed based on judgement of an expert clinician (Sahrmann). The fundamental assumption underlying the system is that people with low back pain tend to move one or more lumbar joints more readily than other adjacent joints. This tendency is thought to be the result of movements and alignments repeatedly performed in the same direction(s) (flexion, extension, rotation or some combination) across a person's day. A person's direction-related tendency is (1) evidenced by specific patterns of altered movements and postures during examination tests and with functional activities and (2) associated with symptoms. The proposed MSI subgroups include lumbar (1) flexion, (2) extension, (3) rotation, (4) rotation with flexion and (5) rotation with extension. Each subgroup is named for the specific direction(s) of movements and alignments considered to contribute to the patient's low back pain. The MSI system is intended to be used with patients with low back pain with or without radiating symptoms, in any stage of acuity, and those with specific low back as well as non-specific low back pain.

The five MSI subgroups are identified based on findings from the examination. The examination includes tests in which patients perform single trunk and limb movements or assume different positions while symptoms are assessed. Tests that increase symptoms are followed by a test in which the patient's preferred movement or alignment strategy is systematically modified. The effect on symptoms of modifying a test is assessed. Additionally, judgements are made of the amount and relative timing of spine and proximal limb joint movements during tests. Neurological screening (including neural tension) is also conducted.

The reliability of examiners to classify patients with the MSI system has been examined in four studies. Van Dillen et al. (1998) examined inter-rater reliability of five physical therapists to perform test items from the examination and make judgements of low back pain subgroup.

Ninety-five patients in various stages of acuity (72% chronic) participated. The therapists were involved in the original development of the system. Agreement was 78% and the kappa value was 0.57 (Norton et al. 2004). A follow-up study examined the inter-rater reliability of two physical therapists: one was involved in the original development and the other was not (Harris-Hayes and Van Dillen 2009). The second therapist was trained in the examination and classification rules. Thirty patients (93% chronic) were examined and classified. The authors reported better reliability than the original study, i.e. 83% agreement and a kappa value of 0.75. Two physical therapists outside of the original development group classified 24 patients with chronic low back pain (Trudelle-Jackson et al. 2008). Both attended continuing education and participated in sessions to practise procedures and decision-making of the classification system. Their reliability was similar to the prior studies with an agreement value of 75% and a kappa value of 0.61. Finally, 13 therapists with moderate to no prior experience with the MSI system attended a two-day workshop (Henry et al. 2009). Therapists classified 21 vignettes. Ninety per cent agreement and a kappa value of 0.81 were attained. Thus, with training physical therapists can attain fair to excellent reliability to classify patients based on the MSI system.

Four development and validation studies have been conducted focusing on whether there are unique low back pain subgroups consistent with the original descriptions. An early study used a confirmatory factor analysis with a split sample cross-validation procedure on examination findings obtained from 188 patients with low back pain (72% chronic) (Van Dillen et al. 2003). Three specific clusters of alignment and movement tests consistent with three of the five proposed low back pain subgroups were identified in both datasets, providing preliminary evidence for the classification system. Additional evidence has been provided based on the findings from laboratory-based studies. Norton et al. (2004) measured lumbar curvature in two low back pain subgroups, rotation with flexion and rotation with extension, and in a group of people without low back pain. There were no differences between the people without low back pain and *all* patients with low back pain. The rotation with extension subgroup, however, stood in more lumbar extension than the rotation with flexion subgroup and the people without low back pain. Thus, there were predictable differences in lumbar curvature between patients in different low back pain subgroups and people without low back pain that could only be detected if the patients were classified. Gombatto et al. (2007) compared the symmetry of passive tissue characteristics of the trunk in 22 patients with chronic or recurrent low back pain in the rotation with extension subgroup and nineteen people without low back pain when the trunk was moved passively in the frontal plane. As predicted, there was more asymmetry in passive elastic energy in the low back pain subgroup than

in the people without low back pain. Another two studies examined movement patterns between patients with chronic or recurrent low back pain classified into the rotation with extension subgroup or the rotation subgroup. It was predicted that patients in the rotation with extension subgroup would display earlier and more asymmetric lumbopelvic movement than patients in the rotation subgroup. Gombatto et al. (2007) examined the lumbopelvic movement patterns during trunk lateral bending in 44 patients classified according to the MSI system. Compared to the rotation subgroup, the rotation with extension subgroup displayed earlier and more asymmetric lumbopelvic movement with trunk lateral bending. Similar findings were obtained in a study of 39 patients when lumbopelvic movement was examined during hip lateral rotation (Van Dillen et al. 2007). Together these studies provide data to support the validity of some of the proposed subgroups of the MSI system. They also provide insight into the potential mechanical factors underlying the different subgroups. To date no randomized controlled trial has been completed that examines whether treatment matched to a person's classification results in larger treatment effects than an alternative treatment. These studies are currently under way.

O'Sullivan classification system

A complete description of the O'Sullivan classification system was published in 2005 (O'Sullivan 2005). The system includes both biomedical and psychosocial characteristics to determine a patient's classification. There are three proposed subgroups: patients with (1) an adaptive/protective altered motor response to an underlying pathological process, (2) an altered motor response and centrally mediated pain secondary to dominant psychosocial factors, or (3) a maladaptive movement impairment or motor control impairment that drives the pain disorder. The third subgroup is considered to be the largest and most amenable to conservative management. Patients with a movement impairment present with pain associated with loss of normal active and passive movement, muscle guarding and excessive stability, and fear of movement. Patients with motor control impairment demonstrate deficits in control of the symptom-provoking spinal segment related to the movement direction that is painful. The control impairment is evident as difficulty with functional control of the neutral zone resulting from poor motor control of the spinal stabilizing muscles. Both the movement and control impairment subgroups can present with an impairment in a specific direction (flexion, extension, rotation, side bending) as well as an impairment associated with combinations of directions (multidirectional impairment). The proposed subgroups are considered to exist in the specific and non-specific low back pain classifications. The system is intended for use with patients with chronic low back pain.

Classification in the OS system is based on findings from (1) a screening protocol, (2) paraclinical and clinical examination tests (history and physical examination) and (3) psychosocial measures. The system was developed by Peter O'Sullivan, a clinical expert (O'Sullivan 2000, 2004, 2005). The physical examination includes analysis of movements and postures in various positions and functional tasks, tests of passive intervertebral motion, neural tension, muscle function, motor control and spinal proprioception. Symptoms are assessed during tests of movement (active and passive), posture and functional tasks. Similar to the MSI examination, select tests that increase symptoms are systematically modified to determine the effect on symptoms. In general, treatment consists of normalizing the primary movement or motor control impairment while addressing the patient's psychosocial characteristics (O'Sullivan 2005).

Reliability testing has been conducted to examine physical therapists' ability to classify patients with low back pain. All patient samples had chronic low back pain. In a two-part study by Dankaerts et al. (2006a), 35 patients who were proposed to have motor control impairment were independently examined by two expert physical therapists, one of whom was the system developer. Patients were assigned to one of the five proposed motor control impairment subgroups. A kappa value of 0.96 and an agreement value of 97% were attained. As a follow-up 13 clinicians (physical therapists and physicians) with varying levels of experience with the OS system were provided with an instruction packet and two days of training. Twenty-five vignettes and videotapes were created from patients from the first study. The clinicians first classified the vignettes and then viewed videotapes of the same patients participating in some examination tests. They assigned a second classification. Clinicians achieved good reliability when the classification was based on history and videotape information; mean kappa value of 0.61 and mean agreement 70%. Finally, Fersum et al. (2009) had four physical therapists independently examine and classify 26 patients with low back pain. One therapist was the developer of the system. All therapists had used the OS system in practice and had extensive experience in orthopedics and training in the system before the study. Agreement was examined comparing each of the three therapists to the developer's assessment. Therapists attained good to excellent reliability across levels of decisions (mean kappa value = 0.74; mean agreement = 94%).

A number of laboratory-based studies have been conducted to test the validity of some of the proposed OS subgroups. The majority of studies have compared patients with chronic low back pain in the motor control impairment subgroups, either flexion or active extension, to people without low back pain. O'Sullivan et al. (2003) examined proprioceptive ability in sitting with 15 patients in the flexion subgroup and 15 people without low back pain. After 5 seconds of sitting in full lumbar flexion,

participants were asked to find their neutral spine position. Patients in the flexion subgroup were less accurate in repositioning than people without low back pain. In a study by Burnett et al. (2004) spinal kinematics and trunk muscle activity were compared while nine cyclists classified in the flexion subgroup and nine cyclists without low back pain cycled to their tolerance level. Compared to those without low back pain, the flexion subgroup tended towards greater lower lumbar flexion and rotation and less co-contraction of the lower lumbar mutifidus muscles. Similar findings were reported in a study of industrial workers with low back pain classified in the flexion subgroup (O'Sullivan et al. 2006). Workers with and without low back pain were measured during postures and activities associated with lumbar flexion. The flexion subgroup displayed more flexion-related findings than the people without low back pain with their usual sitting and maximal slumped sitting. Three additional studies of the same cohort of subjects compared (1) 34 people without low back pain, (2) 20 patients in the flexion subgroup and (3) 13 patients in the active extension subgroup during functional tests of movement and posture (Dankaerts et al. 2006b, 2006c, 2009). Compared to people without low back pain, the active extension subgroup sat in more lower lumbar extension and the flexion subgroup sat in more lumbar flexion with usual sitting. During both usual and slumped sitting the active extension subgroup displayed more muscle activity in the superficial lumbar mutifidus, iliocostalis lumborum pars thoracis and transverse fibres of the internal oblique muscles than the other two groups. Finally, a stepwise linear discriminant analysis was performed using muscle activation and kinematic variables to develop a statistical model to classify the patients with low back pain. Classifications based on clinical examination data were compared to classifications using the statistical model; 96.4% of the cases were correctly classified with the derived model. Overall, these validation studies provide evidence to support the proposed flexion and active extension subgroups of the OS classification system and provide insight into potential contributing factors. However, at present no randomized controlled trial has been published that examines the effectiveness of the OS system.

CURRENT ISSUES

There is an interest in establishing a classification system useful for multiple disciplines. Such a system would allow a common method of communication among people involved in the care of, as well as the study of patients with low back pain. Before such a system can be adopted, however, there are some issues regarding the current state of low back pain classification that merit discussion.

These issues are related to the classification process and to methodology used in the development and testing of classification systems.

Classification process

A primary issue is the lack of an accepted basis for separating patients into clinically relevant subgroups. The lack of agreement is, in large part, the result of the differing perspectives of the developers of the systems. Based on their perspective, each developer has described the subgroups believed to be the most prevalent and the tests needed to identify these subgroups. Depending on the perspective, some systems focus solely on biomedical characteristics, others focus solely on psychosocial characteristics. Very few systems consider both domains. Within the biomedical and psychosocial domains there is also variability in the types of tests to be performed to determine a patient's classification. Common to the described systems is the assessment of symptoms with mechanically based tests, i.e. movements and alignments with standardized examination tests and/or functional activities. The specific movement and alignment tests, however, as well as the variables measured with each test differ among systems. For example, the McKenzie examination includes tests of both single and repeated trunk movements. The emphasis during these tests is on the assessment of symptoms and the amount of trunk motion achieved; particularly the change in trunk motion and symptoms as the patient performs repetitions of movement. On the other hand, the MSI examination includes tests of single movements of the trunk and the limbs. The emphasis of the assessment during these tests is on the symptoms and quality of trunk movement, i.e. motor control. Symptomatic test movements are systematically modified to try to change the trunk movement control and improve the symptoms. In the McKenzie system the symptoms and *mechanical* response to *repetitive* trunk motions are fundamental to deciding a patient's classification and treatment. In the MSI system improving the *control* of trunk movement during *single* trunk and limb movements is an essential component used in the decision making and treatment.

A related issue is the lack of information about how subgroups in various classification systems are related to each other. There are some commonalities in the types of subgroups proposed across the four classification systems we have described. In particular, each system describes groups of patients with low back pain who are intolerant to specific directions of trunk movements and postures. For example, all of the systems describe a subgroup of patients who worsen with flexion-related movements and postures. What is not known is if the patient identified as flexion-intolerant in the McKenzie system would be similarly identified with the tests and classification algorithms of the TBC, MSI or OS systems. To date, there has been no systematic examination of the relationships among tests

from the different systems considered to capture the same behaviour, for example, flexion. There also has been no systematic examination of the relationships among subgroups across classification systems. Such an endeavour could begin to clarify the most prevalent subgroups and the most important tests to identify the subgroups.

An additional issue is the lack of uniformity in the types of patients with low back pain to which the different classification systems can be applied. Each of the four systems we have detailed is intended for use with patients with a non-specific low back pain diagnosis (e.g. lumbar muscle strain, lumbago). The systems can be applied to some specific low back pain diagnoses but these specific diagnoses differ from one system to another. The systems also vary in their application to patients of differing stages of acuity. The McKenzie and MSI systems are proposed to be used with patients of all stages of acuity, i.e. acute, subacute or chronic. The TBC system has been described for patients in an acute exacerbation who have substantial pain and disability. Finally, the OS system is applicable to patients with chronic low back pain. The operational definition for each of these stages of acuity also can vary. Overall, a greater understanding is needed of whether a patient with low back pain (1) needs to be classified into different subgroups during different stages of acuity, or (2) presents with the same classification across stages of acuity but the emphasis of treatment varies depending on acuity status.

Methodological issues

One issue is that the methods used for determining the characteristics that describe the subgroups within a classification system vary among systems. Each of the four classification systems described were initially developed based on *a priori* judgement of expert clinicians and, to varying degrees, guided by individual conceptual models. One advantage of a conceptual model is that it provides a framework for how a group of factors could contribute to a condition based on logic and current empirical evidence. The subgroups defined in each of the four systems were those considered by the developers to be the most prevalent and distinct, i.e. mutually exclusive subgroups. More recently, clinical prediction rule (CPR) methodology has been used as an alternate method to assist the identification of the characteristics of the subgroups. In the current context, a CPR is a process of statistically combining variables to predict the likelihood of a specific outcome (Wasson et al. 1985; Laupacis et al. 1997). For example, in place of the original expert-guided subgroup descriptions, researchers of the TBC system have derived CPRs to assist in identifying factors likely to have a good prognosis for manipulation (Flynn et al. 2002) and stabilization (Hicks et al. 2005). The prognostic factors identified in these CPRs could provide potential characteristics that identify a unique subgroup of patients with low back pain.

Whether the subgroup of patients identified with a CPR influences treatment effects, however, has to be tested in a randomized controlled trial that tests for the interaction of subgroup and treatment condition (Hancock et al., 2009; Kamper et al. 2010). One initial validation study has been conducted for the TBC stabilization subgroup (Childs et al. 2004). Whether the characteristics identified in a CPR are those also considered to contribute to the person's low back pain condition is uncertain. This would depend, in part, on the process used to identify variables to include in the initial development. Treatment based on information about what contributes to a condition is usually considered more effective than treating individual clinical characteristics (Zimny 2004). Given that most of the classification systems available at this point in time are in the development and early validation stages, the value of any one method over another is not known. A combination of methodologies will likely provide the best outcome. Replication of subgroups with different methodologies will increase confidence that the subgroups exist in the low back pain population.

A second issue is that there is variability in the methods and amount of testing of the measurement attributes (reliability and validity) of most classification systems. The four systems we have described each have been examined for reliability of clinicians to assign a classification. The majority of the testing has been conducted within the research group involved in the development of the specific system, and with clinicians with variable amounts of specialty training. Overall, physical therapists familiar with the system (provided with specific training, have several years of clinical experience or have used the system in the clinic or research), appear to be able to attain clinically acceptable reliability (Cicchetti and Sparrow 1981). The results of reliability studies of more novice therapists to classify are not as consistent. The amount of training and the effect of prior clinical experience on ability to make decisions consistently currently is not known. The reliability of clinicians to classify people with low back pain may be enhanced by using a standardized manual of operations and procedures that includes the classification algorithm, and provide standardized training and evaluation of knowledge level before conducting the formal reliability testing.

Many of the systems for classifying low back pain are in the development phase with minimal validity testing (Billis et al. 2007; Kamper et al. 2010). As outlined, the four classification systems we have described have been examined for some aspects of validity. The emphasis of this testing, however, has differed among the systems. Some validation of the TBC, MSI and the OS system has been through the use of multivariate statistical approaches using prospective study designs (Delitto et al. 1992; Van Dillen et al. 2003; Dankaerts et al. 2009). The goal of these studies has been to examine data from tests of patients with low back pain to determine whether there

are distinct clusters of findings consistent with the proposed low back pain subgroups. Cross-sectional, laboratory-based studies have also been conducted to determine if some of the subgroups of the MSI and OS systems exist in the low back pain population, and if they differ from people without low back pain. Both approaches to validation have provided information that has been used to (1) refine the description of the characteristics of the proposed subgroups, and (2) understand potential factors contributing to a particular low back pain subgroup to assist in treatment direction. Validation of the McKenzie and the TBC system has primarily been based on results of randomized controlled trials. The basic design of the trials is one in which subgroups are identified *a priori* and then patients are randomized to a matched treatment or some alternative treatment(s). Validation of a particular subgroup or the classification system as a whole is provided when there is an interaction of subgroup and treatment condition; the matched treatment results in a greater improvement in outcome than an alternative treatment.

Some additional issues are of relevance to the discussion of methods for testing classification systems. One issue is that it is not clear what constitutes an appropriate control condition in randomized controlled trials that examine whether subgrouping patients with low back pain influences the effect of treatment. One option is for the control condition to reflect current clinical practice. This comparison provides information about whether matched treatment provides a greater benefit than other kinds of treatment commonly provided in clinical practice. The majority of randomized controlled trials examining the effect of matching treatment to a person's classification have used these kinds of control conditions. A second option is for the control condition to reflect best evidence based on findings from studies of patients with low back pain who have not been classified. Such a comparison condition may not reflect how clinicians practise; however, this comparison would begin to address the question of whether treatment matched to a patient's classification provides a large enough benefit to warrant implementing the classification process in clinical practice. A second issue is that post hoc subgroup analyses are often performed, particularly in randomized controlled trials where an overall treatment effect is not detected. Such analyses are not recommended (Rothwell 2005). The analyses can often include subgroups that are not based on characteristics present prior to randomization. Thus, the subgroups can be the result of aspects of the treatment provided rather than truly distinct subgroups that respond differentially to treatment (Klebanoff 2007). The analyses also often result in subgroup effects due merely to chance or underestimate effects because the post hoc subgroups are too small to provide sufficient statistical power (Rothwell 2005). A final issue is that there is minimal replication of findings outside the group of researchers involved in the initial development and validation studies. Replication is needed to begin to provide evidence of the generalizability of a particular classification system to clinical practice.

No patient management system should be considered static and it is necessary to incorporate new evidence into existing systems; concepts emerge from research in the field; clinical practice is dynamic, changing in response to emerging evidence. Probably the most important issue at this time is to identify the types of people with LBP and then test the interventions that would be directed at that particular problem. Classification should improve the size of treatment effects currently documented since the classification process is, in part, used to match people to the most appropriate treatments.

CONCLUSION

After decades of low back pain research and many randomized controlled trials on effectiveness of therapeutic interventions, it seems that we still do not know how commonly used low back pain treatments work and for whom. Randomized trials have not shown the effects that we had expected or would like to see. Study populations may not have been adequately selected and too heterogeneous, or interventions may not have been adequately developed. A randomized trial should not be a purpose on its own, but should answer a clinically relevant question about effectiveness of an intervention for which it is plausible that it is effective for that specific population. Many trials have compared different treatments in heterogeneous populations of 'non-specific' low back pain patients. Maybe we should stop doing these trials. For example, it doesn't seem relevant to conduct a trial on proprioception exercises if you don't know how to measure proprioception and as long as you don't know if there is a causal association between proprioception and low back pain. There seems to be consensus that interventions should be better targeted at specific subgroups of patients. Trials of non-specific low back pain that fail to consider the heterogeneity of back pain presentation should be discouraged. To be able to reach this goal, we may need to reconceptualize the research framework in the field of low back pain. A stepwise multidisciplinary approach might be useful that includes:

- *Basic research* on cadavers, animals and humans should provide an empirical basis for plausible working mechanisms regarding a specific type of exercise for a specific and well-defined subgroup of low back pain patients.
- *Observational studies* in patients should assess the safety of the intervention.
- Efficacy should be assessed in an *explanatory randomized trial* in an experimental setting.
- Effectiveness should be assessed in a *pragmatic randomized trial* in clinical practice.
- Cost-effectiveness should be evaluated in an *economic evaluation.*
- *Implementation* of the intervention is the final step to ensure its uptake in clinical practice. Development of an adequate implementation plan and evaluation of process and patient outcomes are essential.

REFERENCES

Abraham, I., Killackey-Jones, B., 2002. Lack of evidence-based research for idiopathic low back pain: the importance of a specific diagnosis. Arch Intern Med 162, 1442–1444.

Billis, E.V., McCarthy, C.J., Oldham, J.A., 2007. Subclassification of low back pain: a cross-country comparison. Eur Spine J 16, 865–879.

Borkan, J.M., Cherkin, D.C., 1996. An agenda for primary care research on low back pain. Spine 21, 2880–2884.

Bouter, L.M., Pennick, V., Bombardier, C., 2003. Cochrane Back Review Group. Spine 28, 1215–1218.

Brennan, G.P., Fritz, J.M., Hunter, S.J., Thackeray, A., Delitto, A., Erhard,

R.E., 2006. Identifying subgroups of patients with acute/subacute 'nonspecific' low back pain: results of a randomized clinical trial. Spine 31, 623–631.

Browder, D.A., Childs, J.D., Cleland, J.A., Fritz, J.M., 2007. Effectiveness of an extension-oriented treatment approach in a subgroup of subjects with low back pain: a randomized clinical trial. Phys Ther 87, 1608–1618.

Burnett, A.F., Cornelius, M.W., Dankaerts, W., O'Sullivan, P.B., 2004. Spinal kinematics and trunk muscle activity in cyclists: a comparison between healthy controls and non-specific chronic low back pain

subjects – a pilot investigation. Man Ther 9, 211–219.

Cherkin, D.C., Deyo, R.A., Battie, M., Street, J., Barlow, W., 1998. A comparison of physical therapy, chiropractic manipulation, and provision of an educational booklet for the treatment of patients with low-back pain. N Engl J Med 339, 1021–1029.

Childs, J.D., Fritz, J.M., Flynn, T.W., Irrgang, J.J., Johnson, K.K., Majkowski, G.R., et al., 2004. A clinical prediction rule to identify patients with low back pain most likely to benefit from spinal manipulation: a validation study. Ann Intern Med 141, 920–928.

Cicchetti, D.V., Sparrow, S.A., 1981. Developing criteria for establishing interrater reliability of specific items: applications to assessment of adaptive behavior. Am J Ment Defic 86, 127–137.

Clare, H.A., Adams, R., Maher, C.G., 2004. A systematic review of efficacy of McKenzie therapy for spinal pain. Aust J Physiother 50, 209–216.

Clare, H.A., Adams, R., Maher, C.G., 2005. Reliability of McKenzie classification of patients with cervical or lumbar pain. J Manipulative Physiol Ther 28, 122–127.

Dankaerts, W., O'Sullivan, P., Burnett, A., Straker, L., Davey, P., Gupta, R., 2009. Discriminating healthy controls and two clinical subgroups of nonspecific chronic low back pain patients using trunk muscle activation and lumbosacral kinematics of postures and movements: a statistical classification model. Spine 34, 1610–1618.

Dankaerts, W., O'Sullivan, P., Burnett, A., Straker, L., 2006c. Altered patterns of superficial trunk muscle activation during sitting in nonspecific chronic low back pain patients: importance of subclassification. Spine 31, 2017–2023.

Dankaerts, W., O'Sullivan, P., Burnett, A., Straker, L., 2006b. Differences in sitting postures are associated with nonspecific chronic low back pain disorders when patients are subclassified. Spine 31, 698–704.

Dankaerts, W., O'Sullivan, P.B., Straker, L.M., Burnett, A.F., Skouen, J.S., 2006a. The inter-examiner reliability of a classification method for non-specific chronic low back pain patients with motor control impairment. Man Ther 11, 28–39.

Delitto, A., Cibulka, M.T., Erhard, R.E., Bowling, R.W., Tenhula, J.A., 1993. Evidence for use of an extension-mobilization category in acute low back syndrome: a prescriptive validation pilot study. Phys Ther 73, 216–222.

Delitto, A., Erhard, R.E., Bowling, R.W., 1995. A treatment-based classification approach to low back syndrome: identifying and staging patients for conservative treatment. Phys Ther 75, 470–485.

Delitto, A., Shulman, A.D., Rose, S.J., Strube, M.J., Erhard, R.E., Bowling, R.W., et al., 1992. Reliability of a clinical examination to classify patients with low back syndrome. Phys Ther Pract 1, 1–9.

Delitto, A., Shulman, A.D., Rose, S.J., 1989. On developing expert-based decision-support systems in physical therapy: the NIOSH low back atlas. Phys Ther 69, 554–558.

Fersum, V.K., O'Sullivan, P.B., Kvale, A., Skouen, J.S., 2009. Inter-examiner reliability of a classification system for patients with non-specific low back pain. Man Ther 14, 555–561.

Flynn, T., Fritz, J., Whitman, J., Wainner, R., Magel, J., Rendeiro, D., et al., 2002. A clinical prediction rule for classifying patients with low back pain who demonstrate short-term improvement with spinal manipulation. Spine 27, 2835–2843.

Fritz, J.M., Brennan, G.P., Clifford, S.N., Hunter, S.J., Thackeray, A., 2006. An examination of the reliability of a classification algorithm for subgrouping patients with low back pain. Spine 31, 77–82.

Fritz, J.M., Childs, J.D., Flynn, T.W., 2005. Pragmatic application of a clinical prediction rule in primary care to identify patients with low back pain with a good prognosis following a brief spinal manipulation intervention. BMC Fam Pract 6, 29.

Fritz, J.M., Cleland, J.A., Childs, J.D., 2007. Subgrouping patients with low back pain: evolution of a classification approach to physical therapy. J Orthop Sports Phys Ther 37, 290–302.

Fritz, J.M., Delitto, A., Erhard, R.E., 2003. Comparison of classification-based physical therapy with therapy based on clinical practice guidelines for patients with acute low back pain: a randomized clinical trial. Spine 28, 1363–1371.

Fritz, J.M., George, S., 2000. The use of a classification approach to identify subgroups of patients with acute low back pain. Interrater reliability and short-term treatment outcomes. Spine 25, 106–114.

Fritz, J.M., Lindsay, W., Matheson, J.W., Brennan, G.P., Hunter, S.J., Moffit, S.D., et al., 2007a. Is there a subgroup of patients with low back pain likely to benefit from mechanical traction? Results of a randomized clinical trial and subgrouping analysis. Spine 32, E793–E800.

Fritz, J.M., Whitman, J.M., Childs, J.D., 2005. Lumbar spine segmental mobility assessment: an examination of validity for determining intervention strategies in patients with low back pain. Arch Phys Med Rehabil 89, 1745–1752.

Gatchel, R.J., 2001. A biopsychosocial overview of pretreatment screening of patients with pain. Clin J Pain 17, 192–199.

Gombatto, S.P., Collins, D.R., Engsberg, J.R., Sahrmann, S.A., Van Dillen, L.R., 2007. Patterns of lumbar region movement during trunk lateral bending in two different subgroups of people with low back pain. Phys Ther 87, 441–454.

Hancock, M., Herbert, R.D., Maher, C.G., 2009. A guide to interpretation of studies investigating subgroups of responders to physical therapy interventions. Phys Ther 89, 698–704.

Harris-Hayes, M., Van Dillen, L.R., 2009. Inter-tester reliability of physical therapists classifying low back pain problems based on the movement system impairment classification system. Phys Med Rehabil 1, 117–126.

Heiss, D.G., Fitch, D.S., Fritz, J.M., Sanchez, W.J., Roberts, K.E., Buford, J.A., 2004. The interrater reliability among physical therapists newly trained in a classification system for acute low back pain. J Orthop Sports Phys Ther 34, 430–439.

Henry, S.M., Van Dillen, L.R., Trombley, A.L., Dee, J.M., Bunn, J.Y., 2009. Reliability of novice raters in using the movement system impairment approach to subgroup people with low back pain. Man Ther http://dx.doi.org/10.1016/j.math.2012.06.008 (accessed February 2013).

Hicks, G.E., Fritz, J.M., Delitto, A., McGill, S.M., 2005. Preliminary development of a clinical prediction rule for determining which patients with low back pain will respond to a stabilization exercise program. Arch Phys Med Rehabil 86, 1753–1762.

Kamper, S.J., Maher, C.G., Hancock, M.J., Koes, B.W., Croft, P.R., Hay, E., 2010. Treatment-based subgroups of low back pain: a guide to appraisal of research studies and a summary of current evidence. Best Pract Res Clin Rheumatol 24, 181–191.

Kiesel, K.B., Underwood, F.B., Mattacola, C.G., Nitz, A.J., Malone, T.R., 2007. A comparison of select trunk muscle thickness change between subjects with low back pain classified in the treatment-based classification system and asymptomatic controls. J Orthop Sports Phys Ther 37, 596–607.

Kilby, J., Stigant, M., Roberts, A., 1990. The reliability of back pain assessment by physiotherapists, using a 'McKenzie algorithm'. Physiother 76, 579–583.

Klebanoff, M.A., 2007. Subgroup analysis in obstetrics clinical trials. Am J Obstet Gynecol 119–122.

Laupacis, A., Sekar, N., Stiell, I.G., 1997. Clinical prediction rules. A review and suggested modifications of methodological standards. JAMA 277, 488–494.

Long, A., Donelson, R., Fung, T., 2004. Does it matter which exercise? A randomized control trial of exercise for low back pain. Spine 29, 2593–2602.

McKenzie, R., May, S., 2003. The lumbar spine. Mechanical diagnosis and therapy, 2nd edn. Spinal Publications New Zealand Ltd, Waikanae.

McKenzie, R.A., 1981. The lumbar spine: mechanical diagnosis and therapy. Spinal Publications, Waikanae, New Zealand.

Norton, B.J., Sahrmann, S.A., Van Dillen, L.R., 2004. Differences in measurements of lumbar curvature related to gender and low back pain. J Orthop Sports Phys Ther 34, 524–534.

O'Sullivan, P.B., Burnett, A., Floyd, A.N., Gadsdon, K., Logiudice, J., Miller, D., et al., 2003. Lumbar repositioning deficit in a specific low back pain population. Spine 28, 1074–1079.

O'Sullivan, P.B., Mitchell, T., Bulich, P., Waller, R., Holte, J., 2006. The relationship beween posture and back muscle endurance in industrial workers with flexion-related low back pain. Man Ther 11, 264–271.

O'Sullivan, P.B., 2004. 'Clinical instability' of the lumbar Spine: its pathological basis, diagnosis and conservative management. In Boyling, J.D., Jull, G.A. (eds), Grieves Modern Manual Therapy, 3rd edn. Elsevier, Edinburgh, pp. 311–322.

O'Sullivan, P.B., 2005. Diagnosis and classification of chronic low back pain disorders: maladaptive movement and motor control impairments as underlying mechanism. Man Ther 10, 242–255.

O'Sullivan, P.B., 2000. Lumbar segmental 'instability': clinical presentation and specific stabilizing exercise management. Man Ther 5, 2–12.

Petersen, T., Kryger, P., Ekdahl, C., Olsen, S., Jacobsen, S., 2002. The effect of McKenzie therapy as compared with that of intensive strengthening training for the treatment of patients with subacute or chronic low back pain: a randomized controlled trial. Spine 27, 1702–1709.

Poitras, S., Blais, R., Swaine, B., Rossignol, M., 2005. Management of work-related low back pain: a population-based survey of physical therapists. Phys Ther 85, 1168–1181.

Razmjou, H., Kramer, J.F., Yamada, R., 2000. Intertester reliability of the McKenzie evaluation in assessing patients with mechanical low-back pain. J Orthop Sports Phys Ther 30, 368–383.

Reesor, K.A., Craig, K.D., 1988. Medically incongruent chronic back pain: physical limitations, suffering, and ineffective coping. Pain 32, 35–45.

Riddle, D.L., Rothstein, J.M., 1993. Intertester reliability of McKenzie's classifications of the syndrome types present in patients with low back pain. Spine 18, 133–1344.

Rothwell, P.M., 2005. Treating individuals 2: Subgroup analysis in randomised controlled trials: importance, indications and interpretation. Lancet 365, 176–186.

Sahrmann, S.A., 2002. Diagnosis and Treatment of Movement Impairment Syndromes. Mosby, St Louis, MO.

Schenk, R., Jozefczyk, C., Kopf, A., 2003. A randomized trial comparing interventions in patients with lumbar posterior derangement. J Man Manip Ther 11, 95–102.

Silfies, S.P., Mehta, R., Smith, S.S., Karduna, A.R., 2009. Differences in feedforward trunk muscle activity in subgroups of patients with mechanical low back pain. Arch Phys Med Rehabil 90, 1159–1169.

Stankovic, R., Johnell, O., 1990. Conservative treatment of acute low-back pain. A prospective randomized trial: McKenzie method of treatment versus patient education in 'mini back school'. Spine 15, 120–123.

Trudelle-Jackson, E., Sarvaiya-Shah, S.A., Wang, S.S., 2008. Interrater reliability of a movement impairment-based classification system for lumbar spine syndromes in patients with chronic low back pain. J Orthop Sports Phys Ther 38, 371–376.

Turk, D.C., 2002. Clinical effectiveness and cost-effectiveness of treatments for patients with chronic pain. Clin J Pain 18, 355–365.

Van Dillen, L.R., Gombatto, S.P., Collins, D.R., Engsberg, J.R., Sahrmann, S.A., 2007. Symmetry of timing of hip and lumbopelvic rotation motion in 2 different subgroups of people with low back pain. Arch Phys Med Rehabil 88, 351–360.

Van Dillen, L.R., Sahrmann, S.A., Norton, B.J., Caldwell, C.A., Fleming, D.A., McDonnell, M.K., et al., 1998. Reliability of physical examination items used for classification of patients with low back pain. Phys Ther 78, 979–988.

Van Dillen, L.R., Sahrmann, S.A., Norton, B.J., Caldwell, C.A., McDonnell, M.K., Bloom, N.J., 2003. Movement system impairment-based categories for low back pain: stage 1 validation. J Orthop Sports Phys Ther 33, 126–142.

Waddell, G., McCulloch, J.A., Kummel, E., Venner, R.M., 1980. Nonorganic physical signs in low-back pain. Spine 5, 117–125.

Waddell, G., 2005. Subgroups within 'nonspecific' low back pain. J Rheumatol 32, 395–396.

Wand, B.M., O'Connell, N.E., 2008. Chronic non-specific low back pain – sub-groups or a single mechanism? BMC Musculoskelet Disord 9, 11.

Wasson, J.H., Sox, H.C., Neff, R.K., Goldman, L., 1985. Clinical prediction rules. Applications and methodological standards. N Engl J Med 313, 793–799.

Zimny, N.J., 2004. Diagnostic classification and orthopaedic physical therapy practice: what we can learn from medicine. J Orthop Sports Phys Ther 34, 105–109.

Chapter |18|

Motor control changes and low back pain: cause or effect?

Jaap H. van Dieën*, G. Lorimer Moseley[†] and Paul W. Hodges[‡]
*MOVE Research Institute Amsterdam, Faculty of Human Movement Sciences, VU University Amsterdam, Amsterdam, The Netherlands, [†]Sansom Institute for Health Research, University of South Australia, Adelaide, and Neuroscience Research Australia, Sydney, Australia, and [‡]NHMRC Centre of Clinical Research Excellence in Spinal Pain, Injury and Health, School of Health and Rehabilitation Sciences, University of Queensland, Brisbane, Queensland, Australia

INTRODUCTION

The objective of this chapter is to present a state-of-the-art overview on the question whether motor control changes are a cause and/or an effect of low back pain (LBP). It is based on a discussion among all the authors of this volume and a review of the literature. We have attempted to avoid overlap with the preceding chapters as much as

possible, but have found it necessary in some places to repeat arguments made there or refer to data reported there.

The question at hand has obvious implications for the feasibility of motor control training as an approach to primary and/or secondary prevention of LBP. However, it should be kept in mind that even when, for example, poor motor control can cause LBP, this does not necessarily imply that motor control training is an effective, let alone the most effective, approach to primary prevention.

The first section of this chapter reviews observations on motor behaviour in individuals with LBP. In the second section, we discuss the evidence that motor control changes can be a primary cause of LBP. In the third section, we discuss evidence that LBP causes changes in motor control. Subsequently, we address the question whether these changes are adaptive, i.e. help the individual to deal with LBP-related impairments, or maladaptive, i.e. contribute to the transition to chronic pain and/or recurrence of pain. The final section summarizes the main conclusions and presents implications for clinical research and practice.

MOTOR BEHAVIOUR IN LBP

The available data on motor behaviour in LBP are predominantly cross-sectional in nature. It is therefore unknown whether differences in motor behaviour between individuals with and without LBP are a cause or a consequence of their LBP. The issue is not moot, however, because the nature of the differences may help to inform us as to the *likely* nature of the relationship between LBP and motor behaviour.

Muscle activity

Differences in muscle activity between patients with LBP and healthy control subjects are quite inconsistent between studies (van Dieën et al. 2003b). In fact, a recent animal experiment suggests that excitatory and inhibitory effects on the control of the same muscle may co-exist at different levels of the motor control system (Hodges et al. 2009).

Most research in this area has focused on activity of the lumbar erector spinae muscle (LES). A review thereof showed that results were highly inconsistent, with some studies showing more activity in patients than in healthy controls, and other studies showing less (van Dieën et al. 2003b). For two classes of motor tasks, fairly consistent evidence was found for increased LES activation in LBP patients, i.e. in rest postures and in full flexion of the trunk. In rest postures such as upright standing and sitting, none of the studies reviewed reported decreased activity, but whether or not increased activity was found varied between postures, even when studied within the same group of subjects (Arena et al. 1989, 1991). In full flexion, most healthy subjects show flexion–relaxation, a complete electromyographical silence of the LES. This phenomenon is absent in many patients with LBP and this absence was associated with reduced intervertebral motion (Kaigle et al. 1998). In some motor tasks, particularly in submaximal isometric contractions, fairly consistent evidence for reduced activation was found. In dynamic conditions, some studies found increased, while other studies found decreased activity in LBP patients.

LES responses to sudden loading in quiet upright stance were shown to be delayed in LBP patients (Alexiev 1994; Magnusson et al. 1996). On the other hand, LBP patients also de-activated the extensor muscles later after a sudden release following isometric extensor contraction (Radebold et al. 2000; Reeves et al. 2005). These studies thus indicate a delayed response to perturbations irrespective of whether the LES turns on or off in this response, suggesting that the delay is not due to decreased LES excitability.

Other extensor muscles have been much less studied than LES. One study showed that LBP patients activated the thoracic erector spinae (TES) at a relatively low level compared to the LES (van Dieën et al. 2003a, see also Chapter 5). However, a study on a larger population showed that the opposite pattern was also found in a subgroup of patients (Reeves et al. 2006). Activity of the multifidus muscle (MU) was decreased relative to the superficial muscles in concentric activity (Lindgren et al. 1993) and LBP patients were less well able to isometrically contract the muscle under visual (ultrasound-based) feedback than controls (Wallwork et al. 2009). In addition, activation of the deep, short-fibred part of the MU after self-induced perturbations was delayed in patients with recurrent LBP during remission (MacDonald et al. 2009).

Several studies have found activity of the extensor muscles to be more asymmetric in subjects with LBP than in those without LBP (Hoyt et al. 1981; Triano and Luttges 1985; Grabiner et al. 1992; Alexiev 1994), whereas other studies reported only a non-significant trend (Cram and Steger 1983), or no effect of LBP on symmetry of extensor muscle activity (Reeves et al. 2006). Finally, some studies report more 'erratic' temporal variation in activity of the extensor muscles in LBP patients than controls (Grabiner et al. 1992; Lamoth et al. 2006b).

Among the abdominal muscles, the rectus abdominus muscle (RA) was found to be more active during gait in patients with LBP than in healthy controls (van der Hulst et al. 2010a, 2010b). During an exercise called 'abdominal hollowing', activation levels of the internal oblique (IO) and RA muscles were not different between patients and controls, but the ratio of the two was different with a higher activation of RA relative to IO in the patient group (O'Sullivan et al. 1997). This finding was, however, not confirmed during free planar motions through the upright posture and during ramp contractions (van Dieën et al. 2003a).

Transversus abdominus muscle activity has been investigated in a range of studies (for reviews see Hodges 1999; Hodges and Moseley 2003 and Chapter 6). Generally its activity in self-induced perturbations was delayed and activity levels were reduced. The delayed activity was associated with a reorganization of the motor cortex (Tsao et al. 2008). In addition, activation of this muscle in relation to a self-induced perturbation appeared less variable in timing in LBP patients than in healthy controls (Jacobs et al. 2009b), which may be suggestive of increased conscious control in the patient group (Jacobs et al. 2009a).

Trunk kinematics and kinetics

Most studies on trunk kinematics in LBP have focused on the range of motion of the trunk during forward bending. Comparisons of hip and lumbar contributions to forward bending yielded conflicting results (Mayer et al. 1984; Paquet et al. 1994; Esola et al. 1996; Porter and Wilkinson 1997; Commissaris et al. 2002), which may be due to the fact that hip mobility is impaired in a subgroup of LBP patients (Wong and Lee 2004). In a wheel-turning task, limited contributions of lumbar and hip motions were compensated for by arm movements (Rudy et al. 1995). While total range of motion of the spine is not consistently reduced in LBP patients (Marras et al. 1995; Lehman 2004), some studies have demonstrated limited motion in one or more segments of the spine that could be compensated for at other levels (Jayaraman et al. 1994; Kaigle et al. 1998; Cox et al. 2000).

Generally, velocity of lumbar motion, rather than range of lumbar motion, appears to better discriminate LBP patients from healthy individuals (Marras et al. 1995,

1999). Lumbar motion occurs more slowly in LBP patients (Boston et al. 1993, 1995; Marras et al. 1995, 1999, 2005; Wong and Lee 2004). Data available on relative timing of lumbar and hip motion are inconsistent (Boston et al. 1993, 1995; Commissaris et al. 2002; Wong and Lee 2004).

Several studies have assessed trunk rotations in the transverse plane during walking. At increasing speed, healthy controls switch from in-phase to out-of-phase transverse rotations of the pelvis and thorax, whereas in LBP patients rotations remain more in-phase (Selles et al. 2001; Lamoth et al. 2002, 2006a, 2006b). This pattern would seem consistent with either an attempt to limit the range and velocity of lumbar rotation, or a consequence of increased rotational stiffness of the lumbar spine.

The literature indicates a reduced precision of trunk postural control in LBP patients. For example, after being trained to move their trunk to a target position, LBP patients were as accurate as controls. However, they did not perform the task in the same way – they used an increased deceleration time, which is consistent with a greater reliance on closed-loop (feedback) control to compensate for reduced precision (Descarreaux et al. 2005b). Furthermore, control of balance in sitting appeared less adequate in subjects with LBP, with one study reporting larger and faster sway (Radebold et al. 2001) and another study reporting reduced sway frequency (van Dieën et al. 2010). In standing, postural sway and time to recover balance after a perturbation are increased with LBP and this coincides with reduced trunk movements (Mok et al. 2007).

Conclusion

From the literature reviewed it is evident that motor control and motor behaviour are different in patients with LBP from healthy controls. However, there appears to exist substantial variability in motor behaviour between subjects with LBP, sometimes with opposite differences to healthy controls in different subgroups of patients. That is, it seems that although people without LBP pain move and control their back in a similar fashion, those with LBP often have a different way of moving and controlling their back and the manner in which it is different seems to vary widely between individuals. This variability may account for the lack of consensus between studies as to the characteristic movement and control patterns in people with LBP.

CAUSE

To determine if motor control changes can cause LBP, one would have to manipulate motor control (and nothing else) and wait to see if LBP would result. Apart from practical problems, obvious ethical limitations would preclude such experiments in humans. To our knowledge, animal experiments, while feasible, have not been performed. Strictly speaking therefore, causality cannot be proven. We thus discuss the feasibility of a causal relationship between motor control and LBP. This discussion is based on associations determined in observational studies and based on experimental studies that interrogate potential mechanisms through which motor control might cause LBP.

A potential mechanism for motor control to cause LBP is through the effects that motor control has on tissue loading. This is perhaps the most intuitive and attractive theory because the idea that self-generated forces can damage tissue is well established and accepted, and even sub-failure injuries of tissue activate nociceptors and set off inflammatory responses. Indeed, inflammatory processes can be set in train purely by ongoing noxious stimulation even without sub-failure tissue injury – activation of nociceptors signals the release of peptidergic inflammatory mediators in the immediate area, which have the potential to engage the full spectrum of local and adaptive inflammatory responses (Lynn 1996). The role of (subfailure) mechanical tissue injury in LBP is indirectly supported by a range of clinical, epidemiological and experimental studies (see van Dieën and van der Beek 2009 for an extensive review). It is very difficult, however, to confirm the presence of microtrauma or sub-injury noxious activity in the back, which makes the theory impossible to substantiate, at least with current investigative technologies. As yet, the literature provides no solid proof that motor control changes cause LBP and at present only potential scenarios of how motor control *could* cause LBP can be proposed.

There is a large amount of theoretical literature that proposes instability of the spine to be a cause of high tissue strains and/or impingements, thereby causing injury and pain (Panjabi 1992a, 1992b). Given that the osteoligamentous spine is inherently unstable, loss of control over spinal curvature or spinal movement, due to motor control errors, could theoretically lead to instability (see Chapter 5 and Cholewicki and McGill 1996a). The probability of such motor control errors is likely dependent on the individual quality of motor control (motor skill) as a variable trait as well as on situational factors.

Cadaver testing has shown that high and repetitive compression on, and bending and torsion of the spine can cause injuries, and such injuries may *in vivo* be a cause of LBP (van Dieën et al. 1999; van Dieën and van der Beek 2009). Specific motor habits, such as a habitually flexed posture, might cause such unnecessarily high, sustained or repeated loading and thus contribute to LBP (see also Chapters 7 and 8). Also, habitually increased levels of trunk muscle co-activation may induce unnecessarily high loading without visible changes in motor behaviour.

Below we will first review the epidemiological support for the two mechanisms (instability and high spinal loading) by which motor control might play a role in the causation of LBP. Subsequently, we discuss experimental studies that have attempted to demonstrate proof for (parts of) the chain of events by which motor control could cause LBP.

Epidemiological evidence

One epidemiological study has associated balance loss to LBP (Manning and Shannon 1981). Reeves et al. (2006) studied differences in relative activation of LES and TES as described above in a longitudinal study. Activation imbalance between erector spinae activity at different levels was similar for individuals who did not get LBP and those who sustained first time LBP, which suggests that imbalance does not cause LBP. A preliminary study in people with neck pain but no back pain demonstrated those with poor ability to perform a voluntary activation of the lower abdominal muscles, poor performance on which is associated with abnormal postural activation of transversus abdominis during arm movements (Hodges et al. 1996), were 3–6 times more likely to develop persistent or recurrent LBP in the following two years than those who performed well on this task (Moseley 2004b).

Cholewicki et al. (2005) found evidence for a weakly increased risk of LBP in athletes with slower responses of trunk muscles to sudden postural perturbations. Takala and Viikari-Juntura (2000) reported that poor balance control was a weak predictor of future LBP in a working population. In contrast, trunk position sense (Silfies et al. 2007) and seated balancing performance (Cholewicki et al. 2005) were not predictive of future LBP among athletes. Other studies have addressed personal traits that might be reflective of poor trunk control. For example, the absence of the normal flexion–relaxation response in people with back pain was positively related to self-efficacy and fear avoidance beliefs (Watson et al. 1997) and double dissociation experiments show that range of trunk movement can be altered in people with LBP by purely cognitive interventions in a manner that is consistent with a relationship between movement and perceived threat of injury (Moseley 2004a).

There are data that suggest that athletes are less likely to get LBP than non-athletes (Videman et al. 1995), which might support a protective role of motor skill. However, it might also implicate a role of strength, activity pattern and level, psychological and behavioural factors. Moreover, high incidences of LBP have been reported in specific populations with relatively good motor skills, such as physical education teachers (Tsuboi et al. 2002; Stergioulas et al. 2004) and athletes (Sward et al. 1990, 1991).

To our knowledge no major prospective epidemiological studies on inefficient motor habits and LBP have been performed. However, some indirect evidence comes from occupational epidemiology, showing that for example frequent trunk bending and twisting (Punnett et al. 1991; Hoogendoorn et al. 1999, 2000; Lotters et al. 2003) are associated with LBP. It can be questioned, however, whether the contrasts in exposure levels in such studies (e.g. the degree and frequency of trunk bending in different occupations) are not much larger than the effect on exposure that inefficient motor habits might have (e.g. the difference in trunk bending between individuals based on their motor habits).

Experimental evidence

A modelling study indicated that spinal instability may occur in tasks that impose low mechanical loads on the spine, while the spine would be stable in tasks imposing high mechanical loading (Cholewicki and McGill 1996b). However, it was later shown that the latter conclusion depends on the assumed relation between muscle stiffness and force, suggesting that spine instability might also occur in tasks that impose very high loads on the spine (Brown et al. 2005). However, perturbation experiments in lifting from ground level indicate a high robustness of trunk control in these demanding tasks (van der Burg et al. 2000) due to the intrinsic stiffness of the musculature and the fact that ample time for feedback corrections is available, because the perturbation force usually applies at distal segments (van der Burg et al. 2005a). Indications of a loss of control over spinal posture were found in less demanding, upright standing lifting tasks (van der Burg et al. 2003, 2004), probably due to lower pre-activation of trunk muscles (Cholewicki and McGill 1996b; Cholewicki et al. 2000; Stokes et al. 2000).

In addition to external perturbations, changes in the neuromusculoskeletal system may increase the probability of spinal instability. Theoretical considerations indicate that the probability of a loss of control over segmental motion in the spinal column increases when degenerative changes or spinal injury have caused a segmental loss of stiffness (Panjabi 1992a, 1992b and see Chapter 5). In addition, experimental data suggest that the probability of a loss of control over trunk motion might increase with additional challenges, such as when breathing is challenged (McGill et al. 1995; Hodges et al. 2001), when a cognitive dual task is performed (Brereton and McGill 1999), after sustained trunk bending has caused ligament creep (Sanchez-Zuriaga et al. 2010, see also Chapter 14), or when trunk muscles are fatigued (van Dieën 1996; van Dieën et al. 1998; Granata and Gottipati 2008).

In addition to instability, perturbations of trunk posture and motion have been associated with high tissue loading. High spinal loading due to vigorous muscular responses has been shown to occur when mechanical perturbations cause balance loss (Oddsson et al. 1999; Mannion et al. 2000; van der Burg et al. 2005b), in line with the epidemiological association between balance loss and LBP.

Differences in motor behaviour during a given task have been shown to have potent effects on spinal loading. To give some examples:

- The use of strategies such as tilting and sliding of loads and use of hand support during lifting can strongly affect back loads (Faber et al. 2007).
- Speed of movement has a strong effect on back load in lifting (Davis and Marras 2000).
- Sustained trunk bending, for example in slouched sitting, induces ligament creep, which has been associated with ligamentous injury in animal experiments (Solomonow et al. 2003, see also Chapter 14).
- Increased co-activation of trunk muscles has been shown to have substantial effects on spinal compression and shear forces in lifting tasks (Granata and Marras 1995; van Dieën and de Looze 1999; de Looze et al. 1999).

Conclusion

We contend that the data reviewed above suggest that it is feasible that the way we move and control our trunk muscles might cause excessive strains of spinal tissues, and thus contribute to the development of LBP. The probability of such a loss of control would be determined by both individual traits (i.e. motor skill) and situational factors (e.g. presence of degenerative changes, fatigue and task demands). The literature reviewed also indicates that 'inefficient' motor control strategies may cause unnecessarily high, frequent, or sustained loading and that such loading can be a cause of LBP. At present, we can conclude that causal relationships are biologically plausible but far from proven.

EFFECT

To determine if LBP causes motor control changes, one would have to manipulate pain (and nothing else). This is, however, difficult if not impossible. The most obvious approach is to use a noxious stimulus such as an injection of hypertonic saline into the low back musculature. However, motor control changes might be a result of the nociceptive signal itself, of pain, or of associated cognitive factors such as fear (see Chapter 11). In light of the fact that nociception is a potent modulator of pain (although it is neither sufficient nor necessary), and for the sake of synthesizing the relevant work into one overview, we will use 'pain' to encompass nociception, pain and pain-related cognitions.

Two models that predict effects of pain on motor control have gained substantial influence in science and clinical practice: the pain–spasm–pain model (Travell et al. 1942;

Wyke 1987; Johansson and Sojka 1991) and the pain-adaptation model (Lund et al. 1991). Both propose that pain results in predictable (though different) changes in motor behaviour through simple 'hard-wired' mechanisms. As is evident from the large variability in findings reviewed above, predictions of these models with respect to LBP are not confirmed by experimental data on clinical pain (van Dieën et al. 2003b).

In this section, we first review effects of experimentally delivered noxious stimuli, and next consider studies on clinical LBP with a focus on the time course of pain and motor control changes. The latter might provide support for a causal relationship between pain and motor control, where differences in motor control between patients and healthy controls do not exist prior to the incidence of LBP, and where differences in motor control disappear when pain disappears.

Motor control and experimentally induced pain

Pain induced through injection of hypertonic saline in the LES coincided with an increase in LES activity in sitting, which appeared to be correlated with pain intensity (Cobb et al. 1975). Experimentally induced pain also coincided with an increased activity of the LES during gait, a pattern of activation similar to that observed in people with chronic LBP (Arendt-Nielsen et al. 1996; Lamoth et al. 2004). Furthermore, and again similar to changes in clinical studies, increased LES activity in end-of-range flexion was found (Zedka et al. 1999). However, Zedka et al. (1999) found no effects on LES stretch reflex amplitude, no changes during trunk bending movements and even a reduced LES activity during trunk extension movements. In a recent, unpublished experiment, induced pain had variable effects on the instant of activation of several superficial trunk muscles in self-induced perturbations. There was a tendency for all participants to have increased activity of at least one of the superficial muscles, but which muscles varied between participants. However, the activation of the TA muscle appeared to be consistently delayed during voluntary arm movements, again in a manner similar to that observed in people with chronic LBP (Hodges et al. 2003; Moseley et al. 2004b).

With induced pain, trunk muscle activation times became less variable over repeated self-induced perturbations in a subgroup of subjects and this effect was associated with negative pain-related cognitions (Moseley and Hodges 2006). In apparent contrast with induced pain, trunk muscle activity was found to be more variable over stride cycles in gait (Lamoth et al. 2004). In addition, force variability in isometric trunk extensions increased with experimentally induced pain through electrical stimulation of the skin, although only at high (75% of maximum) force levels (Descarreaux et al. 2005a). Trunk kinematics in gait were not affected by experimentally induced LBP (Lamoth et al. 2004), while trunk motions in standing sway were decreased coinciding with compensatory increases in knee motion to control postural sway (Smith et al. 2005).

Motor control during remission or after recovery from LBP

Only very few longitudinal studies on motor control in relation to LBP are available. In a study by Reeves et al. (2006), it was found that imbalance in activation between LES and TES was not manifest before the onset of LBP, suggesting that this imbalance was a consequence rather than a cause of LBP. On the other hand, the imbalance remained after recovery from LBP, indicating that the presence of pain does not directly determine this change in motor control.

Cholewicki et al. (2002) studied trunk muscle responses to perturbations of trunk posture. Delayed responses were present after recovery from LBP, but a later study (Cholewicki et al. 2005) revealed that these delayed responses were also predictive of future LBP, suggesting that the changes are a cause a rather than an effect of LBP, although it should be noted that only a small number of the participants had not previously suffered LBP.

Hodges and Richardson (1996) studied transverse abdominus muscle activation in response to self-induced perturbations in subjects with a history of LBP. They found delayed activation of the muscle relative to the onset of the perturbation. Similarly, MacDonald et al. (2009) studied extensor muscle activation in response to self-induced and externally induced, unpredictable (Macdonald et al. 2010) trunk perturbations during remission of LBP. The deep parts of the multifidus muscle were active earlier than the more superficial parts in the healthy participants and on the non-painful side in the remission group, but not on the previously painful side in the remission group. Thus, activity of deep back muscles is different in people with a recurrent unilateral LBP, despite the resolution of symptoms.

Conclusion

The replication of some of the findings from clinical studies in experiments with induced pain strongly supports the idea that noxious stimulation, or pain, or cognitive variables associated with both, or any combination of these three, causes changes in motor control. The literature also shows some disparities between motor control changes in clinical, chronic LBP and in experimentally induced LBP, but given the inconsistencies among clinical studies these disparities are difficult to interpret. Longitudinal studies show that some motor control changes may linger after pain has disappeared or is in remission. This indicates that these motor control changes are not direct

effects of the presence of pain, but leaves the possibility that they are triggered by pain to then remain in place, that they are effects of noxious stimulation (which can occur without pain), or effects of cognitions often associated with pain. Although effects of experimentally induced and clinical pain were not replicated by performance of a cognitive stressful task (Moseley et al. 2004b), anticipated experimental back pain did replicate the effect of pain, at least with regard to postural activation of the trunk muscles during voluntary arm movements (Moseley et al. 2004a). In further support of an indirect relationship between pain and motor control changes through pain-related cognitions is the finding that pain coping strategies – catastrophizing and distraction – relate to motor control changes in people with LBP (van der Hulst et al. 2010c), but pain intensity does not (van der Hulst et al. 2010b).

ARE MOTOR CONTROL CHANGES THAT COINCIDE WITH LBP ADAPTIVE OR MALADAPTIVE?

Generally, human motor control rapidly adapts to changing circumstances and there is little reason to assume to that the presence of pain would not be a very strong stimulus for motor control changes. Motor control changes may thus reflect adaptive responses triggered by noxious stimulation, pain, or by pain-related cognitions. Like pain itself, these responses may be functional, but also like pain, they may persist beyond the need for them to do so.

Chapters 5 and 6 have extensively discussed the question of the adaptive value of motor control changes with LBP. These chapters have emphasized adaptive aspects in providing a more robust control (van Dieën et al. 2003a), but also indicate that these changes may have adverse long-term consequences, such as increased joint loading (Marras et al. 2001, 2004; Healey et al. 2005), increased muscle fatigue (van Dieën et al. 2009), and impaired balance control (Mok et al. 2004, 2007). Furthermore, pain may coincide with a reduction in motor variability (Moseley and Hodges 2006; Jacobs et al. 2009a), which may hamper behavioural flexibility and re-learning of normal control. Chapter 11 proposed that, insofar as acute pain is often adaptive and helpful but chronic pain is often not, motor control changes may be similarly helpful in the short term but problematic later.

The variance of motor control changes between LBP patients may also be relevant clinically. Some adaptive responses may be more effective than other responses and also differences in adverse side effects may be present. This may suggest approaches for sub-grouping of patients for motor control interventions. Finally, an important question will be whether an underlying disorder (still) requires motor control adaptations in an individual patient or whether alternative control strategies can, and should, be explored.

CONCLUSIONS AND CLINICAL IMPLICATIONS

Poor motor control may play a role in causation of LBP, but the relationship with LBP incidence requires further confirmation. Furthermore, the evidence suggests a limited contribution of individual motor skill and hence primary prevention efforts through motor control training are unlikely to be cost-effective. However, in secondary prevention, there may well be a role for motor control training to avoid loss of control and to redress inefficient control strategies. Furthermore, because motor control changes appear to be caused by noxious stimulation, pain, pain-related cognitions, or all three, there may be a role for motor control training in secondary prevention to either enhance adaptive changes or to de-learn such previously adaptive changes, when these are no longer needed. To support clinical decision-making, longitudinal studies are needed to disentangle the adaptive and maladaptive aspects of motor control changes that coincide with pain.

REFERENCES

Alexiev, A.R., 1994. Some differences of the electromyographic erector spinae activity between normal subjects and low back pain patients during the generation of isometric trunk torque. Electromyogr Clin Neurophysiol 34, 495–499.

Arena, J.G., Sherman, R.A., Bruno, G.M., Young, T.R., 1989. Electromyographic recordings of 5 types of low back pain subjects and non-pain controls in different positions. Pain 37, 57–65.

Arena, J.G., Sherman, R.A., Bruno, G.M., Young, T.R., 1991. Electromyographic recordings of low back pain subjects and non-pain controls in six different positions: effect of pain levels. Pain 45, 23–28.

Arendt-Nielsen, L., Graven-Nielsen, T., Svarrer, H., Svensson, P., 1996. The influence of low back pain on muscle activity and coordination during gait: a clinical and experimental study. Pain 64, 231–240.

Boston, J.R., Rudy, T.E., Lieber, S.J., Stacey, B.R., 1995. Measuring treatment effects on repetitive lifting for patients with chronic low back pain: speed, style, and coordination. J Spinal Disord 8, 342–351.

Boston, J.R., Rudy, T.E., Mercer, S.R., Kubinski, J.A., 1993. A measure of body movement coordination during repetitive dynamic lifting. IEEE Trans Rehabil Eng 1, 137–144.

Brereton, L.C., McGill, S.M., 1999. Effects of physical fatigue and cognitive challenges on the potential for low back injury. Hum Move Sci 18, 839–857.

Brown, S.H., Howarth, S.J., McGill, S.M., 2005. Spine stability and the role of many muscles. Arch Phys Med Rehabil 86, 1890; author reply 1890–1891.

Cholewicki, J., Greene, H.S., Polzhofer, G.K., Galloway, M.T., Shah, R.A., Radebold, A., 2002. Neuromuscular function in athletes following recovery from a recent acute low back injury. Journal of Orthopaedic & Sports Physical Therapy 32, 568–575.

Cholewicki, J., McGill, S.M., 1996a. Mechanical stability of the in vivo lumbar spine: implications for injury and chronic low back pain. Clin Biomech (Bristol, Avon) 11, 1–15.

Cholewicki, J., McGill, S.M., 1996b. Mechanical stability of the in-vivo lumbar spine – implications for injury and chronic low-back-pain. Clinical Biomechanics 11, 1–15.

Cholewicki, J., Silfies, S.P., Shah, R.A., Greene, H.S., Reeves, N.P., Alvi, K., et al., 2005. Delayed trunk muscle reflex responses increase the risk of low back injuries. Spine 30, 2614–2620.

Cholewicki, J., Simons, A.P.D., Radebold, A., 2000. Effects of external trunk loads on lumbar spine stability. J Biomech 33, 1377–1385.

Cobb, C.R., DeVries, H.A., Urban, R.T., Luekens, C.A., Bagg, R.J., 1975. Electrical activity in muscle pain. Am J Phys Med 54, 80–87.

Commissaris, D.A.C.M., Nilsson-Wikmar, L.B., van Dieën, J.H., Hirschfeld, H., 2002. Joint co-ordination during whole-body lifting in women with low-back pain following pregnancy. Arch Phys Med Rehabil 83, 1279–1289.

Cox, M.E., Asselin, S., Gracovetsky, S.A., Richards, M.P., Newman, N.M., Karakusevic, V., et al., 2000. Relationship between functional evaluation measures and self-assessment in nonacute low back pain. Spine 25, 1817–1826.

Cram, J.R., Steger, J.C., 1983. EMG scanning in the diagnosis of chronic pain. Biofeed Self-Reg 8, 229–241.

Davis, K.G., Marras, W.S., 2000. The effects of motion on trunk biomechanics. Clin Biomech 15, 703–717.

Descarreaux, M., Blouin, J.S., Teasdale, N., 2005a. Isometric force production parameters during normal and experimental low back pain conditions. BMC Musculoskeletal Disord 6.

Descarreaux, M., Blouin, J.S., Teasdale, N., 2005b. Repositioning accuracy and movement parameters in low back pain subjects and healthy control subjects. Eur Spine J 14, 185–191.

Esola, M.A., Mcclure, P.W., Fitzgerald, G.K., Siegler, S., 1996. Analysis of lumbar spine and hip motion during forward bending in subjects with and without a history of low-back-pain. Spine 21, 71–78.

Faber, G., Kingma, I., van Dieën, J.H., 2007. The effects of ergonomic interventions on low back moments are attenuated by changes in lifting behaviour. Ergonomics 50, 1377–1391.

Grabiner, M.D., Koh, T.J., El Ghazawi, A., 1992. Decoupling of bilateral paraspinal excitation in subjects with low back pain. Spine 17, 1219–1223.

Granata, K.P., Gottipati, P., 2008. Fatigue influences the dynamic stability of the torso. Ergonomics 51, 1258–1271.

Granata, K.P., Marras, W.S., 1995. The influence of trunk muscle coactivity on dynamic spinal loads. Spine 20, 913–919.

Healey, E.L., Fowler, N.E., Burden, A.M., McEwan, I.M., 2005. Raised paraspinal muscle activity reduces rate of stature recovery after loaded exercise in individuals with chronic low back pain. Arch Phys Med Rehabil 86, 710–715.

Hodges, P., Richardson, C., Jull, G., 1996. Evaluation of the relationship between laboratory and clinical tests of transversus abdominis function. Physiother Res Int 1, 30–40.

Hodges, P.W., 1999. Is there a role for transversus abdominis in lumbopelvic stability? Man Ther 4, 74–86.

Hodges, P.W., Galea, M.P., Holm, S., Holm, A.K., 2009. Corticomotor excitability of back muscles is affected by intervertebral disc lesion in pigs. Eur J Neurosci 29, 1490–1500.

Hodges, P.W., Heijnen, I., Gandevia, S.C., 2001. Postural activity of the diaphragm is reduced in humans when respiratory demand increases. J Physiol 37, 99–1008.

Hodges, P.W., Moseley, G.L., 2003. Pain and motor control of the lumbopelvic region: effect and possible mechanisms. J Electromyogr Kinesiol 13, 361–370.

Hodges, P.W., Moseley, G.L., Gabrielsson, A., Gandevia, S.C., 2003. Experimental muscle pain changes feedforward postural responses of the trunk muscles. Exper Brain Res 151, 262–271.

Hodges, P.W., Richardson, C.A., 1996. Inefficient muscular stabilization of the lumbar spine associated with low back pain. A motor control evaluation of transversus abdominis. Spine 21, 2640–2650.

Hoogendoorn, W.E., Bongers, P.M., de Vet, H.C., Douwes, M., Koes, B.W., Miedema, M.C., et al., 2000. Flexion and rotation of the trunk and lifting at work are risk factors for low back pain: results of a prospective cohort study. Spine 25, 3087–3092.

Hoogendoorn, W.E., van Poppel, M.N.M., Bongers, P.M., Koes, B.W., Bouter, L.M., 1999. Physical load during work and leisure time as risk factors for back pain. Scand J Work, Environ Health 25, 387–403.

Hoyt, W.H., Hunt Jr., H.H., De Pauw, M.A., Bard, D., Shaffer, F., Passias, J.N., et al., 1981. Electromyographic assessment of chronic low-back pain syndrome. J Am Osteopath Assoc 80, 728–730.

Jacobs, J., Henry, S., Nagle, K., 2009a. Low back pain associates with altered activity of the cerebral cortex prior to amr movements that require anticipatory postural adjustments of the trunk. In: Chiari, L., Nardone, A. (eds), XIX Conference of the International Society for Posture & Gait Research. DEIS – Universita di Bolhna, Bologna, p. 184.

Jacobs, J.V., Henry, S.M., Nagle, K.J., 2009b. People with chronic low back pain exhibit decreased variability in the timing of their anticipatory postural adjustments. Behav Neurosci 123, 455–458.

Jayaraman, G., Nazre, A., McCann, V., Redford, J., 1994. A computerized technique for analyzing lateral bending of subjects with normal and impaired lumbar spine. Spine 19, 824–832.

Johansson, H., Sojka, P., 1991. Pathophysiological mechanisms involved in genesis and spread of muscular tension in occupational muscle pain and in chronic musculoskeletal pain syndromes. A hypothesis. Med Hypotheses 35, 196–203.

Kaigle, A.M., Wessberg, P., Hansson, T.H., 1998. Muscular and kinematic behavior of the lumbar spine during flexion-extension. J Spinal Dis 11, 163–174.

Lamoth, C.J., Daffertshofer, A., Meijer, O.G., Beek, P.J., 2006a. How do persons with chronic low back pain speed up and slow down? Trunk–pelvis coordination and lumbar erector spinae activity during gait. Gait Posture 23, 230–239.

Lamoth, C.J., Daffertshofer, A., Meijer, O.G., Lorimer Moseley, G., Wuisman, P.I., Beek, P.J., 2004. Effects of experimentally induced pain and fear of pain on trunk coordination and back muscle activity during walking. Clin Biomech 19, 551–563.

Lamoth, C.J., Meijer, O.G., Daffertshofer, A., Wuisman, P.I., Beek, P.J., 2006b. Effects of chronic low back pain on trunk coordination and back muscle activity during walking: changes in motor control. Eur Spine J 15, 23–40.

Lamoth, C.J.C., Meijer, O.G., Wuisman, P.I.J.M., van Dieën, J.H., Levin, M.F., Beek, P.J., 2002. Pelvis-thorax coordination in the transversal plane during walking in subjects with non-specific low back pain. Spine 27, E92–E99.

Lehman, G.J., 2004. Biomechanical assessments of lumbar spinal function. How low back pain sufferers differ from normals. Implications for outcome measures research. Part I: Kinematic assessments of lumbar function. J Manipulative Physiol Ther 27, 57–62.

Lindgren, K., Sihvonen, T., Leino, E., Pitkanen, M., 1993. Exercise therapy effects on functional radiographic findings and segmental electromyographic activity in lumbar spine instability. Arch Phys Med Rehabil 74, 933–939.

de Looze, M.P., Groen, H., Horemans, H., Kingma, I., van Dieën, J.H., 1999. Abdominal muscles contribute in a minor way to peak spinal compression in lifting. J Biomech 32, 655–662.

Lotters, F., Burdorf, A., Kuiper, J., Miedema, H., 2003. Model for the work-relatedness of low-back pain. Scand J Work, Environ Health 29, 431–440.

Lund, J.P., Donga, R., Widmer, C.G., Stohler, C.S., 1991. The pain-adaptation model: a discussion of the relationship between chronic musculoskeletal pain and motor activity. Canad J Physiol Pharmacol 69, 683–694.

Lynn, B., 1996. Neurogenic inflammation caused by cutaneous polymodal receptors. Prog Brain Res 113, 361–368.

MacDonald, D., Moseley, G.L., Hodges, P.W., 2009. Why do some patients keep hurting their back? Evidence of ongoing back muscle dysfunction during remission from recurrent back pain. Pain 142, 183–188.

Macdonald, D., Moseley, G.L., Hodges, P.W., 2010. People with recurrent low back pain respond differently to trunk loading despite remission from symptoms. Spine 35, 818–824.

Magnusson, M.L., Aleksiev, A.R., Wilder, D.G., Pope, M.H., Spratt, K.F., Lee, S.H., et al., 1996. Unexpected load and asymmetric posture as etiologic factors in low back pain. Eur Spine J 5, 23–35.

Manning, D.P., Shannon, H.S., 1981. Slipping accidents causing low-back pain in a gearbox factory. Spine 6, 70–72.

Mannion, A.F., Adams, M.A., Dolan, P., 2000. Sudden and unexpected loading generates high forces on the lumbar spine. Spine 25, 842–852.

Marras, W.S., Davis, K.G., Ferguson, S.A., Lucas, B.R., Gupta, P., 2001. Spine loading characteristics of patients with low back pain compared with asymptomatic individuals. Spine 26, 2566–2574.

Marras, W.S., Ferguson, S.A., Burr, D., Davis, K.G., Gupta, P., 2004. Spine loading in patients with low back pain during asymmetric lifting exertions. Spine J 4, 64–75.

Marras, W.S., Ferguson, S.A., Burr, D., Davis, K.G., Gupta, P., 2005. Functional impairment as a predictor of spine loading. Spine 30, 729–737.

Marras, W.S., Ferguson, S.A., Gupta, P., Bose, S., Parnianpour, M., Kim, J.Y., et al., 1999. The quantification of low back disorder using motion measures. Methodology and validation. Spine 24, 2091–2100.

Marras, W.S., Parnianpour, M., Ferguson, S.A., Kim, J.Y., Crowell, R.R., Bose, S., et al., 1995. The classification of anatomic- and symptom-based low back disorders using motion measure models. Spine 20, 2531–2546.

Mayer, T.G., Tencer, A.F., Kristoferson, S., Mooney, V., 1984. Use of non-invasive techniques for quantification of spinal range of motion in normal subjects and chronic low-back dysfunction patients. Spine 9, 588–595.

McGill, S.M., Sharratt, M.T., Seguin, J.P., 1995. Loads on spinal tissues during simultaneous lifting and ventilatory challenge. Ergonomics 38, 1772–1792.

Mok, N.W., Brauer, S.G., Hodges, P.W., 2004. Hip strategy for balance control in quiet standing is reduced in people with low back pain. Spine 29, E107–E112.

Mok, N.W., Brauer, S.G., Hodges, P.W., 2007. Failure to use movement in postural strategies leads to increased spinal displacement in low back pain. Spine (Phila PA 1976) 32, E537–E543.

Moseley, G.L., 2004a. Evidence for a direct relationship between cognitive and physical change during an education intervention in people with chronic low back pain. Eur J Pain 8, 39–45.

Moseley, G.L., 2004b. Impaired trunk muscle function in sub-acute neck pain: etiologic in the subsequent development of low back pain? Man Ther 9, 157–163.

Moseley, G.L., Hodges, P.W., 2006. Reduced variability of postural strategy prevents normalization of motor changes induced by back pain: a risk factor for chronic trouble? Behav Neurosci 120, 474–476.

Moseley, G.L., Nicholas, M.K., Hodges, P.W., 2004a. Does anticipation of back pain predispose to back trouble? Brain 127, 2339–2347.

Moseley, G.L., Nicholas, M.K., Hodges, P.W., 2004b. Pain differs from non-painful attention-demanding or stressful tasks in its effect on postural control patterns of trunk muscles. Exp Brain Res 156, 64–71.

O'Sullivan, P., Twomey, L., Allison, G., Sinclair, J., Miller, K., 1997. Altered patterns of abdominal muscle activation in patients with chronic low back pain. Aust J Physiother 43, 91–98.

Oddsson, L.I.E., Persson, T., Cresswell, A.G., Thorstensson, A., 1999. Interaction between voluntary and postural motor commands during perturbed lifting. Spine 24, 545–552.

Panjabi, M.M., 1992a. The stabilizing system of the spine. Part I. Function, dysfunction, adaptation, and enhancement. J Spinal Disord 5, 383–389; discussion 397.

Panjabi, M.M., 1992b. The stabilizing system of the spine. Part II. Neutral zone and instability hypothesis. J Spinal Disord 5, 390–397.

Paquet, N., Malouin, F., Richards, C.L., 1994. Hip–spine movement interaction and muscle activation patterns during sagittal trunk movements in low back pain patients. Spine 19, 596–603.

Porter, J.L., Wilkinson, A., 1997. Lumbar–hip flexion motion. A comparative study between asymptomatic and chronic low back pain in 18- to 36-year old men. Spine 22, 1508–1514.

Punnett, L., Fine, L.J., Keyserling, W.M., Herrin, G.D., Chaffin, D.B., 1991. Back disorders and nonneutral trunk postures of automobile assembly workers. Scand J Work, Environ Health 17, 337–346.

Radebold, A., Cholewicki, J., Panjabi, M.M., Patel, T.C., 2000. Muscle response pattern to sudden trunk loading in healthy individuals and in patients with chronic low back pain. Spine 25, 947–954.

Radebold, A., Cholewicki, J., Polzhofer, G.K., Greene, H.S., 2001. Impaired postural control of the lumbar spine is associated with delayed muscle response times in patients with chronic idiopathic low back pain. Spine 26, 724–730.

Reeves, N.P., Cholewicki, J., Milner, T.E., 2005. Muscle reflex classification of low-back pain. J Electromyogr Kinesiol 15, 53–60.

Reeves, N.P., Cholewicki, J., Silfies, S.P., 2006. Muscle activation imbalance and low-back injury in varsity athletes. J Electromyogr Kinesiol 16, 264–272.

Rudy, T.E., Boston, J.R., Lieber, S.J., Kubinski, J.A., Delitto, A., 1995. Body motion patterns during a novel repetitive wheel-rotation task – a comparative-study of healthy-subjects and patients with low-back-pain. Spine 20, 2547–2554.

Sanchez-Zuriaga, D., Adams, M.A., Dolan, P., 2010. Is activation of the back muscles impaired by creep or muscle fatigue? Spine 35, 517–525.

Selles, R.W., Wagenaar, R.C., Smit, T.H., Wuisman, P.I., 2001. Disorders in trunk rotation during walking in patients with low back pain: a dynamical systems approach. Clin Biomech 16, 175–181.

Silfies, S.P., Cholewicki, J., Reeves, N.P., Greene, H.S., 2007. Lumbar position sense and the risk of low back injuries in college athletes: a prospective cohort study. BMC Musculoskelet Disorders 8.

Smith, M., Coppieters, M.W., Hodges, P.W., 2005. Effect of experimentally induced low back pain on postural sway with breathing. Exper Brain Res 166, 109–117.

Solomonow, M., Baratta, R.V., Zhou, B.-H., Burger, E., Zieske, A., Gedalia, A., 2003. Muscular dysfunction elicited by creep of lumbar viscoelastic tissues. J Electromyogr Kinesiol 13, 381–396.

Stergioulas, A., Filippou, D.K., Triga, A., Grigoriadis, E., Shipkov, C.D., 2004. Low back pain in physical education teachers. Folia Med (Plovdiv) 46, 51–55.

Stokes, I.A.F., Gardner-Morse, M., Henry, S.M., Badger, G.J., 2000. Decrease in trunk muscular response to perturbation with preactivation of lumbar spinal musculature. Spine 25, 1957–1964.

Sward, L., Hellstrom, M., Jacobsson, B., Nyman, R., Peterson, L., 1991. Disc degeneration and associated abnormalities of the spine in elite gymnasts. A magnetic resonance imaging study. Spine (Phila PA 1976) 16, 437–443.

Sward, L., Hellstrom, M., Jacobsson, B., Peterson, L., 1990. Back pain and radiologic changes in the thoracolumbar spine of athletes. Spine (Phila PA 1976) 15, 124–129.

Takala, E.P., Viikari-Juntura, E., 2000. Do functional test predict low back pain? Spine 25, 2126–2132.

Travell, J., Rinzter, S., Herman, M., 1942. Pain and disability of the shoulder and arm. JAMA 120, 417–422.

Triano, J.J., Luttges, M., 1985. Myoelectric paraspinal response to spinal loads: potential for monitoring low back pain. J Manip Physiol Ther 8, 17–145.

Tsao, H., Galea, M.P., Hodges, P.W., 2008. Reorganization of the motor cortex is associated with postural control deficits in recurrent low back pain. Brain 131, 2161–2171.

Tsuboi, H., Takeuchi, K., Watanabe, M., Hori, R., Kobayashi, F., 2002. Psychosocial factors related to low back pain among school personnel in Nagoya, Japan. Ind Health 40, 266–271.

van der Burg, J.C.E., Casius, L.J.R., Kingma, I., van Dieën, J.H., van Soest, A.J., 2005a. Factors underlying the perturbation resistance of the trunk in the first part of a lifting movement. Biol Cybernet 93, 54–62.

van der Burg, J.C.E., van Dieën, J.H., Toussaint, H.M., 2000. Lifting an unexpectedly heavy object: the effects on low-back loading and control of balance. Clin Biomech 15, 469–477.

van der Burg, J.C.E., Kingma, I., van Dieën, J.H., 2003. Effects of unexpected lateral mass placement on trunk loading in lifting. Spine 28, 764–770.

van der Burg, J.C.E., Kingma, I., van Dieën, J.H., 2004. Is the trunk movement more perturbed after an asymmetric than after a symmetric perturbation during lifting? J Biomech 37, 1071–1077.

van der Burg, J.C.E., Pijnappels, M., van Dieën, J.H., 2005b. Out-of-plane trunk movements and trunk muscle activity after a trip during walking. Exper Brain Res, 165, 407–412.

van der Hulst, M., Vollenbroek-Hutten, M.M., Rietman, J.S., Hermens, H.J., 2010a. Lumbar and abdominal muscle activity during walking in subjects with chronic low back pain: support of the 'guarding' hypothesis? J Electromyogr Kinesiol 20, 31–38.

van der Hulst, M., Vollenbroek-Hutten, M.M., Rietrnan, J.S., Schaake, L., Groothuis-Oudshoorn, K.G., Hermens, H.J., 2010b. Back muscle activation patterns in chronic low back pain during walking: a 'guarding' hypothesis. Clin J Pain 26, 30–37.

van der Hulst, M., Vollenbroek-Hutten, M.M., Schreurs, K.M., Rietman, J.S., Hermens, H.J., 2010c. Relationships between coping strategies and lumbar muscle activity in subjects with chronic low back pain. Eur J Pain 14, 640–647.

van Dieën, J.H., 1996. Asymmetry of erector spinae muscle-activity in twisted postures and consistency of muscle activation patterns across subjects. Spine 21, 2651–2661.

van Dieën, J.H., Cholewicki, J., Radebold, A., 2003a. Trunk muscle recruitment patterns in patients with low back pain enhance the stability of the lumbar spine. Spine 28, 834–841.

van Dieën, J.H., Koppes, L., Twisk, J., 2010. Low-back pain history and postural sway in unstable sitting. Spine 35, 812–817.

van Dieën, J.H., van der Beek, A.J., 2009. Work-related low-back pain: biomechanical factors and primary prevention. In: Shrawan, Kumar (ed.), Ergonomics for Rehabilitation Professionals. CRC Press, Boca Raton, FL, pp. 359–395.

van Dieën, J.H., van der Burg, P., Raaijmakers, T.A.J., Toussaint, H.M., 1998. Effects of repetitive lifting on the kinematics, inadequate anticipatory control or adaptive changes? J Motor Behav 30, 20–32.

van Dieën, J.H., de Looze, M.P., 1999. Sensitivity of single-equivalent trunk extensor muscle models to anatomical and functional assumptions. J Biomech 32, 195–198.

van Dieën, J.H., Selen, L.P.J., Cholewicki, J., 2003. Trunk muscle activation in low-back pain patients, an analysis of the literature. J Electromyogr Kinesiol 13, 333–351.

van Dieën, J.H., Weinans, H., Toussaint, H.M., 1999. Fractures of the lumbar vertebral endplate in the etiology of low back pain. A hypothesis on the causative role of spinal compression in aspecific low back pain. Medical Hypotheses 53, 246–252.

van Dieën, J.H., Westebring-van der Putten, E., Kingma, I., de Looze, M.P., 2009. Low-level activity of trunk extensor muscles causes electromyographic manifestations of fatigue in absence of decreased oxygenation. J Electromyogr Kinesiol 19, 398–406.

Videman, T., Sarna, S., Battie, M.C., Koskinen, S., Gill, K., Paananen, H., et al., 1995. The long-term effects of physical loading and exercise lifestyles on back-related symptoms, disability, and spinal pathology among men. Spine (Phila PA 1976) 20, 699–709.

Wallwork, T.L., Stanton, W.R., Freke, M., Hides, J.A., 2009. The effect of chronic low back pain on size and contraction of the lumbar multifidus muscle. Man Ther 14, 496–500.

Watson, P.J., Booker, C.K., Main, C.J., 1997. Evidence for the role of psychological factors in abnormal paraspinal activity in patients with chronic low back pain. J Musculo Pain 5, 41–56.

Wong, T.K.T., Lee, R.Y.W., 2004. Effects of low back pain on the relationship between the movements of the lumbar spine and hip. Hum Move Sci 23, 21–34.

Wyke, B.D., 1987. The neurology of back pain. In: Jayson, M.I.V. (ed), The Lumbar Spine and Back Pain. Churchill Livingstone, Edinburgh.

Zedka, M., Prochazka, A., Knight, B., Gillard, D., Gauthier, M., 1999. Voluntary and reflex control of human back muscles during induced pain. J Physiol 520, 591–604.

Chapter |19|

What is the relation between proprioception and low back pain?

Simon Brumagne*, Patricia Dolan† and Joel G. Pickar‡
*Department of Rehabilitation Sciences, University of Leuven, Leuven, Belgium, †Centre for Comparative and Clinical Anatomy, University of Bristol, Bristol, UK, and ‡Palmer Center for Chiropractic Research, Palmer College of Chiropractic, Davenport, Iowa, USA

INTRODUCTION

This chapter focuses on the role of proprioception in sensorimotor control of the spine and considers the specific contribution of its sensory components in preventing tissue overload and injury. The importance of impaired proprioception in individuals with low back pain is discussed, as are the methods used to evaluate its effects. The final section considers whether proprioception can be improved by training, and discusses the potential benefits this may have for patients with low back pain.

DEFINITION OF PROPRIOCEPTION

The somatosensory system conveys information about touch and proprioception. While touch is a straightforward sensation familiar to us as clinicians and scientists, proprioception is a mysterious sense, because we are largely unaware of it during activities of daily living. Only in certain conditions does this sensation become conscious (e.g. kinaesthetic illusions during muscle vibration). However, the term 'proprioception', first used by Sherrington at the start of the twentieth century (Sherrington 1900), is generally used to describe 'the unconscious perception of movement and spatial orientation arising from stimuli within the body' (*Stedman's Medical Dictionary* 2002).

Based upon neurophysiological studies, convention has identified four components of proprioception: (i) the kinaesthetic sense or kinaesthesia (i.e. sense of position and movement sense) (Bastian 1888); (ii) sense of tension or force; (iii) sense of balance; and (iv) sense of effort or heaviness (Proske 2005). In the literature and in the clinic, most attention is focused on the kinaesthetic sense, namely that of position and movement.

The current (but not universal) view is that kinaesthetic sense is provided predominantly by muscle spindles with some contribution from skin and joint receptors; the sensation of force is provided by Golgi tendon organs; and the sense of balance is provided by the vestibular system. Sense of effort, which should be distinguished from the peripheral sense of force, is thought to be a central phenomenon that is generated somewhere upstream of the motor cortex (Gandevia et al. 1992; Gandevia 1996; Proske 2005; Proske and Gandevia 2009).

Evidently some proprioceptors such as the muscle spindles and Golgi tendon organs can act in isolation to produce spinal reflexes without the need for any higher input. This enables them to initiate rapid and forceful muscle contractions in response to sudden perturbations in order to prevent tissue injury. However, proprioceptors also play a central role in the maintenance of posture and in the control of voluntary movement. This relies upon intricate and complex circuitry in both the spinal cord and higher centres for these afferent inputs which must be integrated and processed in order to produce the most appropriate motor response. A strong relation therefore exists between the somatosensory system and the motor control system, hence the term sensorimotor control, which is now used frequently to describe the interplay between these two systems. However, it might be important and fruitful to look at the specific contribution from the sensory part, if it is possible to disentangle the sensory from the motor component.

THE PROPRIOCEPTORS IMPORTANT FOR MOTOR CONTROL OF THE SPINE

Our knowledge of peripheral proprioceptive pathways has developed predominantly from studies in the limbs. While muscle, skin and joint receptors are thought to contribute to the sense of position and movement, current opinion considers the muscle spindle as the most important source for proprioceptive feedback, in particular for detecting the direction of movement. The relative contributions of skin and joint receptors may vary between different regions of the body (Collins et al. 2005). Muscle spindles in particular may provide a reliable source of proprioceptive information for joints crossed by uni-articular muscles.

Based upon the muscle vibration studies of Goodwin et al. (1972), position sense and movement sense in the limbs are derived primarily from muscle spindles and not from joint receptors, as previously believed. In principle, activation of low threshold, mechanically sensitive joint receptors could serve a proprioceptive function if their discharge depended upon the degree to which the joint capsule is loaded over the range of physiological movement. Unless the capsule is mechanically loaded, there is no reason to expect that embedded receptive endings would evoke a neural signal. A substantial number of studies in the limb joints show that very few joint receptors respond in the mid-range of movement whereas most are responsive at the extremes of joint position and thus serve as limit detectors (reviewed in Gandevia 1996). At finger and elbow joints, the joint capsule does not deform during flexion movements and therefore is not the likely source of information enabling individuals to detect the direction of movement (Hall and McCloskey 1983).

It may not be appropriate to generalize conclusions regarding the proprioceptive role of joint receptors based upon studies of limb joints. In the lumbar spine, the facet capsule is preloaded in the neutral position and can therefore deform without buckling during physiological motion (Ianuzzi et al. 2004). Although it is difficult to record specifically from facet joint capsule afferents in the lumbar spine, a small group of studies suggests that lumbar movement which is not at the extremes of intervertebral joint position can activate facet joint receptors (Pickar and McLain 1995; Yamashita et al. 1990). Facet joint receptors in the lumbar spine may therefore serve a proprioceptive function within the physiological range of movement.

Muscle spindles in the dorsal paraspinal muscles are clearly loaded within the physiological range of low back movement (Cao et al. 2009a). Spindles in the lumbar longissimus and multifidus muscles are more sensitive to vertebral position and to the velocity of vertebral movement than spindles in the arm and leg muscles are to limb position and movement (Cao, et al. 2009a, 2009b). Position sense of the trunk appears at least comparable if not better than that of the appendicular skeleton depending upon the positioning task (Jakobs et al. 1985; Taylor and McCloskey, 1990; Ashton-Miller et al. 1992). The back actually has substantial proprioceptive acuity exhibiting repositioning errors of less than 1 degree in flexion–extension tasks (Jakobs et al. 1985; Ashton-Miller et al. 1992; Brumagne et al. 2000). Rotational repositioning of the trunk appears even more accurate than that in the neck (Taylor and McCloskey 1990) despite neck muscles having the highest density of spindles (Richmond and Abrahams 1975).

Experimentally, muscle vibration is a strong stimulus for muscle spindles evoking not only reflex motor responses (tonic vibration reflex, antagonist vibration reflex) but also sensory effects (illusion of joint movement, muscle lengthening). The sensory effects demonstrate that some muscle spindle input projects to the sensory cortex and evokes conscious awareness. In the limbs, muscle spindles tend to concentrate in the deeper and central portions of muscles, where oxidative extrafusal fibres predominate. In cases where oxidative fibres predominate in the superficial muscle layer, muscle spindles are also located superficially (Kokkorogiannis 2008). In the lumbar spine, examination of fetal tissue indicates that more muscle spindles are located in the intermediate than in either the medial or lateral portion of the low back musculature (Amonoo-Kuofi 1982). On average, the spindles may be superficially located, lying less than a millimetre below the dorsal surface of the back. The number of spindles in the lumbar region appears higher than in the thoracic region but when normalized for muscle area, spindle density is lower in the lumbar region compared to either the thoracic or cervical regions due to the muscle bulk in the lumbar spine (Amonoo-Kuofi 1982, 1983).

In the spine, the small intervertebral muscles, which are mechanically weak and act with short lever arms about the centre of rotation, have a much higher density of muscle spindles compared to the more superficial polysegmental muscles (Nitz and Peck 1986), suggesting that their main role is sensory. The short fibres of these muscles, which run between the spinous and mammillary or transverse processes of adjacent vertebrae, will be subjected to higher relative strains during spinal motion when compared to the long fibres of the paraspinal muscles. Spindles lying within them are likely to be activated more strongly providing greater sensitivity to intervertebral motion. Afferents in these muscles may also initiate efferent activity in motor neurones at neighbouring levels, and the presence of intersegmental reflexes in the lumbar spine (Kang et al. 2002) would help coordinate responses at multiple spinal levels.

While muscle spindles are now thought to be the most important receptors involved in kinaesthesia, cutaneous receptors and joint receptors may also play a role. The contribution from cutaneous receptors appears to be particularly important in some joints, such as those in the fingers, where the muscles controlling their movement lie some distance away. Here, the tendons must cross more than one joint, and it has been suggested that this could lead to less reliable input from muscle receptors (Proske and Gandevia 2009). Under these circumstances, there may be increased dependence upon skin receptors which can monitor joint movement more directly (Collins et al. 2005). The importance of cutaneous receptors in spinal proprioception has received little investigation although a recent study found that tactile stimulation in the neck improved position sense in the cervical spine (Pinsault et al. 2010). It is possible that similar effects may operate in the low back.

Based upon studies in the appendicular skeleton, current thinking concerning joint and ligament receptors is that they probably make only a minor contribution to position sense and movement sense under normal circumstances because the vast majority of them are strongly activated only towards the limit of normal movement when tension within the ligament or capsule is high (Burgess and Clark 1969; Sjölander et al. 2002). However, several studies have identified the presence of low threshold receptors in ligaments and joint capsules that are activated throughout the normal range of movement (Ferrell 1980; Ferrell et al. 1987; Burke et al. 1988). Ligament afferents are known to synapse with spinal motor neurones through interneurones (Sjölander et al. 2002). There is also evidence that they have strong supraspinal projections, including to the cortex (Pitman et al. 1992; Lavender et al. 1999) giving them the capacity to influence both reflex and voluntary control of movement. These findings suggest that ligamentous receptors fulfil several roles, with low threshold receptors providing information to the central nervous system (CNS) about joint position and movement during normal motion, and high threshold receptors acting as limit detectors that help to protect the joint from excessive movement.

In the spine, sensory receptors have been identified in ligaments (Rhalmi et al. 1993), thoracolumbar fascia (Yahia et al. 1992), apophyseal joint capsules (McLain and Pickar 1998) and intervertebral discs (Yamashita et al. 1993a; Roberts et al. 1995). All may potentially contribute to proprioception. Receptors in the thoracolumbar fascia have been little investigated although a recent study found

that removal of the fascia in anaesthetised cats had no mechanical effect on proprioceptive signalling from lumbar paraspinal muscle spindles, at least during small passive vertebral movements (Cao and Pickar 2009). Receptors in the disc (Yamashita et al. 1993a) and a majority of those in the joint capsule (Yamashita et al. 1990, Cavanaugh et al. 1997) are reported to have high mechanical thresholds, suggesting they more likely act as nociceptors when loading is extreme. However, lower threshold mechanosensitive afferents have been identified in the joint capsule, as well as in muscle and tendon (Yamashita et al. 1993a, 1993b), suggesting a role in proprioception. Spinal ligaments have been the subject of considerable interest in recent years and the presence of a specific ligamentomuscular reflex induced by large stretches of the supraspinous ligament has been confirmed in anaesthetized patients and animals (Solomonow et al. 1998). These findings suggest that afferent input from spinal ligaments may be integrated into the proprioceptive input arising from primary and secondary muscle spindle afferents, and in this way may initiate reflex muscle activation via its influence on the gamma-motoneurone-muscle spindle system (Sjölander et al. 2002).

Understanding where in a causal chain proprioceptive deficits related to the muscle spindle can occur is complicated by the fact that muscle spindles are the only somatosensory receptor whose mechanical sensitivity can be adjusted by the CNS. Intrafusal fibres of the muscle spindle apparatus are innervated by gamma-motoneurones whose discharge causes these fibres to contract thereby maintaining the sensitivity of the spindle to stretch. Gamma-motoneurones are thought to be coactivated with the alpha-motoneurones although there is evidence for independent action. During co-activation, despite shortening of the spindle apparatus as the whole muscle shortens, the spindle can remain responsive as the gamma-motoneurones continue to activate the intrafusal fibres. Consequently, proprioceptive deficits related to the muscle spindle could occur at several different levels of the nervous system: within the sensory region of the spindle apparatus; in the CNS where afferent spindle input is integrated; in the CNS where gamma-motoneurones are controlled; and at the motor endplates of the spindle apparatus.

Dramatic changes in the responsiveness of muscle spindles leading to feedback errors occur in experimental situations following maintained postures or positions. When a limb or limb muscle is held in a fixed position for a short period of time, non-recycling crossbridges form which stiffen the spindle at the new length without developing any active force (Hill 1968; Proske et al. 1993). Subsequent passive shortening excessively slackens and unloads the spindle while lengthening excessively tensions it. The direction of conditioning history relative to a reference position determines whether resting spindle discharge is augmented or diminished when compared to its discharge at the identical but non-conditioned reference position

(Morgan et al. 1984; Gregory et al. 1988). This thixotropic behaviour has also been observed in the lumbar spine (Ge and Pickar 2008). Vertebral positions that lengthen the multifidus or longissimus muscles relative to a previously-held reference position increase spindle discharge whereas positions that shorten these muscles decrease it (Ge et al. 2005). In addition vertebral positions that lengthen the paraspinal muscles also decrease the velocity sensitivity of their spindles (Cao and Pickar 2011).

The significance of this intrafusal fibre thixotropy for motor control may lie in the introduction of unpredictability for the timing and magnitude of central neural responses (Hutton and Atwater 1992; Proske et al. 1993). For example, in the limbs, the error in spindle discharge affects spindle-mediated muscle reflexes (Gregory et al. 1987; Gregory et al. 1990). Conditioning directions which hold the limb muscles long versus short produce opposite effects on the magnitude of both deep tendon and H-reflexes (Gregory et al. 1987; Gregory et al. 1990).

In the spinal column, passive changes in vertebral position which could elicit thixotropic behaviour may be expected for two reasons. Intervertebral motion may contain a neutral zone, a region of the force–displacement curve where the facet joints, ligaments and intervertebral disc produce little resistance to motion (Oxland et al. 1992; Panjabi 1992; Thompson et al. 2003). Second, hysteresis in force-displacement curves for the lumbar spine indicates that there is an indeterminacy to the passive position of a vertebra, despite unchanging internal forces. Both factors suggest that a vertebra's spatial position may not be uniquely determined at low loads.

THE EFFECT OF IMPAIRED PROPRIOCEPTION ON SPINAL CONTROL

Posture and movement depend to a large extent upon the interaction between sensory and motor systems. With sensory signals provided by the somatosensory, vestibular and visual systems, the brain constructs internal representations of our bodies and the external world. Our precise, goal-oriented, purposeful movements can be performed effortlessly because the parts of the brain that control movement have access to these internal representations and to the sensory signals that continuously update them. The strong interactions between each sensory system and the motor control system are embodied in the concept of sensorimotor control. However, we probably cannot fully understand the spinal control problem in back pain unless we better understand the nature and consequences of somatosensory impairment. Therefore, this must be a priority for further study.

Theoretically, proprioception must be important in spinal control. Both clinical and basic research evidence underscore this statement having revealed devastating effects on postural control when proprioception has been lost through large fibre neuropathy (Cole 1995), by cooling ischaemia (Thoumie and Do 1996) or injection of pyridoxine in humans (Stapley et al. 2002; Lockhart and Ting 2007; Ollivier-Lanvin et al. 2010), and by de-afferentiation through dorsal rhizotomy in animals (Polit and Bizzi 1978). For the spine in particular, the visual system provides no direct sensory information about the position or movement of the back.

Proprioceptive feedback seems particularly important for spinal control. In the lumbar spine, its passive tissue properties do not adequately provide stabilization to prevent it from collapsing or buckling (Wilder et al. 1988; Cholewicki and McGill 1996). Consequently, combinations of sensory feedback and feed-forward neural signals must contribute to the control of both intersegmental and regional spinal position and movements (Panjabi 1992; Cholewicki and McGill 1996). Feedback mechanisms are thought to account for 40% of the trunk stiffness that maintains stable posture during sudden loading (Moorhouse and Granata 2007). In contrast to the limbs where co-contraction of appendicular muscles accompanies the need to accomplish accurate and precise movements, precision movements of the trunk appear to rely more on feedback control and less on stiffening by co-contraction arising from feed-forward control (Willigenburg et al. 2010).

In people with low back pain, the loss of proprioceptive information is not complete, i.e. they are not deafferented, yet they demonstrate decreased precision and decreased accuracy of position and movement compared to those without low back pain. However, adverse functional consequences from this may not be guaranteed because people with back pain may be able to adapt their motor control strategies and accommodate for any such impairment. In this section we will consider the observed proprioceptive (sensory) changes in people with low back pain and discuss the factors that may contribute to them. In addition, the impact these changes have on spinal control and low back pain will be evaluated.

Numerous studies have shown that individuals with low back pain have altered (in most studies decreased) lumbosacral position sense when assuming a variety of postures such as standing, sitting and four-point-kneeling, compared to healthy control subjects (e.g. Gill and Callaghan 1998; Brumagne et al. 2000; O'Sullivan et al. 2003). However, some studies show no difference in spine proprioception between individuals with and without low back pain (Descarreaux et al. 2005; Asell et al. 2006) or they show only a direction-specific change in proprioception, e.g. decreased acuity in the direction of flexion but not in spinal extension (Newcomer et al. 2000). Changes in proprioceptive acuity have also been seen in different populations such as young, middle-aged and elderly people, in highly active (e.g. professional ballet dancers) and sedentary individuals, in patients with mild and severe disability, and in patients with non-specific low back pain as well as those with spinal stenosis or disc herniation (e.g. Brumagne et al. 2000; Leinonen et al. 2002, 2003; O'Sullivan et al. 2003; Brumagne et al. 2004a, 2004c, 2008b). While advancing age has also been described as having a negative effect on lumbosacral proprioceptive acuity, this is more manifest in elderly individuals with low back pain (Brumagne et al. 2004a).

Several mechanisms have been described which adversely influence lumbosacral proprioceptive acuity. For one, pain itself can have a direct negative effect on proprioceptive acuity, however the pain cannot solely explain the changes in acuity. Patients with recurrent low back pain tested during pain-free episodes still showed altered proprioception (Brumagne et al. 2008b; Janssens et al. 2010). Moreover, experimentally induced acute, deep back pain in healthy individuals did not change the magnitude of stretch-reflexes from their back muscles (Zedka et al. 1999). Animal studies have similarly indicated that noxious stimulation does not alter proprioceptive signals from lumbar paraspinal muscle spindles (Kang et al. 2001).

In addition to pain, back muscle fatigue and decreased blood supply might have a negative effect on lumbosacral position sense. People with low back pain have been observed to have decreased back muscle endurance (Biering-Sørensen 1984; Brumagne et al. 1999b; Taimela et al. 1999; Johanson et al. 2011) and increased fatigue, which is often associated with ischaemia. The build-up of ischaemic metabolites might negatively affect proprioceptive control (Delliaux and Jammes 2006; Johanson et al. 2011). There is also evidence that loading and/or fatigue of the respiratory muscles may induce an increased reliance on proprioceptive signals from the ankles rather than the back muscles through an elicited metaboreflex that redistributes blood from the trunk muscles to the diaphragm (Janssens et al. 2010, 2012).

Other studies suggest that proprioception may be impaired by action exerted through the sympathetic nervous system on muscle spindle receptors. The sympathetic nervous system may have both an indirect effect on proprioception by decreasing the blood flow to skeletal muscles (Thomas and Segal 2004) and a direct effect on muscle spindles, generally characterized by a depression of their sensitivity to changes in muscle length (Roatta et al. 2002). Moreover, sympathetic activation may also affect basal discharge rate of muscle spindles (Hellström et al. 2005). However, most of these results have yet to be confirmed in the human lumbar spine, since sympathetic modulation of muscle spindle afferent activity is mainly documented in animal studies and related to jaw and neck muscles (Passatore and Roatta 2006).

In addition to studies that have looked specifically at proprioceptive acuity of trunk muscles in people with back pain, others have looked more generally at the effects of back pain on postural control by investigating postural sway. Differences in postural sway between people with low back pain and healthy controls depend upon the postural condition. During simple standing conditions, no differences in postural sway are observed between people with low back pain and healthy controls. If anything, even smaller sways are observed for the patient population (Brumagne et al. 2004a, 2008a, 2008b; Claeys et al. 2011). However, when stance conditions are made more challenging (for example by introducing unstable support surfaces, translating platforms, unipedal stance, or ballistic arm movements) then postural sway increases significantly in people with low back pain compared to healthy individuals (Luoto et al. 1998; Mientjes and Frank 1999; Brumagne et al. 2004a; della Volpe et al. 2006; Henry et al. 2006; Mok et al. 2007; Popa et al. 2007; Brumagne et al. 2008a, 2008b; Claeys et al. 2011). Similar results have been obtained during unstable sitting, where larger sways are observed for people with low back pain compared to healthy controls, especially at the most difficult stability levels (Radebold et al. 2001; Van Daele et al. 2009).

Changes in postural balance in people with low back pain may be related to altered sensory reweighting (e.g. upweighting ankle proprioceptive signals and downweighting back muscle signals) (Brumagne et al. 2004a; della Volpe et al. 2006; Popa et al. 2007; Brumagne et al. 2008b) and to changes in reference frames (e.g. offset in the subjective vertical) (Brumagne et al. 2008a). Accordingly, people with low back pain seem to adopt a rigid postural control strategy in preference to a multi-segmental postural control strategy which may serve its purpose in restricting excessive movement during simple, familiar tasks but then becomes suboptimal under more complex postural conditions when it actually induces larger spinal motions (Brumagne et al. 2008a, 2008b; Claeys et al. 2011; della Volpe et al. 2006; Henry et al. 2006; Mok et al. 2004, 2007; Popa et al. 2007; Van Daele et al. 2009).

The question arises whether the reports on altered lumbosacral proprioception are related to local dysfunction of proprioceptors (e.g. due to disuse or damaged muscle spindles), thus affecting the quality of sensory reception used to track the spine, or to changes in central processing of these proprioceptive signals. In other words, is it a problem of sensory impairment or of impaired sensory integration? Position and movement sense paradigms are more inclined to target the receptor hypothesis. However, recent studies suggest that changes in central processing of proprioceptive signals (i.e. sensory integration) may also play an important role in the observed altered proprioception in patients with low back pain (Brumagne et al. 2004a, 2008b; della Volpe et al. 2006; Popa et al. 2007; Claeys et al. 2011).

For optimal postural control, the CNS must identify and selectively focus on the sensory inputs (visual, vestibular and proprioceptive) which are providing the most functionally reliable input. Presumably, reliability is determined by some kind of comparison with internal representations contained in cortical, subcortical and cerebellar body maps. Through sensory reweighting and gain control, the CNS must integrate incoming sensory signals adaptively to cope with potentially conflicting and complex postural conditions in order to perform the task at hand. If some sensory signals are deemed unreliable, the CNS will increase the gain or upweigh another sensory system (e.g. vision over proprioception) or signals from a location within the proprioceptive system itself (e.g. ankle proprioceptive signals over back proprioceptive signals) and/or downweigh the unreliable sensory system or signals (Brumagne et al. 2004a; Carver et al. 2006). In this way, the proprioceptive system can adapt rapidly to changing conditions in order to coordinate movement and prevent excessive tissue loading.

Finally, proprioception plays an important role in the calibration of internal representations of the body (Gurfinkel et al. 1995; Lackner and DiZio 2000). The same proprioceptive signals may be processed differently depending upon which internal reference frame the CNS chooses at that time. The process involved in selecting a reference frame in order to interpret incoming proprioceptive signals is closely related to the mechanisms of a body scheme (Gurfinkel and Levik 1998). Plastic changes may occur in the brain that alter the perception of body image and body scheme. These may arise due to chronic pain conditions (Maravita et al. 2003; Moseley 2005) or tonic muscle activity as evoked by the Kohnstamm phenomenon or muscle vibration (Gilhodes et al. 1992; Brumagne et al. 2004b; Ivanenko et al. 2006), and as a result proprioceptive signals may be interpreted in a different way resulting in abnormal or impaired motor responses.

TESTING OF PROPRIOCEPTION

The previous discussion raises questions concerning the best methods for testing proprioception in the spine. Most studies on proprioception in healthy individuals and in people with low back pain have focused on repositioning accuracy in tests of spinal position sense (Gill and Callaghan 1998; Swinkels and Dolan 1998; Brumagne et al. 2000; O'Sullivan et al. 2003; Descarreaux et al. 2005; Asell et al. 2006; Silfies et al. 2007). Such tests have some obvious advantages, but also important disadvantages. Evaluations are often performed during simple tasks that involve flexing and extending the trunk either in standing or sitting. They are usually fairly intuitive, and can be performed in a clinical setting. Furthermore, the reliability of the measurements is generally good and can be substantially improved with repeated testing. For this reason, some investigators have advocated performing a minimum number of trial tests before making the actual

measurements. However, this highlights one of the problems with this type of testing because acuity during repeated testing can be improved due to a learning effect. As mentioned earlier, impairments in proprioceptive function in people with back pain often only manifest themselves under more challenging conditions where the person has not been able to learn the most appropriate response. Under normal everyday conditions, the body must continually respond to changing circumstances. Therefore, testing protocols that assess initial responses might be more relevant to the 'real world' and may be better able to demonstrate impairments in people with low back pain. Furthermore, the use of more complex tasks such as sit-to-stand may also prove more useful in this respect (Cordo and Gurfinkel 2004; Claeys et al. 2012).

Movement sense, the second component of kinaesthesia, has also been used to assess spinal proprioception. This is normally assessed using tests of movement detection or movement discrimination, where the former identify thresholds to the detection of motion (Taylor and McCloskey 1990; Parkhurst and Burnett 1994; Taimela et al. 1999; Silfies et al. 2007) and the latter assess the ability to sense movement magnitude or direction (Garn and Newton 1988; Sharma 1999; de Jong et al. 2005). However, in studies of spinal proprioception, movement detection tests have been used more frequently than movement discrimination tests.

In recent years, tests of velocity replication and velocity discrimination have also been reported in the literature (Lönn et al. 2001; Westlake et al. 2007) and it has been suggested that such tests may add to the repertoire of methods available for proprioceptive testing. However, such tests have not as yet been used for assessing spinal proprioception.

The question remains whether tests of position sense, movement sense and velocity sense, whereby individual components of proprioception are assessed separately, are the most appropriate methods for assessing proprioception. An alternative approach is to look more holistically at the system by using postural control or postural balance tasks (Mok et al. 2004; Brumagne et al. 2008b; Claeys et al. 2011). Such assessments can be performed while keeping the signals from the visual and vestibular systems relatively constant (e.g. by blindfolding subjects and removing head accelerations) (Allum et al. 1998), and can also incorporate the effects of sensory weighting by using muscle vibration.

The use of muscle vibration as an experimental probe can help in clarifying proprioceptive control in a more direct manner. Muscle vibration, often mistaken as a disturbance, is a powerful stimulus of muscle spindles and can induce kinaesthetic illusions (Goodwin et al. 1972; Roll and Vedel 1982; Brumagne et al. 1999a; Cordo et al. 2005). Direction-specific responses can be expected if the CNS uses the afference of the stimulated muscles for postural control. Therefore, muscle vibration can be used during experiments using the 'conscious' position sense paradigm (Brumagne et al. 2000) and during experimental set-ups where 'subconscious' proprioceptive control is evaluated such as in postural balance paradigms (Brumagne et al. 2008b, 2012; Claeys et al. 2011).

Currently, only a limited number of studies have investigated central mechanisms (brain mapping) in relation to proprioceptive impairment in low back pain (Flor 2003; Tsao et al. 2008). People with chronic low back pain have been observed to have an altered somatotopic organization within their primary somatosensory cortex (Flor 2003). Representations for the low back were located more inferior and medial, indicating an expansion toward the cortical representation of the leg. According to Flor (2003), these results suggest that chronic pain leads to expansion of the cortical representation zone related to the nociceptive input. An alternative explanation may be that this change in mapping is related to altered proprioceptive weighting, i.e. reweighting of the proprioceptive signals from the ankles at the expense of the lumbosacral afference (Brumagne et al. 2004a, 2008b, 2012; della Volpe et al. 2006). Further investigation of this hypothesis is required. Tsao et al. (2008), using transcranial magnetic stimulation (TMS), showed that the motor cortical map of the trunk muscles is located more posterior and lateral in patients with recurrent low back pain compared to healthy controls. Moreover, the patient group showed greater symmetrical activation during an anticipatory postural control task compared to healthy controls. These results suggest that healthy persons use uncrossed polysynaptic corticospinal pathways that project via regions in the brainstem (Tsao et al. 2008).

Recently, TMS and neuroimaging techniques such as functional magnetic resonance imaging (fMRI) and functional near-infrared spectroscopy (fNIRS) have been used to identify where kinaesthetic signals are processed in the brain, and they have provided evidence that the left cerebellum might act as a processor of sensory signals (Hagura et al. 2009). Neuroimaging techniques can also be used in conjunction with muscle vibration as an alternative approach for the evaluation of sensory and motor functions (Montant et al. 2009; Goble et al. 2011). Use of these novel methods is in its infancy but warrants further investigation.

PROPRIOCEPTIVE TRAINING AND FUTURE DIRECTIONS

For most of us, proprioceptive training is associated with standing or exercising on unstable support surfaces such as a wobble board, a bosu ball, or a trampoline. Such approaches are based on the assumption that unstable support surfaces disturb postural balance and consequently challenge the body's sensory systems including

proprioception. However, a better understanding of this process (e.g. why unstable support surfaces induce complex postural conditions, not only from a mechanical point of view but from a control perspective that may involve weighting mechanisms, gain control etc.) might further enhance the therapeutic interventions for postural control (Kiers et al. 2012). Moreover, taking into account all aspects of proprioception, such 'balance' training might represent only a part of proprioceptive training. Consequently, more specific and direct proprioceptive exercises that are based on *sensing, localizing* and *discriminating* proprioceptive signals of specific trunk muscles during functional activities might be more effective. Preliminary results have shown that patients with recurrent low back pain can change their proprioceptive control strategy through 'cognitive' muscle control exercises (combined with muscle vibration) (Brumagne et al. 2005). Moreover, motor control training has been demonstrated to lead to motor learning of automatic postural control strategies that persist over time (Tsao and Hodges 2008).

Recently, stochastic resonance stimulation of paraspinal muscles evoked improved sitting balance control in patients with chronic low back pain, but no effect was demonstrated on spinal proprioception (i.e., movement sense) (Reeves et al. 2009). Further study is required to clarify this discrepancy and the effects of stochastic resonance stimulation on the sensorimotor system of the spine.

'Proprioceptive' tape and neoprene braces are already used in clinical practice to enhance the patient's awareness of lumbosacral spine position and movement (e.g. McNair and Heine 1999). The question arises whether proprioceptive tape has a real (long term) influence on lumbosacral proprioception or whether it just temporarily enhances awareness through cutaneous input. Moreover, one can argue that if tactile feedback is not the principal source of lumbosacral proprioception, then this type of intervention might have a negative effect on the neural control of posture and movement in the long run when the tape or brace is no longer present (i.e. negative transfer). Further research is necessary to demonstrate the effectiveness of such approaches.

Lastly, motor imagery, a dynamic mental process during which an individual internally simulates a motor action without any apparent motion of the body segments involved in that action, may play an important role in proprioceptive training of patients with low back pain. Motor imagery activates similar brain areas as the actual execution of a movement – the two differ only in the final motor output stage (Jeannerod and Frak 1999; Gerardin et al. 2000; Guillot et al. 2007). Visual motor imagery, already frequently used in neurorehabilitation and sports performance, requires one to imagine seeing oneself performing a motor task. However, the modalities of motor imagery consist of not only visual imagery, but also kinaesthetic imagery (Guillot et al. 2009). Kinaesthetic imagery requires the person to imagine the feeling produced by the actual task performance, e.g. to perceive muscle contractions or stretching of muscles mentally. Kinaesthetic imagery activates similar brain areas as visual motor imagery, although the effects are not completely identical (Guillot et al. 2009). Moreover, a closer coupling in activated brain areas between kinaesthetic imagery and motor execution shows kinaesthetic imagery is a stronger functional equivalent of motor execution than visual imagery (Guillot et al. 2007). These results suggest different roles for the two modalities of motor imagery, and the implications for proprioceptive training warrant further investigation.

Future studies are required to identify those aspects of proprioception that are most often altered in low back pain and to determine if such changes have any influence on spinal function, pain or disability. If specific components of proprioception are impaired in low back pain then it is important to know whether they are a cause or consequence of the pain and whether they can predispose to chronicity.

While there is some evidence that people with poor postural balance (Takala and Viikari-Juntura 2000) and

delayed trunk muscle responses (Cholewicki et al. 2005; Silfies et al. 2007) have an increased risk of developing back pain, information concerning the links between sensorimotor impairment and the development of chronic back pain is lacking. Also, the role of sensorimotor impairment in post-surgical patients has received little attention. Further prospective studies in this area will help to determine the importance of sensorimotor impairment and may help to target future training regimes in order to improve outcome in different patient groups.

Brain imaging techniques such as functional magnetic resonance imaging, diffusion tensor imaging or functional near-infrared spectroscopy may help to improve our understanding of the central mechanisms involved in proprioception (e.g. the role of the cerebellum). Moreover, functional brain imaging techniques may provide a means to disentangle the sensory from the motor influences in determining sensorimotor control of the spine.

Finally, randomized controlled trials of interventions based on the mechanisms of proprioceptive impairment are necessary to demonstrate whether recovery of proprioceptive function improves functional and clinical outcome in patients with low back pain.

REFERENCES

Allum, J.H., Bloem, B.R., Carpenter, M.G., Hulliger, M., Hadders-Algra, M., 1998. Proprioceptive control of posture: a review of new concepts. Gait Posture 8, 214–242.

Amonoo-Kuofi, H.S., 1982. The number and distribution of muscle spindles in human intrinsic postvertebral muscles. J Anat 135, 585–599.

Amonoo-Kuofi, H.S., 1983. The density of muscle spindles in the medial, intermediate and lateral columns of human intrinsic postvertebral muscles. J Anat 136, 509–519.

Asell, M., Sjölander, P., Kerschbaumer, H., Djupsjöbacka, M., 2006. Are lumbar repositioning errors larger among patients with chronic low back pain compared with asymptomatic subjects? Arch Phys Med Rehabil 87, 1170–1176.

Ashton-Miller, J.A., McGlashen, K.M., Schultz, A.B., 1992. Trunk positioning accuracy in children 7–18 years old. J Orthop Res 10, 217–225.

Bastian, H.C., 1888. The 'muscular sense': its nature and cortical localization. Brain 10, 1–137.

Biering-Sørensen, F., 1984. Physical measurements as risk indicators for

low-back trouble over a one-year period. Spine 9, 106–119.

Brumagne, S., Cordo, P., Lysens, R., Swinnen, S., Verschueren, S., 2000. The role of paraspinal muscle spindles in lumbosacral position. Spine 25, 989–994.

Brumagne, S., Cordo, P., Verschueren, S., 2004a. Proprioceptive weighting changes in persons with low back pain and elderly persons during upright standing. Neurosci Lett 366, 63–66.

Brumagne, S., Devos, J., Maes, H., Roelants, M., Delecluse, C., Verschueren, S., 2005. Whole body and local spinal muscle vibration combined with segmental stabilization training improve trunk muscle control and back muscle endurance in persons with recurrent low back pain: a randomized controlled study. Eur Spine J 14, S31–S32.

Brumagne, S., Janssens, L., Janssens, E., Goddyn, L., 2008a. Altered postural control in anticipation of postural instability in persons with recurrent low back pain. Gait & Posture 28, 657–662.

Brumagne, S., Janssens, L., Pijnenburg, M., Claeys, K., 2012. Processing of conflicting proprioceptive signals during standing in people with and without recurrent low back pain. XIX Congress of the International Society of Electrophysiology and Kinesiology, Brisbane.

Brumagne, S., Janssens, L., Süüden-Johanson, E., Claeys, K., Knapen, S., 2008b. Persons with recurrent low back pain exhibit a rigid postural control strategy. Eur Spine J 17, 1177–1184.

Brumagne, S., Lysens, R., Swinnen, S., Charlier, C., 1999b. Effect of exercise-induced fatigue on lumbosacral position sense. Proceedings of the 13th International Congress of the World Confederation for Physical Therapy, Yokohama, p. 171.

Brumagne, S., Lysens, R., Swinnen, S., Verschueren, S., 1999a. Effect of paraspinal muscle vibration on position sense of the lumbosacral spine. Spine 24, 1328–1331.

Brumagne, S., Smets, S., Staes, F., Van Deun, S., Stappaerts, K., 2004b. Paraspinal muscle spasms as a mechanism for an altered internal representation in patients with low back pain. Abstract Book Spineweek SP8.

Brumagne, S., Valckx, R., Staes, F., Van Deun, S., Stappaerts, K., 2004c. Altered proprioceptive postural control in professional classic dancers with low back pain. Abstract Book Spineweek 2004c; P145.

Burgess, P.R., Clark, F.J., 1969. Characteristics of knee joint receptors in the cat. J Physiol 203, 317–335.

Burke, D., Gandevia, S.C., 1988. Interfering cutaneous stimulation and the muscle afferent contribution to cortical potentials. Electroencephalogr Clin Neurophysiol 70, 18–125.

Cao, D.Y., Khalsa, P.S., Pickar, J.G., 2009b. Dynamic responsiveness of lumbar paraspinal muscle spindles during vertebral movement in the cat. Exp Brain Res. 197, 369–377.

Cao, D.Y., Pickar, J.G., 2009. Thoracolumbar fascia does not influence proprioceptive signaling from lumbar paraspinal muscle spindles in the cat. J Anat 215, 417–424.

Cao, D.Y., Pickar, J.G., 2011. Lengthening but not shortening history of paraspinal muscle spindles in the low back alters their dynamic sensitivity. J Neurophysiol. 105, 434–441.

Cao, D.Y., Pickar, J.G., Ge, W., Ianuzzi, A., Khalsa, P.S., 2009a. Position sensitivity of feline paraspinal muscle spindles to vertebral movement in the lumbar spine. J Neurophysiol. 101, 1722–1729.

Carver, S., Kiemel, T., Jeka, J.J., 2006. Modeling the dynamics of sensory reweighting. Biol Cybern. 95, 123–134.

Cavanaugh, J.M., Ozaktay, A.C., Yamashita, T., Avramov, A., Getchell, T.V., King, A.I., 1997. Mechanisms of low back pain: a neurophysiologic and neuroanatomic study. Clin Orthop 335, 166–180.

Cholewicki, J., McGill, S.M., 1996. Mechanical stability of the in vivo lumbar spine: Implications for injury and chronic low back pain. Clin Biomech 11, 1–15.

Cholewicki, J., Silfies, S.P., Shah, R.A., Greene, H.S., Reeves, N.P., Alvi, K., et al., 2005. Delayed trunk muscle reflex responses increase the risk of

low back injuries. Spine 30, 2614–2620.

Claeys, K., Brumagne, S., Dankaerts, W., Kiers, H., Janssens, L., 2011. Decreased variability in proprioceptive postural strategy during standing and sitting in people with recurrent low back pain. Eur J Appl Physiol 111, 115–123.

Claeys, K., Dankaerts, W., Janssens, L., Kiers, H., Brumagne, S., 2012. Altered preparatory pelvic control during the sit-to-stance-to-sit movement in people with non-specific low back pain. J Electromyogr Kinesiol (in press).

Cole, J., 1995. Pride and the Daily Marathon. MIT Press, Boston, MA.

Collins, D.F., Refshauge, K.M., Todd, G., Gandevia, S.C., 2005. Cutaneous receptors contribute to kinesthesia at the index finger, elbow, and knee. J Neurophysiol 94, 1699–1706.

Cordo, P., Gurfinkel, V.S., 2004. Motor coordination can be fully understood only by studying complex movements. Prog Brain Res 143, 29–38.

Cordo, P.J., Gurfinkel, V.S., Brumagne, S., Flores-Vieira, C., 2005. Effect of slow, small movement on the vibration-evoked kinesthetic illusion. Exp Brain Res. 167, 324–334.

de Jong, A.S., Kilbreath, L.,Refshauge, K.M., Adams, R., 2005. Performance in different proprioceptive tests does not correlate in ankles with recurrent ankle sprain. Arch Phys Med Rehabil 86, 2101–2105.

della Volpe, R., Popa, T., Ginanneschi, F., Spidalieri, R., Mazzocchio, R., Rossi, A., 2006. Changes in coordination of postural control during dynamic stance in chronic low back pain patients. Gait & Posture 24, 349–355.

Delliaux, S., Jammes, Y., 2006. Effects of hypoxia on muscle response to tendon vibration in humans. Muscle Nerve 34, 754–761.

Descarreaux, M., Blouin, J.S., Teasdale, N., 2005. Repositioning accuracy and movement parameters in low back pain subjects and healthy control subjects. Eur Spine J 14, 185–191.

Ferrell, W.R., 1980. The adequacy of stretch receptors in the cat knee joint for signalling joint angle throughout a full range of movement. J Physiol 299, 85–99.

Ferrell, W.R., Gandevia, S.C., McCloskey, D.I., 1987. The role of joint receptors in human kinaesthesia when intramuscular receptors cannot contribute. J Physiol 386, 63–71.

Flor, H., 2003. Cortical reorganisation and chronic pain: implications for rehabilitation. J Rehabil Med 41, 66–72.

Gandevia, S.C., 1996. Kinesthesia: roles for afferent signals and motor commands. In: Rowell, L.B., Shepherd, J.T. (Eds.), Handbook of Physiology, section 12 exercise: regulation and integration of multiple systems. Oxford University Press, New York, pp. 128–172.

Gandevia, S.C., McCloskey, D.I., Burke, D., 1992. Kinaesthetic signals and muscle contraction. Trends Neurosci 15, 62–65.

Garn, S.N., Newton, R.A., 1988. Kinesthetic awareness in subjects with multiple ankle sprains. Phys Ther 68, 1667–1671.

Ge, W., Long, C.R., Pickar, J.G., 2005. Vertebral position alters paraspinal muscle spindle responsiveness in the feline spine: effect of positioning duration. J Physiol. 569, 655–665.

Ge, W., Pickar, J.G., 2008. Time course for the development of muscle history in lumbar paraspinal muscle spindles arising from changes in vertebral position. Spine J. 8, 320–328.

Gerardin, E., Sirigu, A., Lehéricy, S., Poline, J.B., Gaymard, B., Marsault, C., et al., 2000. Partially overlapping neural networks for real and imagined hand movements. Cereb Cortex. 10, 1093–1104.

Gilhodes, J.C., Gurfinkel, V.S., Roll, J.P., 1992. Role of Ia muscle spindle afferents in post-contraction and post-vibration motor effect genesis. Neurosci Lett 135, 247–251.

Gill, K.P., Callaghan, M.J., 1998. The measurement of lumbar proprioception in individuals with and without low back pain. Spine 23, 371–377.

Goble, D.J., Coxon, J.P., Van Impe, A., Geurts, M., Doumas, M., Wenderoth, N., et al., 2011. Brain activity during ankle proprioceptive stimulation predicts balance performance in young and older adults. J Neurosci 31, 16344–16352.

Goodwin, G.M., McCloskey, D.I., Matthews, P.B.C., 1972. The

contribution of muscle afferents to kinesthesia shown by vibration induced illusions of movement and by the effects of paralysing joint afferents. Brain 95, 705–748.

Gregory, J.E., Morgan, D.L., Proske, U., 1987. Changes in size of the stretch reflex of cat and man attributed to aftereffects in muscle spindles. J Neurophysiol. 58, 628–640.

Gregory, J.E., Morgan, D.L., Proske, U., 1988. Responses of muscle spindles depend on their history of activation and movement. Progr Brain Res. 74, 85–90.

Gregory, J.E., Mark, R.F., Morgan, D.L., Patak, A., Polus, B., Proske, U., 1990. Effects of muscle history on the stretch reflex in cat and man. J Physiol. 424, 93–107.

Guillot, A., Collet, C., Nguyen, V.A., Malouin, F., Richards, C., Doyon, J., 2009. Brain activity during visual versus kinesthetic imagery: an fMRI study. Hum Brain Mapp 30, 2157–2172.

Guillot, A., Lebon, F., Rouffet, D., Champely, S., Doyon, J., Collet, C., 2007. Muscular responses during motor imagery as a function of muscle contraction types. Int J Psychophysiol. 66, 18–27.

Gurfinkel, V.S., Ivanenko, Y.P., Levik, Y.S., Babakova, I.A., 1995. Kinesthetic reference for human orthograde posture. Neurosci 68, 229–243.

Gurfinkel, V.S., Levik, Y.S., 1998. Reference systems and interpretation of proprioceptive signals. Fiziol Cheloveka. 24, 53–63.

Hagura, N., Oouchida, Y., Aramaki, Y., Okada, T., Matsumura, M., Sadato, N., et al., 2009. Visuokinesthetic perception of hand movement is mediated by cerebro-cerebellar interaction between the left cerebellum and right parietal cortex. Cereb Cortex 19, 176–186.

Hall, L.A., McCloskey, D.I., 1983. Detections of movements imposed on finger, elbow and shoulder joints. J Physiol 335, 519–533.

Hellström, F., Roatta, S., Thunberg, J., Passatore, M., Djupsjöbacka, M., 2005. Responses of muscle spindles in feline dorsal neck muscles to electrical stimulation of the cervical sympathetic nerve. Exp Brain Res 165, 328–342.

Henry, S.M., Hitt, J.R., Jones, S.L., Bunn, J.Y., 2006. Decreased limits of stability in response to postural perturbations in subjects with low back pain. Clin Biomech 21, 881–892.

Hill, D.K., 1968. Tension due to interaction between the sliding filaments in resting striated muscle. The effect of stimulation. J Physiol. 199, 637–684.

Hutton, R.S., Atwater, 1992. Acute and chronic adaptations of muscle proprioceptors in response to increased use. Sports Med 14, 406–421.

Ianuzzi, A., Little, J.S., Chiu, J.B., Baitner, A., Kawchuk, G., Khalsa, P.S., 2004. Human lumbar facet joint capsule strains: I. During physiological motions. Spine J 4, 141–152.

Ivanenko, Y.P., Wright, W.G., Gurfinkel, V.S., Horak, F., Cordo, P., 2006. Interaction of involuntary post-contraction activity with locomotor movements. Exp Brain Res 169, 255–260.

Jakobs, T., Miller, J.A., Schultz, A.B., 1985. Trunk position sense in the frontal plane. Exp Neurol 90, 129–138.

Janssens, L., Troosters, T., McConnell, A., Raymaekers, J., Goossens, N., Pijnenburg, M., et al., 2012. Suboptimal postural strategy and back muscle oxygenation during inspiratory resistive loading. Med Sci Sports Exerc, in press.

Janssens, L., Brumagne, S., Polspoel, K., Troosters, T., McConnell, A., 2010. The effect of inspiratory muscles fatigue on postural control in people with and without recurrent low back pain. Spine 35, 1088–1094.

Jeannerod, M., Frak, V., 1999. Mental imaging of motor activity in humans. Curr Opin Neurobiol. 9, 735–739.

Johanson, E., Brumagne, S., Janssens, L., Pijnenburg, M., Claeys, K., Pääsuke, M., 2011. The effect of acute back muscles fatigue on postural control in individuals with and without recurrent low back pain. Eur Spine J 20, 2152–2159.

Kang, Y.M., Choi, W.S., Pickar, J.G., 2002. Electrophysiologic evidence for an intersegmental reflex pathway between lumbar paraspinal tissues. Spine 27, E56–E63.

Kang, Y.M., Wheeler, J.D., Pickar, J.G., 2001. Stimulation of chemosensitive afferents from multifidus muscle does not sensitize multifidus muscle spindles to vertebral loads in the lumbar spine of the cat. Spine 26, 1528–1536.

Kiers, H., Brumagne, S., Van Dieen, J., vander Wees, P., Vanhees, L., 2012. Ankle proprioception is not targeted by exercises on an unstable surface. Eur J Appl Physiol 112, 1577–1585.

Kokkorogiannis, T., 2008. Two enigmas in proprioception: abundance and location of muscle spindles. Brain Res Bull. 75, 495–496.

Lackner, J.R., DiZio, P.A., 2000. Aspects of body self-calibration. Trends Cogn Sci 4, 279–288.

Lavender, A., Laurence, A.S., Bangash, I.H., Smith, R.B., 1999. Cortical evoked potentials in the ruptured anterior cruciate ligament. Knee Surg Sports Traumatol Arthrosc 7, 98–101.

Leinonen, V., Kankaanpää, M., Luukkonen, M., Kansanen, M., Hänninen, O., Airaksinen, O., et al., 2003. Lumbar paraspinal muscle function, perception of lumbar position, and postural control in disc herniation-related back pain. Spine 28, 842–848.

Leinonen, V., Määttä, S., Taimela, S., Herno, A., Kankaanpää, M., Partanen, J., et al., 2002. Impaired lumbar movement perception in association with postural stability and motor- and somatosensory-evoked potentials in lumbar spinal stenosis. Spine 27, 975–983.

Lockhart, D.B., Ting, L.H., 2007. Optimal sensorimotor transformations for balance. Nat Neurosci. 10, 1329–1336.

Lönn, J.M., Djupsjöbacka, M., Johansson, H., 2001. Replication and discrimination of limb movement velocity. Somatosens Motor Res 18, 76–82.

Luoto, S., Aalto, H., Taimela, S., Hurri, H., Pyykkö, I., Alaranta, H., 1998. One-footed and externally disturbed two-footed postural control in patients with chronic low back pain and healthy control subjects: A controlled study with follow-up. Spine 23, 2081–2090.

Maravita, A., Spence, C., Driver, J., 2003. Multisensory integration and the body schema: close to hand and within reach. Curr Biol 13, R531–R539.

McLain, R.F., Pickar, J.G., 1998. Mechanoreceptor endings in human thoracic and lumbar facet joints. Spine 23, 168–173.

McNair, P.J., Heine, P.J., 1999. Trunk proprioception: Enhancement through lumbar bracing. Arch Phys Med Rehabil 80, 96–99.

Mientjes, M.I., Frank, J.S., 1999. Balance in chronic low back pain patients compared to healthy people under various conditions in upright standing. Clin Biomech 14, 710–716.

Mok, N.W., Brauer, S.G., Hodges, P.W., 2004. Hip strategy for balance control in quiet standing is reduced in people with low back pain. Spine 29, E107–E112.

Mok, N.W., Brauer, S.G., Hodges, P.W., 2007. Failure to use movement in postural strategies leads to increased spinal displacement in low back pain. Spine 32, E537–E543.

Montant, M., Romaiguère, P., Roll, J.P., 2009. A new vibrator to stimulate muscle proprioceptors in fMRI. Hum Brain Mapp. 30, 990–997.

Moorhouse, K.M., Granata, K.P., 2007. Role of reflex dynamics in spinal stability: intrinsic muscle stiffness alone is insufficient for stability. J Biomech. 40, 1058–1065.

Morgan, D.L., Prochazka, A., Proske, U., 1984. The after-effects of stretch and fusimotor stimulation on the responses of primary endings of cat muscle spindles. J Physiol 356, 465–477.

Moseley, G.L., 2005. Distorted body image in complex regional pain syndrome. Neurology. 65, 773.

Newcomer, K.L., Laskowski, E.R., Yu, B., Johnson, J.C., An, K.N., 2000. Differences in repositioning error among patients with low back pain compared with control subjects. Spine 25, 2488–2493.

Nitz, A.J., Peck, D., 1986. Comparison of muscle spindle concentrations in large and small human epaxial muscles acting in parallel combinations. Am Surg 52, 273–277.

Ollivier-Lanvin, K., Keeler, B.E., Siegfried, R., Houlé, J.D., Lemay, M.A., 2010. Proprioceptive neuropathy affects normalization of the H-reflex by exercise after spinal cord injury. Exp Neurol. 221, 198–205.

O'Sullivan, P.B., Burnett, A., Floyd, A.N., Gadsdon, K., Logiudice, J., Miller, D., et al., 2003. Lumbar repositioning deficit in a specific low back pain population. Spine 28, 1074–1079.

Oxland, T.R., Crisco, J.J., Panjabi, M.M., Yamamoto, I., 1992. The effect of injury on rotational coupling at the lumbosacral joint: A biomechanical investigation. Spine 17, 74–80.

Panjabi, M.M., 1992. The stabilizing system of the spine: Part I. Function, dysfunction, adaptation, and enhancement. J Spinal Disord 5, 383–389.

Parkhurst, T.M., Burnett, C.N., 1994. Injury and proprioception in the lower back. J Orthop Sports Phys Ther 4, 282–295.

Passatore, M., Roatta, S., 2006. Influence of sympathetic nervous system on sensorimotor function: whiplash associated disorders (WAD) as a model. Eur J Appl Physiol 98, 423–449.

Pickar, J.G., McLain, R.F., 1995. Responses of mechanosensitive afferents to manipulation of the lumbar facet in the cat. Spine 20, 2379–2385.

Pinsault, N., Bouvier, B., Sarrazin, Y., Vuillerme, N., 2010. Effects of vision and tactile stimulation of the neck on postural control during unperturbed stance and cervical joint position sense in young asymptomatic adults. Spine 35, 1589–1594.

Pitman, M.I., Nainzadeh, N., Menche, D., Gasalberti, R., Song, E.K., 1992. The intraoperative evaluation of the neurosensory function of the anterior cruciate ligament in humans using somatosensory evoked potentials. Arthroscopy 8, 442–447.

Polit, A., Bizzi, E., 1978. Processes controlling arm movements in monkeys. Science 201, 1235–1237.

Popa, T., Bonifazi, M., Della Volpe, R., Rossi, A., Mazzocchio, R., 2007. Adaptive changes in postural strategy selection in chronic low back pain. Exp Brain Res 177, 411–418.

Proske, U., 2005. What is the role of muscle receptors in proprioception? Muscle Nerve 31, 780–787.

Proske, U., Gandevia, S.C., 2009. The kinaesthetic senses. J Physiol. 587, 4139–4146.

Proske, U., Morgan, D.L., Gregory, J.E., 1993. Thixotropy in skeletal muscle

and in muscle spindles: A review. Prog Neurobiol. 41, 705–721.

Radebold, A., Cholewicki, J., Polzhofer, G.K., Greene, H.S., 2001. Impaired postural control of the lumbar spine is associated with delayed muscle response times in patients with chronic idiopathic low back pain. Spine 26, 724–730.

Reeves, N.P., Cholewicki, J., Lee, A.S., Mysliwiec, L.W., 2009. The effects of stochastic resonance stimulation on spine proprioception and postural control in chronic low back pain patients. Spine 34, 316–321.

Rhalmi, S., Yahia, L.H., Newman, N., Isler, M., 1993. Immunohistochemical study of nerves in lumbar spine ligaments. Spine 18, 264–267.

Richmond, F.J.R., Abrahams, V.C., 1975. Morphology and distribution of muscle spindles in dorsal muscles of cat neck. J Neurophysiol 38, 1322–1339.

Roatta, S., Windhorst, U., Ljubisavljevic, M., Johansson, H., Passatore, M., 2002. Sympathetic modulation of muscle spindle afferent sensitivity to stretch in rabbit jaw closing muscles. J Physiol 540, 237–248.

Roberts, S., Eisenstein, S.M., Menage, J., Evans, E.H., Ashton, I.K., 1995. Mechanoreceptors in intervertebral discs. Morphology, distribution, and neuropeptides. Spine 20, 2645–2651.

Roll, J.P., Vedel, J.P., 1982. Kinaesthetic role of muscle afferents in man, studied by tendon vibration and microneurography. Exp Brain Res. 47, 177–190.

Sharma, L., 1999. Proprioceptive impairment in knee osteoarthritis. Rheum Dis Clin North Am 25, 299–314.

Sherrington, C.S., 1900. The muscular sense. In: Scafer, E.A. (Ed.), Textbook of Physiology, Vol. 2. Pentland, Edinburgh, pp. 1002–1025.

Silfies, S.P., Cholewicki, J., Reeves, N.P., Greene, H.S., 2007. Lumbar position sense and the risk of low back injuries in college athletes: a prospective cohort study. BMC Musculoskelet Disord. 8, 129.

Sjölander, P., Johansson, H., Djupsjöbacka, M., 2002. Spinal and supraspinal effects of activity in ligament afferents. J Electromyogr Kinesiol 12, 167–176.

Solomonow, M., Zhou, B.H., Harris, M., Lu, Y., Baratta, R.V., 1998. The ligamento-muscular stabilizing system of the spine. Spine 23, 2552–2562.

Stapley, P.J., Ting, L.H., Hulliger, M., Macpherson, J.M., 2002. Automatic postural responses are delayed by pyridoxine-induced somatosensory loss. J Neurosci. 22, 5803–5807.

Stedman's Medical Dictionary, 2002. Houghton Mifflin Company, Boston, MA.

Swinkels, A., Dolan, P., 1998. Regional assessment of joint position sense in the spine. Spine 23, 590–597.

Taimela, S., Kankaanpää, M., Luoto, S., 1999. The effect of lumbar fatigue on the ability to sense a change in lumbar position: a controlled study. Spine 24, 1322–1327.

Takala, E.P., Viikari-Juntura, E., 2000. Do functional tests predict low back pain? Spine 25, 2126–2132.

Taylor, J.L., McCloskey, D.I., 1990. Proprioceptive sensation in rotation of the trunk. Exp Brain Res 81, 413–416.

Thomas, G.D., Segal, S.S., 2004. Neural control of muscle blood flow during exercise. J Appl Physiol 97, 731–738.

Thompson, R.E., Barker, T.M., Pearcy, M.J., 2003. Defining the neutral zone of sheep intervertebral joints during dynamic motions: an in vitro study. Clin Biomech 18, 89–98.

Thoumie, P., Do, M.C., 1996. Changes in motor activity and biomechanics during balance recovery following cutaneous and muscular deafferentation. Exp Brain Res. 110, 289–297.

Tsao, H., Galea, M.P., Hodges, P.W., 2008. Reorganization of the motor cortex is associated with postural control deficits in recurrent low back pain. Brain. 131, 2161–2171.

Tsao, H., Hodges, P.W., 2008. Persistence of improvements in postural strategies following motor control training in people with recurrent low back pain. J Electromyogr Kinesiol 18, 559–567.

Van Daele, U., Hagman, F., Truijen, S., Vorlat, P., Van Gheluwe, B., Vaes, P., 2009. Differences in balance strategies between nonspecific chronic low back pain patients and healthy control subjects during unstable sitting. Spine 34, 1233–1238.

Westlake, K.P., Wu, Y., Culham, E.G., 2007. Velocity discrimination: reliability and construct validity in older adults. Hum Move Sci 26, 443–456.

Wilder, D.G., Pope, M.H., Frymoyer, J.W., 1988. The biomechanics of lumbar disc herniation and the effect of overload and instability. J Spinal Disord. 1, 16–32.

Willigenburg, N.W., Kingma, I., van Dieën, J.H., 2010. How is precision regulated in maintaining trunk posture? Exp Brain Res 203, 39–49.

Yahia, L., Rhalmi, S., Newman, N., Isler, M., 1992. Sensory innervation of human thoracolumbar fascia. An immunohistochemical study. Acta Orthop Scand 63, 195–197.

Yamashita, T., Cavanaugh, J.M., el-Bohy, A.A., Getchell, T.V., King, A.I., 1990. Mechanosensitive afferent units in the lumbar facet joint. J Bone Joint Surg Am 72, 865–870.

Yamashita, T., Cavanaugh, J.M., Ozaktay, A.C., Avramov, A.I., Getchell, T.V., King, A.I., 1993b. Effect of substance P on mechanosensitive units of tissues around and in the lumbar facet joint. J Orthop Res 11, 205–214.

Yamashita, T., Minaki, Y., Oota, I., Yokogushi, K., Ishii, S., 1993a. Mechanosensitive afferent units in the lumbar intervertebral disc and adjacent muscle. Spine 18, 2252–2256.

Zedka, M., Prochazka, A., Knight, B., Gillard, D., Gauthier, M., 1999. Voluntary and reflex control of human back muscles during induced pain. J Physiol 520, 591–604.

|20|

Motor control of the spine and changes in pain: debate about the extrapolation from research observations of motor control strategies to effective treatments for back pain

Paul W. Hodges*, Stuart McGill[†] and Julie A. Hides[‡]

*NHMRC Centre of Clinical Research Excellence in Spinal Pain, Injury and Health, School of Health and Rehabilitation Sciences, University of Queensland, Brisbane, Queensland, Australia, [†]Department of Kinesiology, Faculty of Applied Health Sciences, University of Waterloo, Waterloo, Ontario, Canada, and [‡]School of Physiotherapy, Australian Catholic University, McAuley Campus, Banyo, Queensland, Australia

CHAPTER CONTENTS

Introduction 231

Issues with consensus of opinion 231

The spine is controlled by a complex interplay of many muscles (i.e. no single muscle is the most important for spine control) 232

Changing the manner in which a patient controls the spine and pelvis is likely to be beneficial in management of back pain 233

Motor control can be changed with treatment/exercise 234

Treatment involves consideration of more than a uni-dimensional focus on a single muscle or muscle activation strategy 235

Treatment requires progression to enhanced execution of activities of daily living 236

Issues with difference in opinion 236

Control of deeper muscles of the trunk, including TrA and LM, should be assessed and addressed if dysfunction is identified 236

Conclusion 237

References 237

INTRODUCTION

An issue of hot debate is how to extrapolate findings from research related to spine control into effective interventions. As stated in Chapters 2, 5–10, there are differing views of the components of the optimal strategy to control the spine for function and how this changes with pain/injury/dysfunction. This underpins different approaches to exercise rehabilitation of people with low back and pelvic pain. This chapter considers: (i) the issues for which there is consensus of opinion; (ii) the issues where opinions differ; (iii) the relevance of this debate for rehabilitation of low back and pelvic pain; and (iv) the questions that need to be addressed as a matter of priority to resolve the differences.

ISSUES WITH CONSENSUS OF OPINION

Despite the apparent divergence of opinion related to different approaches to understanding normal and abnormal spine control, and the extrapolation to design of clinical interventions to optimize control, there is in fact considerable agreement on fundamental concepts that underpin back pain management using approaches that target restoration of motor control of the spine. Key points of agreement are:

1. The spine is controlled by a complex interplay of many muscles (i.e. no single muscle is the most important for spine control).
2. Changing the manner in which a patient controls the spine and pelvis is likely to be beneficial in management of back pain.
3. Motor control of the spine can be changed with treatment/exercise.
4. Treatment involves consideration of more than a uni-dimensional focus on a single muscle or muscle activation strategy.
5. Treatment requires progression to enhanced execution of activities of daily living.

The following sections discuss the current state-of-understanding related to each of these issues of consensus and considers several issues that require further investigation.

The spine is controlled by a complex interplay of many muscles (i.e. no single muscle is the most important for spine control)

One issue that is often debated relates to which muscles provide the *greatest* contribution to stability for the spine and pelvis. There is consensus that this is the wrong question. It is clear that each muscle of the complex array of muscles that surrounds or attaches to the spine and pelvis or adjacent regions provides a contribution to the control of lumbopelvic movement and stiffness. There is no doubt that back function requires an integrated contribution of a range of muscles (Cholewicki et al. 1997; Hodges and Richardson 1997; McGill et al. 2003) and this has been a consistent observation throughout the range of tasks that have been studied. However this fact has often been lost in the recounting of research observations. For instance, although early studies of the postural adjustment associated with arm movement are often cited as evidence that transversus abdominis (TrA) (Hodges and Richardson 1997), lumbar multifidus (LM) (Moseley et al. 2002), diaphragm (Hodges et al. 1997) and pelvic floor muscles (Hodges et al. 2007) have a unique contribution to spine control, these studies also provide evidence of the important contribution of the many other abdominal and back muscles. These other muscles act predictably to control the spine and pelvis in a manner primarily linked to the direction of reactive moments. Rather than consider which muscle is most important, it appears more appropriate to consider that an array of muscles is necessary to meet the demands of function. However, alteration of how the multiple muscles interact in functional tasks may have consequences for the loading on the spine.

In basic terms it is essential to consider that the spine is controlled dynamically by the interplay of activity of the multiple muscles. The control operates at two levels: one is control of the body segments that influences joint loading resulting from posture and movement choice; the other is control to stiffen spinal joints (such as those experiencing aberrant micro-movements from tissue damage with the potential to irritate nociceptors). Optimal spine control requires a balance between stiffness and movement and this balance will depend on the task. Although the demands of some tasks will be optimally met by increased stiffness (control of displacement), the demands of another may be better served by dynamic solution, such as optimized damping (control of velocity). These strategies require different muscle activation strategies. Failure to match the right solution or a less than ideal solution to a specific context (which may involve too much or too little activity of a range of muscles) is unlikely to be ideal and may be a potential target for rehabilitation. This view is agreed.

Both extremes of compromised morphology and behaviour of a range of muscles, and conversely, augmented activation of muscles could negatively impact lumbopelvic health. In both cases the argument can be reduced to consideration of suboptimal loading of the tissues. Reduced or compromised activity may lead to increased load as a result of less than ideal control of motion or insufficient stiffness. Reduced contribution of a range of muscles has been presented in the literature, including TrA (Hodges et al. 2007), LM (MacDonald et al. 2009), psoas (Ploumis et al. 2011), gluteus maximus (Hungerford et al. 2003), to name a few, although some appear prevalent in the back pain population, it is likely that many or most of these changes will be specific to subpopulations of people with low back and pelvic pain. For example, recent results suggest inhibition of gluteal muscles with experimentally induced hip pain and capsule pressure that is reversed by reduction of pain and pressure (Freeman and McGill, in press). In the case of increased activity, the load on the spinal structures may be increased via factors such as greater compressive force, excessive stiffening, altered damping (control of velocity) or compromised shock absorption. There is considerable evidence that people with low back and pelvic pain have increased muscle activity, but this varies between individuals (Hodges et al. 2003, 2013; van Dieën et al. 2003). An important consideration is whether the increased activity is required (to compensate for decreased passive control of the spine leading to aberrant joint motion, perhaps due to injury (Panjabi, 1992)) or is problematic (with the additional load a cause of persistence or recurrence of pain (Hides et al. 2001; Hodges and Tucker, 2011)). Both alternatives may be plausible but the relative balance between positive and negative effects may depend on the individual patient. Each patient has different compressive load tolerance, bending motion tolerance, joint laxity and therapeutic stiffening/compliance requirements that must be considered in treatment planning.

Issues that require further investigation include identification of the scope of changes that are present in low back and pelvic pain, and the specificity of changes to specific groups within the heterogeneous back pain population. Whether identification of subgroups is helpful for treatment guidance and efficacy is discussed in detail in Chapter 17.

Changing the manner in which a patient controls the spine and pelvis is likely to be beneficial in management of back pain

A fundamental concept that is almost universally agreed by protagonists of motor control training approaches is that clinical benefit can be gained if motor control can be changed to optimize the load on structures of the spine and pelvis and stiffness between them. Although additional load enhances stiffness in one patient, the load may not be tolerated in another. A key message is that optimization of loading, and therefore, back pain rehabilitation, is not about training to improve coordination/strength/endurance/etc. of a single muscle, or of a single strategy. Instead the approach aims to change the function of whichever aspect of the motor control system is responsible for suboptimal loading or insufficient stiffness in the unique individual. Focus on a specific muscle or multiple muscle co-activation strategy is not the sole intervention, but may be an important *component* of restoring ideal motor control. It makes biological sense that management should require careful consideration of all aspects of control, including posture, movement and muscle activation strategies, identification of the aspects that require correction, and then implementation of a rehabilitation program to achieve/restore/rectify this control.

The biological model implies that suboptimal loading of spinal and/or pelvic structures is relevant for, and may underpin, nociceptor input that contributes to low back and pelvic pain. It follows that lumbopelvic control is likely to be less than optimal when the contribution of any muscle is decreased, or in fact, if it is increased, or when the posture and/or movement of the spine loads structures in a manner that is not ideal (e.g. increased, decreased, sustained, etc.) or even aberrant. However, the ideal pattern of muscle activity, posture and movement, and any compromise or dysfunction, will be task-specific (e.g. the recruitment of a pattern of muscle that provides a substantial contribution to stability in one specific set of conditions may not be ideal in another). A solution that may be ideal to maintain stability of the spine in a static upright posture may not be ideal to maintain stability when the spine is dynamically moving between points. Thus, the consideration of effect of changes in muscle activity in lumbopelvic pain is most likely to be effective if addressed in a manner that is specific to the task, specific to the individual, and also specific to the environmental context.

A further point of consensus is that rehabilitation should follow a progression beginning with refinement/restoration of the strategy for control of muscle activation, posture and movement. This early phase could involve identification of the most appropriate patterns of muscle activation, posture and/or movement that eliminate/reduce pain. For example, pain may be controlled by encouraging a specific patient to maintain a lumbar lordosis with appropriate co-activation of deep and superficial muscles of the lumbar spine during trunk flexion, or the exact opposite, encouraging a patient to allow spine flexion during this task, with the strategy that is selected based on the presenting features of the patient's pain pattern. It is emphatically agreed that this necessitates comprehensive assessment to identify the patterns that could both be responsible for generation/perpetuation of nociceptive input to the central nervous system and be a candidate parameter that may have the potential to eliminate this contribution to pain.

The initial step is to identify which aspects of movement, posture and muscle activation may be relevant to symptoms. The next is to find the optimal solution to change these aspects in a way that is matched in an individualized manner to the patient and their functional requirements. It follows that there is unlikely to be any single aspect of motor control that should be universally targeted in exercise management, although some features may need to be addressed more commonly than others (e.g. control of motion in a specific direction; control of a specific component of the spine; activation or deactivation of specific muscles or muscle groups). What remains is disagreement about some of the features of muscle activation that should be assessed and targeted with intervention. A key aspect of this disagreement is whether attention should be placed on assessment and training of some of the deeper muscles of the trunk, e.g. TrA, LM, pelvic floor and diaphragm muscles, which forms a basic part of treatment programmes described by some authors (Richardson et al. 1999; Hides et al. 2001; Ferreira et al. 2007) but not by others (McGill 2002). Or whether attention should be focussed on exercises that encourage specific patterns of activation of muscle groups (e.g. bracing of the trunk muscles), again emphasized by some authors (McGill, 2002), but not by others (Richardson et al. 1999). Aspects of this divergence of opinion are considered in detail later in this chapter under the heading 'Issues with difference in opinion'.

An important consideration is that the biological contribution of abnormal loading to persistence/recurrence of pain is not a universally held opinion. Although many agree that mechanical loading may be responsible for the initiation of a painful episode, e.g. the cause of an injury that initiates nociceptive input or reactivates nociceptive input or a 'memory' of such, it is not universally agreed that repeated/ongoing discharge of nociceptive afferents is the mechanism that underpins ongoing pain. As discussed in Chapter 11, one interpretation of changes in motor control is that they may simply be considered as epiphenomena, i.e. observations that co-exist with the pain but are neither sufficient nor necessary for the perpetuation of symptoms. Although there is evidence that changes in movement, posture and muscle activation induce changes in load on spinal structures and can lead to injury, there is, as yet, limited data confirming a direct relationship between this dysfunction and pain. A recent report of four case studies documented immediate relief of pain by 'tuning' spine loading and stiffness by adjustment to muscular bracing patterns and spine and hip postures/movements (Ikeda and McGill, 2012). Although there are data to suggest pain is not contingent upon the presence of poor control, there is insufficient evidence to discount the view that poor control contributes. The major reason for the absence of definitive evidence of a relationship between suboptimal loading and pain is that a causal link is very difficult to confirm *in vivo* in humans as it is unethical to induce poor loading in humans, and suboptimal loading is likely to require time and repetition before problems develop. It is difficult to develop definitive animal muscles, as it is difficult to measure pain (as opposed to nociceptive activity) in animals. Unfortunately, the clinical observation of a reduction in pain after implementing a change in motor control with a therapeutic intervention does not confirm that the change in mechanics was the critical feature. This is because many other explanations can be provided from the literature. Resolution of debate regarding the relevance of biological changes in loading and pain is fundamentally important to progress work in this field. Priority needs to be placed on finding methods to assess the relevance of suboptimal loading, secondary to suboptimal motor control, and its restoration to the development, persistence, recurrence and resolution of low back and pelvic pain.

Even if a biological link can be confirmed, a critical element that must be considered is that persistent or recurrent lumbopelvic pain is multi-factorial and the biological aspects must be considered in a biopsychosocial framework, and the relative importance of biological, psychological and social aspects must be considered as potentially individual-specific. Although restoration of optimal mechanical control of the lumbar spine and pelvis may be a primary target in one individual, it may have a less important role in another individual who has a dominant contribution of unhealthy attitudes about pain such as fear avoidance, or dominant social features. Thus, characterization of patients across multiple domains and judgement of the relative importance of each for their presentation is essential for development of a multi-disciplinary rehabilitation programme. Although this proposal makes logical sense, research is required to clarify such a targeted treatment approach and its efficacy. A

further issue to consider is that the domains are not independent. For instance, attitudes and beliefs about pain can moderate the effect of pain on motor control parameters (Moseley et al. 2004). Interdependence of the biopsychosocial domains in low back pain is only beginning to be understood and should be a focus of future investigation.

Motor control can be changed with treatment/exercise

Although the specific features of motor control that are addressed in different approaches may differ, there is agreement in the opinion that motor control can be changed with exercise and that improvements in motor control can be translated to function. Evidence is emerging to confirm that this is the case (Scannell and McGill 2003; Tsao and Hodges 2007) and other work is beginning to highlight the neural processes that may underpin this recovery (Tsao, Galea et al. 2010).

One issue of some debate is how to best achieve restoration/modification of motor control strategies. Several options have been presented, and these include: (i) practice of complex functional tasks with correction of the component considered to be 'faulty' (O'Sullivan 2005); (ii) attention to specific muscles (e.g. selective deep muscle contraction (Richardson et al. 1999)) or muscle activation strategies (e.g. coached movement (McGill, 2002)); (iii) indirect training using automatic strategies (e.g. walking on unstable surfaces to encourage changes in motor patterns of proximal muscles (Bullock-Saxton et al. 1993)); (iv) identifying the painful movement and altering the movement pattern coupled with muscular bracing to reduce reported pain (Ikeda and McGill, 2012); or (iv) that this can be achieved with encouragement to return to function without specific attention to correction of muscle activation, posture or movement. The question of which intervention is most effective and whether the most effective intervention differs between individuals has not been completely resolved. However, there is evidence for some of these approaches. For instance, specific attention to muscle activation can change motor control in terms of the augmented (Tsao and Hodges, 2007) or reduced (Tsao, Druitt et al. 2010) activation of those muscles in a functional task. At this point it is important to reinforce that although this strategy can change muscle activation, this is never intended to be the complete intervention and other strategies must be utilized as part of a comprehensive treatment package to restore other aspects of motor function (e.g. correction of postural dysfunction).

One issue to consider further is that although practice of voluntary contraction of specific muscles or patterns of muscle activity has been shown to change motor control, this voluntary approach has been criticized on two grounds. First, one argument is stated that the brain controls muscles rather than movements and focus on muscle is a fundamental departure from this property of central nervous system organization. This argument can be countered by evidence that the nervous system organizes motor control both in terms of movements and muscles (Kakei et al. 1999). Second, it is argued that control of the trunk is normally coordinated automatically without the requirement for conscious input, and by inference, the argument has been put forward that practice of voluntary contraction involving input from primary motor cortex is unlikely to influence postural strategies. Yet there is sound evidence that inputs from the primary motor cortex contribute to control of the postural function (Gahéry and Nieoullon 1978) and it has been shown in a number of studies with a range of experimental methods including investigation of temporal parameters of automatic activation of the deep muscles in association with arm movements (Tsao and Hodges 2007), spatial features of trunk muscle activity in gait (Tsao and Hodges 2008), and organization of neurone networks in the motor cortex (Tsao, Galea et al. 2010) that motor control can be resolved by repeated voluntary muscle activation. This highlights that the cognitive approach of voluntary practice of a task leads to improved control, and this is associated with clinical improvement (Ferreira et al. 2010). This does not exclude the possibility that other techniques could also achieve a change, although other interventions must be subjected to evaluation. It is likely that a range of approaches will be required to change control depending on the individual patient, the nature of their change in control, and the specific motor tasks that are affected.

A feature common to different motor control approaches is the use of multiple methods to enhance the restoration of control of posture, movement and muscle activation. In addition to voluntary correction of aspects that are considered to be 'faulty', training may include other techniques such as application of tape to the skin, use of exercise equipment to enhance challenge, electrical stimulation of muscle, soft tissue techniques and manual therapy, etc. Many questions remain unresolved about the efficacy of many of these adjunctive treatments.

Treatment involves consideration of more than a uni-dimensional focus on a single muscle or muscle activation strategy

A common misconception presented in the lay literature is that some exercise approaches have a universal and uni-dimensional focus on a single solution for the management of low back pain. This is a common misconception of the place of 'bracing' or 'isolation of deep muscle activation/hollowing' in treatment. This misconception is likely to be founded on several issues. First, the protagonists of each approach often aim to emphasize the aspects

of their approach that differ from others in order to highlight unique aspects. Unfortunately this can lead to the assumption that the highlighted component is the 'whole approach' and other aspects are excluded. Second, some degree of reductionism is commonplace in the lay literature to efficiently translate a message to clinical practice or common use and it is common for the media (e.g. magazine articles of 'core stability' exercise) to present the 'best' exercise, and this could never replicate the complexity of a comprehensive rehabilitation approach. It is when it becomes assumed that this is the 'whole' approach that the issues arise. Third, authors aiming to discredit a management philosophy often use the technique of oversimplification in order to undermine the intellectual integrity of an approach (e.g. Lederman 2010; see critique by McGill 2011).

An extrapolation of these reductionist views is that it is assumed that the protagonists of the approaches advocate the use of the 'universal solution' to trunk control for function. For instance, it has been suggested that the intention of training a patient to isolate TrA activation from the other abdominal muscles is for this to be the strategy trained for function, i.e. for patients to attempt to isolate TrA when lifting a mass from the floor. This is not the intention of training independent activation of TrA (Richardson et al. 1999) and isolated activation of this muscle has been shown to compromise spine control (see Chapter 7). Instead, the intention of training independent TrA activation is purported to be to train the activation of this muscle, such that it can then be incorporated in function, as a component of the complex interaction of multiple muscles (Tsao and Hodges 2007). Likewise, the suggestion to encourage abdominal bracing to 30% of a maximal effort (McGill 2002) was not intended to imply that patients should maintain this level of activation throughout all functions; this is neither attainable or sustainable. Contraction of this intensity cannot be maintained beyond a timescale of seconds (Bjorksten and Jonsson 1977). Yet training such activation as a component of an exercise programme is intended to make this muscle activation pattern *available* for function and to enhance the capacity for its use as demanded by the function.

It is almost universally agreed that it is unlikely that rehabilitation of a single or few muscles will be sufficient to rehabilitate low back and pelvic pain. Although the observation of changes in the deep muscles is common, this does not diminish the likely importance of changes in other parts of the system – other muscles, postural changes and movement patterns. Although there may be some consistency in the adaptation of the deep muscles, there are unique individual-specific changes in the other aspects of the system. As highlighted above this may include increased or reduced activity of other muscles; changes in the coordination between hip and spine motion (Van Dillen et al. 2007); or changes in movement or posture (Mitchell et al. 2008). There is considerable evidence that many or most of these factors are specific to individuals/subgroups. Some have been related to clinically identified subgroups of people with spinal pain (Astfalck et al. 2010). It appears reasonable to conclude that rehabilitation of the whole system will be ideal, that this would need to be individualized to the patient, and that attempts to increase and decrease activation of specific muscles may be important components of a comprehensive approach. Furthermore, different strategies are likely to be important for different tasks. Higher load tasks that require restriction of spine movement may require greater co-contraction of large trunk muscles and with specific alignment of the spine, whereas dynamic control of the spine during functions such as gait is likely to require another solution, and these may need to be trained specifically.

Treatment requires progression to enhanced execution of activities of daily living

It is well known that better transfer to function is achieved with practice of the task as close as possible to the 'real life' situation (Shumway-Cook and Woollacott, 2006). It follows that early phases of rehabilitation of motor control of the trunk for treatment of low back and pelvic pain are followed by progression beyond the retraining of optimal control strategies, to complex function. This necessitates not only the reinforcement of use of ideal strategies of muscle activation, posture and movement in function, but also improvement in the capacity of the system to meet higher functional loads (e.g. muscle strength, muscle endurance, cardiovascular fitness).

The progression eventually incorporates enhancement of skilled execution of activities of daily living and these tasks are different for each individual, thus each individual will have a different rehabilitation 'end point'. The progression to this functional level necessitates consideration of other aspects relevant to function such as resolution of psychosocial elements relevant to perpetuation of symptoms such as fear of movement/pain/(re)injury, catastrophization and other biological aspects such as balance and sensory function. These factors may be addressed by functional training or may require specific attention with separate interventions incorporated into the comprehensive management of the patient.

ISSUES WITH DIFFERENCE IN OPINION

Although the fundamental basis for extrapolation of research observations into clinical practice is agreed, as

outlined above, there remains a major point of difference of opinion. The detail of the divergent viewpoints has been outlined in individual chapters (including Chapters 6 and 7), but can be summarized as follows below.

Control of deeper muscles of the trunk, including TrA and LM, should be assessed and addressed if dysfunction is identified

This issue is a major point of departure from consensus of opinion in the literature. Although it is generally agreed that aspects of motor control modified in a patient with low back pain should be addressed in exercise interventions, opinion does not converge whether activation of the deeper muscles forms part of this consideration. One viewpoint is that changes in the deeper muscles of the trunk are common (Hodges and Richardson 1996; Hides et al. 2008), that changes in the activation of these muscles contributes to a compromise in the quality of control of the load on spinal and pelvic structures (Hodges, Kaigle-Holm et al. 2003), that control of these elements of the system can be restored with exercise interventions (Tsao and Hodges 2007; Tsao and Hodges 2008), and that restoration of control of these muscles contributes to recovery of pain and disability (Ferreira et al. 2010). The alternative view is that these muscles are no more important to consider than any other, and that the control of these muscles is not necessary to address in patients with pain, not possible to address in patients with pain, and potentially counterproductive if addressed in patients with pain (see Chapter 7).

These divergent opinions are considered in detail in preceding chapters and this will not be repeated here. Instead it is important to consider how to resolve the debate. Although on the surface the most obvious study design would be to compare the outcome of interventions that do and do not include training of TrA and LM, this is unlikely to be fruitful as many components require consideration in complete treatment and the contribution of one element will be difficult to extract. Clinical trials are known to have relatively blunt outcomes and rarely find differences between treatments (Macedo et al. 2009). The current status of evidence from systematic reviews concludes that training that *includes* attention focussed to activation of the deep muscles reduces pain and disability and decreases recurrence of pain (Ferreira et al. 2006) and is more effective than placebo treatment (Costa et al. 2009). However, there is limited evidence that this type of intervention is better than other interventions. Importantly, although large effects have been identified in specific subgroups of lumbopelvic pain (O'Sullivan et al. 1997; Hides et al. 2001; Stuge et al. 2004), smaller effects have been identified in non-specific low back pain groups and it is this latter group that has been used to compare interventions. Future work may identify characteristics of individuals who respond best to motor control treatments and how it is best targeted to the individual. There is preliminary evidence that poor control of deep muscles predicts good response to motor control interventions (Ferreira et al. 2010; Unsgaard-Tondel et al. 2012).

One key issue that requires resolution is to investigate the prevalence of changes in control of TrA and LM in the people with low back and pelvic pain, and those without pain. Although it is assumed that these changes are prevalent, and this is revealed by clinical assessment (Richardson et al. 2004), this issue has not been studied consistently in a large population and although it would be surprising to be uniform across the back pain population, it is a common observation in small groups with pain (Hides et al. 1994; Hodges and Richardson 1996) and is consistently identified in response to experimentally induced pain in humans (Hodges et al. 2003; Kiesel et al. 2008), and following experimental injuries in animals (Hodges et al. 2006). Some work has identified differences between patient subgroups (Kiesel et al. 2007). Thus, further work is required to determine whether reduced contribution of TrA and LM leads to changes in the health of the spine such as injury and pain and to identify the prevalence of changes in morphology and behaviour of these muscles in people with low back and pelvic pain. This latter issue requires the development of less invasive and easier methods to study the morphology and behaviour of these muscles. This is a topic of interest for many groups internationally (Ferreira et al. 2004; Kiesel et al. 2007; Mannion et al. 2008; Vasseljen et al. 2009).

CONCLUSION

This chapter aimed to summarize current points of consensus and divergence of opinion regarding the extrapolation of research regarding the control of the spine and pelvis in a healthy context and in the presence of pain to the design of effective interventions for low back and pelvic pain. Consideration of the debate reveals a perhaps surprising degree of agreement regarding the fundamental concepts that underpin this extrapolation, but areas of divergence remain. The biological plausibility of the arguments is clear and the review has highlighted areas that could be considered priorities for future research to test the foundation of the application of training of motor control to changing biology and to optimize its application to clinical management of people in pain. The clear consensus is that intervention is likely to be best when all aspects in a patient's presentation (e.g. posture, movement and muscle activation, as well as psychological and social aspects) are considered and a treatment plan is developed with consideration across the domains that have the potential to contribute to the individual's pain experience. Many questions remain to be answered, but the data so far continue to be promising.

REFERENCES

Astfalck, RG., O'Sullivan, P.B., Straker, L.M., Smith, A.J., Burnett, A., Caneiro, J.P., et al., 2010. Sitting postures and trunk muscle activity in adolescents with and without nonspecific chronic low back pain: an analysis based on subclassification. Spine 35, 1387–1395.

Bjorksten, M., Jonsson, B., 1977. Endurance limit of force in long-term intermittent static contractions. Scand J Work Environ Health 3, 23–27.

Bullock-Saxton, J.E., Janda, V., Bullock, M.I., 1993. Reflex activation of gluteal muscles in walking with balance shoes: an approach to restoration of function for chronic low back pain patients. Spine 18, 704–708.

Cholewicki, J., Panjabi, M.M., Khacha-tryan, A., 1997. Stabilizing function

of trunk flexor-extensor muscles around a neutral spine posture. Spine 22, 2207–2212.

Costa, L.O., Maher, C.G., Latimer, J., Hodges, P.W., Herbert, R.D., Refshauge, K.M., et al., 2009. Motor control exercise for chronic low back pain: a randomized placebo-controlled trial. Phys Ther 89, 1275–1286.

Ferreira, P., Ferreira, M., Hodges, P., 2004. Changes to recruitment of the abdominal muscles in people with low back pain: ultrasound measurement of muscle activity. Spine 29, 2560–2566.

Ferreira, M.L., Ferreira, P.H., Latimer, J., Herbert, R.D., Hodges, P.W., Jennings, M.D., et al., 2007. Comparison of general exercise, motor control exercise and spinal manipulative therapy for chronic low

back pain: a randomized trial. Pain 131, 31–37.

Ferreira, P.H., Ferreira, M.L., Maher, C.G., Herbert, R.D., Refshauge, K., 2006. Specific stabilisation exercise for spinal and pelvic pain: a systematic review. Aust J Physiother 52, 79–88.

Ferreira, P., Ferreira, M., Maher, C., Refshauge, K., Herbert, R., Hodges, P., 2010. Changes in recruitment of transversus abdominis correlate with disability in people with chronic low back pain. Br J Sports Med 44, 1166–1172.

Freeman, S., McGill, S.M., 2013. Arthrogenic neuromuscular inhibition: a foundational investigation of existence in the hip joint. Clin Biomech (in press).

Gahéry, Y., Nieoullon, A., 1978. Postural and kinetic co-ordination following cortical stimuli which induce flexion movements in the cat's limbs. Brain Res 155, 25–37.

Hides, J., Gilmore, C., Stanton, W., Bohlscheid, E., 2008. Multifidus size and symmetry among chronic LBP and healthy asymptomatic subjects. Man Ther 13, 43–49.

Hides, J.A., Jull, G.A., Richardson, C.A., 2001. Long term effects of specific stabilizing exercises for first episode low back pain. Spine 26, 243–248.

Hides, J.A., Stokes, M.J., Saide, M., Jull, G.A., Cooper, D.H., 1994. Evidence of lumbar multifidus muscle wasting ipsilateral to symptoms in patients with acute/subacute low back pain. Spine 19, 165–177.

Hodges, P., Tucker, K., 2011. Moving differently in pain: a new theory to explain the adaptation to pain. Pain 152, S90–S98.

Hodges, P.W., Butler, J.E., McKenzie, D., Gandevia, S.C., 1997. Contraction of the human diaphragm during postural adjustments. J Physiol 505, 239–248.

Hodges, P.W., KaigleHolm, A., Hansson, T., Holm, S., 2006. Rapid atrophy of the lumbar multifidus follows experimental disc or nerve root injury. Spine 31, 2926–2933.

Hodges, P., Kaigle Holm, A., Holm, S., Ekstrom, L., Cresswell, A., Hansson, T., et al., 2003. Intervertebral stiffness of the spine is increased by evoked contraction of transversus abdominis and the diaphragm: in vivo porcine studies. Spine 28, 2594–2601.

Hodges, P.W., Moseley, G.L., Gabrielsson, A., Gandevia, S.C., 2003. Experimental muscle pain changes feedforward postural responses of the trunk muscles. Exp Brain Res 151, 262–271.

Hodges, P.W., Pengel, H.M., Sapsford, R., 2007. Postural and respiratory functions of the pelvic floor muscles. Neurourol Urodyn 26, 362–371.

Hodges, P.W., Richardson, C.A., 1996. Inefficient muscular stabilisation of the lumbar spine associated with low back pain: a motor control evaluation of transversus abdominis. Spine 21, 2640–2650.

Hodges, P.W., Richardson, C.A., 1997. Feedforward contraction of transversus abdominis in not influenced by the direction of arm movement. Exp Brain Res 114, 362–370.

Hodges, P.W., Coppieters, M.W., Macdonald, D., Cholewicki, J., 2013. New insight into motor adaptation to pain revealed by a combination of modelling and empirical approaches. Eur J Pain. doi: 10.1002/j.1532-2149. 2013.00286.x.

Hungerford, B., Hodges, P., Gilleard, W., 2003. Evidence of altered lumbopelvic muscle recruitment in the presence of sacroiliac joint pain. Spine 28, 1593–1600.

Ikeda, D., McGill, S.M., 2012. Can altering motions, postures and loads provide immediate low back pain relief? Spine 37, E1469–E1475.

Kakei, S., Hoffman, D.S., Strick, P.L., 1999. Muscle and movement representations in the primary motor cortex. Science 285, 2136–2139.

Kiesel, K.B., Uhl, T., Underwood, F.B., Nitz, A.J., 2008. Rehabilitative ultrasound measurement of select trunk muscle activation during induced pain. Man Ther 13, 132–138.

Kiesel, K.B., Underwood, F.B., Mattacola, C.G., Nitz, A.J., Malone, T.R., 2007. A comparison of select trunk muscle thickness change between subjects with low back pain classified in the treatment-based classification system and asymptomatic controls. J Orthop Sports Phys Ther 37, 596–607.

Lederman, E., 2010. The myth of core stability. J Bodywork Movement Ther [Review] 14, 84–98.

MacDonald, D., Moseley, G.L., Hodges, P.W., 2009. Why do some patients keep hurting their back? Evidence of ongoing back muscle dysfunction during remission from recurrent back pain. Pain 142, 183–188.

Macedo, L.G., Maher, C.G., Latimer, J., McAuley, J.H., 2009. Motor control exercise for persistent, nonspecific low back pain: a systematic review. Phys Ther 89, 9–25.

Mannion, A.F., Pulkovski, N., Schenk, P., Hodges, P.W., Gerber, H., Loupas, T., et al., 2008. A new method for the noninvasive determination of abdominal muscle feedforward activity based on tissue velocity information from tissue Doppler imaging. J Appl Physiol 104, 1192–1201.

McGill, S., 2002. Low back disorders: Evidence Based Prevention and Rehabilitation. Human Kinetics Publishers, Champaign, IL.

McGill, S., 2011. Invited response. J Bodywork Movement Ther [Comment] 15, 150–152.

McGill, S.M., Grenier, S., Kavcic, N., Cholewicki, J., 2003. Coordination of muscle activity to assure stability of the lumbar spine. J Electromyogr Kinesiol 13, 353–359.

Mitchell, T., O'Sullivan, P.B., Burnett, A.F., Straker, L., Smith, A., 2008. Regional differences in lumbar spinal posture and the influence of low back pain. BMC Musculoskelet Disord 9, 152.

Moseley, G.L., Hodges, P.W., Gandevia, S.C., 2002. Deep and superficial fibers of lumbar multifidus are differentially active during voluntary arm movements. Spine 27, E29–E36.

Moseley, G.L., Nicholas, M.K., Hodges, P.W., 2004. Does anticipation of back pain predispose to back trouble? Brain 127, 2339–2347.

O'Sullivan, P., 2005. Diagnosis and classification of chronic low back pain disorders: maladaptive movement and motor control impairments as underlying mechanism. Man Ther 10, 242–255.

O'Sullivan, P.B., Twomey, L.T., Allison, G.T., 1997. Evaluation of specific stabilizing exercise in the treatment of chronic low back pain with radiologic diagnosis of spondylolysis or spondylolisthesis. Spine 22, 2959–2967.

Panjabi, M.M., 1992. The stabilizing system of the spine. Part I. Function, dysfunction, adaptation, and enhancement. J Spinal Dis 5, 383–389.

Ploumis, A., Michailidis, N., Christodoulou, P., Kalaitzoglou, I., Gouvas, G., Beris, A., 2011. Ipsilateral atrophy of paraspinal and psoas muscle in unilateral back pain patients with monosegmental degenerative disc disease. Br J Radiol 84, 709–713.

Richardson, C.A., Hodges, P.W., Hides, J.A., 2004. Therapeutic Exercise for Lumbopelvic Stabilisation: a motor control approach for the treatment and prevention of low back pain. Churchill Livingstone, Edinburgh.

Richardson, C.A., Jull, G.A., Hodges, P.W., Hides, J.A., 1999. Therapeutic Exercise for Spinal Segmental Stabilisation in Low Back Pain: scientific basis and clinical approach. Churchill Livingstone, Edinburgh.

Scannell, J.P., McGill, S.M., 2003. Lumbar posture – should it, and can it, be modified? A study of passive tissue stiffness and lumbar position during activities of daily living. Phys Ther [Research Support, Non-US Govt] 83, 907–917.

Shumway-Cook, A., Woollacott, M., 2006. Motor Control: translating research into clinical practice, 3rd edn. Lippincott Williams & Wilkins, Philadelphia, PA.

Stuge, B., Laerum, E., Kirkesola, G., Vollestad, N., 2004. The efficacy of a treatment program focusing on specific stabilizing exercises for pelvic girdle pain after pregnancy: a randomized controlled trial. Spine 29, 351–359.

Tsao, H., Hodges, P.W., 2007. Immediate changes in feedforward postural adjustments following voluntary motor training. Exp Brain Res 181, 537–546.

Tsao, H., Hodges, P., 2008. Persistence of improvements in postural strategies following motor control training in people with recurrent low back pain. J Electromyogr Kinesiol 18, 559–567.

Tsao, H., Galea, M.P., Hodges, P.W., 2010. Driving plasticity in the motor cortex in recurrent low back pain. Eur J Pain 14, 832–839.

Tsao, H., Druitt, T.R., Schollum, T.M., Hodges, P.W., 2010. Motor training of the lumbar paraspinal muscles induces immediate changes in motor coordination in patients with recurrent low back pain. J Pain [Research Support, Non-U.S. Govt] 11, 1120–1128.

Unsgaard-Tondel, M., Lund Nilsen, T.I., Magnussen, J., Vasseljen, O., 2012. Is activation of transversus abdominis and obliquus internus abdominis associated with long-term changes in chronic low back pain? A prospective study with 1-year follow-up. Br J Sports Med 46, 729–734.

van Dieën, J.H., Selen, L.P., Cholewicki, J., 2003. Trunk muscle activation in low-back pain patients, an analysis of the literature. J Electromyogr Kinesiol 13, 333–351.

Van Dillen, L.R., Gombatto, S.P., Collins, D.R., Engsberg, J.R., Sahrmann, SA., 2007. Symmetry of timing of hip and lumbopelvic rotation motion in 2 different subgroups of people with low back pain. Arch Phys Med Rehabil 88, 351–360.

Vasseljen, O., Fladmark, A.M., Westad, C., Torp, H.G., 2009. Onset in abdominal muscles recorded simultaneously by ultrasound imaging and intramuscular electromyography. J Electromyogr Kinesiol 19, e23–e31.

Part 6

State-of-the-art approach to clinical rehabilitation of low back and pelvic pain

Chapter |21|

Integrated clinical approach to motor control interventions in low back and pelvic pain

Paul W. Hodges*, Linda R. Van Dillen†, Stuart McGill‡, Simon Brumagne§, Julie A. Hides‖ and G. Lorimer Moseley¶
*NHMRC Centre of Clinical Research Excellence in Spinal Pain, Injury and Health, School of Health and Rehabilitation Sciences, University of Queensland, Brisbane, Queensland, Australia, †Program in Physical Therapy and Department of Orthopaedic Surgery, Washington University School of Medicine at Washington University Medical Center, St Louis, Missouri, USA, ‡Department of Kinesiology, Faculty of Applied Health Sciences, University of Waterloo, Waterloo, Ontario, Canada, §Department of Rehabilitation Sciences, University of Leuven, Leuven, Belgium, ‖School of Physiotherapy, Australian Catholic University, McAuley Campus, Banyo, Queensland, Australia, and ¶Sansom Institute for Health Research, University of South Australia, Adelaide, South Australia and Neuroscience Research Australia, Sydney, Australia

INTRODUCTION

At first glance the different approaches to exercise management of low back and pelvic pain can seem divergent with mutually exclusive elements. For instance, some approaches highlight the evaluation and activation of the deeper muscles of the trunk (Richardson et al. 2004; Hodges et al. 2009), whereas others consider this aspect of the system to be either corrected automatically by management of

other aspects such as correction of movement 'faults' or 'alteration' (Sahrmann 2002; McGill 2007). Further, some approaches focus on cognitive correction (explicit learning) whereas others rely on more automatic solutions (implicit learning) without cognitive attention to muscles or movements (Janda 1996). Despite these apparent areas of difference in opinion, on closer examination, there is far greater convergence than divergence in the recommendations for treatment. It is just the *emphasis* that differs between approaches. Many authors and protagonists for specific approaches tend to highlight aspects that may receive limited attention in other approaches. This chapter aims to bring together the contemporary views in the field related to rehabilitation of motor control for the management of low back and pelvic pain and presents a framework for an integrated approach that provides insight into how the multiple different approaches fit together. The chapter also aims to consider the interaction between this approach and other interventions in the broader multidisciplinary biopsychosocial framework with consideration of the interaction between motor control and the other domains of low back and pelvic pain in assessment and treatment. An important distinction between this chapter and the other sections of this book is that many of the ideas presented here have clinical observations as their basis and have not been subjected to rigorous testing. However, this does not detract from their importance in understanding contemporary views of spine control as a focus of clinical management, and where evidence is available this is highlighted. In the context of this chapter the term 'motor control' interventions/treatments/exercise is used to describe treatment that aims to change the manner in which patients maintain posture/alignment, movement and muscle activation to change loading on lumbopelvic structures for the purpose of reducing pain and dysfunction. The term 'spine control' is used broadly to encompass the mechanisms used control movement and stiffness of the spine and pelvis.

KEY ISSUES IN APPLICATION OF EXERCISE INTERVENTIONS FOR LOW BACK AND PELVIC PAIN

A basic premise that underlies motor control approaches for the management of low back and pelvic pain is the objective to optimize *load* on the spine and pelvis to manage the biological contribution to pain that may arise from a peripheral contribution to nociceptive input as a result of tissue loading. Optimization of load may aim to reduce or remove: (i) mechanical irritation of lumbopelvic structures and discharge of nociceptive afferents (at least in the early acute phase); (ii) the potential for ongoing or recurring irritation; (iii) up-regulation of the inflammatory response; and (iv) peripheral sensitization with sub-failure damage or frank injury to spinal structures. The contemporary concept of suboptimal loading goes further than Panjabi's early ideas of 'clinical instability' (Panjabi 1992). In that early framework it was considered that pain would be explained by any deficit in the active (muscle), passive (non-contractile elements of the spine such as ligaments; joint orientation) or control (including contributions from the sensory input from the periphery and control of output by the nervous system) subsystems leading to increased movement (particularly within the 'neutral zone'). The contemporary view is that problems may arise if there is change in any aspect of the system that compromises the *optimal* control of the spine leaving the system less 'robust' (less able to tolerate load and adapt to change), and this may be related to too much or too little control.

In the acute or recurring acute phase there may be a reasonably direct relationship between peripheral events, nociceptor discharge and the pain experience, although the pain experience will be dependent on a spectrum of other factors that influence the magnitude of pain such as cognitive (e.g. catastrophizing) and other experiential aspects. In the chronic/maintained phase the relationship between peripheral events may be less clear as a result of further secondary central biological changes (central sensitization) and psychosocial aspects that lead to a mismatch between the events in the periphery and the experience of pain. However, the peripheral input from discharge of nociceptors can persist and can plausibly be considered to remain relevant in many patients. Figure 21.1 shows a biological model that provides a foundation to understand the potential basis for suboptimal loading

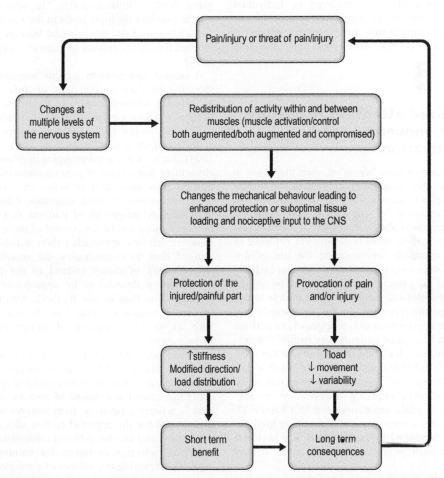

Figure 21.1 Physiological model of the relationship between pain/injury and motor control. This model provides a basis to interpret many of the changes that present in muscle activation, posture and movement and provides a foundation to understand the place for intervention for low back and pelvic pain that targets motor control of this region. Intervention can be targeted at multiple steps in the path, from reduction of the threat-value of pain/injury to reduction of pain-provocative adaptations.

and the role for motor control changes in the biological aspects of low back and pelvic pain.

Optimization of loading for tissue health can be achieved by changing: (i) posture/alignment, (ii) movement and/or (iii) muscle activation. Such optimization requires individualization to the specific features of the patient's pain presentation (e.g. aspects that are provocative or relieving for the patient, and the patient's functional demand) and balanced against other features that may contribute to the pain experience (e.g. cognitions and beliefs about pain (see 'Fitting training of spine control into the biopsychosocial framework')) or features that interact with the spine control and increase the complexity of training (e.g. respiratory and continence functions of trunk muscles (see 'Clinical application of strategies to manage barriers to recovery')). The relative emphasis placed on when and how posture/alignment, movement and muscle activation are considered in individual approaches varies, but all are considered to some extent. A key issue to recognize is that these three elements interact and attempts to change one element will necessarily affect the others.

Individualized attention to posture/alignment, movement and muscle activation

Motor control interventions, in general, share the common aim to modify posture/alignment, movement and muscle activation strategies to achieve the goal of optimization of load (via optimization of movement and stiffness). However, as mentioned above, the *targets* or *priorities* vary between approaches. As there is insufficient evidence to argue for one approach over another, the aim of this chapter is to present an integrated approach that includes consideration of the principles underlying the rehabilitation of posture/alignment, movement and muscle activation in different interventions. In future, research may highlight greater effectiveness of one approach, or perhaps more likely, that individual patients may require different approaches. Future work should determine whether identification of such individual differences and possible classification into 'subgroups' leads to improved outcomes. Issues associated with targeting interventions to subgroups in clinical trials are considered in Chapter 17. Table 21.1 provides a summary of subgrouping methods that have been developed for patients with low back and pelvic pain that include consideration of motor control training.

Most, if not all, clinical approaches focused on motor control advocate tailoring of rehabilitation strategies to individual patients based on assessment findings. Several approaches to individualization have been developed and adopted to varying degrees. One approach aims to assign patients to categories or diagnostic subgroups based on similarities in features of their presentation (e.g. movements or postures that are provocative/relieving) (Janda 1996; Sahrmann 2002; Kendall 2005; O'Sullivan 2005). This approach can be helpful to communicate assessment findings between health care providers and aims to assist the therapist in the process of selecting treatments for individual patients. Currently there is no dominant paradigm amongst the methods used to subgroup on the basis of posture/movement and there are important differences amongst the approaches in terms of the strategy for allocation for subgrouping. Some approaches aim to select specific patients with specific features from the heterogeneous group of people with back pain (e.g. distal cross syndrome – Janda 1996), whereas others aim to allocate all patients to one of a range of mutually exclusive categories (Sahrmann 2002; O'Sullivan 2005). The approaches may or may not involve multiple levels in the assessment, such as consideration of the psychosocial features, as well as the biological features related to motor control (O'Sullivan 2005).

A second approach to patient subgrouping involves grouping patients on the basis of their responsiveness to different interventions (e.g. Treatment Based Classification – Delitto et al. 1995) or on identification of structures thought to be the pain source (e.g. Petersen et al. 2003) or a combination of both (e.g. McKenzie 2003). Each of these subgrouping methods includes an element of assessment of posture, movement (e.g. direction of movement that provokes or relieves pain) or muscle activation. The basic emphasis of these approaches is to identify subgroups of patients that could benefit from rehabilitation of the control of the spine. However, in several of these approaches there is limited consideration of how to individualize the specific strategy for rehabilitation of motor control to the patient within the subgroup deemed to be appropriate for this type of treatment. That is, the methods identify responders to motor control training, but do not provide guidance as to what features of motor control require management.

A third approach advocates that treatment should be guided by assessment findings without explicit allocation to a subgroup. These assessment-guided approaches generally use careful assessment of posture, movement and muscle activation (sharing many features with the assessments used for the approaches that allocate patients to subgroups) and use the obtained information to guide the individual selection of targets for training, rather than explicitly allocating the patient to a subgroup (Lee 2004; Richardson et al. 2004; McGill 2007). One approach is to modify postures, motions and loads, to identify those which provoke or exacerbate pain (several examples are shown in Fig. 21.2) (Van Dillen et al. 2003a, 2009).

Table 21.1 Common approaches to subgrouping patients with low back and pelvic pain that are used to guide rehabilitation of spine control

Approach	Sub-groups	Key features
Classification based on movement/posture		
Kendall postural classification (Kendall 2005)	1. Kyphosis–lordosis posture 2. Sway-back posture 3. Military-type posture 4. Flat-back posture	Posture assessed by lateral assessment of landmarks relative to a plumb line
Movement system impairment syndromes (MSI) (Sahrmann 2002)	1. Lumbar rotation-extension syndrome 2. Lumbar extension syndrome 3. Lumbar rotation syndrome 4. Lumbar rotation–flexion syndrome 5. Lumbar flexion syndrome	Multiple specific movement and posture/alignment tests. Key features of assessment include: direction of symptom provocation; dissociation between adjacent segments (e.g. hip and spine); muscle stiffness at adjacent joints
O'Sullivan classification system (O'Sullivan 2005)	Control disorder 1. Multidirectional 2. Flexion 3. Lateral shift 4. Active extension 5. Passive extension Movement disorder 1. Flexion 2. Extension 3. Flexion with rotation/side bending 4. Extension with rotation/side bending Pelvic girdle pain 1. Form closure 2. Force closure	Aims to identify the underlying mechanisms considered to drive pain. Multiple specific movement and posture/alignment tests. Key features of assessment include: direction of symptom provocation; control of specific spine segments/regions. Consideration of pain avoidance, pain provocative behaviour and peripheral and central pain mechanisms
Distal cross syndrome (Janda 1996)	Distal cross syndrome	Specific subgroup within the heterogeneous back pain population based on posture and muscle activity/length
McGill approach to identification of pain-provoking motions, postures and loads (McGill 2007)	1. Compression load intolerant 2. Shear load intolerant 3. Flexion motion intolerant 4. Extension motion intolerant 5. Twist motion intolerant 6. Multiple mode intolerant 7. Other subgroups	Battery of provocative tests used to identify exacerbating postures together with the current tolerance of the patient to load and activity capacity. This directs the development of a progressive program of corrective exercise followed by training to create balance between several variables and pain-free tolerance to activity. Stiffening patterns or compliant movements are 'tuned' to reduce or eliminate pain

Continued

Table 21.1 Common approaches to subgrouping patients with low back and pelvic pain that are used to guide rehabilitation of spine control—cont'd

Approach	Sub-groups	Key features
Classification based on response to treatment		

Treatment-based classification (TBC) (Delitto et al. 1995)	Specific exercise
	  1. Flexion
	  2. Extension
	  3. Lateral shift/side-gliding
	Manipulation
	Stabilization
	Traction
		Subgrouping based on the likelihood of response to specific intervention. Assessment based on demographic and questionnaire-based outcomes in addition to evaluation of physical tests (e.g. response to repeated movement, manual joint testing). Involves use of a clinical prediction rule

Classification based on identification of pain source		

Pathoanatomic-based classification (Petersen et al. 2003)	Disc syndrome
	  1. Reducible
	  2. Irreducible
	  3. Non-mechanical
	  4. Nerve root compression
	Spinal stenosis
	Zygopophyseal joint
	Postural
	Sacroiliac joint
	Dysfunction
	Myofascial pain
	Adverse neural tension
	Abnormal pain
	Inconclusive
		Subgrouping method based on identification of the likely source of pain by use of a range of orthopaedic tests. Syndromes are defined by symptom location and effect of mechanical loading

Mixed-method classification approach		

Mechanical diagnosis and treatment (McKenzie and May 2003)	Derangement syndrome
	  1. Central and symmetrical
	  2. Unilateral and proximal to knee
	  3. Unilateral and distal to knee
	Dysfunction syndrome
	  1. Flexion
	  2. Extension
	  3. Lateral shift/side-gliding
	  4. Adherent nerve root
	Postural syndrome
	Other
	  1. Stenosis
	  2. Hip
	  3. Sacroiliac joint
	  4. Mechanically inconclusive
	  5. Spondylolisthesis
	  6. Chronic pain state
		Multiple tests including response to repeated loading. Aims to determine if LBP symptoms can be abolished or reduced through application of direction-specific, repeated lumbar spine movements or sustained postures. 'Derangement syndromes' thought to relate to internal intervertebral disc displacement; relate to tissue that has undergone 'contraction, scarring, adherence, adaptive shortening, or imperfect repair'. 'Postural syndrome' is assumed to arise from joint capsule and ligament ischemia due to prolonged spinal end range positioning

These variables are then removed by modification of the exacerbating movement and muscle activation patterns, and replaced with tolerable patterns that broaden the potential for pain-free performance. This approach relies on good clinical reasoning of specific assessment of features of the patient's presentation, and then targeting intervention to those features. These features include any aspect of posture, movement and muscle activation that the clinician identified to be related to the patient's symptoms. This approach enables similar individualization of treatment to subgroupings of patients with common features. A key advantage of clustering of features

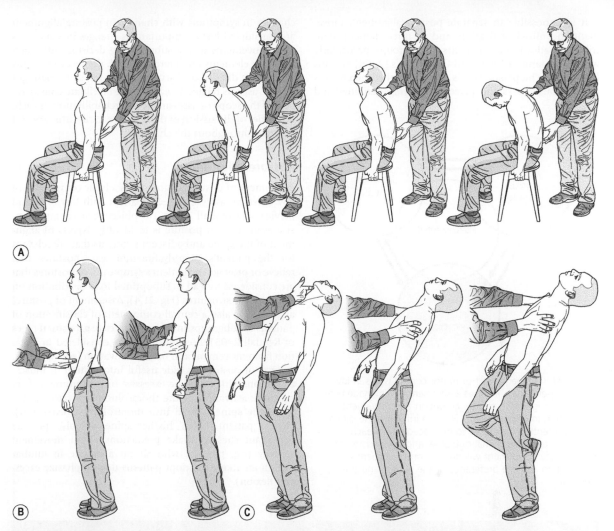

Figure 21.2 Examples of provocative testing in sitting and standing used by McGill. (A) The patient compresses the spine by grabbing the side edges of the seat and pulling down. First the spine is postured upright and the torso stiffened with muscle activity. The test is then repeated in a slouched posture where discomfort in this position as compared to an upright back shows a lower tolerance when the spine is flexed (in a flexion-intolerant patient). Then neural tensions are assessed with changes in cervical spine posture. (B) The 'standing drop test' is performed starting on the balls of the feet and dropping down abruptly onto the heels with the muscles relaxed to determine whether pain is provoked from ballistic compressive load. Control is adjusted by focusing on abdominal bracing, or latissimus/pectoral muscle stiffening, or postural adjustments to ascertain whether pain can be reduced or eliminated. (C) Extension of the spine in standing is assessed for pain provocation. This is then combined with rotation (no pain is thought to exclude the facet joints as pain generators). The test is repeated while standing on one leg, which adds stiffness and control. This stiffness is evaluated as a candidate strategy for pain control.

into subgroups is that it may facilitate the training of clinicians to select appropriate treatments. This would be particularly important for novice clinicians who are learning how to recognize patterns, a feature of skilled clinical reasoning (Jones and Rivett 2004). However, in the clinical-reasoning approach, the clinician is not 'biased' to expect a specific combination of features,

viewing each patient as an individual. Although aided by pattern recognition, this clinical reasoning approach emphasizes the uniqueness of an individual's presentation across multiple domains and is used in many contemporary clinical approaches to motor control training for low back and pelvic pain (e.g. Lee 2004; Richardson et al. 2004; McGill 2007).

It is impossible to separate posture/alignment, movement and muscle activation, and all three elements contribute to allocation of patients to subgroups, particularly with Sahrmann's (2002) and O'Sullivan's (2005) systems (Fig. 21.3). The perspective is that the limited behaviours are obvious across the person's everyday activities and

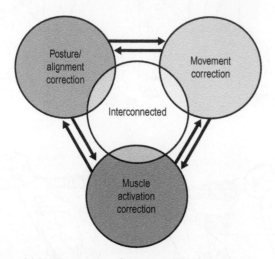

Figure 21.3 Management of motor control issues in low back and pelvic pain involves assessment and management of posture/alignment, muscle activation and movement. Intervention in one domain is likely to influence the others. Specific attention may need to be placed within each domain to achieve optimal outcome, and the decision of where to start treatment will depend on the patient's presentation and the preference of the patient and the therapist.

changes in symptoms with changes in posture/alignment are considered just as important as changes in symptoms with movements to the subgrouping decision. Although the three elements are interconnected, the sections of this chapter are divided to discuss each separately to highlight unique aspects related to each, and to facilitate consideration of the scope of assessment and rehabilitation of each. The order of discussion of these is necessarily arbitrary and is varied throughout the chapter.

Posture/alignment

Assessment of posture/alignment is a basic component of any objective assessment of a patient with low back and pelvic pain (Kendall 2005). The objective of a comprehensive evaluation of posture is to identify aspects of alignment of the spine and adjacent segments that are relevant for the patient's pain/dysfunction, e.g., postures that relieve or provoke the patient's symptoms, or postures that are considered to lead to suboptimal load distribution on lumbopelvic structures (Fig. 21.4). Assessment of posture/alignment is also a central component of classification of patients to subgroups in some schemes (e.g. postural types of Kendall 2005). Posture cannot be considered in isolation from movement and muscle activation (see Fig. 21.3). Aspects of posture provide useful information of muscle activation, which may be excessive or compromised (e.g. excessive activation of the thoracolumbar erector spinae when the spine is held into thoracolumbar extension). How a patient 'holds' his/her spine will also provide important cues to make predictions about movement strategy (e.g. patients who sit on a bicycle in lumbar flexion are likely to adopt patterns that emphasize excessive flexion).

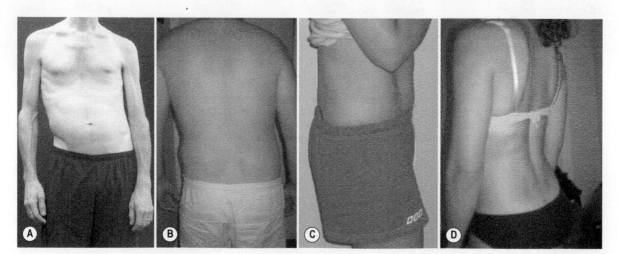

Figure 21.4 Common postural/alignment 'faults' in acute low back pain (LBP). (A) and (B) Acute lumbar list. (C) Lumbar kyphosis in acute LBP. Note increased activity of oblique abdominal muscles. (D) Increased activity of thoracic and lumbar erector spinae. Note long lordosis extending up to mid-thoracic spine.

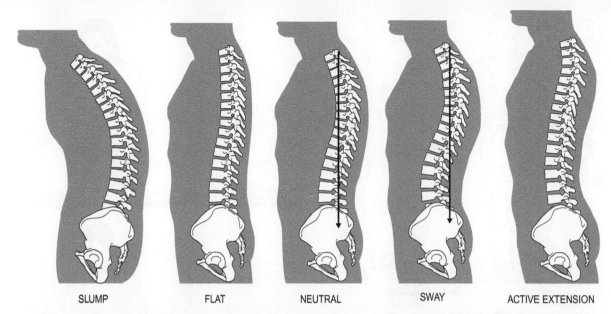

SLUMP   FLAT   NEUTRAL   SWAY   ACTIVE EXTENSION

Figure 21.5 Common spinal postures adopted in standing. Postures are shown from the most flexed to the most extended. The 'Neutral' position is a mid-range position that involves neutral or slight anterior tilt of the pelvis, gentle lumbar lordosis and thoracic kyphosis with a smooth transition in the thoracolumbar junction, cervical lordosis and level head. In this posture sagittal alignment is shown with the arrow. This neutral position is considered as a blueprint for ideal, but may not be ideal for all patients and should not be considered as a static position, but more a functional range of motion.

Most approaches aim to change posture towards some proposed ideal posture. The basis for selecting a specific posture as 'ideal' involves a blend between (i) the posture that relieves symptoms and (ii) the posture that is argued in a specific approach to: optimize the load distribution on the spine; optimize the orientation of muscle anatomy to resist control load and movement (McGill 2007); rely on minimal muscle activation or a more optimal muscle activation pattern (Richardson et al. 2004; Claus et al. 2009a); and/or enhance activation of specific muscles (Sapsford et al. 2001; Sapsford et al. 2008; Claus et al. 2009a). There has been considerable debate regarding the ideal posture. Based on the posture that is considered 'normal' from radiological data, some defend a posture with a neutral pelvic tilt, lumbar lordosis with smooth transition at the thoracolumbar junction to a gentle kyphosis in the thoracic spine and lordosis in the cervical spine (Richardson et al. 2004) (Fig. 21.5). Others defend postures with a flat lumbar spine with or without posterior pelvic tilt (Kendall 2005; Magee 2006), or greater thoracolumbar extension (Sprague 2001). McGill seeks to find a posture that reduces static erector spinae muscle activity to reduce the risk of 'muscle cramps' from continual activation and the associated occlusion of muscle blood flow (see Fig. 21.6). Regardless of the approach, a critical consideration is that the 'ideal' posture is unlikely to be a fixed

position, but rather a 'zone' away from end range. Moreover, posture 'change' may be as important as an 'ideal' posture, which highlights the necessity to consider posture and movement together.

There is no definitive link between posture and pain. For every aspect of posture that is considered to be suboptimal there will always be examples of individuals who frequently use the posture, without reporting symptoms. Although, this has been used as evidence of lack of relevance of postural deviations to pain, it is often argued in ergonomics that whether a deficit becomes problematic depends on the demands the individual places on their body. A suboptimal loading strategy may only lead to pain if the individual undertakes activities that place sufficient load on the tissues to exceed tolerance. This will depend on both the demand exposure and individual's tissue properties. Postural deviations may also be a precursor for future pain.

Despite considerable research investigating the theories underpinning the selection of ideal posture, there are limited data from clinical trials to confirm that one ideal leads to better outcomes than others. This aside, it would seem reasonable to assume that there will be no one 'ideal' posture for all individuals. This would be likely to be influenced by pathology (e.g. patients with spinal stenosis are likely to achieve greater comfort in a position with less

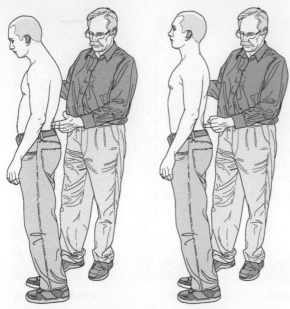

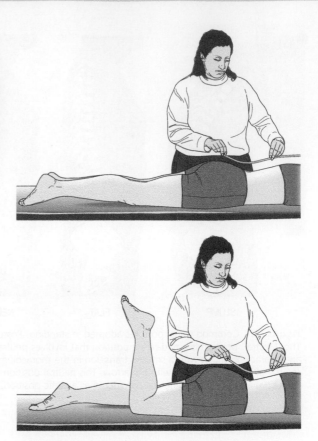

Figure 21.6 Identification of a control strategy to reduce pain in standing. Poor standing posture in this patient compromises pain-free training capacity. Here the lower erector spinae muscles are palpated to determine whether they are chronically active (which may lead to painful muscle cramps). Posture is adjusted (in this case by chin retraction and modification of shoulder alignment) until the back muscles relax. If pain is relieved, the pain-relieving control strategy is taught to the patient.

Figure 21.7 Exaggerated anterior pelvic tilt with lumbar extension early in the range of active knee flexion.
Reproduced from Sahrmann, S., 2002. Diagnosis and Treatment of Movement Impairment Syndromes. *Mosby, with permission of Elsevier.*

extension); functional demand; and other individual factors such as joint range of motion, muscle length and anthropometric features, each of which would influence what is achievable and helpful. Although there are data that provide evidence that posture can be trained (Falla et al. 2007) and that treatments that include posture correction are effective (Costa et al. 2009), there are many remaining questions. A critical element that remains unanswered is confirmation of the most effective methods to achieve change in posture. Current approaches use cognitive learning (e.g. correction of aspects that are deemed inappropriate), manual techniques, sensory feedback, and a range of other tools/techniques (see 'Clinical application of motor control training of posture/alignment').

Movement

Movement is evaluated in most motor control approaches and may be considered as motion of the spine in space (e.g. trunk flexion or extension), motion of regions of the spine (e.g. flexion of the lumbar spine), relative motion of adjacent regions (e.g. lumbar spine relative to thoracolumbar junction, or hip relative to lumbar spine), or

motion of intervertebral segments (e.g. hinge-like motion at a specific spinal segment, or excessive translation at a segment). The emphasis placed on these different components varies between approaches. Some place specific emphasis on the interaction between hip and spine/pelvic motion (Sahrmann 2002; Gombatto et al. 2006; Van Dillen et al. 2007; Scholtes et al. 2009) with the argument that back pain is often associated with motion of the spine too early after the initiation of hip motion (i.e. poor dissociation of movement of hip from spine) and that this, if performed regularly will excessively load the spine (Fig. 21.7). Other approaches place greater emphasis on the motion of specific regions of the spine and identification of segments/regions that have greater or lesser motion (O'Sullivan 2005) (Fig. 21.8). Still others place emphasis on whether repeated loading of the spine in a specific direction increases or decreases pain/pain patterns (McKenzie and May 2003). These concepts are not

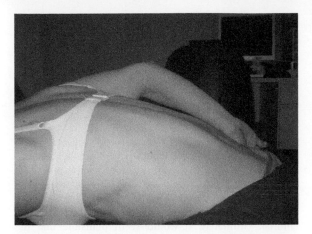

Figure 21.8 Common movement 'fault' during trunk flexion. Increased recruitment of erector spinae muscles in association with stiff thoracic spine and hypermobile lumbosacral junction.

mutually exclusive, and although the emphasis is different, each approach includes consideration of the other aspect of movement. Regardless of the emphasis, movements are considered relevant if they either provoke or relieve pain, or those that are associated with greater or lesser loading of the spine or pelvis.

Treatment of movement aims to either 'optimize' distribution of spine loading (by increasing or decreasing motion of the spine or the adjacent segments) or to use repeated movement to alleviate pain. However, movement cannot be considered independently from posture and muscle activation. These three components are inextricably linked (see Fig. 21.3); the manner in which a patient moves depends on lumbopelvic posture/curvature (which influence available motion) and muscle activity (which may restrict motion or allow/encourage excessive motion). In fact, movement is likely to provide useful insight into aspects of posture/alignment and muscle activation that are likely to be relevant for the patient's pain.

There is considerable debate regarding the best method(s) to change movement. Although some approaches use skill/motor learning strategies to encourage patients to learn to change the manner in which they move, a whole spectrum of other options are employed such as techniques to compel a patient to move the spine (e.g. placing a patient on an unstable surface that encourages motion of the spine to maintain balance); techniques that enhance sensory input (e.g. application of a brace to the back (McNair and Heine 1999)); walking on balance shoes (Bullock-Saxton et al. 1993; Janda 1996); manual therapy techniques; and many other options (see 'Clinical application of motor control training of movement' for further examples).

Muscle activation

Muscle activation strategies are generally considered relevant to the presentation of back pain in two extremes – muscle activity that may be less than, or greater than that considered to be ideal for optimal function of the spine and pelvis. This may present as clinically determined 'under-' or 'over-activity' of a specific muscle or group of muscles, or the adoption of muscle activation patterns that are considered to be inappropriate for optimal loading. Muscle activation is challenging to assess for several reasons. First, the specific pattern of muscle changes are generally unique to the individual patient, and within the individual they may be unique to the movement, posture or task that is assessed. There will not be one strategy of muscle activation that is universally ideal for control of the spine and pelvis, and not one strategy universally adopted by all patients in pain. A range of muscle activation solutions along a spectrum is required for optimal function (Hodges and Cholewicki 2007). At one end of the spectrum are strategies that aim to stiffen the spine to maintain an optimal alignment through co-contraction of large muscles (e.g. bracing). At the other end are more dynamic solutions that encourage movement. The nervous system will select strategies based on demands of the task (Fig. 21.9). Assessment and rehabilitation of motor control of the spine requires consideration of this spectrum of motor control choices, and evaluation of whether the muscle activation strategy matches the demands of the task and the needs of the patient's system.

Second, there are limited methods available to make objective judgements of muscle activation and most have some limitations for interpretation. Some standard options include manual muscle tests, observation and palpation (of muscle activity directly, or estimation of muscle activation based on observation/palpation of posture and movement), electromyography, ultrasound imaging, and numerous other tools such as standardized clinical tests of control, e.g. control of the spine with incremental increases in leg load (Sahrmann 2002); holding time for specific postures such as a side-bridge (McGill 2007); ability to contract one muscle independently from others (Richardson et al. 2004), or in patterns of activation (McGill 2007). Although tests that provide basic information of strength of major muscles that cross the region are available, there are many other muscles and aspects of muscle function that may be important to consider. These include aspects such as the timing of activation, the relative activity of different muscles, and the ability to recruit a muscle in a specific pattern, or in a specific manner during function.

The aims for treatment of *muscle activation* are variable. In some cases the target is to reduce excessive activity (Richardson et al. 2004). The intention is not to completely relax these muscles, but instead to optimize their activity to match the demands of the task, in combination

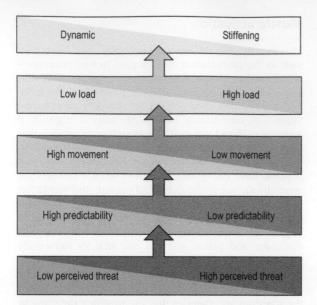

Figure 21.9 Selection of muscle activation strategy based on functional demands. The central nervous system will select a strategy for control of the spine and pelvis from a spectrum ranging from stiffening to more dynamic solutions. Selection of strategy depends on many features of a task including the load, the requirement to restrict or allow movement, and the predictability of the task. Many issues will impact on this decision, such as the threat value placed on the nervous system for a particular task; more threatening tasks (e.g. greater risk of pain provocation) are likely to be associated with a more protective solution for spine control.

with augmentation of activity of any muscle that is considered to be compromised. Other approaches aim to encourage augmented activity of specific muscles (Richardson et al. 2004) or specific patterns of muscle activity to control motion (McGill 2007). Another alternative is the encouragement of movement and posture without attention to specific muscle activation patterns, but with the expectation that the muscle activation will self-organize (Sahrmann 2002). Implicit in this approach is the aim to optimize muscle activity by attention to the quality of control of the other components (e.g. control of pelvic alignment during rotation or sagittal motion of the hip (Sahrmann 2002; Scholtes et al. 2010; Hoffman et al. 2011) and to the control symptoms). Regardless of the approach, individual patients are treated as 'case studies' and any modification, whether by targeting muscle directly or indirectly via movement and posture changes, requires reassessment to determine whether a change has been achieved. For example, if abdominal bracing is used in the McGill approach (McGill 2007) to enhance trunk stiffness, its effect is monitored. Although it may reduce symptoms

in some, it may cause pain in others. Although the augmented stiffness may be beneficial for this individual, the associated compressive loading may be beyond the compression load tolerance of that particular spine. Another stiffening pattern can be attempted to reduce the pain, such as a co-activation pattern of pectoral and latissimus muscles advocated by McGill. The key is to 'tune' the pattern to the individual via a process of trial and error as an 'experiment in progress'.

It is clear that changes in movement, posture and muscle activity are common in low back pain; but where should intervention begin? Different clinical approaches place different emphasis on the three. Currently the decision of which component to address first or emphasize is largely based on the approach/system with which the clinician is familiar. Ultimately, it would seem plausible that the choice of strategy to optimize control should be that which is likely to achieve the greatest change and in the shortest period of time. This could vary between individuals on the basis of many issues including: (i) their pain presentation/movement dysfunction; (ii) their response; and (iii) their preference. Future tools may guide clinical decisions regarding which component(s) to target first. Regardless, it is critical to remember that the movement, posture and muscle activation are inextricably linked (see Fig. 21.3) and it is impossible to change one without an effect on the others. But specific attention to each is probably required to varying degrees.

Assessment

One area where consensus has not yet been reached relates to which tests should be included in an assessment. The approaches converge in the view that assessment needs to be comprehensive and extend across a number of domains of movement, posture and muscle activation in addition to features such as sensory function and psychosocial issues. However, the tests that are used to interpret motor control, and to make clinical decisions for management differ vastly. This is generally related to the bias that each approach places on specific aspects of motor control. For instance, the Sahrmann (2002) approach includes a range of tests that evaluate the interaction between the movement of the extremities and spine (see Fig. 21.4) and the interaction of movement of different regions of the spine (e.g. upper lumbar vs. lower lumbar movement during a trunk lateral bend to the right vs. the left (Fig. 21.10)); whereas other approaches have a greater focus on evaluation of specific patterns of muscle recruitment in order to gain an interpretation of the quality of muscle control (Richardson et al. 2004; Hodges et al. 2009) (Fig. 21.11). Further, even when similar tasks are used, different interpretations can be made based on the target feature being assessed (e.g. approaches differ in the regions of the spine emphasized

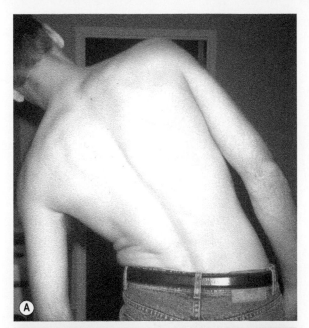

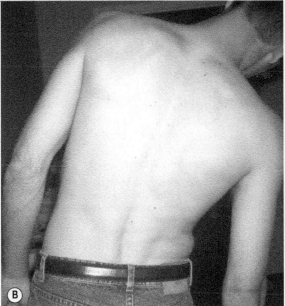

Figure 21.10 Asymmetric and impaired lateral bending. The subject is able to laterally bend to the left but the motion appears to be occurring primarily in the lower lumbar spine, in particular, L5–S1 intervertebral joint (A). The subject displays limited lateral bend to the right, but more motion occurs *across* the lumbar region compared to lateral bend to the left (B). *Reproduced from Sahrmann, S., 2002.* Diagnosis and Treatment of Movement Impairment Syndromes. *Mosby, with permission of Elsevier.*

when evaluating spine curvature during assessment of posture in standing (thoracolumbar junction vs. lumbar lordosis)).

There is no current minimum set of measures that can be advocated. In many cases the specific tests incorporated in an approach are specific for identification of the subgroup that a patient may be allocated to. As the features used to distinguish subgroups differ between approaches this will underpin the argument for a specific comprehensive test battery for each subgrouping method. Further work is necessary to define a minimum set of measures that may be helpful to guide management. However, this needs to be considered on multiple levels that include:

1. Tests to determine whether a patient is appropriate for management using a motor control approach – is motor control the right intervention? This is the basis for the test battery used in the Treatment Based Classification Scheme (Delitto et al. 1995) for identification of patients considered most likely to respond to a range of treatment paths, including 'stabilization' exercise (a term often used to describe motor control exercise).

2. If motor control training is considered appropriate for a patient, a further layer of assessment is required to determine how to tailor the intervention to the individual. In some approaches this involves application of a battery of tests to identify features that cluster patients together into subgroups (Sahrmann 2002; Van Dillen et al. 2003b; O'Sullivan 2005). Other assessment-guided approaches that do not specifically aim to allocate patients to subgroups rely on *clinical reasoning* to guide selection of a battery of tests that are applied to identify features to be individually targeted with treatment. The clinical reasoning-based approach is almost identical to the subgrouping approach, except it does not allocate the patient to a subgroup and, therefore, does not benefit from the guidance that subgrouping can provide towards pattern recognition and identification of treatment priorities. On the other hand, a clinical reasoning-based approach can allow more attention to unique characteristics for an individual patient.

3. Assessment also involves consideration of the patient interview in addition to the physical examination. Examples of important information obtained from the patient interview include information on the age of the patient, length of history, pain levels, types of low back and pelvic pain (e.g. continual low level pain vs. episodic recurrent), history of surgery, conditions (e.g. spondylolisthesis, spinal stenosis, osteoporosis) history of trauma and what kinds of treatments have been tried and successful (or unsuccessful) in the

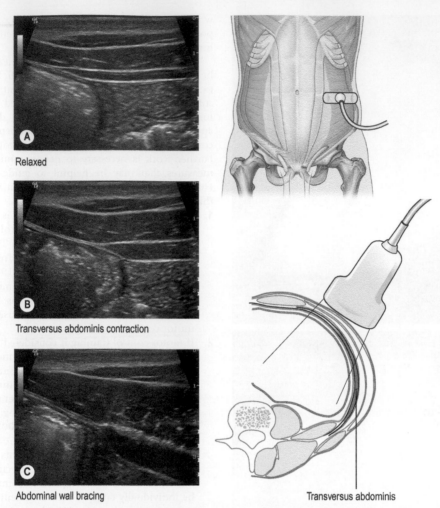

Relaxed

Transversus abdominis contraction

Abdominal wall bracing

Transversus abdominis

Figure 21.11 Assessment of independent activation of the transversus abdominis with ultrasound imaging. Position of the ultrasound transducer and imaging method are shown on the right. Ultrasound images show relaxed abdominal muscles (A); increased thickness and shortening of transversus abdominis without change in the other abdominal muscles with an independent contraction of the muscle (B); bracing contraction of all abdominal muscles with increased thickness of transversus abdominis and obliquus internus abdominis (C).

past. It is also important to determine why the patient has presented, their occupational and recreational activities, and their expectations of the treatment. This is a problem-solving approach, and includes consideration of many factors as well as synthesis of a large amount of information. For first-contact practitioners, the clinical reasoning approach also includes exclusion of red flags (or serious non-mechanical pathology). It is also important to view imaging studies. For the muscle system, magnetic resonance imaging and computed tomography images contain a large amount of information on the muscles of the trunk, such as muscle size and fatty infiltration.

4. A final level of assessment is the inclusion of measures to be used to judge outcome. These can be specifically targeted to determine whether treatment has changed the parameter addressed in the training, or a gross assessment of motor performance.

Training approach

There is considerable convergence in the techniques used for training. Although the emphasis on specific targets for treatment may differ between approaches, there are similarities between the techniques often employed (Fig. 21.12). Across approaches there is a general trend towards application of a motor learning approach where

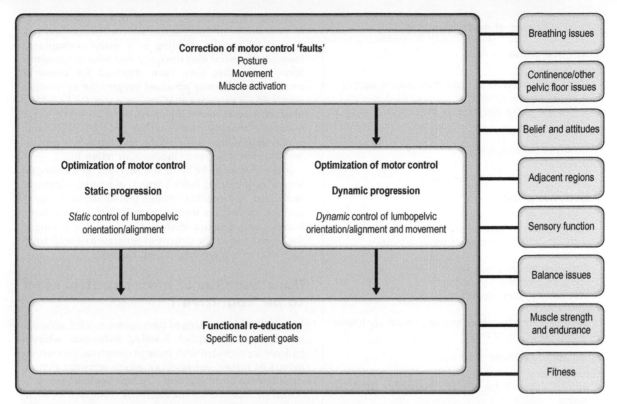

Figure 21.12 Integrated model of motor control intervention for low back and pelvic pain. The boxed area (left) provides an overview of the basic process of progression from initial goal of correction of faults in muscle activation, posture and movement to functional re-education and the intervening steps through static and dynamic training. On the right are the additional issues that are necessary to consider in a case-by-case manner. These issues may present as barriers to recovery for individual patients and are considered to differing degrees within different approaches to management of motor control in low back and pelvic pain.

the specific deficit in posture, movement and muscle activation is highlighted and the performance is corrected with techniques such as a combination of verbal/visual instruction, feedback and manual guidance. This is followed by progression into increasingly challenging situations towards full function. Some approaches highlight the necessity to incorporate other interventions to facilitate this process. Examples include: the use of tape for feedback and to modify movement, posture or muscle activation; application of manual therapy techniques to treat pain and movement dysfunction; techniques to reduce muscle activity such as manual therapies and dry needling; and electrical muscle stimulation to enhance learning of muscle activation. An important consideration is that motor learning requires a change of the concept of 'exercise' in both patients and therapists, from the common conventional interpretation of 'strength and endurance training' to one of 'control, coordination and precision'.

Motor learning involves achievement of permanent change in motor control. Traditionally motor learning has been considered in terms of rehabilitation of movement and posture in patients with neurological disorders, and skill training for sports performance. Increasingly motor learning principles are being applied to management of musculoskeletal pain and dysfunction (Hodges et al. 2009; Tsao et al. 2010). Although motor learning principles have been applied using different clinical models the basic strategy involves transition through three clinical phases: an initial 'cognitive' phase with conscious attention to detail and correction of errors; an 'associative' phase with attention to consistency of performance in more challenging contexts; and an 'autonomous' phase where transfer to automatic control is encouraged Box 21.1 (Fitts and Posner 1967). Underpinning this motor learning strategy are clinical principles that are commonly used to facilitate learning. These include principles such as 'segmentation' (practise of individual components of a task before practise of the whole task), 'simplification' (practise with reduced demand to enable better quality performance) and use of 'augmented feedback' (Hodges et al. 2009).

Recommended dosage of exercise differs between approaches, ranging from frequent short periods of training to a smaller number of longer sessions with focus on quality. Both approaches may lead to motor learning and different patients may respond better to one approach than another.

Ultimately, the success of motor learning will depend on the patient's adherence to the intervention and progression of the intervention as far as necessary for the patient to meet his/her functional demands. It is necessary to use whatever means necessary to encourage commitment of the patient to high quality and frequent practise with attention to quality of performance. Multiple methods

have been suggested, such as design of a treatment package to maintain motivation with frequent updates and progression of exercise, training in a group environment, intermittent review after discharge and other mechanisms. Some approaches have been criticized for failure to emphasize sufficiently advanced progression to function. Advanced progressions that are necessary for individual patients may involve implementation of strength and endurance training protocols (see 'Strength and endurance'), depending on the ability and functional demand that the patient hopes to maintain or return to.

It is the responsibility of the therapist to identify the objectives of training (which aspects of posture/alignment, movement, and muscle activation that should be changed), find the appropriate training approach to achieve motor learning and design a treatment package that maintains the motivation of the patient to progress to a sufficiently high level to achieve long-lasting change.

Does training of motor control need to be 'cognitive'?

Most approaches aiming to train motor control, although not all, rely on explicit learning techniques whereby patients are provided with tools to consciously correct the aspects of *posture*, *movement* or *muscle activation* that are considered to be problematic. This approach is often questioned because the motor system is controlled by many regions of the brain, including subcortical structures such as the more primitive brain stem mechanisms, in addition to the cortical motor areas that are involved in voluntary control of movement (Gahery and Massion 1981). However, it is clear from a range of studies that cortical brain regions such as the primary motor cortex are involved in generation and control of postural adjustments (Gahery and Massion 1981) (see also Chapter 20). Further it is often commented that activation of individual muscles is unfounded as it is often suggested by clinicians that the brain controls 'movement and not muscles'. As argued in Chapter 20, the latter point is not accurate as the brain, including the motor cortex, control both movements *and* muscles (Evarts 1967). The evidence for use of a cognitive approach is that: (i) clinical trials show that cognitive training is associated with changes in activation of trunk muscles in untrained postural and gait tasks (Tsao and Hodges 2007, 2008) and changes in organization of the motor map on the cortex (Tsao et al. 2010); (ii) cognitive attention to correction of muscle activation induces greater change in behaviour of the muscle (Tsao and Hodges 2007) and cortical brain map organization (Tsao et al. 2010) than exercise that activates the muscles to a similar amplitude, but without any conscious attention to the muscle, or without cognitive intention to change the behaviour/recruitment of the muscle (e.g. simple activation during a simple sit-up or during walking, rather than targeted attention to modify the recruitment in a specific manner); and (iii) skill training with attention to a task leads to greater cortical changes than strength training (Remple et al. 2001). Strategies that involve cognitive training of muscle activation, posture or movement are in-keeping with well-established skill learning strategies (Fitts and Posner 1967). Theories of skill learning argue for an initial phase of cognitive learning prior to more automatic training (Fitts and Posner 1967). Gentile (1987) described this phase as 'getting the idea' of the task prior to integration into function. Recent work has highlighted that although functional automatic training with attention to overall performance (e.g. load lifted, distance a ball is kicked) may be suitable for individuals who have already gained basic abilities (McNevin et al. 2003; Perkins-Ceccato et al. 2003), those with more novice performance skills benefit from attention to detail (Perkins-Ceccato et al. 2003), such as specific features of muscle activation, posture and movement. The use of conscious attention to control of posture, movement and muscle activation appears to be a reasonable and effective approach to treatment. This does not mean that cognitive attention is the *only* way to change control, but it does indicate that this approach is one way that is known to be able to achieve change.

If it is accepted that cognitive skill-training strategies are appropriate for changing motor control then it is worthy to consider the most ideal methods to enhance motor learning in this framework. The literature provides a wealth of clinical guidance on issues such as: *segmentation* (practise of components of function before incorporation into the 'whole' task), *simplification* (practise of task elements in a simplified context, such as slower speed, greater body support, etc.), *feedback* (consideration of which type of feedback is most helpful at a specific phase in recovery of function; knowledge of performance or knowledge of results), *dosage* (how much and whether this should be applied as few long sessions or many short sessions) and methods to optimize *transfer* to function (transfer is better when the exercise is closely aligned to the function being trained). Numerous texts have been written on this topic that provide a helpful resource for planning effective treatments (e.g. Magill 2001; Shumway-Cook and Woollacott 2006).

An alternative approach would be to find methods that change motor control strategies in a more 'implicit' manner without attention to error correction by the patient. Janda (1996) used sensory stimulation (e.g. walking on unstable shoes) with the intention to change recruitment of proximal muscles. Others train higher-level tasks such as sitting on balls or functional movements. There is some evidence that these strategies can lead to changes in muscle activation (Bullock-Saxton et al. 1993), but it is unclear whether these changes are meaningful. Some work has aimed to investigate whether passive techniques, such as joint mobilization and manipulation, induce recovery of motor function (Fritz et al. 2011). Although there are data of small immediate improvements in specific aspects of motor control (Marshall and Murphy 2006), this has not been observed in all studies (Ferreira et al. 2007a) and large-scale clinical trials have not supported the assumption that passive treatment leads to recovery of motor control behaviour (Ferreira et al. 2009). A future challenge is to identify whether these more implicit/automatic methods can be identified that change the function of the motor system in a manner that leads to improved spine control for a patient, and whether there are specific groups who would benefit from this intervention.

Who benefits from rehabilitation of spine control?

As yet the answer to the question of who benefits from interventions that aim to rehabilitate the motor control of the spine and pelvis remains unclear. Some groups have proposed that patients may be selected on the basis of clinical issues that suggest 'instability' (Hicks et al. 2005; Kiesel et al. 2007). The factors proposed to identify this group include a 'prone shear instability test', hypermobility (Fig. 21.13), tests of joints, and questionnaires such as that developed by a process of expert consensus to establish features considered to be related to 'clinical instability' (Cook et al. 2006). There are some data to show that people who satisfy such criteria fare better than others when treated with exercise aimed at optimizing motor control of the spine and pelvis (Hicks et al. 2005). As mentioned earlier, a contemporary view held by many is that motor control training approaches may be appropriate not only for individuals who are considered to have too little stability, but for a range of patients who may suboptimally load the tissues of their spine and pelvis, whether that be too little or too much (Hodges and Cholewicki 2007). O'Sullivan (2005) argues that appropriateness for such intervention depends on exclusion of psychosocial features as a dominant aspect of their presentation. This issue is central to consideration of whether a patient may benefit from allocation to a treatment that targets motor control issues, such as those advocated for and described in this chapter, or one that has a focus in the psychosocial domain such as graded activity using the principles of cognitive behavioural therapy (Macedo et al. 2012). Although the outcomes of each of these treatments are similar when they are applied generically across a non-specific low back pain group, it is reasonable to speculate that there will be individuals who respond better to one or other approach. Current work aims to identify baseline features that may predict the responsiveness in this context (Macedo et al. 2008). A key issue from the clinical trials literature is that when motor control interventions for

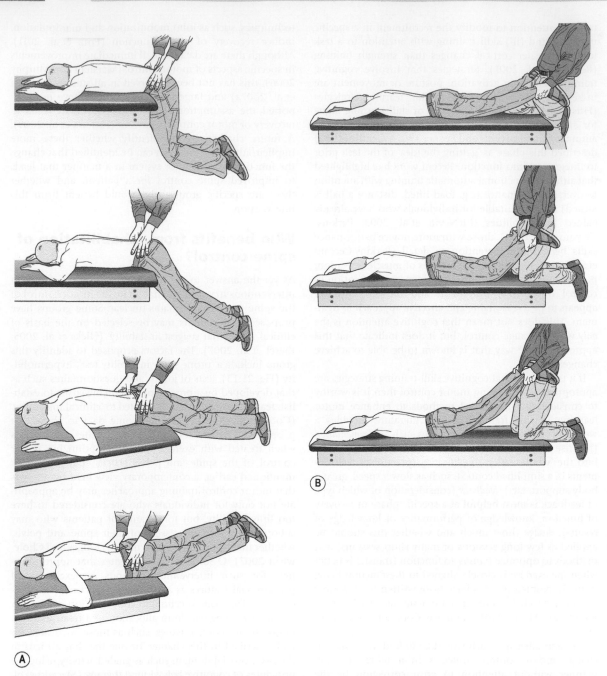

Figure 21.13 Examples of provocative testing in the prone positions used by McGill. (A) The 'prone shear stability test' begins with the patient relaxed on the table and feet on the floor. Poor posturing (panel 2) can create pain simply through flexion intolerance giving a false sign. Manual load (about 2 kg) is applied to each posterior spinous process to locate sensitive and pain-producing segments. Then the legs are extended which activates the extensor muscles stiffening the spine in a shear mode. The height of the legs is adjusted to find the posture of best pain relief or most tolerance. Note this may increase pain in some patients, but cueing different postures and loads identifies this. (B) The 'prone leg raise' assesses the response to traction and then to a load that is directed to exacerbate pain thought to arise from a spondylolisthesis as the thighs are lifted off the table. Increase in pain is interpreted to suggest intolerance to an anterior shear load (spondylolisthesis), whereas relief is interpreted to suggest a mechanism-related pain generation via retrolisthesis.

control of the spine and pelvis are applied to non-specific back pain groups the size of the clinical effect is smaller (Goldby et al. 2006; Ferreira et al. 2007b) than when the intervention is applied to specific subgroups (e.g. acute unilateral low back pain (Hides et al. 2001), spondylolisthesis (O'Sullivan et al. 1997), pregnancy-related pelvic girdle pain (Stuge et al. 2004)). There is a clear challenge for the future to identify which patients may benefit from rehabilitation of motor control of the spine and pelvis.

It is important to recognize that there are two layers to the question of matching the intervention to the patient. First, which patients are likely to benefit from an approach targeted at improving motor control, and second, in those who are predicted to benefit, how should the intervention be applied (i.e. in a generic manner to all, or in a targeted manner) within the group? The issues surrounding subgrouping in low back pain are discussed in Chapter 17 and other sections of this chapter (see 'Assessment', p. 255). Evidence is emerging that treatment targeted to the individual based on their movement subgroup leads to better outcomes (Fersum et al. 2010).

A critical consideration of subgrouping and targeting of interventions is the relative weighting of biological and psychosocial elements in a patient's presentation, and within the biological component, the relative weighting of biomechanical elements (e.g. aberrant motion or excessive loading leading to nociceptor stimulation) vs. biological changes that underpin changes in pain system function (e.g. peripheral and central sensitization; inflammatory system responses). The relative importance of each of these aspects is likely to influence the responsiveness to intervention and treatment is likely to be more effective if intervention is targeted to the individual across the different domains. This will necessitate the use of informative assessments that build the picture of the individual patient and the aspects of his/her presentation that should be prioritized to achieve the greatest change, and this may vary over time as the patient progresses.

There will always be people who do not benefit from motor control training. This may be because suboptimal loading is not a major contributor to their symptoms (e.g. highly sensitized nervous system), the motor control system may not have the capacity to modify the loading (e.g. in the presence of a structural deficit), or the patient may be unable to modify motor control to optimize the loading (e.g. insufficient motivation to take responsibility for changing control; therapist unable to find the optimal solution to training). In these cases, motor control may not be the complete answer, but may provide sufficient functional improvement to improve a patient's quality of life, or it may not be appropriate. The therapist should always remain responsive to indications that including treatments that can influence the function of the spine and pelvis (e.g. manual therapy, etc.), and function of the pain system, could be beneficial.

Fitting training of spine control into the biopsychosocial framework

As alluded to in the preceding sections of this chapter and other chapters in this book (see Chapter 11), a critical issue is that low back and pelvic pain is a biopsychosocial problem that requires a biopsychosocial intervention. Furthermore, it must be recognized that these three aspects – the 'bio', the 'psycho' and the 'social' – do not exist in 'silos'. In fact, the biopsychosocial framework emphasizes the integration rather than separation of these three aspects. For instance, motor control can be influenced by psychosocial variables, just as low back pain can (see Chapters 6 and 11). The biopsychosocial nature of both pain and motor control of the spine and pelvis can be appreciated by remembering that both are emergent properties, not cortical inputs (see also below), and the influence of a biopsychosocial framework can be observed both in the assessment and management of someone with low back and pelvic pain.

As far as assessment is concerned, psychosocial elements cannot really be removed from any patient's presentation, but their impact is often predictable, and helpful for the goal of recovery. However, in many patients, it is necessary to consider psychosocial elements that might be less predictable and unhelpful – how do they contribute to pain, behaviour, motor outputs and, most pertinent here, spinal control? One might suggest that the aim of a comprehensive assessment is to identify the extent to which there are contributions from each domain. The nature of a patient's pain can give important clues to the relative involvement of nociceptive and non-nociceptive contributions (see Fig. 21.14). Beyond gaining a clear understanding of the contributions to a patient's pain, a comprehensive assessment will also evaluate the behavioural consequences of pain. This distinction is critical – whereas psychosocial factors can modulate pain and motor control directly, they can also modulate the impact of their pain on their work and social life, the manner in which they cope with their pain and their choices in overcoming it.

When non-nociceptive contributions exist or predominate, and psychosocial factors also impact on pain, spinal control, behaviour and well-being, the clinician faces a daunting task – to prioritize targets for intervention and identify the best methods to address them. Sometimes this will require an advanced understanding of the interaction between domains. For example, cognitive variables such as the conviction that the spine is vulnerable when it is moving, may limit gains of an otherwise appropriate motor-control target. Conversely, motor strategies may lead to provocation of pain while attempting an appropriate task. Either situation requires a flexible and multimodal clinical approach.

Ideally, the process of identifying treatment priorities should be undertaken with a focus on what the patient is aiming at – what do they see as the most important short

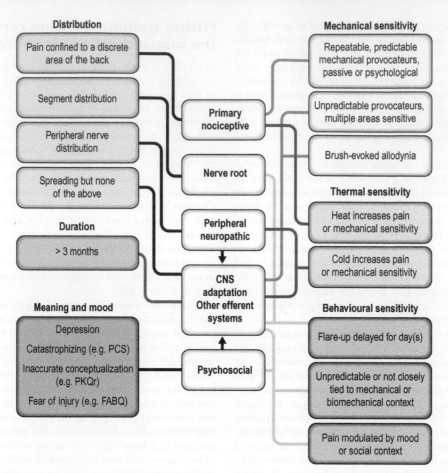

Figure 21.14 Some general guides for interpretation of a comprehensive assessment to identify contributions to a pain state from nociceptive and non-nociceptive domains. Patterns are consistent with contribution of biological mechanisms (primary nociceptive, nerve root (also dorsal root ganglion-evoked nociceptive discharge), peripheral neuropathic and central nervous system, immune, autonomic and endocrine contributions). Psychosocial contributions clearly have their effect on the CNS but are not biological contributions. PCS = Pain Catastrophizing Scale (Sullivan et al. 1995); PKQr = Revised Pain Knowledge Questionnaire (Parkitny et al. – http://www.bodyinmind.org/resources/posters/iasp-2012/rasch-analysis-of-neurophysiology-of-pain-questionnaire/); FABQ = Fear Avoidance Beliefs Questionnaire (Waddell et al. 1993).

term and long term goal? What are their expectations of treatment? What are their resources for achieving those goals? However, this process is also dependent on the knowledge and skill set of the clinician, the context of the intervention, the patient-clinician alliance, and the time and economic constraints of the interaction.

A critical consideration is that there is rarely a case where the issue of 'presence' or 'not' of certain nociceptive or psychosocial elements is black-and-white. All features operate along a sliding scale and some element of change is likely within each domain. That is, features within the psychological domain are relevant for many patients, not only those with chronic unremitting low back pain and high scores on clinical scales of catastrophizing, etc. It is

the challenge for the clinician to judge the relative importance of issues across domains and identify what he/she may consider to be the best route to change the system. In one patient this may be to change the biomechanics of movement (improve muscle activation, posture and movement to optimize loading on the tissues). In another patient it may be to instigate a graded activity approach to encourage the patient to return to function using the principles of cognitive behavioural therapy, without specific attention to the pain or the biomechanical issues that provoke it (Macedo et al. 2012). In general, it seems logical that the optimal outcome may be achieved by implementation of a package of intervention that incorporates aspects that address all domains. Although logical, this requires careful consideration, as some aspects may be mutually exclusive; for instance graded activity encourages patients to *ignore* the pain, and increase function. Motor control interventions, on the other hand, generally aim to encourage patients to adjust movement, posture and muscle activation in a manner that prevents pain provocation, and this necessitates *attention* to pain and the actions that provoke and relieve it. Thus, although combined approaches may be optimal, some important questions require consideration for the individual patient. Some current work aims to identify whether baseline features can assist in the prediction of which patients are likely to respond better to which intervention.

Two very important issues require further consideration. First, pain is an emergent experience related to the implicit perception of threat to body tissue, and is not linearly related to activity in nociceptive afferents (the threat receptors) (Butler and Moseley 2003; Woolf 2011). Mechanisms within the peripheral and central nervous system can upregulate the nociceptive input, as can other efferent systems and psychosocial elements. Therefore, if the aim of modifying spinal control is to reduce activation of nociceptive afferents, then one cannot expect an isomorphic relationship between improved control and pain reduction. This highlights the difficulty of relying on reported symptoms to evaluate the quality of spinal control. That is, if a modification to motor control does not change pain, this does not confirm that it was irrelevant. Second and conversely, training spinal control cannot exclusively train motor pathways. For example, the simple command to 'activate your corset muscle' carries with it potential potent inputs that imply support and safety for the spine. Therefore, the reduction of pain with motor control training is not necessarily due to changes in motor output.

Figure 21.14 shows characteristic patterns associated with various nociceptive and non-nociceptive contributions to pain. Neuropathic pain, which is pain arising directly from damage or disease of the nervous system, CNS adaptation and involvement of other efferent systems, is less likely to be responsive to changes in spinal control. In low back pain, neuropathic pain has been limited to sciatica, but emerging data suggest it may be more common and not necessarily involving leg pain. This is important because when the primary nociceptor is not making a significant contribution to a patient's pain state, any treatment that targets it is not indicated. Importantly, however, one might argue that this does not preclude motor control training, which may be an important vehicle to address cognitive and systemic contributions.

It is reasonable to suggest that the more complex a patient's presentation, the more likely psychosocial elements are making important contributions. There are established treatments that directly target psychosocial elements and the interested reader is referred elsewhere for more extensive coverage. For example, pain biology education (so-called 'Explain pain') (Butler and Moseley 2003), cognitive behavioural management (Nicholas et al. 2002), fear exposure therapy and conditioning paradigms (Turk and Flor 2006).

MOTOR CONTROL APPROACH TO MANAGEMENT OF LOW BACK AND PELVIC PAIN

The key aim of this section is to provide an overall framework within which to consider the management of motor control of the lumbopelvic region for treatment of low back and pelvic pain, and to discuss key concepts related to the clinical application of motor control training. The objective is to present a model that can aid interpretation of how the many different approaches to motor control training may interweave together. The resulting comprehensive approach incorporates a range of different strategies that can be viewed as tools in an eclectic toolbox providing options for the unique individuals that present clinically. There are numerous factors that can influence the selection of a specific clinical route. This will include the experience and biases of the clinician, the experience and preferences of the patient, and the characteristics of the patient, which may be more suited to one clinical approach than another. Just as much as different approaches suit different patients, different clinicians suit different approaches. There is no doubt some clinicians will always do better using one specific system or combination of systems while others will get better results with another system on the same clinical population, and this needs to be considered in the selection of treatment.

The second aim of this section is to provide a summary, although not exhaustive, of clinical techniques that are available for the assessment and management of parameters considered to be relevant to the patient's presentation. In many cases the techniques are derived from clinical experience and are not yet tested, or for some there is emerging evidence.

Overall framework for motor control training in low back and pelvic pain

Figure 21.12 presents a framework designed to provide a somewhat sequential pathway of steps for motor control training. The framework is inclusive of the paths defined in many of the approaches that have been presented for designing treatment programmes for motor control training, as well as provide a structure to consider how the various treatment options or specific forms of exercise intervention may fit together. The boxed section on the left provides the primary pathway from 'correction'

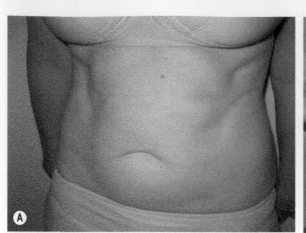 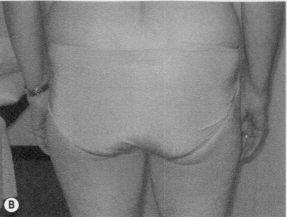

Figure 21.15 Common muscle activation 'faults' in low back pain. (A) Increased recruitment of the oblique abdominal muscles in low back pain. (B) Atrophy of the right side gluteus maximus in a patient with low back pain.

of motor control deficits at the initiation of treatment, through to 'functional rehabilitation' via progression through 'static' and 'dynamic' focussed training. The boxes to the right indicate additional issues that may require consideration in treatment planning, because they: (i) are central to the patient's presentation (e.g. modified trunk muscle activity based on the presence of a respiratory disease; or changes in mobility of the hip, which impact on the necessity to use motion of the lumbar spine in function), (ii) provide barriers for progression of exercise, or (iii) are necessary to consider in order to return the patient to full function, regardless of whether or not there is a direct relationship to pain (e.g. cardiovascular fitness, balance performance, etc.).

The following sections describe the basic process for guiding a patient through the framework with consideration of the various treatment approaches that have been presented in the literature. The subsequent sections provide the clinical 'pearls' of how this model can be practically applied to the management of patients with low back and pelvic pain.

Correction of motor control 'faults'

The first step in planning and implementing a motor control training programme for a patient with low back and pelvic pain is the identification of which features, if any, of *posture*, *movement* and *muscle activation* are considered relevant for the patient's presentation and require consideration in treatment. The underlying premise of this phase of rehabilitation is identification of features of physical presentation that, if changed, would alter the presence, perpetuation or recurrence of pain and dysfunction. As highlighted in an earlier section, the emphasis placed on specific features differs between motor control approaches.

For instance, Sahrmann's (2002) approach places emphasis on consideration of the relative flexibility of adjacent regions (e.g. does the spine rotate too early during rotation of the hip?), or to change the timing of movement of segments participating in the overall movement or change the extent of the total range of motion used to assume and maintain a posture, Richardson et al (2004) place (among other things) emphasis on evaluation of activation of muscles (e.g. identification of excessive activity of muscles such as the obliquus externus abdominis or muscles with reduced activity (Fig. 21.15)), and O'Sullivan's approach emphasizes correction of postures and movements including those that may be provocative of pain (Fig. 21.16). In McGill's approach, provocative testing is performed to identify the motions, postures and loads that exacerbate pain (see Figs 21.2, 21.13, 21.17), with the first objective being to identify these to the patient and assist them in creating strategies to avoid them. Corrective exercises to facilitate pain-free postures and movements are then devised. This does not mean that each approach only considers those aspects, but that the approach favours assessment and training of these components early in management, if they are present.

The basic objective of this initial phase of motor control assessment and training is similar across approaches; as a result of careful assessment (the elements of which vary between approaches) a clinical picture is built of the presentation of the patient in the aspects of posture, movement and muscle activation that are considered relevant for the patient's presentation, and a treatment plan is developed to correct these features. A range of clinical assessments is available, with specific tests designed to evaluate the components considered important by each approach. These tests have been subject to varying levels of research in terms of validation, assessment of approach as a basis for targeting specific deficits in motor control.

There is again a range of treatment approaches available and many specific exercise tasks have been developed with the intention of correcting the features of motor control that are considered relevant. If the patient has been 'subgrouped', this may assist the clinician to identify and prioritize the elements of the intervention. If the approach is based on 'clinical reasoning' (without aiming to place the patient into a category/subgroup) the specific individual deficits and their combination is taken into account to design the treatment for the individual patient. The major difference between approaches is not the individualization of treatment, but the guidance provided by the approach. Subgrouping has the advantage of providing the novice therapist with guidance for 'pattern recognition'; whereas the more eclectic clinical reasoning approach relies on the experience of the therapist. Another advantage of subgrouping is that it could assist with communication between therapists, as long as they are all familiar with the subgrouping method. An advantage of the individual clinical reasoning approach is that it can allow the therapist to be more sensitive to unique characteristics of the patient in front of them, rather than being biased by expected features of a subgroup. Although many patients are neatly classifiable into a subgroup in one approach or another, others do not so easily fit within the expectations of an approach.

A critical aspect of this initial phase of motor control training is the necessity to evaluate the outcome achieved by changing a specific feature of a motor control strategy. This involves two components: first, evaluation of the success in changing the aspect of motor control that has been targeted (i.e. does the patient perform the task differently?), and second, evaluation of the success in reducing the symptoms (i.e. did it help the symptoms?). The first component is straightforward and depends on ongoing and repeated assessment. The second is straightforward for some aspects of motor control, but not others. For instance, if a patient provokes his/her symptoms by flexion of the lumbar spine during sitting, correction of this 'fault' by training more optimal alignment in upright sitting should lead to decreased pain. However, for some aspects the relationship between correction of the 'fault' and change in clinical symptoms may not be as clear. For instance, improvement of the activation of transversus abdominis may improve the quality of spine control by enabling a reduction of dependence on over-activation of the larger more superficial muscles, but correction of this fault may not lead directly to a reduction in pain. In this latter case, improved performance is the key criterion for evaluating improvement. Another issue to consider, as discussed earlier (see 'Fitting training of spine control into the biopsychosocial framework'), is that there may not be a linear relationship between mechanical aspects of tissue loading (at its most basic level, presumably leading to

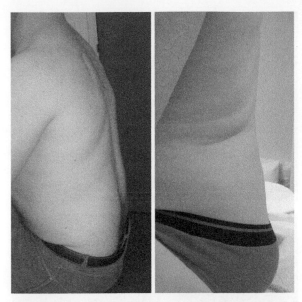

Figure 21.16 Common postural/alignment 'faults' in sitting. Flexed lumbosacral junction in sitting with long lordosis above this.

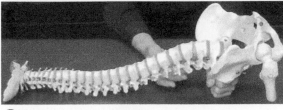

(A)

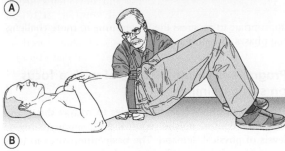

(B)

Figure 21.17 Example of provocative testing in supine used by McGill. A fist is placed under the sacrum and then 'pulsed' to evaluate the SI joints provoked in shear. Posture is adjusted with the other hand along with instructions to the patient to adjust muscular control patterns in order to determine whether a pain-relieving control strategy can be identified.

repeatability, sensitivity and specificity. Some of these research findings are discussed in subsequent sections of this chapter. The outcome of the assessment may lead to classification of the patient to a specific subgroup, or the collected information may be used in a clinical reasoning

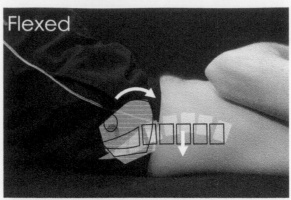

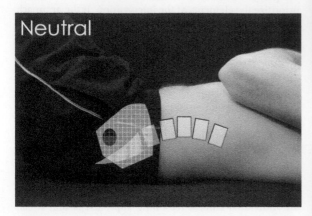

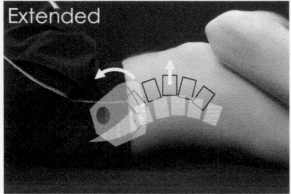

Figure 21.18 Assessment of control of spinal and pelvic alignment during leg loading task. Loss of alignment may be identified by increased or decreased lumbar lordosis with anterior or posterior pelvic tilt respectively.

increased nociceptor discharge) and the pain the patient experiences. Determination of the appropriateness of a change in motor control and a change in the patient's pain is not watertight. A patient may report no benefit of a potentially ideal correction or a large benefit from changing an aspect unrelated to his/her presentation as a result of having 'taken action' to relieve pain (see Chapter 11). Thus, response to correction must be considered along with other information when determining the appropriateness of a correction and also the response over time, not simply the immediate response.

The ultimate outcome or endpoint for the first phase of training is the establishment of an improved motor pattern. That is, the patient has *learnt the skills to correct the features of motor control considered to be relevant to his/her symptoms*. This may be achieved rapidly, or take considerable time, depending on the patient, the status of his/her system, their motivation, the accuracy of exercise implementation by the treating clinician, and many other factors. Once learnt, and the patient has both the capacity to *confidently* correct the significant features, and to *sense* when he/she has not controlled this feature, it is then

appropriate to progress the programme to more challenging phases of training.

Progression of motor control with a focus on static training

Once a patient has learnt strategies to correct the 'faults' in motor control he/she requires progression to higher levels of physical demand. The basic objective is to train correction of the specific features of motor control that have been identified as problematic in the initial phase, in situations of increased physical demand (e.g. load, speed, duration, etc.). Many approaches have been developed for implementation of this phase of training. One major distinction between approaches is whether they focus on *static control of alignment of the spine and pelvis* (Fig. 21.18), or whether they encourage more *dynamic control during movement* (i.e. control of lumbopelvic movement and control of the lumbar spine and pelvis during whole body movement). Both options are likely to be necessary, as function requires the opportunity to select a motor strategy across the spectrum from more static solutions to more dynamic solutions, depending on the demands/features of the task. The following discussion in this section is focussed on options for progression of *static* control of orientation and alignment of the spine and pelvis for progression. As mentioned earlier, the standard is a neutral alignment or as close to that as possible but there are many possible structural changes in the spine, so a position away from the range of the alignment that is symptom-provoking to one that provides control of symptoms is the goal, and this may not necessarily be neutral. As this component of training requires tracking of the quality of control of a single element (i.e. spinal alignment), its application is relatively straightforward, unlike dynamic control where the aspects monitored to judge success differ between tasks and require understanding of ideal and suboptimal performance in a case by case manner. The relative simplicity of the philosophy of static training, combined with the plethora of approaches that have been designed to target this aspect and the simplistic philosophy that 'more' control of the spine is the goal, has led this type of training to become almost synonymous with motor control or, to use an older term, spine stability training. This is a problem, as it has led individuals to believe, inaccurately, that training aimed at enhancing static control of the trunk is the sole target of treatment and is the 'whole' approach, rather than just one part of a more comprehensive intervention that aims to individually optimize dynamic control with consideration of posture, movement and muscle activation. The reductionist interpretation of the approach has led to the publication of misguided critiques of basis for motor control training (e.g. Lederman 2010).

Static progression of control generally involves training a patient to control a specific alignment of the spine and pelvis while he/she adds load to the system via movement of limbs (e.g. leg loading from Sahrmann's approach (2002)) or application of force to the body (e.g. rhythmic stabilizations from proprioceptive neuromuscular facilitation (PNF)). A major distinction between some approaches to motor control training is that some clinical programmes *begin* the intervention for the patient with this type of training *without* prior assessment and learning of strategies to correct posture, movement and muscle activation 'faults'. In that case, and to varying degrees, it is assumed that implementation of static training encourages *automatic* correction of motor control 'faults' without the requirement to specifically address them. Although there is some evidence that such approaches (without specific attention to correction of patient-specific motor control faults) do not automatically restore muscle activation patterns (Hall et al. 2009), there is no current evidence from clinical trials that outcomes differ between these viewpoints. However, it is broadly considered that specific attention to correction of motor control faults is likely to achieve the greatest change, and is advocated in this volume.

Control of the static alignment of the spine and pelvis requires activation of a whole system of muscles. Although sometimes purported clinically, it is mechanically impossible for isolated activation of the deeper trunk muscles to achieve this task, with an additional contribution of the more superficial muscles that have appropriate moment arms to oppose external and internal forces. The specific pattern of muscle activation depends on the direction of torque that is applied to the trunk. For instance, with a patient in supine lying with the knees and hips flexed (crook lying), for him/her to be able to maintain/control the static position of the pelvis and spine when one leg is lifted or the hip abducted and externally rotated with the foot in contact with the table, it is necessary to activate a specific pattern of abdominal and back extensor muscles that oppose the rotary torque on the trunk. Although different exercise approaches may advocate different target postures to be controlled in supine lying (e.g. flat lumbar spine and posteriorly tilted pelvis vs. maintenance of a lumbar lordosis), different methods of application of load (force applied to the trunk vs. limb load), different methods of evaluation of the success (e.g. monitoring of lumbopelvic position with pressure cuff placed under the spine (Richardson et al. 2004)) and other unique features (e.g. coordination with expiration in some version of 'Pilates' exercise), the basic objective of all approaches is to control alignment when challenged by additional load. The effectiveness of the intervention, to varying degrees, is considered to depend on the attention placed on evaluation of the 'success' in terms of the patient's ability to control the alignment and to control the symptoms by controlling the alignment.

Assessment in this phase revolves around identification of: (i) the threshold loads/forces that can be applied before the patient can no longer maintain the pelvic and lumbar alignment; (ii) asymmetry in the ability to control alignment when force is applied in opposite directions; or (iii) specific directions/planes of force that present a specific challenge to the patient. Identification of these features guides the planning of treatment for selection of appropriate exercises (that challenge the threshold for control and specific directions/planes of force) and guidance for progression of exercise. Assessment can involve specific assessment tasks (e.g. formal sequence of incremental loads) or can be undertaken by evaluation of response to loading in an individualized manner matched to the needs of the patient.

It is common, but not universal, to implement *static* training before progression to *dynamic* training as it is generally easier for a patient to assess his/her success (easier to identify loss of control of a specific alignment, than complex features of a movement response). However, many approaches encourage a combination of static and dynamic training exercises.

Progression of static training can involve incremental increases in loading (increasing lever arm length,

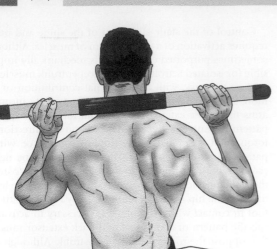
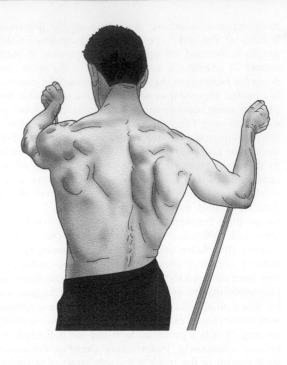

Figure 21.19 Training of thoracic rotation on stable lumbar base.

increasing load) or by making the control of alignment more challenging by modifications such as reduction of the support provided to the body (e.g. leg loading from a bridged position, or progression from supine to sitting). Many exercise devices are available for progression of load including devices that provide resistance to limbs (e.g. elasticized bands) or devices that apply force of differing amplitude when moved at different speeds (Fig. 21.19). It is unlikely to be sufficient to focus solely on exercises on static control of the spine in supine lying as static control of the spine is necessary in weight-bearing (standing and sitting) positions and this is likely to involve recruitment of different muscles and different patterns of muscle activation.

Progression of motor control with a focus on dynamic training

Progression to *dynamic* control is a critical aspect of training for most/many patients. Rehabilitation of control of *movement* of the spine and pelvis is critical as the spine must move through a trajectory for most functions (as opposed to maintaining a fixed orientation, which is required for some activities, such as heavy lifting, but not all functions), as well as for shock absorption, load transfer, and for the spine to contribute to other functions such as breathing and balance control (Hodges and Cholewicki 2007). Dynamic

control includes two main issues: (i) control of dynamic movement of the spine itself (Fig. 21.20) and (ii) control of the spine during movement of the whole body. In the former, the spine and pelvis may be required to move more or less, depending on the function. In the latter, the spine deals with aspects such as load transfer and segmental control, but may not require considerable motion (e.g. running, which involves controlled rotation and lateral flexion of the spine within a small range, but with large demand for load transfer/shock absorption).

Two key strategies are commonly used to encourage dynamic control. First, patients can be specifically instructed to increase or decrease motion (as guided by the specific deficits that are identified in the patient's presentation) during either: (i) regimented exercise progressions, or (ii) during performance of the functional tasks the patient had indicated he/she finds problematic. Second, patients can be progressed to dynamic control by maintaining balance on unstable surfaces. When standing on a balance board or sitting on a ball it is impossible to maintain balance with the trunk held rigidly erect. Maintenance of balance in these situations can be used to gradually encourage motion, and it is the therapist's responsibility to ensure that the challenge is adequately matched to the patient, i.e., it does not exceed his/her ability, and appropriately challenges him/her in specific directions and amplitude of instability.

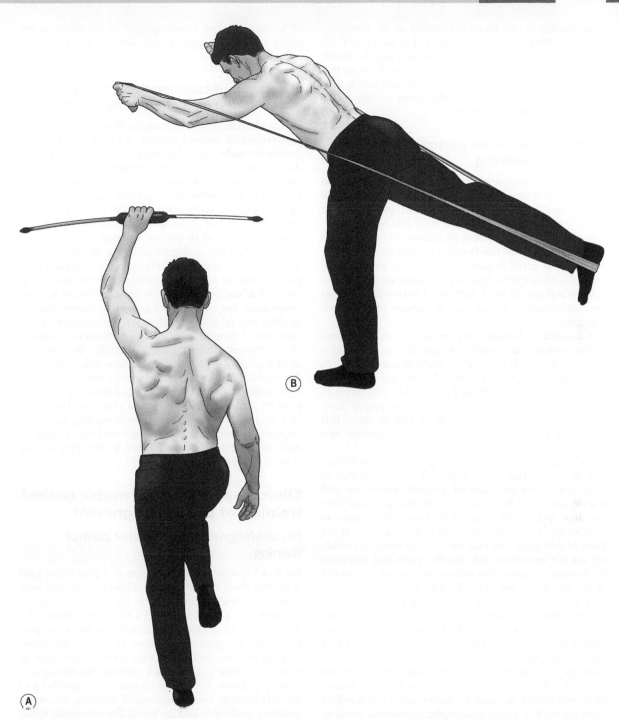

Figure 21.20 Advanced training involving whole kinetic chain using equipment to apply additional load. (A) Bodyblade®; (B) Thera-Band®.

Assessment in this phase is focussed on the identification of threshold dynamic demand that the patient can tolerate, the identification of asymmetries, and the identification of specific directions/planes of motion that present an issue. Treatment planning involves selection of appropriate tasks to challenge the issues specific to the individual patient's presentation.

Progression of motor control to high level functional retraining

As transfer to function is most likely to be optimal when practise is performed as close to the function as possible (Shumway-Cook and Woollacott 2006), progression to functional exercise is critical. The basic principle is correction of the 'faults' in posture, movement and muscle activation in the specific functional tasks that the patient has identified as most important. Again, the principles of motor learning can be applied (e.g. segmentation, simplification and provision of augmented feedback) to change the motor control strategy that is adopted in functional contexts.

Assessment techniques vary, but are commonly limited to observation of the 'quality' of control of the spine. Such tests are necessarily subjective, although some new tools are being developed such as light, wireless movement sensors that can be applied to the spine and pelvis to monitor control of lumbopelvic motion during functional tasks, and even over long periods of time. This is an area that is likely to progress rapidly over the next few years.

Training in this phase is unique to the individual patient and is dependent on the skills of the clinician to determine when elements of posture, movement and muscle activation have not been ideally integrated into function, and identification of an appropriate means to address the lack of integration. The means to achieve the goals of this phase can take the form of either: (i) breaking up the movement into smaller parts and practising the specific elements with enhanced awareness of control of the specific motor control 'fault' (i.e. motor learning principle of 'segmentation'); (ii) practise of the function in a manner that makes it easier to perform with correction of the motor control 'fault', such as performance with reduced speed, increased stability of the base of support, decreased range of motion (i.e. motor learning principle of 'simplification') or augmentation of the patient's ability to sense whether he/she has been successful in controlling the fault by use of additional feedback methods such as electromyography, ultrasound imaging, movement sensors (i.e. motor learning principle of 'augmented feedback'). All the techniques that are used to enhance learning of the skills for correction of motor control 'faults' for the first three phases of training can be continued into the functional retraining phase (e.g. tape applied to the lumbar region to enhance feedback of lumbar position, hands applied to the sternum and pelvis to evaluate sagittal alignment of the spine and pelvis).

Integration of consideration of 'additional issues' in development of a treatment plan

Design of a comprehensive package of treatment to ensure achievement of optimal control of the spine and pelvis requires consideration of a range of issues in addition to the primary progression from 'correction of motor control faults' to 'function'. These issues may present as: (i) barriers to further improvement in control: e.g. biomechanical issues at adjacent joints that prevent or compromise optimization of control at the spine, such as excessively pronated feet that lead to internal rotation of the legs and anterior pelvic tilt; or augmentation of the activation of the abdominal muscles for enhancement of expiration in people with co-morbid respiratory conditions; or (ii) issues that are not necessarily linked directly to pain provocation, but are necessary to train to ensure return to function (e.g. cardiovascular fitness). The inclusion of consideration of these issues in the treatment package depends on the clinical picture determined by the therapist. The relative priority placed on these aspects will change over the course of treatment. The section entitled 'Clinical application of strategies to manage barriers to recovery' provides a comprehensive review of a range of these issues that are important to consider (with varying degrees of emphasis for different clinical approaches), a range of methods to assess their relevance to the patient, and options for training.

Clinical application of motor control training of posture/alignment

Posture/alignment and motor control training

The link between posture and pain at a population level is unclear; there are few aspects of posture that have been linked to pain or future pain (Griffith et al. 2012). However, at an individual level a somewhat clearer relationship can be observed in clinical practice: some postures provoke pain and others relieve it for many individuals. The lack of a significant relationship of postural features to pain when patients are viewed as a larger population is likely to be due to the specificity of the relationship within individual patients, no single posture is uniformly 'bad' or 'good'. The other issue is that back pain is multi-factorial and posture will interact with other aspects. Some examples include the pathology (e.g. spinal stenosis is often associated with pain in lumbar extension), psychosocial issues such as self-efficacy (O'Sullivan 2005), and stress of work environment (Marras et al. 2004), to name a few. A specific posture may only be relevant once accompanied by other elements, which 'push' the patient over some threshold to develop pain or to be considered a dysfunction.

Evaluation of posture is a conventional part of clinical objective assessment of low back and pelvic pain and involves identification of aspects that could be related to pain presentation, such as spinal curvature (e.g. is the position provocative?) or muscle activation (e.g. is the activity excessive, leading to excessive loading of the thoracolumbar region into extension?; or too little, leading to excessive loading of the spine into flexion by slumping?). There is no reason to expect that posture will be identical for sitting, standing and other functional positions. Central to the analysis of posture is determination of what is ideal posture. The clinical literature defines a range of postures as a 'neutral spine' posture (for review see Claus et al. 2009b). This ranges from 'flat', to a posture that approximates the curves identified in standing with cervical lordosis, thoracic kyphosis, lumbar lordosis, neutral pelvic tilt (Fig. 21.7). Why is this posture considered to be ideal? This is argued on the basis of a number of issues: (i) it provides more optimal loading of spinal structures (McGill 1992); (ii) it avoids 'creep' of viscoelastic tissues into flexion and extension; (iii) it is associated with less overactivity of large, more superficial trunk muscles, which would be required to overcome gravity if the sagittal balance is biased towards anterior or posterior placement of the centre of mass of the trunk or to maintain an extreme position of the spine (Dankaerts et al. 2006; Claus et al. 2009a); (iv) it is thought to encourage greater activity of the deeper muscles of the trunk (Claus et al. 2009a); (v) it is associated with a breathing pattern that is argued to be more relaxed with greater mechanical efficiency (Lee et al. 2010), and (vi) it is related to greater activity of other muscles thought to contribute to lumbopelvic control, such as the pelvic floor muscles (Sapsford et al. 2008). This aside, it is important to consider that the ideal spinal posture will not be the same for all individuals as it will depend on pathology (e.g. spinal stenosis), spinal mobility, positions and movements that are provocative of pain, function, habitual postures and movements, anthropometric features (e.g. lumbosacral angle), and many other issues. Further, ideal posture cannot be a single static position but a posture that is moved into and out of, and used in specific tasks (e.g. more optimal loading during lifting and tasks that require static positions for a sustained period).

As would be predicted, posture has a strong association with muscle activity. Sitting with a lumbar lordosis and a smooth transition to kyphosis at the thoracolumbar junction is associated with greater activation of multifidus and the lower regions of transversus abdominis and obliquus internus abdominis than flat postures; thoracolumbar extension is associated with greater thoracic erector spinae and obliquus externus abdominis muscle activity than sitting in a more neutrally aligned spine and pelvis; and

slumped sitting is associated with minimal activity of the extensor muscles (Claus et al. 2009a; O'Sullivan et al. 2006). In a sway back position there may be a tendency to 'hang' on the obliquus externus abdominis muscle as a result of the more posterior alignment of the upper trunk relative to the pelvis.

The key to correction of posture relies on careful assessment of posture, the identification of features that are considered relevant to the patient's symptoms, and the evaluation of the outcome for his/her symptoms when specific features are modified. Many techniques have been proposed to assist the patient to correct motor control 'faults' in posture and a trial and error approach to find the best solution is optimal.

Assessment of posture/alignment

Posture is assessed in a range of positions, but most commonly in the early phases it is assessed in sitting and standing. Different approaches to training have different priorities for assessment and different features that are considered ideal or clinically relevant. Here we present an overview of the breadth of features that are considered, without placing specific emphasis on one approach. The sequence of postural assessment can include a range of features that are listed in Box 21.2. Some common postural types in standing are presented in Fig. 21.5. The relevance of a specific feature of posture for the patient's presentation can be supported if changing the feature leads to a positive change in symptoms, although this will not always be expected (see 'Fitting training of spine control into the biopsychosocial framework').

Goals of training posture/alignment correction

Use of strategies to change posture has many goals: these include, but are not limited to, changing posture to avoid those that are provocative or associated with excessive or reduced muscle activity. Box 21.3 includes a summary of the multiple goals that may be targeted with correction of posture, each with varying relevance for individual patients.

Techniques to train posture/alignment correction

The basic goal in treatment planning is to find a strategy to change posture. Once a technique has been trialled it is critical to evaluate the outcome. It is acceptable for the new posture to feel 'odd' or 'awkward', but it should not be painful or difficult to hold (i.e. muscle activity required to maintain the posture should not be excessive). As mentioned above, the target posture needs to be considered with respect to pathology if it is known (e.g. symptoms in patients with advanced spinal stenosis will unlikely be

---

Box 21.2 Postural correction: Assessment

Evaluation in multiple positions

Sitting – unsupported and supported
Standing
During functional task

Identification of provocative/suboptimal elements

Presence of pain in naturally selected posture – location and response to change in posture (e.g. effect of lumbar support)

Evaluation of sagittal alignment/sagittal balance

Alignment relative to plumb line using traditional reference points
   Upright, sway (thorax posterior to pelvis), kyphotic (thorax forward of the pelvis)

Evaluation of spinal curvature

Approximate level of start and finish of sagittal spinal curves and depth of curves
   Lumbar lordosis
   Thoracic kyphosis
   Transition between thoracic kyphosis and lumbar lordosis – flat, flexed or extended at the thoracolumbar junction
   Cervical lordosis and head position
Segmental changes – e.g. segmental lordosis, segmental lumbar kyphosis (flexion at lumbosacral junction) with long lordosis above this
Pelvic position
   Anterior/posterior tilt
   Rotation

Frontal plane (front/back)

   Lateral shift/list upper trunk
   Lateral tilt pelvis
   Right/left weight bearing
   Scoliosis
   Infra-sternal angle symmetry

Evaluation of muscle activity

Palpation, observation, electromyography, ultrasound imaging
   Hypertrophy/atrophy
   Hyperactivity/underactivity
   Asymmetry

Evaluation of posture of adjacent segments

Lower limb, including the feet
   Hip angle – flexed, neutral, extended, adducted, rotated
   Knee angle – flexed, neutral, (hyper)extended, internal/external rotation
   Foot/ankle – pronated/supinated
Shoulder girdle
Neck/thorax

Effect of correction of postural 'fault(s)' on pain and muscle activity

Evaluation of response to sit erect
Evaluation of response to slump
Evaluation of response to change/correction curvature/alignment

Differentiation of structural abnormalities that cannot change

e.g. Assessment of structural scoliosis – evaluation of 'rib hump' with forward flexion test

---

Box 21.3 Postural correction: Training goals

Optimize lumbopelvic loading

Avoid provocative postures
Encourage relieving postures
Correct asymmetry
Minimize activity of overactive muscles (often superficial/global muscles)
Enhance activity of underactive muscles (often deep/local muscles, but not limited to these muscles)
Avoid prolonged postures or *encourage* posture change

Optimize respiratory pattern

Optimize control of pelvic floor muscles

reduced by adoption of a lordotic lumbar curve) and the individual patient's motor control presentation. Once the optimal posture is identified along with a technique that the patient can use to effectively achieve this change, training may be started with a few sessions throughout the day as a home programme to learn to change posture, with progression towards adoption of this posture frequently throughout the day as required by the functions being performed. Finding a strategy to keep reminding a person to correct posture, such as correction of posture each time the telephone rings, can be helpful. Patients should be instructed that they will need to develop endurance in the appropriate muscles to allow them to adopt postures for any length of time. Box 21.4 presents a range of strategies that are used across a range of clinical approaches to modify posture.

Box 21.4 **Postural correction: Techniques**

Cognitive correction
Instructions
Use of verbal instruction to guide a patient to make an adjustment to a specific feature of their posture
- e.g. 'Roll forwards on tailbone' to improve anterior tilt and increase lordosis of the lumbar spine, 'breathe into base of ribs' to remove excessive extension of the thoracolumbar junction
- e.g. 'Grow tall'
- e.g. 'Position (or lift) ischial tuberosities while sitting, avoiding flexion at the lumbosacral junction'
- e.g. 'Check that the shoulder girdle is relaxed'

Imagery (visual and proprioceptive)
Identification of a 'mental image' that aids a patient to understand the change that is required
- e.g. image of 'lengthening' the spine to reduce thoracic kyphosis

Manual guidance
Placement of treating clinician's hands or patient's hands on the body to provide guidance towards the corrected position
- e.g. hand on sacrum to provide guidance of anterior rotation of pelvis (see Fig. 21.21); hand on the thoracolumbar junction to provide guidance to relax into flattening in this region

Manual cues
Placement of hands on key landmarks of the body to provide a reference to monitor position or alignment
- e.g. little finger and thumb of one hand on the xiphoid and navel to monitor the distance between these two landmarks as indirect feedback of changes in the angle of the thoracolumbar junction (distance reduces and increases with thoracolumbar flexion and extension) (Fig. 21.22)

'Dissociation' tasks
Attention to change the relative motion of adjacent body regions
- e.g. 'Waiters bow' exercise to teach a patient to flex at the hips rather than the lumbar spine; attention to control of thoracolumbar junction curvature while rotating the pelvic and lower lumbar spine (Fig. 21.23)

Muscle activation
Change muscle activation to assist with change in posture – either increase activity of a specific muscle to aid movement to a new position or decrease activity of a specific muscle to aid movement from a specific posture
- e.g. augmented feedback of muscle activity to aid increase or decrease in activity (palpation, observation, electromyography, ultrasound imaging for biofeedback); application of techniques to directly/indirectly change activity such as manual therapies (articular mobilization; connective tissue massage)
- e.g. use of serratus anterior activation (reversed origin insertion) to facilitate a thoracic kyphosis (Fig. 21.24)

Cues/reminders
Provision of inputs/stimuli to provide reminder when postural correction is no longer maintained or to remind a patient to frequently adopt the corrected position
- e.g. application of therapeutic tape to the spine when in a lordotic position to provide stretch if curvature flattens; a software program that flashes a reminder on the computer screen at predetermined intervals
- e.g. photos taken to show patient his/her posture in different positions. Sticky dots can be placed over the tragus, middle of the shoulder (anteroposterior), middle of the hip, middle of the knee and anterior to the lateral malleolus to demonstrate the appropriate line of gravity

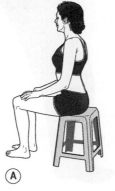 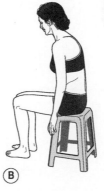 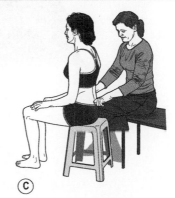

Figure 21.21 Correction of sitting posture/alignment: (A) thoracolumbar extension; (B) flexed lumbosacral junction; and (C) correcting sitting posture (lumbar lordosis and thoracic kyphosis).

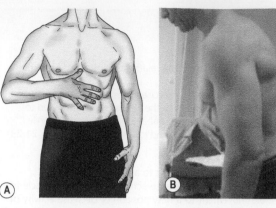

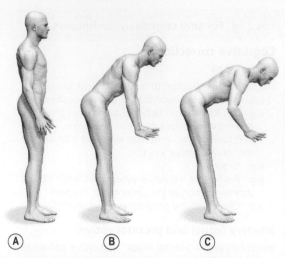

Figure 21.22 Use of manual feedback (little finger on umbilicus and thumb on sternum) to provide feedback of control of thoracolumbar junction to train dissociation of hip movement from lumbopelvic movement. (A) Hand position. (B) Patient using manual feedback to monitor control of the thoracolumbar junction while bending forward.

Figure 21.23 Forward bending with hip flexion and a flat lumbar region. The person is instructed to place his/her hands on a flat surface (A) and put the weight of the trunk on his/her hands (B). The person is to bend in the hip joints by 'thinking about sticking your seat out'. The person is told not to bend in his back (C). *Reproduced from Sahrmann, S., 2002. Diagnosis and Treatment of Movement Impairment Syndromes. Mosby, with permission of Elsevier.*

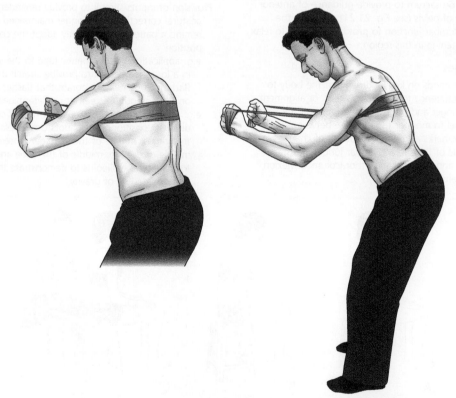

Figure 21.24 Use of Thera-Band® to train 'reverse origin and insertion' action of the serratus anterior muscle to encourage control of the thoracic kyphosis.

Clinical application of motor control training of *movement*

Movement and motor control training

Like posture correction, correction of motor control 'faults' in movement aims to change aspects of movement considered to be relevant for a patient's symptoms either because it is provocative or loads the tissues inappropriately because of too much or too little control. This may be because of poor interaction between adjacent body regions, suboptimal postures, suboptimal muscle activation, etc. In many ways the principles for consideration of suboptimal movement are similar to those outlined when considering posture, only in this case it is the movement trajectory while changing position (posture) that is being considered for relevance to the patient's symptoms. Faults in movement control share many features with postural faults in: (i) the absence of any one feature of movement that is suboptimal in all patients (the specific features relevant for a patient's symptoms must be identified individually); (ii) the relevance of a movement feature must be considered in the effect of changing this parameter on the symptoms; (iii) different approaches have different priority movement features that they address; (iv) there is a strong association between movement and muscle activation strategy; and (v) the challenge is to find a tool/technique to aid a patient to change the feature that is considered to be relevant to his/her symptoms and then integrate this into more challenging dynamic contexts. Thus, as with all features of motor control training, the key to successful correction of movement is the accuracy of the assessment of the motor control fault (is the movement fault relevant to symptoms?) and the assessment of the outcome of the application of a treatment technique (has the technique made a difference to movement?).

Assessment of movement

Evaluation of movement is a usual component of assessment of any patient with low back or pelvic pain. Information gained from range of motion and directions of provocation are important features. In motor control intervention, the focus of movement assessment is investigation of the strategy of movement and its relevance to suboptimal loading of the tissues in a manner that could be responsible for the development, provocation or maintenance of symptoms. This involves assessment of the pain response to individual tests along with quality of movement. An important consideration again is the inherent connection between posture and movement. Of special note is the possibility that the movement is affected by the starting posture/position (e.g. motion of the lumbar spine during a function will differ depending on whether the lumbar region starts in a position of flexion or extension) or changes in preparatory control during the initial posture. Box 21.5 provides a summary of key principles of assessment of movement and key features that are 'searched' for in different approaches.

Goals of training movement correction

Again, like posture correction, strategies to change movement have many goals, and these include, but are not limited to, changing movement to avoid those that are provocative. Again the key distinction is that for movement correction the objective is to change aspects that load the tissues suboptimally in a dynamic sense as the spine and pelvis move through a trajectory. Box 21.6 includes a summary of the multiple goals that may be targeted with correction of movement, each with varying relevance for individual patients.

Techniques to train movement correction

The basic goal in treatment planning is to find a strategy to change movement such that it is performed in a manner that more optimally loads the tissues. Once a technique has been trialled it is critical to identify the outcome. It is acceptable for the new movement to feel 'odd' or 'awkward', but it should not be painful or difficult to maintain (i.e. muscle activity required to control the movement should not be excessive). As mentioned above, the target movement needs to be considered with respect to pathology if it is known and the individual patient's motor control presentation. Once the optimal movement pattern is identified, along with a technique that the patient can use to effectively achieve this change, then training may be started with a few sessions throughout the day as a home programme to learn to change the movement. A progression would be to adopt the movement pattern as required by the functions being performed. Box 21.7 presents a range of categories of strategy that are used across a range of clinical approaches to modify movement and these are similar to those used to modify posture.

Clinical application of motor control training of muscle activation strategy

Muscle activation strategy and motor control training

Central to the control of posture and movement is the activation of muscles of the lumbopelvic region. Correction of muscle control faults can be the first line treatment to change posture and movement; or correction of faults in posture and movement can be initiated with an objective to change muscle activation. It is well known that muscle activation can be changed with motor control training, and there is evidence that parameters of muscle activation strategy at baseline are related to the responsiveness of an individual patient to a motor control intervention

Box 21.5 Movement control: Assessment

Evaluation in multiple tasks

Basic physiological movements – flexion, extension, etc. – provides information of multiple components including segmental motion (joint function) and guides muscle assessment (e.g. a block of many segments in lateral flexion may be due to tightness/stiffness of the quadratus lumborum muscle)

Standardized functional movement – sit-to-stand, etc.

During functional tasks identified by the patient in subjective assessment (e.g. lifting)

Specific movement tests

Identification of provocative/suboptimal elements

Evaluation of changes in sagittal/frontal/ transverse alignment during movement

Timing

Amplitude

Sequence

Evaluation of muscle activity

Palpation, observation, electromyography, ultrasound imaging

Evaluation of posture/movement of adjacent segments and ability to dissociate movement of lumbopelvic region from adjacent segments

Lumbar vs. hip

Lumbar vs. thoracolumbar junction

Lower limb and feet

Shoulder girdle

Neck/thorax

Specific movement tests

Sitting

Slump/rock backward

Knee extension with ankle dorsiflexion

- Observe for – inability to dissociate hip from spine (Fig. 21.25)

Neutral repositioning test

- Place in neutral, fully slump and return – observe for flexion at symptomatic segment
- Bend forward as maintaining neutral position – observe for flexion at symptomatic segment

Sit upright/erect

- Observe for – inability to move lumbar spine and pelvis independently from thoracolumbar regions

Sit-to-stand

Stand after placing spine in neutral

- Observe ability to maintain lumbar lordosis – observe for where the movement is initiated, increased lumbar flexion, decreased lumbar extension, increased thoracolumbar extension, increased posterior pelvic tilt, anterior pelvic sway, medial hip rotation, relationship between hip and lumbar motion

Standing

Flexion

- Observe for – loss of motion, increased lumbar flexion/lateral shift, increased lumbar extension, increased thoracolumbar extension, increased posterior/anterior pelvic tilt, relationship between hip and lumbar motion (Fig. 21.26)

Return from flexion

- Observe for – relationship between hip and lumbar motion, increased thoracolumbar extension, anterior pelvic sway, increased or decreased extension, anterior pelvic rotation

Extension

Side bending (lateral flexion)

Side 'glide'

Rotation

Response to axial loading

Squat

Observe ability to maintain lumbar lordosis: observe for – increased lumbar flexion, decreased lumbar extension, increased thoracolumbar extension, increased posterior pelvic tilt, medial hip rotation, relationship between hip and lumbar motion

Include single leg squat and mini-squat

Single leg stand (Fig. 21.27)

Observe ability to control pelvic/trunk control during single leg stance: observe for – Trendelenberg sign (drop of pelvis on side of lifted leg), lateral shift of thorax/lateral flexion, medial hip rotation, pelvic sway

Pelvic rotation

Weight through heels not toes

Supine

Position and effect of support to hip/lumbar spine

Hip and knee flexion

- Observe for – lumbar flexion, pelvic rotation with lumbar extension

Anterior pelvic rotation

- Observe for – ability to rotate pelvis and extend lumbar spine independent of thoracolumbar junction

Posterior pelvic rotation

- Observe for – ability to rotate pelvis and extend lumbar spine independent of hip

Lateral pelvic rotation

- Observe for – ability to rotate pelvis independent of thoracolumbar junction and hip

Hip abduction/lateral rotation with hips and knees flexed

- Observe for – ability to move hip independently of lumbar spine and pelvis, asymmetry

Muscle length tests

- Tensor fascia latae, rectus femoris, psoas
- Hamstrings
- Paraspinal muscles

Box 21.5 **Movement control: Assessment—cont'd**

Side lying
  Rolling
    • Observe rotation of trunk and effect of control of
      rotation of trunk
  Hip abduction/lateral rotation
  Muscle length tests
    • Tensor fascia latae/iliotibial band
Prone
  Knee flexion (active and passive)
    • Observe for – pelvic rotation, anterior pelvic tilt
  Hip rotation – medial and lateral (active and passive)
    • Observe for – pelvic rotation
  Hip and knee extension
    • Observe for – excessive lumbar extension or
      segmental extension, absence of gluteal muscle
      activation, excessive trunk rotation
Four point kneeling
  Rock back and forward
    • Observe for – relative motion of hips and lumbar
      spine, hip motion independent of thoracolumbar
      junction, lateral deviation of pelvis, lumbar rotation

Arm lift
    • Observe for – lumbar rotation
Anterior and posterior pelvic tilt
    • Observe for – relative motion of lumbar spine
      and thoracolumbar junction, lateral deviation
Gait
  Observe for – symmetry between sides, decreased
    motion, excessive pelvic rotation, relationship
    between hip and lumbar motion, increased lumbar
    flexion/lateral shift, increased thoracolumbar
    extension, increased anterior/posterior pelvic rotation,
    lack of thoracic rotation, limping

Effect of repeated loading

Extension in prone
Flexion in supine

Effect of correction of postural 'fault(s)' on pain and muscle activity

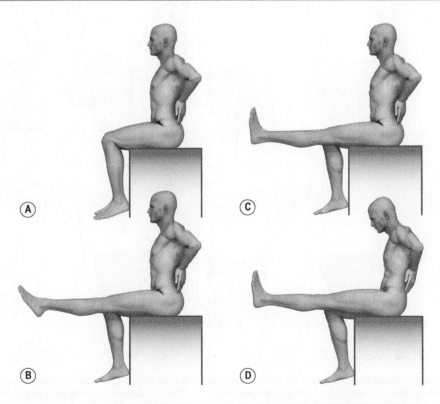

Figure 21.25 Knee extension with ankle dorsiflexion. The person should be able to fully extend the knee and dorsiflex the ankle while maintaining the hip at 90 degrees and the shoulders in line with the hips (A–C). (D) The person flexes the lumbar region with knee extension and ankle dorsiflexion. *Reproduced from Sahrmann, S., 2002.* Diagnosis and Treatment of Movement Impairment Syndromes. *Mosby, with permission of Elsevier.*

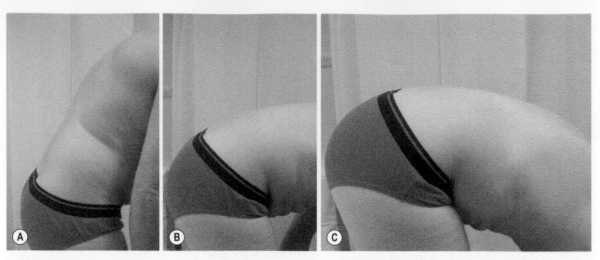

Figure 21.26 Flexion movement sequence. Movement initiated at the lumbosacral junction.

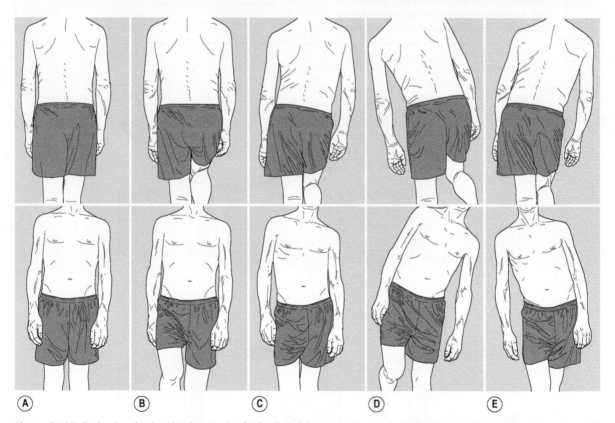

Figure 21.27 Optimal and suboptimal strategies for lumbopelvic control during single leg stance. (A) Bipedal start position. (B) Single leg stance with control of frontal plane lumbopelvic alignment. (C) Poor lumbopelvic control with loss of frontal alignment of pelvis, hip medial rotation, anterior pelvic tilt and lateral flexion of trunk. (D) Poor lumbopelvic control with lateral flexion of trunk over stance leg. (E) Poor lumbopelvic control with lateral flexion of trunk over lifted leg and shift of pelvis over the stance leg.

Box 21.6 **Movement correction: Training goals**

Optimize lumbopelvic loading

Avoid provocative movements
Encourage relieving movements
Correct specific faults in movement
    Dissociation between regions
    Poor control at a specific segment/region
    Maintain spinal alignment (lumbar lordosis, thoracic
      kyphosis and cervical lordosis)
    Avoid breath holding
Encourage sharing of load between adjacent regions
Correct asymmetry
Encourage functional use of improved muscle activation
  patterns
    Minimize activity of overactive muscles (often
      superficial/global muscles)
    Enhance activity of underactive muscles (often deep/
      local muscles)
    Can also use to train endurance (e.g. sit-to-stand,
      pauses just after lift-off from bed)

Box 21.7 **Movement correction: Techniques**

Techniques to correct individual specific faults in movement

Cognitive correction
Instructions (e.g. hold lordosis when bending)
Imagery (visual and proprioceptive)
Manual guidance (e.g. hand on sacrum to facilitate
  anterior rotation of pelvis)
Manual cues (e.g. finger on xiphoid and navel to control
  thoracolumbar junction)
Dissociation tasks (e.g. separate lumbar from
  thoracolumbar junction motion, 'waiter's bow')
Muscle activation (e.g. palpation, observation, EMG
  biofeedback)
Cues/reminders (e.g. taping)

(Ferreira et al. 2009; Unsgaard-Tondel et al. 2012); and change in muscle activation strategy is related to clinical improvement (Ferreira et al. 2009; Unsgaard-Tondel et al. 2012; Vasseljen and Fladmark 2010). These outcomes highlight the potential relevance of rehabilitation of muscle activation strategy as a priority in motor control training. As highlighted in other sections of this book, muscle activation may be either too much or too little, and both of these extremes are commonly present in the same patient, but with considerable variation between individuals in terms of the muscles that may be modified. An additional consideration is that although the coordination of recruitment of the muscle by the nervous system is the emphasis of the muscle activation strategies described here, it is also important to evaluate other aspects that affect the ability of a muscle to meet its demands in function. This includes the strength and endurance of the muscle, and structural issues such as muscle size and tissue changes such as fat infiltration, both of which will affect the performance of the muscle in function. In general it is important to correct the pattern first, then load the muscle to induce change in strength, endurance and structure (Danneels et al. 2001).

Like the other aspects of motor control training, the key to inclusion of retraining of muscle activation strategy in a motor control approach is the identification of potential deficits in muscle activation, and the determination of the relevance of these changes to the patient's symptoms. The challenge then is to find a technique to encourage change in muscle recruitment that can be transferred to function.

Assessment of muscle activation strategy

Assessment of muscle activation strategy is complicated by difficulty in accurately assessing muscle function in clinical practice as outlined in the section on muscle activation (see p. 253). In general every time a patient moves and every posture he/she adopts will provide some information of muscle activation strategies. The specific features of posture and movement that provide insight into muscle activation strategy are outlined respectively in 'Assessment of posture/alignment' and 'Assessment of movement'. This section provides detail of assessments that are directed to assess a patient's ability to activate specific muscles or their automatic activation in specific tasks (see Box 21.8). Additional information of muscle activation is also gleaned from assessment of the ability to control alignment of the spine and pelvis during tasks that challenge the static control of the spine. These tests are discussed in 'Clinical application of motor control training of static control of spine and pelvis'.

Goals of training muscle activation strategy

The goal of training muscle activation strategy is to encourage control of optimal load on the spine and pelvis, by a combination of increasing and decreasing muscle activity. Again, the specific features that need to be trained are individual-specific, and treatment must be targeted to the changes identified in the individual patient and then confirmed to be relevant to his/her presentation. Box 21.9 summarizes the various specific goals that underpin optimization of loading.

Techniques to train muscle activation strategy

Ultimately, every technique applied to change motor control will influence muscle activation. It is by changing muscle activation that posture and movement corrections are enacted. However, a range of techniques have been

Box 21.8 Muscle activation: Assessment

Interpretation from posture and movement

See 'Clinical application of motor control training of posture/alignment' and 'Clinical application of motor control training of movement' for guidance to interpretation of muscle activity from assessment of these features

Specific muscle activation tests

Tests of 'independent' activation of muscles

Test principle

Evaluate ability to activate short/deep muscles independently from long/superficial muscles – outcome is related to quality of control of the muscle in function (e.g. Hodges et al. 1996)

Task

Ability to cognitively perform the motor skill of contraction of transversus abdominis or multifidus independently from the other superficial trunk muscles. Assessments have also been devised along similar principles for psoas and pelvic floor muscles, to name a few

Measure

Precision
   Which muscles – observation, palpation (Fig. 21.28), electromyography, ultrasound imaging (Figs 21.11, 21.29–31)
   What sequence
   What quality – smooth, symmetrical, slow
Ideal response
   Palpable slow gentle increase in tension (Hides et al. 2000)
   Co-contraction with other deep muscles
   No/little activity of superficial muscles

Symmetrical
Smooth and sustained (not jerky)
Normal breathing
Repeat multiple contractions (up to $10 \times 10\,s$)

Interpretation

Ability to activate specific deep muscles = well controlled in function with relevance for predicting treatment efficacy (Ferreira et al. 2009)

Strategy of overactivity of superficial trunk muscles (combine with observation from movement and posture assessment) – this generally forms the foundation (in addition to information gleaned from assessment of posture and movement) of identification of the muscles that may require reduction in activity to optimize load on the spine/pelvis

Other muscle activation tests

Assess whether strategy to stiffen the spine increases or decreases pain – strategies are tuned to optimize the pain control

Assessment of control of static alignment in static progressions (see 'Clinical application of motor control training of static control of spine and pelvis')
   Tests of 'quality' of control of static spinal/pelvic alignment – see static assessment
   • load tolerance
   • symmetry
   • dissociation of movement of limbs from trunk

Active straight leg raise (Mens et al. 2002)
   Perceived ease of lifting leg – greater heaviness in presence of pelvic girdle dysfunction
   Affect of contraction of deep muscles or manual compression on perceived ease can be assessed

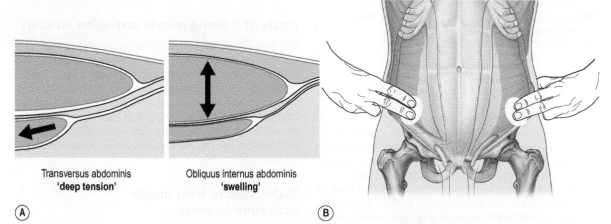

Transversus abdominis
'deep tension'

Obliquus internus abdominis
'swelling'

(A)   (B)

Figure 21.28 Technique for palpation of independent contraction of transversus abdominis (Hides et al. 2000). (A) During transversus abdominis contraction a deep tensioning should be palpated as the anterior fascias are tensioned by contraction of the muscle, whereas a superficial bulge will be palpated during contraction of obliquus internus abdominis. (B) Finger placement for palpation of independent activation of transversus abdominis contraction.

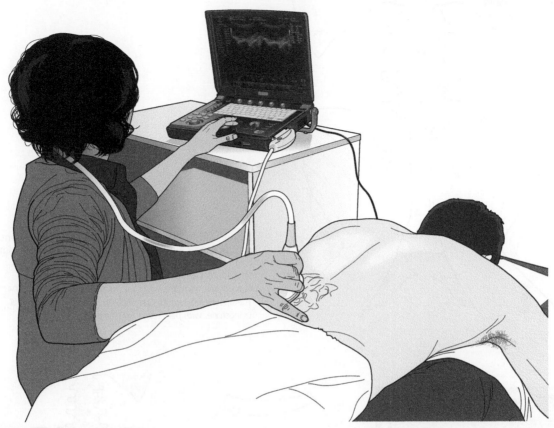

Figure 21.29 Use of ultrasound imaging to measure voluntary contraction of the multifidus muscle.

Box 21.9 **Muscle activation: Training goals**

Optimize lumbopelvic loading

Avoid provocative muscle activity
  e.g. discourage muscle activity that overloads tissues/
  muscle activity that prevents an ideal posture or
  motion path
Encourage muscle activity that improves control
  e.g. encourage muscle activity the controls aberrant
  motion; encourage muscle activity that enables a
  more ideal loading strategy of posture or movement
Correct asymmetry
Encourage variation in muscle activation strategy to 'share
  the load'
Encourage functional use of improved muscle activation
  patterns in postures and movements

Minimize activity of overactive muscles (often
  superficial/global muscles)
Enhance activity of underactive muscles (often deep/
  local muscles, but not limited to these muscles, e.g.
  common presentation of 'inhibition' of the gluteal
  muscles that is commonly discussed in Janda's
  approach (Janda 1996))

Optimize breathing pattern
Optimize control of pelvic floor muscles
Aim to increase endurance in muscles that control spinal posture

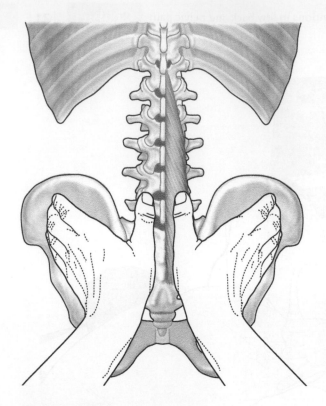

Figure 21.30 Technique for palpation of independent contraction of lumbar multifidus. During lumbar multifidus contraction a bilateral, symmetrical deep tensioning should be palpated close to the midline.
Reproduced from Richardson, C., Hodges, P., Hides, J., 2004. Therapeutic Exercise for Lumbopelvic Stabilization. Churchill Livingstone, with permission from Elsevier.

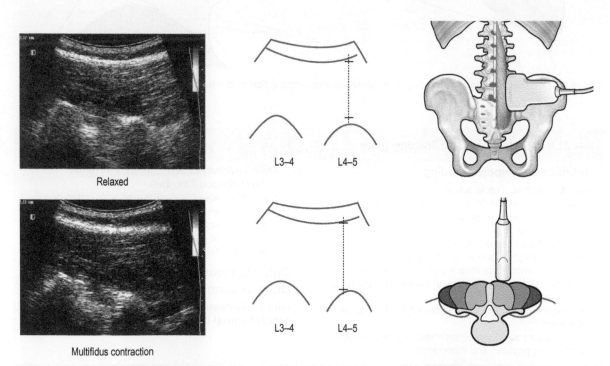

Relaxed

L3–4   L4–5

Multifidus contraction

L3–4   L4–5

Figure 21.31 Assessment of activation of the lumbar multifidus with ultrasound imaging. Position of the ultrasound transducer and imaging method are shown on the right. Ultrasound images on the left show relaxed and contracted multifidus muscle. Activation can be observed with thickening of the muscle and movement of the muscle fascicles, observable as displacement of the white connective tissue planes that are identifiable longitudinally in the muscle.
Reproduced from Richardson, C., Hodges, P., Hides, J., 2004. Therapeutic Exercise for Lumbopelvic Stabilization. Churchill Livingstone, with permission from Elsevier.

Box 21.10 **Muscle activation: Techniques**

Techniques to reduce activity of overactive lumbopelvic muscles

Whole body posture (in general more activity requires more support to encourage reduction)
Spinal posture (in general 'neutral' spinal alignment involves less activity of superficial muscles)
Instruction
Breathing techniques
Feedback (EMG, palpation)
Decrease effort
Connective tissue techniques, trigger point, dry needling
Inhibitory taping
Imagery

Techniques to increase activity of underactive lumbopelvic muscles

Whole body posture (stretch on muscle)
Spinal posture (greater activity in neutral)
Instruction
Co-contraction with other muscles to facilitate contraction (e.g. pelvic floor muscles can be used to encourage improved contraction of transversus abdominis (Sapsford et al. 2001))
Manual facilitation
Imagery
Feedback (observation, palpation, ultrasound)
Taping

Techniques to train co-contraction strategies to control lumbopelvic pelvic alignment

See 'Clinical application of motor control training of static control of spine and pelvis'

Box 21.11 **Muscle activation: Treatment planning**

Three critical questions

1. What strategy works best for the patient?
   Find a strategy that gives best contraction of underactive components
   Find a strategy to reduce overactive components
2. How can you be sure that the patient will practise the correct exercise at home?
   Find a (feedback) technique to ensure correct practise
3. What would the home programme be?
   Indicate number of contractions and duration
   2–3 sessions per day initially

Treatment progression

Increase hold time, repetitions
Decrease feedback, facilitation strategies
Aim for 'confident' correction
   Independent
   Cognitive
   Minimal feedback
   Minimal effort
   10 s hold
   Ideal to be able to breathe

---

used in clinical practice with the explicit aim to change muscle activation as a primary outcome to modify the load on the tissues of the spine and pelvis; either by enhancing muscle activation to improve control of aberrant movement or reducing muscle activation to decrease overload. Box 21.10 provides a summary of a range of techniques that are commonly used to train increased or decreased muscle activity and Box 21.11 provides guidance for treatment progression and planning.

Clinical application of motor control training of static control of spine and pelvis

Static control of the spine and pelvis and motor control training

As outlined in 'Progression of motor control with a focus on static training', there are many clinical approaches that have been designed to train control of static alignment of

the spine and pelvis. In fact this type of training (in which a patient is encouraged to maintain a specific alignment while load is applied to the trunk either directly or via limb movement or loading) has become somewhat synonymous with the approach and has led to the misconception that motor control training aims to train static control of the spine and pelvis as an end point, rather than a focus on optimal dynamic control of the spine. Although there are many clinicians and researchers who advocate this component as the entirety of motor control training, the prevailing contemporary view expressed throughout this book is that this component is part of the training, and not the whole. It is our contention that optimal application of this component of training depends on when and how it is applied and this should be: (i) *after* the patient has learnt the skill of correction of the motor control faults that are considered relevant for his/her presentation; and (ii) in combination with a progression of exercise that aims to encourage movement of the spine and pelvis for dynamic control. This section highlights the guiding principles of assessment and training that cut across the various approaches that have been advocated in clinical practice.

Assessment of static control of the spine and pelvis

Assessment of static control basically involves determination of the ability of a patient to maintain an alignment of the spine and pelvis. This can be assessed during formal assessment tasks that involve a standardized sequence of incremental loads (as outlined in Box 21.12); by careful evaluation of response to loading in an individualized manner matched to the needs of the patient (loads applied in specific directions and with specific loads that challenge performance); or by careful analysis of functions that include static alignment as one component (e.g. static control during weight lifting). One consideration for this phase of training is that although movements are commonly initiated from the extremities rather than the spine, many tasks involve a combination of both. For example, to kick a ball, the movement is initiated from the hip (with a maintained lumbar lordosis), but for full range in this

---

Box 21.12 Static control: Assessment

Assessment principle

Evaluate control of orientation/alignment of spine and pelvis during loading or limb movement

Components

Evaluation of muscle activation strategy – pattern, co-activation of deep and superficial muscles

Evaluation of the threshold loads/forces (amplitude and direction) that can be tolerated before lumbopelvic alignment is lost

Evaluation of symmetry/asymmetry of control – asymmetry of control of rotation is common

Evaluate dissociation of movement of limb from spine

Assessment task

Control of static orientation of spine and pelvic position during addition of load to limbs/trunk that aims to challenge the control of orientation – many options are available

Leg loading exercise (Sahrmann 2002)

Ball exercise

Pilates

Proprioceptive neuromuscular facilitation – rhythmic stabilization (Voss et al. 1985)

Limb loading

Thoracic rotation (sitting or standing, with or without resistance)

Upper limb tasks

Loading in weight bearing: e.g. dead lifts, upright row

Standing, hip flexion, abduction or extension

Can add perturbations to upper limb, e.g. FLEXI-BAR® or Bodyblade®, observe curves and muscle activation strategies

Assess muscle length/stiffness (e.g. tight hamstrings leading to inability to fully extend knee in sitting if lumbar region is not allowed to move (Fig 21.32), or tight latissimus dorsi increasing the lumbar lordosis with overhead tasks)

Assess response to correction of 'fault' in posture, movement, muscle activation

Assess for lack of endurance (unable to maintain spinal curves)

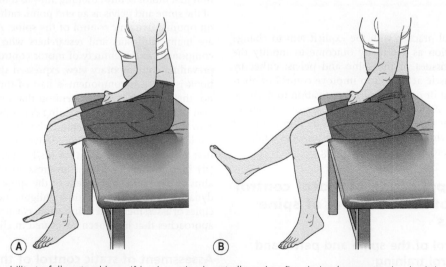

Figure 21.32 Inability to fully extend knee if lumbar spine is not allowed to flex during knee extension in sitting. The person's preferred alignment in sitting is lumbar flexion (A). The person is unable to fully extend the knee and dorsiflex the ankle when the person is not allowed to flex the lumbar spine (B). *Reproduced from Sahrmann, S., 2002.* Diagnosis and Treatment of Movement Impairment Syndromes. *Mosby, with permission of Elsevier.*

activity, the lumbar spine will be required to flex, and therefore is more closely aligned with dynamic control training. A key consideration in that task is that the movement is not initiated from the spine.

Goals of training static control of the spine and pelvis

The goals of static training are common across the various programmes developed to address this component of training and are outlined in Box 21.13.

Techniques to train static control of the spine and pelvis

The specific techniques used to challenge and train static alignment depend on the training and preferences of the treating clinician, the preferences of the patient, and the potential for the patient to apply the intervention as a component of a home programme (this may limit the use of equipment). One feature that varies between approaches is the specific alignment that the patient is encouraged to adopt and maintain during the application of the load. This is still the subject of debate, although the 'neutral' alignment defined in 'Assessment of posture/alignment' is commonly accepted in contemporary practice and advocated by the authors of this chapter. Choice of position of exercise is an important consideration. This will lead to variation in the strategy of muscle recruitment. For example, in supine lying, there may be a bias towards recruitment of the abdominal (and psoas major) muscles rather than trunk extensor muscles as a result of the gravity vector and because the thoracic spine/rib cage and pelvis are in contact with the bed. Upright forward leaning positions may bias recruitment towards the trunk extensor

muscles. In the latter position, patients may find it challenging to maintain the thoracic kyphosis, which may require activation of additional muscles such as the serratus anterior muscle acting in a reversed origin and insertion manner for control. Endurance and observation of muscle fatigue is crucial in this phase of training. Box 21.14 summarizes key features of application of training to control of static alignment and Box 21.15 provides guidance for treatment planning.

Clinical application of motor control training of dynamic control of spine and pelvis

Dynamic control of the spine and pelvis and motor control training

Training of dynamic control of the spine and pelvis is more complicated than training of static alignment as there is not a single goal (e.g. maintenance of a static

---

Box 21.13 Static control: Training goals

Correct faults into more challenging situations – static

Train integration of correct muscle activation
Train integration of correct posture (Fig. 21.33)
Train integration of correct movement (e.g. dissociation of hip from spine)

Focus on improved static control of lumbopelvic orientation/alignment

Increase threshold load amplitude before loss of control of alignment
Restore symmetry of control of alignment
Target the functional needs of the patient
Train endurance
Teach patients to identify when they are fatigued, and not to push through fatigue

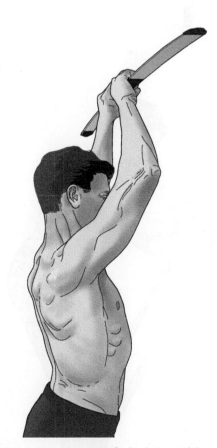

Figure 21.33 Common alignment 'fault' during training. Increased thoracolumbar extension during overhead exercise using Bodyblade®.

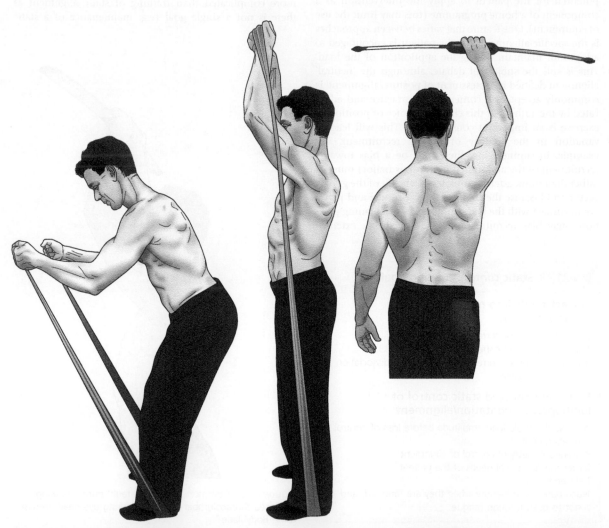

Figure 21.34 Advanced training of spine alignment using Thera-Band® and Bodyblade®. Training is reliant on maintenance of optimal spinal alignment and breathing. Ultrasound imaging can be used to provide feedback of control of the lumbar lordosis and contraction/fatigue of the lumbar multifidus muscle. Thera-Band® can be placed under heels and through heel of hand.

Box 21.15 **Static control: Treatment planning**

Target to functional needs of patient

Select approach that patient can use frequently

Target specific deficits in muscle system – target asymmetries in large superficial torque producers

Monitor posture, movement, muscle activation strategies

Progression

Load
  ↑ lever length
  ↑ load/resistance
Position
  Supported
  Unsupported
Dynamics
  ↑ speed of movement
  ↑ instability
Mental challenge
  Dual task
  Psychological challenge (e.g. fear of movement)

Box 21.16 **Dynamic control: Assessment**

Assessment principle

Evaluation of ability to maintain control of muscle activation, posture and movement during movement
Consideration of two components of dynamic control:
- movement of the spine and pelvis
- control of the spine and pelvis during movement of the whole body

Components

Ability to maintain correction of motor control faults* during formal movement tests
  As described for 'Movement correction: assessment' (see p. 275)
Ability to maintain correction of motor control faults* during functional movement
Ability to maintain correction of motor control faults* on unstable base

Task

Formal movement assessment task (e.g. flexion in standing with attention to sharing of load between lumbar and hip regions)
Any movement of relevance to the patient's presentation – requires understanding of the optimal performance of the task and consideration of control of the motor control faults* within the context of the movement task

Assess response to correction

*Faults in posture (alignment/symmetry/etc.), muscle activation (excessive/compromised/pattern/etc.) and movement (dissociation/excessive/restricted/etc.).

alignment) that needs to be monitored to ensure accuracy of the performance. Instead the clinician must have an understanding of the ideal and suboptimal features of a specific task and monitor those features during the performance of the task. The features of interest depend both on the presentation of the patient (i.e. the motor control 'faults' that are specific to the patient) and the components of the dynamic task (e.g. control of lumbar lordosis during thorax rotation). An important consideration is that although the term 'dynamic' implies movement, the amount of movement varies between tasks and its distribution between the individual planes. Some tasks involve more or less motion and this motion may be restricted to one of two planes. For instance, running involves transfer of load through the spine, this involves some rotation and lateral flexion, but with less motion in the sagittal plane (Saunders et al. 2005), which contrasts with hurdling, where the spine must undergo greater flexion.

The features that are the target of the progression and require careful monitoring during training are generally those that were highlighted at the initial phase of training as the motor control 'faults' apparent in the function of the individual patient. Thus, training of dynamic control requires an individualized approach and requires greater skill of assessment and training to be able to ensure that the patient is successful and that he/she is sufficiently challenged. It is no doubt due to this increment in complexity, beyond that required to train control of static

alignment, that underpins the less frequent discussion and application of training to a dynamic level.

Assessment of dynamic control of the spine and pelvis

Assessment of dynamic control is complicated as the feature that is assessed depends on the presentation of the patient. That is, the assessment aims to determine the success with which the patient is able to correct a specific motor control 'fault' during performance of a task that involves movement. This will be difficult to apply in an objective manner and often depends on assessment of the quality based on observation or methods that are difficult to quantify. Box 21.16 defines the principles of assessment of dynamic control. Problems in dynamic control may involve too much movement, too little movement, suboptimal trajectory of movement, poor quality of movement, excessive out of plane movement, etc.

Box 21.17 Dynamic control: Training goals

Correct faults into more challenging situations – dynamic

Train integration of correct muscle activation
Train integration of correct posture
Train integration of correct movement

Focus on dynamic control of lumbopelvic orientation/alignment

Train control during changes in lumbopelvic position

Train incorporation of lumbopelvic movement into simple dynamic functions

Goals of training dynamic control of the spine and pelvis

The goal of dynamic training may be straightforward, but its application to patients may be complex. The underlying objective is to correct the motor control faults that have been identified as relevant for a patient's presentation in a dynamic situation. This may involve increased, decreased or modified movement trajectory or quality during the dynamic task. This may involve control of the spine and pelvis as they move, and control of movement of the spine and pelvis in the context of whole body function. Box 21.17 summarizes key guiding principles related to this goal.

Techniques to train dynamic control of the spine and pelvis

Although the goal of dynamic training is straightforward (i.e., to correct the motor control faults that have been identified as relevant for a patient's presentation in a dynamic context) the methods to achieve this are complex and individual-specific. Box 21.18 presents a range of clinical techniques and principles that can be applied to train more optimal motor control in dynamic contexts, and guidelines for planning treatment are provided in Box 21.19.

Clinical application of motor control training of function

Functional retraining of control of the spine and pelvis and motor control training

The phase of functional retraining in a motor control approach is an extension of the dynamic and static training phases discussed in the preceding sections, with the exception that the objective is to work towards practising integration of correction of motor control faults in the tasks (movements/functions) that have been identified by

Box 21.18 Dynamic control: Techniques

Train control of posture, movement and muscle activity *during lumbopelvic movement and during movement of the whole body*

Correct motor control faults* in dynamic situation
Monitor lumbopelvic alignment in one plane while moving in another – rotation in neutral sagittal alignment
    e.g. control of sagittal alignment/posture during practise of counter-rotation of the thorax and pelvis (rotation of the spine in the transverse plane) in standing or standing with tandem stance in preparation for walking

Train control of movement, posture and muscle activity on *unstable surfaces*

This task can be useful to initiate training of dynamic control as it is impossible to maintain balance if the spine is held rigidly; instead motion must occur to maintain body equilibrium. This requires careful assessment of the patient's ability to meet the demands of a specific degree of instability (e.g. height of balance board, curvature of surface, amplitude of available motion)

Sequence

Ensure correct posture
Ensure correct muscle activation
Monitor lumbar and pelvic position and motion
    e.g. pressure biofeedback, hand, mirror
Cognitive correction if motor control fault*
    e.g. instructions, manual guidance, etc.

Techniques for correction of motor control faults*

Manual guidance
Manual cues
Dissociation tasks
Muscle activation
Cues/reminders

*Faults in posture (alignment/symmetry/etc.), muscle activation (excessive/compromised/pattern/etc.) and movement (dissociation/excessive/restricted/etc.).

the patient as those that are of particular relevance for him/her. This relevance may either be that the tasks are those the patient reports to be associated with pain, or tasks that the patient wants to be able to perform but is restricted from achieving for some reason, which may be related to pain. Of particular note, the basic features of the task may be focussed on static or dynamic features. Like dynamic training, this component of the progression requires the treating clinician to be able to analyze the task to determine which aspects are critical to retrain (e.g. static

Box 21.19 Dynamic control: Treatment planning

Target to functional needs of patient

Target specific deficits in neuromuscular system – target asymmetries

Combine with static control exercise

Monitor posture/alignment, movement, muscle activation strategies

Progression

Load
  ↑ lever length
  ↑ load/resistance
Position
  Supported
  Unsupported
Dynamics
  ↑ speed of movement
  ↑ instability
Mental challenge
  Dual task
  Psychological challenge (e.g. fear of movement)

Box 21.20 Functional retraining: Assessment

Assessment principle

Evaluation of ability to maintain control of muscle activation, posture and movement during movement of the lumbar spine and pelvis

Components

Ability to maintain correction of motor control faults* during complex functional movements that have been identified by the patient as a priority

Assess response to correction

*Faults in posture (alignment/symmetry/etc.), muscle activation (excessive/compromised/pattern/etc.) and movement (dissociation/excessive/restricted/etc.).

Box 21.21 Functional retraining: Training goals

Correct motor control faults during function

Train integration of correct muscle activation
Train integration of correct posture
Train integration of correct movement

Specific to patient presentation

Priority tasks (functions that are compromised by pain and/or dysfunction)

Use principles of motor learning

Segmentation – practise parts before practise of the whole task
Simplification – modify task with reduced/simplified speed, position, load to enable optimal performance with progression as skill improves
Feedback – of specific elements that are to be corrected during performance of the 'part' then 'whole' task
Move from internal focus of attention (attention to detail of motor control) to external focus of attention (attention to outcome of movement)

Focus on transfer of motor control skills into function – practise exercise that is as close to function as possible

Consider the potential for loss of control at the onset of fatigue

Consideration of need for basic elements of athleticism (i.e. range of motion, endurance, strength, speed, power, etc.)

Goals of training control of the spine and pelvis in function

The goals of functional retraining in the context of motor control training are similar to those defined for dynamic control and are summarized in Box 21.21.

Techniques to train control of the spine and pelvis in function

Techniques applied for retraining control of a motor control 'fault' in function are defined in Box 21.22. The techniques used for a specific patient require careful consideration to ensure the accuracy of correction of the fault in a complex functional task. The accuracy is a result of the skills of the treating clinician to evaluate the success of the technique and to be able to identify a relevant technique that is most likely to be effective for the individual patient.

Similar to the phase of dynamic control, it is essential to both consider control of motion of the spine and pelvis, and control of the spine and pelvis during motion of the whole body. The elements of this phase can be considered

control of alignment, or control of movement trajectory, or a combination of both) and then to monitor the success in achievement and improvement of control of this aspect.

Assessment of control of the spine and pelvis in function

The assessment principles for functional retraining are outlined in Box 21.20 and are similar to those defined for dynamic training with a key focus on evaluation of control of the motor control 'fault' that has been identified for the patient throughout the period of training.

Box 21.22 Functional retraining: Techniques

Train control of movement, posture and muscle activity in a functional task

Correct motor control faults* in functional situation – requires understanding of the requirement/components of the task

Sequence

Correct posture
Correct muscle activation
Monitor lumbar and pelvic position and motion
Cognitive correction if motor control fault*

Techniques for correction of motor control faults*

Use of any technique that can guide the acquisition/correction/reinforcement of an improved motor control strategy is advocated. Examples include:
manual guidance
manual cues
dissociation tasks
muscle activation
cues/reminders

*Faults in posture (alignment/symmetry/etc.), muscle activation (excessive/compromised/pattern/etc.) and movement (dissociation/excessive/restricted/etc.).

using the example of a runner. Optimal function and functional training of a runner who suffers low back pain involves consideration of multiple aspects. These include spinal loading, impact and the transmission and dissipation of forces. Dynamic alignment and biomechanical interaction of the hips, knees and feet of the lower limbs are also critical to consider. As running involves the entire kinetic chain, a motor control problem anywhere along the chain could contribute to the patient's clinical presentation/symptoms. There is emerging evidence that the relationship between adjacent regions has consequences in both directions; limb dysfunction has implications for the spine; and lumbopelvic dysfunction has implications for the lower limb. With respect to the latter issue, prospective studies have identified that altered control of the spine in response to perturbation is predictive of future lower limb injuries in collegiate female athletes (Zazulak et al. 2007). Issues such as hip adduction, internal rotation and knee valgus are consistently related to lower limb injuries. Consideration of the interaction between trunk and lower limb is particularly relevant for the relationship between the lumbopelvic region and any muscle that attaches from the lower limb to the pelvis. For example, tight/stiff hamstrings and poor endurance of the multifidus muscle could relate to the adoption (either as cause or effect) of a position of posterior tilt during running. Coordination of respiration (see the section on

'Breathing' below), thoracic rotation/mobility, symmetry, running technique and cardiovascular fitness (see the section on 'Fitness' below) are also important fundamental issues underlying optimal running performance. Careful assessment of each of these elements and consideration of their relevance for the patient's symptoms is necessary. Attention to specific individual aspects is required. For instance, it may be important to consider when the patient begins to tire when running as this may be the point at which load transfer is modified. Subtle observations may highlight problems in control. For instance the lateral head wobble reported by some runners may be explained by excess trunk stiffness, possibly explained by over-recruitment of the quadratus lumborum muscle that would block lateral flexion of the spine, limiting normal frontal plane movement of the lumbar spine during running. As illustrated in this example the phase of functional training requires consideration of the patient individually and holistically to ensure optimal control of load on lumbopelvic structures for the management of the biological contribution to his/her symptoms.

Clinical application of strategies to manage barriers to recovery

The preceding sections highlight the basic clinical sequence in planning and implementation of training of motor control for people with lumbopelvic pain, but comprehensive management of a patient's symptoms requires consideration of a range of other issues that may present to a greater or lesser degree for each individual patient. In some cases these additional issues may have a minor impact on presentation and recovery, and require either no change or a simple modification to exercise prescription. In others they may form a major barrier and require detailed assessment and treatment. It is when these issues present as a barrier to recovery that they are most obvious and generally require attention in order to achieve the optimal outcome for the patient. The challenge for the clinician is to evaluate the relative importance of each and to determine the amount of time and effort to devote to assessment and management. The following section briefly summarizes the major elements of the relationship of the most common 'barriers' to recovery of optimal motor control. This is presented along with tabulated summaries of the major treatment goals, assessment tools and strategies, and a selection of contemporary treatment techniques. For each issue, assessment is critical in order to determine treatment goals and select treatment techniques.

In addition to the *potentially modifiable* barriers highlighted in this section, there are, of course, a number of barriers that may limit the potential for motor control training to make any impact on symptoms. For instance, some specific pathologies will limit the potential for improvements in motor control to change symptoms.

Examples could include some post-surgical patients when the potential to change control may be limited by disruption to muscle and fascia, and scarring; diseases that change structural mobility (significant structural scoliosis); and the presence of pain of neuropathic origin (see 'Fitting training of spine control into the biopsychosocial framework').

Beliefs, attitudes and neurobiology of pain

Broader dimensions of pain, beyond the contribution of nociceptive input from the periphery, have been detailed elsewhere in this chapter and this book (see Chapter 11) and are critical to consider in all patients with pain. The importance will vary depending on the individual patient and aspects of his/her presentation. A key issue is the interaction between psychosocial and biological issues; that is, a person's beliefs and attitudes have a direct impact on the manner in which he/she holds posture, uses muscles, and moves. It is obvious that these issues and their interactions require consideration. Management may be parallel (targeting motor control and psychosocial issues with separate treatments, but at the same time), concurrent (targeting motor control and psychosocial issues with a combined treatment) or sequential.

Consideration of psychosocial issues related to pain is clearly critical. Pain is an emergent experience produced by the brain. In fact, one might argue that the brain is unable to *produce* pain, and that pain is an emergent property of the entire person (see Thacker and Moseley 2012). Nociception is an important trigger and modulator of pain, but the ultimate experience is dependent on a far more complex evaluation that occurs outside of our consciousness (see Chapter 11). Beliefs about pain, injury, body vulnerability, and possible consequences, are fundamental. A simple rule of thumb is this: if an inaccurate belief increases the perception of threat to body tissue, it will serve to increase pain and is therefore a target for treatment.

Some key training goals, assessments to determine the nature of psychosocial contributors to the pain experience and some considerations for treatment are presented in Boxes 21.23, 21.24 and 21.25, respectively.

Breathing

Breathing involves all muscles of the trunk in one way or the other. This can range from a primary contribution to inspiration by the diaphragm muscle, to an occasional contribution to expiratory effort under situations of increased demand by some regions of the abdominal muscles. Even pelvic floor muscles modulate their activity with respiration to maintain continence with fluctuation in intra-abdominal pressure (Hodges et al. 2007). It is obvious that the contribution of trunk muscles for breathing must be coordinated with the contribution to motor control of the trunk for control of stability (movement and stiffness). There is potential for disruption of this

---

Box 21.23 Beliefs, attitudes and neurobiology of pain: Training goals

Ensure an accurate picture of the state of the tissues

Reduce catastrophization

Reduce kinesiophobia

Train pain coping skills

Gain motivation and resources to self manage

Improve understanding of the biology that underpins pain

Reduce and manage depression

Manage social issues

Manage neuropathic pain

Box 21.24 Beliefs, attitudes and neurobiology of pain: Assessment

Questionnaires

Catastrophizing
   Pain Catastrophizing Scale (PCS)
   Coping Skills Questionnaire (CSQ)
Kinesiophobia
   Tampa Scale for Kinesiophobia (TSK)
   Photograph series of Daily Activities-Short electronic
     Version (PHODA-SeV)
   Fear-Avoidance Beliefs Questionnaire (FABQ)
Pain biology knowledge/conceptualization
Pain Knowledge Questionnaire (revised)
Depression
   Center for Epidemiological Studies-Depression
     Questionnaire (CES-D)
   Hospital Anxiety and Depression Score (HADS)
   Depression Anxiety Symptoms Scale (DASS)
Readiness to change
   Readiness to change questionnaire
Pain coping skills
   Coping Skills Questionnaire (CSQ)
Self efficacy
Pain Self-Efficacy Questionnaire (PSEQ)
General psychosocial aspects
Orebro questionnaire
StarT back screening tool

Assessment of neuropathic pain

LANSS pain scale
Neuropathic pain scale
Neuropathic pain symptom inventory
PainDetect
Quantitative sensory testing

Box 21.25 Beliefs, attitudes and neurobiology of pain: Techniques

Reduce catastrophization and kinesiphobia

Explain pain
Graded exposure
Psychological therapies – cognitive-behavioural therapy, acceptance commitment therapy, operant therapy

Train pain coping skills

Coping skills training, graded exposure, imagery, family involvement

Improve understanding of pain physiology

Explain pain

Manage depression

Psychological therapies
Antidepressant medications
Social and family support and engagement

Manage social issues

Workplace intervention
Psychological therapies
Group interventions

Box 21.26 Breathing: Training goals

Optimize respiratory activity of trunk muscles

Reduce tonic muscle activity that compromises respiratory motion
Reduce excessive respiratory activity of trunk muscles

Optimize respiratory movements

Encourage even distribution of movement between regions
Change breathing pattern to simplify spine control
Train symmetry

Optimize posture to optimize breathing

Optimize thorax dynamic control (thoracic spine and rib cage) to optimize breathing (Lee 2003)

Optimize efficiency of breathing pattern in disease

Assess and train breathing pattern with each progression in the motor control exercise programme

Box 21.27 Breathing: Assessment

Assessment of breathing pattern

Movement
Observation and palpation of breathing movements
- Three components – evenly distributed with no dominance
  - Upper chest
  - Basal chest expansion
  - Abdominal displacement
- Symmetry
Muscle activity
Observation, palpation, electromyography, ultrasound imaging (see Figs 21.35 and 21.36)

Evaluate and manage (if necessary) the effect of correction of motor control 'fault' on the natural breathing pattern

Muscle activation, posture, movement
Implement training if correction negatively interferes with breathing pattern (e.g. redistributes respiratory motion of the chest wall; encourages excessive muscle activity for breathing)

Consider chest wall flexibility and chest wall motor control and their impact on lumbopelvic function (Lee 2003)

coordination to be relevant in the presentation of a patient with pain or a patient with a breathing disorder. Poor ability to coordinate breathing and spine control has been observed in situations of increased respiratory demand (hypercapnoea) (Hodges et al. 2001) and in disease states (chronic airways limitation) (Hodges et al. 2000). There is observation of breathing changes in people with lumbopelvic pain (O'Sullivan et al. 2002). Posture and muscle activity are particularly relevant; even subtle changes in posture affect breathing pattern (Lee et al. 2010), and muscle activation modifies chest wall compliance with effects on respiratory movements.

Although unlikely to be an issue for all patients with lumbopelvic pain, it is reasonable to consider that respiratory issues may contribute to a patient's dysfunction of motor control of the spine and pelvis and may be a barrier to recovery unless addressed. Cycling is a good example of a sport that requires optimal breathing during dynamic function. Competitive cyclists are positioned in spinal flexion, with hip muscles activated in their outer to middle range (not into inner range). Cyclists with low back or pelvic pain tend to clench their oblique abdominal muscles when they tire and this is likely to impede breathing as a result of the restriction to basal rib cage expansion. Cyclists can be taught on their own bike (with the bike fixed) to maintain the correct spinal position and address their breathing pattern.

Methods for assessment of breathing are available and can be used to determine the specific nature of deficits and challenges with which a patient presents. Boxes 21.26, 21.27 and 21.28 summarize the goals of addressing breathing, key assessment methods and techniques to apply clinically to target issues identified in the assessment, respectively.

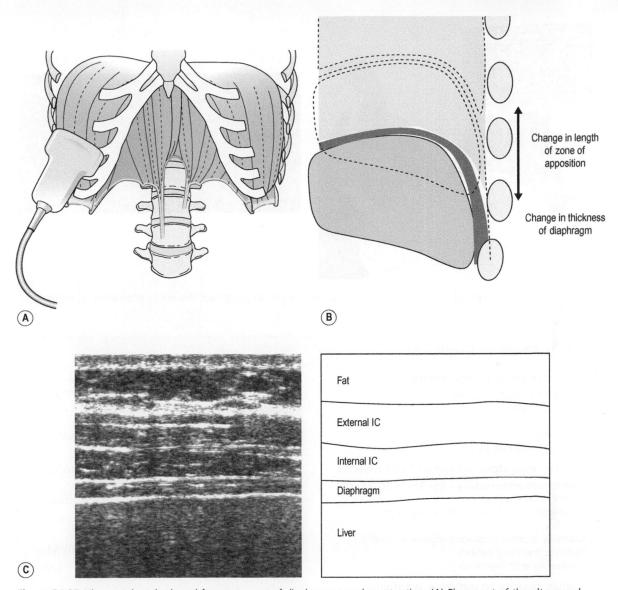

Figure 21.35 Ultrasound method used for assessment of diaphragm muscle contraction. (A) Placement of the ultrasound transducer along the intercostal space. (B) Diaphragm contraction involves shortening of the muscle (reduced length of the zone of apposition) and muscle thickening. (C) Ultrasound image showing the diaphragm and adjacent intercostal (IC) muscles.

Continence

The trunk muscles have an impact on continence. The equation is simple: if the pressure in the bladder exceeds that in the urethra, or the pressure in the rectum exceeds that in the anus, the result will be incontinence. The trunk muscles contribute to this equation in a number of ways. First, the muscles of the pelvic floor and sphincters are important both for maintenance of closure of the urethra

and anus for both continence and to enable intra-abdominal pressure to increase – the latter of which provides a contribution to spine control (Hodges et al. 2007; Smith et al. 2007; Stafford et al. 2012). Second, the muscles of the abdominal wall and the diaphragm muscle increase the bladder pressure (along with contraction of the smooth muscle of the bladder wall, the detrusor) and rectum via elevation of intra-abdominal pressure. Presence of incontinence may impact spine control (by limiting

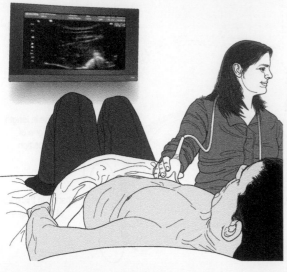

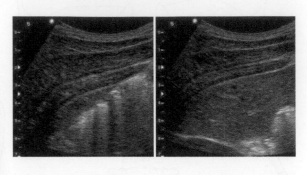

Figure 21.36 Use of ultrasound imaging to provide indirect feedback of diaphragmatic descent by observation of movement of the liver.

Box 21.28 **Breathing: Techniques**

Optimize respiratory movements

Respiratory training techniques
    Manual facilitation
    Quick stretch
    Positioning
    Feedback – manual, elastic

Optimize respiratory activity of trunk muscles

Reduce tonic/excessive activity – see Box 21.10 'Muscle
    activation: Techniques'
Maintain deep muscle activity during respiration
    Feedback
    Gradually increase inspiratory volume to threshold
    Optimize breathing pattern
    Commence with expiration

Optimize posture to optimize breathing

Retrain neutral posture
See 'Posture: techniques'

Optimize thorax dynamic control (thoracic spine and rib cage) to optimize breathing

Thoracic spine mobility/motor control – exercise, manual
    therapy
Rib cage mobility/motor control – exercise, manual
    therapy

Optimize efficiency of breathing pattern in disease

    Optimize breathing movements and muscle activity
    Increase fitness – pulmonary rehabilitation
    Flexibility – muscle length and thorax dynamics

Train breathing pattern with motor control progressions

---

intra-abdominal pressure control via incompetence of the pelvic floor muscles or via effects on abdominal muscle activity). Presence of motor control dysfunction in lumbopelvic pain may impact continence by placing additional challenges on the continence system as a result of augmented trunk muscle activation to protect the trunk. Furthermore, pelvic floor muscle activity is affected by lumbopelvic posture (activation is reduced in a slumped sitting posture) (Sapsford et al. 2008). Other issues of pelvic floor muscle dysfunction are also likely to be

relevant, such as pelvic organ prolapse, which also has potential involvement of compromised support mechanisms (pelvic floor muscle activation) and excessive pressure (abdominal muscle activation), although these have not been well tested. Pelvic floor muscle dysfunction is particularly prevalent after menopause, and this period is associated with other co-morbid spinal conditions such as osteoporosis. The associated thoracic spine crush fractures and an increased thoracic kyphosis, may be relevant. Problems related to hyperactivity of pelvic floor muscles, which is implicated in pelvic pain syndromes (Pool-Goudzwaard et al. 2005), may also be relevant. Furthermore, the natural coordination between the abdominal and pelvic floor muscles that has been reported in functional tasks and with voluntary contractions may be disrupted with resultant effects on efficiency of function.

The potential importance of the interaction between pelvic floor muscle dysfunction (including continence and other conditions) and lumbopelvic pain and/or dysfunction means that assessment of this system is important to consider in many people with lumbopelvic pain. This may range from simple subjective assessment to ascertain potential involvement of pelvic floor muscle dysfunction, to comprehensive specialist assessment and management of a pelvic floor muscle dysfunction. The extent of assessment is limited by the training of the treatment provider. Careful assessment is necessary to ascertain the presence and relevance of dysfunction. This information then needs to be interpreted to determine the most appropriate course of action. Boxes 21.29, 21.30 and 21.31 provide a summary of the key training goals, assessments and treatment techniques that are available.

Box 21.29 Continence: Training goals

Train activation of pelvic floor muscles

Train gentle tightening and elevation of the pelvic floor
Restore symmetry of contraction
Train timing of contraction of pelvic floor muscles
Increase holding time (endurance)
Increase muscle strength
Reduce overactivity (hypertonicity) of pelvic floor muscles that may impair lumbopelvic function

Retrain coordination between pelvic floor and trunk muscles

Reduce overactivity of superficial trunk muscles
Retrain co-activation with deep trunk muscles

Retrain control of pelvic floor muscles with breathing

Box 21.30 Continence: Assessment

Subjective assessment

Evaluate symptoms and type of incontinence
  Do you have any urine loss on exertion, coughing, etc.?
    • Could suggest stress urinary incontinence
  Do you often experience symptoms of urge to urinate?
    • Could suggest urge incontinence
  Do you have any pain/discomfort?
Assess potential to activate pelvic floor muscles
  Can you stop the flow of urine midstream?
    • Ability to activate (avoid for training)
  Do you have difficulty initiating micturition?
    • Could suggest hyperactivity

Assessment of voluntary activation of pelvic floor muscles

Purpose of assessment
  Identify presence of **hypo-/hyper-**activity
  Evaluate **ability** to contract
  Evaluate **quality** of contraction
  Evaluate **symmetry** of contraction
  Evaluate muscle **strength and endurance**
  Evaluate **structural** deficits
Methods for assessment
  Self-assessment
    • External palpation of perineal body (female – elevation; male – tightening)
    • Voluntary stopping flow of urine – avoid for training

Ultrasound imaging
  • **Trans-abdominal** (transverse (assessment of position, elevation and right–left symmetry) and sagittal (assessment of elevation and position)) (Fig. 21.37A) or **trans-perineal** (technique for females is shown in Fig. 21.37B and for males in Fig. 21.38)
  • Provides information of contraction ability, quality, symmetry, direction
Specialized techniques – require additional training
  • Manual palpation of muscle contraction
  • Vaginal/anal EMG
  • Vaginal/anal pressure

Assessment of pelvic floor muscle activity during breathing

Tonic hold with subtle lengthening (expiration) and shortening (inspiration)

Assessment of affect of posture and posture change

Slump → decreased pelvic floor muscle activity; upright → increased pelvic floor muscle activity

Assessment of co-activation of pelvic floor and deep trunk muscles

Assessment of structural deficit of pelvic floor muscles

Manual palpation, ultrasound imaging – additional training required for these techniques

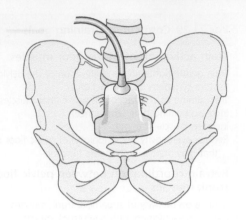

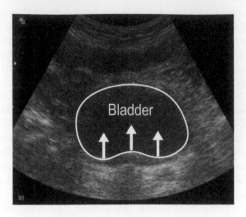

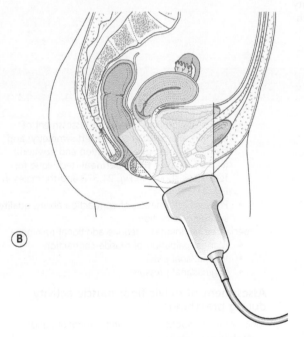

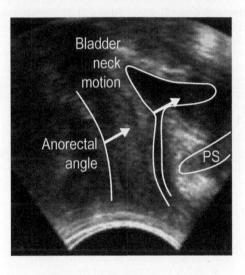

Figure 21.37 Methods for ultrasound assessment of pelvic floor muscle activation. (A) The transabdominal approach involves evaluation of lift of the bladder base observed in an ultrasound image made with the ultrasound transducer placed suprapubically and directed inferiorly to observe the bladder. This method enables observation of elevation of the bladder during pelvic floor muscle contraction, resting position of the bladder base and symmetry of position and contraction. This technique is difficult to interpret when the abdominal wall moves as there is no bony landmark for standardization of the measurements. (B) Transperineal approach to imaging. Measurement is made of motion of the bladder neck and anorectal angle. Measures can be made with respect to the fixed bony landmark of the pubic symphysis (PS).

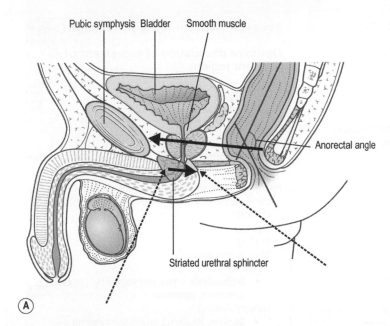
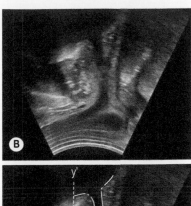
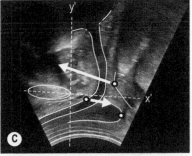

Figure 21.38 Transperineal ultrasound for assessment of pelvic floor muscle activation in males. (A) Anatomy of the male continence mechanism showing the direction of motion generated by contraction of the puborectalis/pubovisceralis muscle (cranio-ventral motion of the anorectal angle) and striated urethral sphincter (posterior motion of the urethra). (B) Ultrasound image made with transperineal placement of the ultrasound transducer and (C) features highlighted for measurement of motion based on the anatomy in (A).

Box 21.31 Continence: Techniques

Train activation of pelvic floor muscles

Education and instruction
Positioning
Feedback
Reduce overactivity of hyperactive pelvic floor muscles
    Requires specialist training
Timing
    Voluntary pre-activation
Strength and endurance training
    Repeated strong contractions – weights/feedback

Retrain coordination between pelvic floor muscles and other trunk muscles

Reduce overactivity of superficial trunk muscles – see Box 21.10 'Muscle activation: Techniques'

Co-activation with deep trunk muscles
    Submaximal/gentle
    Depends on lumbopelvic posture – neutral better

Breathing – see Box 21.28 'Breathing: Techniques'

Optimize breathing pattern → movement and muscle activation
Instruction
Feedback – palpation, observation, EMG, ultrasound

Posture – see Box 21.4 'Postural correction: Techniques'

Optimize posture

Adjacent body regions/segments

Although the contribution of function of adjacent joints to a patient's presentation and the most appropriate strategy to manage their symptoms is discussed elsewhere (e.g. 'Clinical application of motor control training of movement'), it is noteworthy to summarize the training goals

(Box 21.32), assessment (Box 21.33) and treatment techniques (Box 21.34) here to draw together the various ways in which the function of adjacent regions impacts the lumbopelvic region. These considerations include not only the necessity to dissociate the motion of the extremities from the lumbopelvic region, but also the necessity to ensure sufficient 'proximal' stiffness of the lumbopelvic

---

Box 21.32 Adjacent regions: Training goals

Optimize dissociation of movement of adjacent regions

Optimize relative 'stiffness'
   Muscle
   Articular

Correct *biomechanical* influences/interaction between lumbopelvic region and adjacent segments

e.g. hip and lower limb; thorax and thoracic spine; shoulder girdle

Correct *neuromuscular* influences/interaction between lumbopelvic region and adjacent segments

e.g. hip and lower limb; thorax and thoracic spine; shoulder girdle

---

Box 21.33 Adjacent regions: Assessment

Evaluation of dissociation of spine and limbs

Specific tests – see Box 21.5 'Movement control: Assessment'

Evaluation of dissociation between spine regions

Specific tests – see Box 21.5 'Movement control: Assessment'

Evaluation of biomechanical interaction between regions

Consider mechanical interactions between adjacent regions (e.g. association between pronated feet, internal rotation of the legs and anterior tilt)
Careful and detailed observation and palpation of position and movement)

Evaluation of neuromuscular interaction between regions

Consider muscle activity, proprioception

Evaluation of the effect of correction of 'faults' at adjacent segments and lumbopelvic region, on the interaction between segments

---

Box 21.34 Adjacent regions: Techniques

Optimize dissociation of movement of adjacent regions

Consider necessity to optimize muscle length/stiffness
   Control proximally while stretch distally
Manage articular issues
   Manual therapy
   Exercise – control with movement

Correct biomechanical and/or neuromuscular influences/interaction

Hip, knee, foot, shoulder girdle, thorax and thoracic spine, head/neck
   Orthotics
   Taping
   Bracing
   Manual therapy
   Active control
   • Biofeedback – electromyography, ultrasound, palpation, observation
Sensory training
   • Sensing, localizing and discriminating
   • Balance board, taping, repositioning

---

region/trunk to enable better mobility and power generation of the extremities. Like all aspects of motor control training, careful assessment is required to identify the aspects to be addressed in the comprehensive treatment approach. Unless functional deficits in adjacent regions are resolved, optimal function of the lumbar spine and pelvis is unlikely to be achieved.

Balance

Balance is a complex function with motor and sensory components. It is an integral part of human function. As the trunk involves 70% of a person's body weight, and motion of the trunk is a critical aspect of balance recovery mechanisms (Horak and Nashner 1986; Mok et al. 2007), balance training may be required in many individuals with low back and pelvic pain to ensure return to full function. Optimal targeting of a treatment approach is dependent on identification of the basis for postural control deficits. Balance deficits may involve an inability to involve trunk in balance adjustments as a result of pain, poor sensation of spinal position or movement, or reduced ability to move or generate trunk moments (e.g. increased passive stiffness or excessive muscle activation), or balance may be compromised as a result of generalized sensory deficits (visual, vestibular or somatosensory deficits), leg weakness, or poor coordination. Thus, incorporation of balance training into the management of a patient requires careful assessment and targeting of an appropriate treatment technique to overcome the specific deficit affecting balance. Boxes 21.35, 21.36 and 21.37 provide a summary of the key training goals, assessments and treatment techniques that are available.

Sensory function

As outlined in Chapter 19, many patients require consideration of sensory function. Without optimal sensory

---

Box 21.35 **Balance: Training goals**

Encourage incorporation of lumbopelvic movement into balance control strategies

Train hip/trunk strategy (multi-segmental strategy)

Improve quality of balance control for function

Box 21.36 **Balance: Assessment**

Evaluation of balance in function

Comprehensive balance assessment

Standardized clinical balance assessment tasks
    Balance scales – e.g. Berg balance scale
    Static postural stability – e.g. measurement of trunk
        motion with pen attached to pole from spine
Balance performance on unstable surfaces
Instrumented balance assessment
    Balance assessment systems

Evaluation of sensory integration

Effect of vision removal/distortion (e.g. blindfold;
    movement of visual surround)
Effect of stimulation of muscle spindle input (e.g.
    muscle vibration; unstable surface)
Effect of removal of vestibular inputs (e.g. stabilization
    of head)

Box 21.37 **Balance: Techniques**

Incorporation of lumbar spine and pelvis into balance control (Fig. 21.39)

Encourage hip/trunk strategy (multi-segmental strategy)
    Limit contribution of ankle torque to balance
- Stand on unstable base – reduces potential to use ankle torque for balance control, thus encouraging use of spine/hip for balance
    – Single plane progressing to multiple plane
    – Increase range of motion
- Short base (limit ankle contribution)
    Limit sensory signals from ankle muscles
- Stand on foam
Cognitive correction/instructions
Manual guidance
Manual cues
Cues/reminders

Improve quality of balance control

Challenge balance in static and dynamic progression
    tasks
    Balls (unstable surface with inherent flexibility of
        exercise prescription)
    Reduced base of support – e.g. single leg stance
Challenge balance in functional tasks
Challenge balance with dual tasking (e.g. mental tasks)

---

function the potential to adequately control posture, movement and muscle activation will be limited. This may present as a major feature of the patient's presentation with important consequences for motor control (e.g. compromised control as a consequence of poor awareness of position, movement and/or muscle activation), or may be a component that simply requires enhancement and refinement. Most aspects of a motor control approach to rehabilitation have a sensory component. For instance, an essential component of a cognitive approach to correction of motor control faults in the initial phase is the perception of incorrect and correct performance of the retraining task. Sensory function can be improved with training (Jull et al. 2007) and this will have an impact on the quality of motor performance. Boxes 21.38, 21.39 and 21.40 provide a summary of the key training goals, assessments and treatment techniques that are available.

Strength and endurance

In most patients it is necessary to train muscle strength and endurance to some extent. This may involve training these parameters for specific muscles of the trunk control system. It has been confirmed that although atrophy of multifidus can be reversed with gentle voluntary muscle activation in patients after their first episode of acute pain (Hides et al. 1996), resistance training is necessary to reverse atrophy in people with chronic/persistent back pain (Danneels et al. 2001). During the course of progression through static and dynamic training it may be necessary to train specific strength and endurance deficits. This may involve strength for control of a specific direction of lumbopelvic rotation.

It is also necessary to consider motor control of the lumbar spine and pelvis during general strength training for limb and trunk muscles. During performance of conventional paradigms for training hip and knee muscles, for example, it is necessary to monitor and control alignment of the spine and pelvis, with specific attention to the motor control faults that were identified in the initial phases of treatment.

Rehabilitation in terms of strength and endurance is a staged process. Usually a foundation is laid with 'corrective' exercise to establish patterns of muscle activation, posture and movement that conserve/protect the spine. Then regional stability and mobility is enhanced appropriately. It is only on this foundation that considerations for endurance and strength enhancement can begin. Several studies have attempted to quantify the forms of

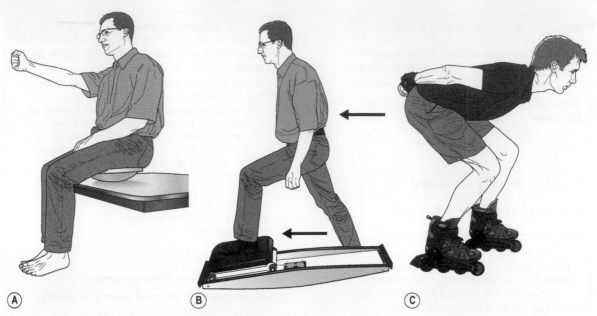

Figure 21.39 Balance training. (A) Challenge balance: sitting on unstable support surface and ballistic arm movement. (B) Encourage hip/trunk strategy (multi-segmental strategy): lunge on unstable support surface. (C) Challenge balance in functional tasks tailored to the individual needs of the patient, e.g. inline skating.

Box 21.38 Sensory function: Training goals

Improve sensory function
Sensing – acuity
Localization
Discrimination

Improve perception of lumbopelvic posture

Improve perception of lumbopelvic movement

Improve perception of muscle activation

Box 21.39 Sensory function: Assessment

Evaluate accuracy of repositioning
Ability to return to previously shown position
Sitting/standing/four point kneeling
Flexion and/or extension

Evaluate sensory acuity
Threshold for detection of motion
Requires use of an assessment device

Evaluate discrimination
Threshold for discrimination between 2 movements of
   different magnitude or direction (75% accuracy)
Requires use of an assessment device

Evaluation of postural control
Whole system assessment – not specific to proprioception
Can include specific assessment of muscle spindles with
   the use of muscle vibration
See Box 21.36 'Balance: Assessment'

---

exercise that spare the spine of exacerbating load and movement, while providing sufficient loading of muscle to enhance endurance and strength. For example, variations of the 'Big 3' stabilization exercises proposed by McGill (modified curl-up, side-bridge and bird dog/quadruped) are used to control the spine while loading the limbs and spine (Fig. 21.41) (Callaghan et al. 1998; Kavcic et al. 2004; McGill et al. 2009; Fenwick et al. 2009).

Endurance is worthy of discussion separately from strength given that spine stability requires co-contraction of trunk muscles for substantial durations, but at relatively low levels. This is an endurance and motor control challenge – not a strength challenge. Generally, the guideline is to constrain the duration of isometric stabilization exercises under 10 seconds, and build endurance with repetitions, not by increasing the duration of the holds. Near

Infrared Spectroscopy (NIRS) of the trunk muscles has shown that this method builds endurance without the muscles cramping that can be experienced with oxygen starvation and acid accumulation (McGill et al. 2000). The 'Russian descending pyramid' is often used in an attempt to preserve exercise technique as fatigue builds. In this

Box 21.40 **Sensory function: Techniques**

Non-specific training methods

Unstable surfaces (balance training)
  Ball, balance board, trampoline – challenge use of
  sensory signals

Training of specific aspects of proprioception
(Fig. 21.40)

Focus attention to sensing, localizing, discriminating
  (position, movement and muscle activation)

Repositioning training
Cognitive control training
  Conscious attention to posture, movement and muscle
  activation
Taping, bracing to enhance somatosensory input
Motor imagery – simulation of motor action with
  attention to 'feeling' of task

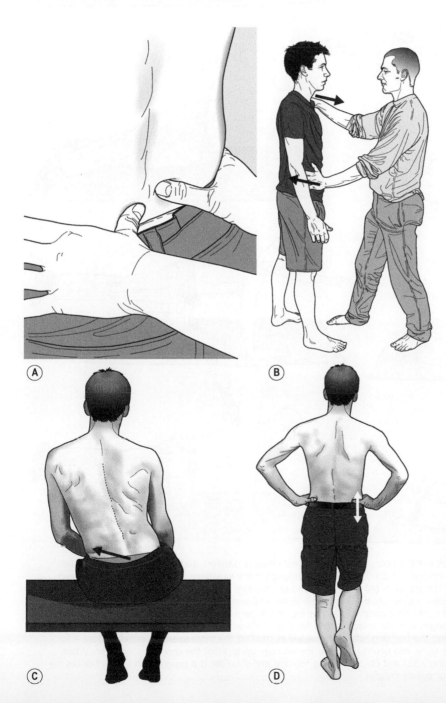

Figure 21.40 Sensory function training. (A) Sensing, localizing and discriminating lumbar multifidus with manual stimulation by therapist (or haptic control by patient). (B) Sensing, localizing and discriminating larger movement patterns with manual stimulation by therapist. (C) Conscious attention to lumbar posture, pelvic movement and muscle activation: slow diagonal pelvic motion pattern during sitting. (D) Conscious attention to lumbar posture, pelvic movement and muscle activation: slow pelvic motion pattern during unipedal stance.

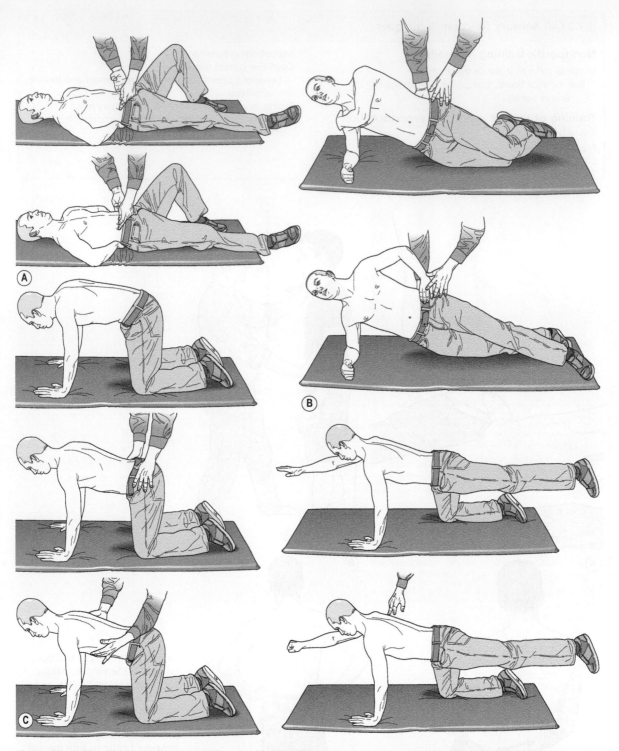

Figure 21.41 The 'Big 3' stabilization exercises used by McGill to create muscle patterns that are considered to ensure stability: (A) the curl-up, (B) the side-bridge and (C) the bird dog. Although many variations and progressions have been quantified, several cues are used for correct form. (A) During the curl-up, the aim is to remove any motion from the lumbar and cervical spines. Progression includes 'tuned' pre-bracing of the abdominal wall, elevating the elbows off the floor, and breathing, to name a few. Note that nearly no motion occurs but the challenge is self-generated from the concomitant 'tuned' abdominal bracing. (B) The beginner's side-bridge is held for sets of 10-seconds contraction before more challenging progressions are attempted. (C) During the bird dog, effort is directed at creating the most tolerable initial posture – for example, in this case, set the lumbar spine into neutral and cue the rib cage up to assist the thoracic alignment. While performing the loaded posture, making a fist and co-contracting the arm and shoulder is a progression that enhances the contraction levels in the upper erector spinae muscles.

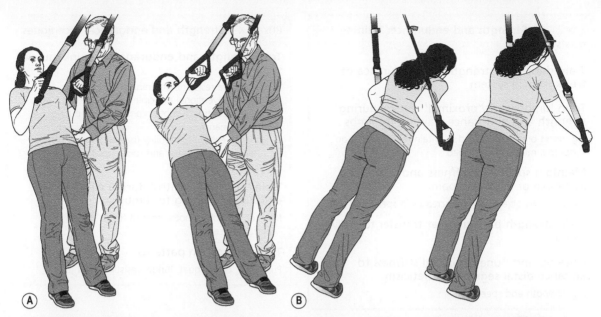

Figure 21.42 Many variations of push/pull exercises are used by McGill. Two beginners' variations illustrated here that have been quantified to neutralize shear load on the spine are (A) 'pull-ups' and (B) 'push-ups' using straps, with the feet on the floor. Control emphasis is placed on stiffening the torso and enhancing the handgrip while focussing motion only about the shoulders and elbows.

approach the repetitions of each exercise are reduced with each subsequent set (McGill 2009). Impeccable form also creates a higher volume of tolerable training because the joints are spared of loading associated with deviated postures and inappropriate muscle activation levels (McGill and Karpowicz 2009).

Endurance has also been suggested by several studies to play some predictive role with respect to individuals who will develop back pain in the future. For example, not only is a lack of extensor endurance predictive (Biering-Sørensen 1984), but also the balance of endurance between the anterior torso muscles and the side and the back muscles is associated with those who have repeated episodes when compared to matched controls without pain (McGill et al. 2003). Imbalances in strength, endurance and range of motion, not surprisingly, have been associated with prediction of many musculoskeletal injury types (Van Dillen et al. 2008; Knapik et al. 1991). Specific tests that measure endurance together with some cut-off scores for different populations have been described by McGill (2007) and colleagues (1999, 2010).

Strengthening of the back muscles is generally approached by loading the back in tasks in which the spine/torso form a link within the entire body. This is done in order to enhance transfer to daily activities. In this way strength may be enhanced in specific patterns such as pushing, pulling (Fig. 21.42), carrying, squatting, lunging, twisting (or resisting applied twisting torque) (McGill

2009). True strengthening for the purpose of enhancing athletic objectives requires muscle overload, is associated with elevated risk, and is not considered for the patient with low back or pelvic pain. Such training is reserved for a time after the pain has been eliminated. Many people, whether they have athletic objectives (such as wanting to play golf) or have physically demanding occupations, will fall into this category. On the other hand, many patients confuse health objectives (minimizing pain, developing joint sparing strategies) with performance objectives (which require risk) and compromise their progress by initiating specific strength training too early in their recovery/rehabilitation. Many exercises typically prescribed to patients with low back and pelvic pain are done so without the clinician having knowledge of the spine load and associated muscle activation levels. For this reason, exercises in McGill's approach have been quantified with respect to load and activation levels to allow evidence-based decisions when planning optimal exercise progressions. Finally, training involving movement patterns creates balances of torso strength and functional capacity. For example, carrying objects in one hand uniquely challenges lateral strength and muscle pairings such as statically contracted quadratus lumborum (proximal stiffness) and the opposite gluteal muscle group (power development) (McGill and Karpowicz 2009).

Any conventional strength or endurance training protocol can be implemented into a motor control approach

Box 21.41 Strength and endurance: Training goals

Train deficits in strength and endurance of trunk muscle system

Train lumbopelvic/'proximal' control during strength and endurance training for limbs

e.g. don't break 'form' and maintain movement in an optimal manner under load

Maintain sufficient stiffness and stability to minimize or eliminate pain

continue this objective with increases in speed and load

Train strength patterns that transfer to daily living

Develop and 'tune' proximal stiffness to enhance distal segment athleticism

e.g. strength and speed

Box 21.43 Strength and endurance: Techniques

Train strength and endurance of trunk muscle system

- Progressive resistance training (PRT)
  Follow conventional principles of PRT
  Monitor control of motor control 'fault' during performance
  Enhance extremity mobility (ball and socket joint – hips and shoulders) and torso stability
- Endurance training

Train 'proximal' control during strength and endurance training for limbs

Monitor control of motor control 'fault' during performance

Train strength in patterns

Push, pull, carry, squat, lunge, resisting twist, etc.

Box 21.42 Strength and endurance: Assessment

Any conventional assessments of strength and endurance

Limit of loading/holding time/number of repetitions is indicated by:
  loss of 'proximal' control or re-emergence of motor control 'fault'
  inability to overcome load
Enhance strategies to spare the spine of load while enhancing strength and endurance of muscles (e.g. McGill's 'big 3 exercises')
Consider models for prescription of exercise for endurance (e.g. Russian descending pyramid)
Every exercise forms a screening test where poor control is recognized and the cause is appropriately corrected

depending on the needs of the patient and the preference of the treatment provider. Whatever approach is implemented, careful attention to detail is required to ensure that patients do not resort to suboptimal postures/alignment, movements and muscle activation patterns. The basic principles of assessment and treatment are highlighted in Boxes 21.41, 21.42 and 21.43.

Fitness

It is not uncommon for patients with low back and pelvic pain to be deconditioned. This may be both a cause of pain (e.g. muscle changes secondary to disuse (Belavý

et al. 2011)) or a consequence of pain (e.g. disuse and inactivity secondary to fear-avoidance beliefs/behaviours (Vlaeyen and Linton 2000)). Regardless of the temporal sequence, this may require specific attention in the design of the optimal treatment package for the patient. Any approach to fitness training can be used, based on the experience of the treatment provider and the needs of the patient (based on assessment findings). Fitness involves many components, including cardiovascular fitness to movement flexibility. Like all other aspects of a motor control training approach, the specific programme implemented for a patient depends on his/her individual functional needs and his/her individual deficits.

Enhancement of fitness requires repeated and prolonged loading to be challenged. This is usually not appropriate until pain control has been mastered. As with all patients with low back or pelvic pain, programmes must be individualized to enhance the load tolerance and the capacity to train. Each individual has a loading *tolerance* which – when exceeded – will cause pain and ultimately tissue damage. For example, a patient may tolerate a 'bird dog' extension posture but not a 'superman' extension over a gym ball, which imposes twice the compressive load on the lumbar spine. A person's *capacity* is the cumulative work that he/she can perform before pain begins. The patient's capacity influences the way he/she can successfully enhance fitness. For example, a patient who can only walk 20 m before pain develops can be considered to have a low capacity. This patient is unlikely to benefit from therapeutic exercise that is performed three times per week; instead, he/she is more likely to benefit from three sessions per day. Corrected walking in three short sessions per day, never exceeding the current tolerance and

---

Box 21.44 **Fitness: Training goals**

Improve fitness to match the functional needs of the patient

Consider all aspects of fitness – e.g. cardiovascular fitness, flexibility

Encourage optimization of motor control during fitness training protocol

---

Box 21.45 **Fitness: Assessment**

Conventional assessments of fitness
Clinical tests
   Not specific for patients with LBP
     • e.g. Shuttle run test
Laboratory tests
   Examples of tests that are not specific to low back and pelvic pain, but could be used to quantify fitness include:
     • Maximal oxygen consumption test (VO_2max)
During assessment of fitness parameters it is essential to monitor:
   Loss of 'proximal' control
   Re-emergence of motor control 'fault'

Box 21.46 **Fitness: Techniques**

Improve fitness
Follow conventional program for training any aspects of fitness that are deemed to be a priority for the patient
   e.g. interval training walking/corrective walking
Attention to motor control 'fault' identified in earlier phases of training and correct if necessary

---

capacity, is likely to be the only tolerable option. Typically, this type of patient will progress to one session per day as their pain-free capacity grows.

There are many options to enhance fitness or total capacity for work. Unfortunately pain may restrict the approach to walking or running, or perhaps using an elliptical trainer. This may be appropriate for one patient but entirely inappropriate for another. For example, elliptical trainers cause higher back load and motion in individuals with reduced hip range of motion, and may therefore increase the potential for pain exacerbation (Moreside and McGill, unpublished data). Interval training can control the exposure and allows quite demanding work rates for repeated bursts. For example hand-over-hand rope pulling may be very appropriate for the person seeking proportionate strength in their upper body with a stiffened and 'buttressed' spine.

For integration into the motor control training approach it is necessary to assess, monitor and train lumbopelvic control during performance of fitness assessment and training tasks. Like other progressions of training this is based on the motor control faults identified throughout the training programme and through careful evaluation during the fitness tasks. Evaluation can be accomplished either through observation or palpation, or by use of additional assessment methods such as electromyography, ultrasound imaging and movement tools. Training goals, and principles for assessment and training are presented in Boxes 21.44, 21.45, and 21.46.

CONCLUSION

The purpose of this chapter was to provide an overview of the basis and application of motor control training to the management of a patient with lumbopelvic pain and dysfunction. It is clear that many issues require consideration in evaluation of the scope and relevance of motor control issues for the presentation of the patient. Design of a motor control training approach depends on careful assessment and targeting of treatment techniques in a package designed to achieve optimal outcomes for the patient. This must be fitted into a biopsychosocial framework to ensure all aspects of the presentation and the interaction among them have been addressed. The many approaches to motor control training that have been presented in the literature share many common features, with variation in: (i) the emphasis on individual issues; (ii) the assessment methods used to define the nature of the problem; and (iii) the specific techniques used to manage the patient. Despite this variation, the basic underlying philosophies are surprisingly similar. Time will tell which approaches are more effective. However, the likely outcome is that a combination of approaches within a clinician's armamentarium will be the most optimal approach as this provides the flexibility to match a package of intervention to the needs and preferences of the patient. As discussed throughout this chapter and the entire book there is considerable evidence for many aspects of the approach, yet there are many questions remaining and it is hoped that this book provides a fruitful foundation for ongoing research to test the efficacy and physiological rationale for the approach, and to refine the implementation of motor control training for low back and pelvic pain, and application of the principles to other regions of the body.

REFERENCES

Belavý, D.L., Armbrecht, G., Richardson, C.A., Felsenberg, D., Hides, J.A., 2011. Muscle atrophy and changes in spinal morphology: is the lumbar spine vulnerable after prolonged bed-rest? Spine 36, 137–145.

Biering-Sørensen, F., 1984. Physical measurements as risk indicators for low-back trouble over a one year period. Spine 9, 106–119.

Bullock-Saxton, J.E., Janda, V., Bullock, M.I., 1993. Reflex activation of gluteal muscles in walking with balance shoe: an approach to restoration of function for chronic low back pain patients. Spine 18, 704–708.

Butler, D., Moseley, G., 2003. Explain pain. NOI Group Publishing, Adelaide.

Callaghan, J.P., Gunning, J.L., McGill, S.M., 1998. The relationship between lumbar spine load and muscle activity during extensor exercises. Phys Ther 78, 8–18.

Claus, A.P., Hides, J.A., Moseley, G.L., Hodges, P.W., 2009a. Different ways to balance the spine: subtle changes in sagittal spinal curves affect regional muscle activity. Spine 34, E208–E214.

Claus, A.P., Hides, J.A., Moseley, G.L., Hodges, P.W., 2009b. Is 'ideal' sitting posture real? Measurement of spinal curves in four sitting postures. Man Ther 14, 404–408.

Cook, C., Brismee, J.M., Sizer Jr., P.S., 2006. Subjective and objective descriptors of clinical lumbar spine instability: a Delphi study. Man Ther 11, 11–21.

Costa, L.O., Maher, C.G., Latimer, J., Hodges, P.W., Herbert, R.D., Refshauge, K.M., et al., 2009. Motor control exercise for chronic low back pain: a randomized placebo-controlled trial. Phys Ther 89, 1275–1286.

Dankaerts, W., O'Sullivan, P., Burnett, A., Straker, L., 2006. Altered patterns of superficial trunk muscle activation during sitting in nonspecific chronic low back pain patients: importance of subclassification. Spine 31, 2017–2023.

Danneels, L., Cools, A., Vanderstraeten, G., Gambier, D., Witrouw, E.,

Bourgois, J., et al., 2001. The effect of 3 different training modalities on the cross sectional area of paravertebral muscles. Scand J Med Sci Sports 11, 335–341.

Delitto, A., Erhard, R.E., Bowling, R.W., 1995. A treatment-based classification approach to low back syndrome: identifying and staging patients for conservative treatment. Phys Ther 75, 470–485; discussion 485–479.

Evarts, E.V., 1967. Representation of movements and muscles by pyramidal tract neurons of the precentral motor cortex. In: Yahr, M.D., Purpura, D.P. (eds), Neurophysiological Basis of Normal and Abnormal Motor Activities. Raven Press, Hewlett, NY, pp. 215–251.

Falla, D., Jull, G., Russell, T., Vicenzino, B., Hodges, P., 2007. Effect of neck exercise on sitting posture in patients with chronic neck pain. Phys Ther 87, 408–417.

Fenwick, C.M., Brown, S.H., McGill, S.M., 2009. Comparison of different rowing exercises: trunk muscle activation and lumbar spine motion, load, and stiffness. J Strength Cond Res 23, 1408–1417.

Ferreira, M.L., Ferreira, P.H., Hodges, P.W., 2007a. Changes in postural activity of the trunk muscles following spinal manipulative therapy. Man Ther 12, 240–248.

Ferreira, M.L., Ferreira, P.H., Latimer, J., Herbert, R.D., Hodges, P.W., Jennings, M.D., et al., 2007b. Comparison of general exercise, motor control exercise and spinal manipulative therapy for chronic low back pain: a randomized trial. Pain 131, 31–37.

Ferreira, P., Ferreira, M., Maher, C., Refshauge, K., Herbert, R., Hodges, P., 2009. Changes in recruitment of transversus abdominis correlate with disability in people with chronic low back pain. Br J Sports Med 44, 1166–1172.

Fersum, K.V., Dankaerts, W., O'Sullivan, P.B., Maes, J., Skouen, J.S., Bjordal, J.M., et al., 2010. Integration of subclassification strategies in randomised controlled clinical trials evaluating manual therapy treatment

and exercise therapy for non-specific chronic low back pain: a systematic review. Br J Sports Med 44, 1054–1062.

Fitts, P.M., Posner, M.I., 1967. Human Performance. Brooks/Cole, Belmont, CA.

Fritz, J.M., Koppenhaver, S.L., Kawchuk, G.N., Teyhen, D.S., Hebert, J.J., Childs, J.D., 2011. Preliminary investigation of the mechanisms underlying the effects of manipulation: exploration of a multivariate model including spinal stiffness, multifidus recruitment, and clinical findings. Spine 36, 1772–1781.

Gahery, Y., Massion, J., 1981. Co-ordination between posture and movement. Trends Neurosci 4, 199–202.

Gentile, A.M., 1987. Skill acquisition: action, movement and neuromuscular processes. In: Carr, J.H., Shepherd, R.B., Gordon, J., Gentile, A.M., Hinds, J.M. (eds), Movement and Science: foundations for physical therapy in rehabilitation. Aspen, Rockville, MD, pp. 93–154.

Goldby, L.J., Moore, A.P., Doust, J., Trew, M.E., 2006. A randomized controlled trial investigating the efficiency of musculoskeletal physiotherapy on chronic low back disorder. Spine 31, 1083–1093.

Gombatto, S.P., Collins, D.R., Sahrmann, S.A., Engsberg, J.R., Van Dillen, L.R., 2006. Gender differences in pattern of hip and lumbopelvic rotation in people with low back pain. Clin Biomech 21, 263–271.

Griffith, L.E., Shannon, H.S., Wells, R.P., Walter, S.D., Cole, D.C., Cote, P., et al., 2012. Individual participant data meta-analysis of mechanical workplace risk factors and low back pain. Am J Publ Health 102, 309–318.

Hall, L., Tsao, H., MacDonald, D., Coppieters, M., Hodges, P.W., 2009. Immediate effects of co-contraction training on motor control of the trunk muscles in people with recurrent low back pain. J Electromyogr Kinesiol 19, 763–773.

Hicks, G.E., Fritz, J.M., Delitto, A., McGill, S.M., 2005. Preliminary development of a clinical prediction rule for determining which patients with low back pain will respond to a stabilization exercise program. Arch Phys Med Rehabil 86, 1753–1762.

Hides, J., Scott, Q., Jull, G., Richardson, C., 2000. A clinical palpation test to check the activation of the deep stabilising muscles of the spine. Int Sportmed J 1.

Hides, J.A., Jull, G.A., Richardson, C.A., 2001. Long term effects of specific stabilizing exercises for first episode low back pain. Spine 26, 243–248.

Hides, J.A., Richardson, C.A., Jull, G.A., 1996. Multifidus muscle recovery is not automatic after resolution of acute, first-episode low back pain. Spine 21, 2763–2769.

Hodges, P., Cholewicki, J., 2007. Functional control of the spine. In: Vleeming, A., Mooney, V., Stoeckart, R. (eds), Movement, Stability and Lumbopelvic Pain. Elsevier, Edinburgh.

Hodges, P., Ferreira, P., Ferreira, M., 2009. Lumbar spine: treatment of instability and disorders of movement control. In: Magee, D., Zachazewski, J., Quillen, W. (eds), Pathology and Intervention in Musculoskeletal Rehabilitation. Saunders Elsevier, St Louis, MO, pp. 389–425.

Hodges, P.W., Heijnen, I., Gandevia, S.C., 2001. Reduced postural activity of the diaphragm in humans when respiratory demand is increased. J Physiol 537, 999–1008.

Hodges, P.W., McKenzie, D.K., Heijnen, I., Gandevia, S.C., 2000. Reduced contribution of the diaphragm to postural control in patients with severe chronic airflow limitation. In: Proceedings of the Annual Sceintific Meeting of the Thoracic Society of Australia and New Zealand, Melbourne, Australia.

Hodges, P.W., Pengel, H.M., Sapsford, R., 2007. Postural and respiratory functions of the pelvic floor muscles. Neurourol Urodyn 26, 362–371.

Hodges, P.W., Richardson, C.A., Jull, G.A., 1996. Evaluation of the relationship between the findings of a laboratory and clinical test of transverus abdominis function. Physiother Res Int 1, 30–40.

Hoffman, S.L., Johnson, M.B., Zou, D., Harris-Hayes, M., Van Dillen, L.R., 2011. Effect of classification-specific treatment on lumbopelvic motion during hip rotation in people with low back pain. Man Ther 16, 344–350.

Horak, F., Nashner, L.M., 1986. Central programming of postural movements: adaptation to altered support-surface configurations. J Neurophysiol 55, 1369–1381.

Janda, V., 1996. Evaluation of muscular imbalances. In: Liebenson, C. (ed.), Rehabilitation of the Spine: a practitioner's manual. Williams and Wilkins, Baltimore, MD, pp. 97–112.

Jones, M., Rivett, D., 2004. Clinical Reasoning for Manual Therapists. Butterworth–Heinemann, Edinburgh.

Jull, G., Falla, D., Treleaven, J., Hodges, P., Vicenzino, B., 2007. Retraining cervical joint position sense: the effect of two exercise regimes. J Orthop Res 25, 404–412.

Kavcic, N., Grenier, S., McGill, S.M., 2004. Quantifying tissue loads and spine stability while performing commonly prescribed low back stabilization exercises. Spine 29, 2319–2329.

Kendall, F., 2005. Muscles: testing and function with posture and pain, 5th edn. Lippincott Williams & Wilkins, Baltimore, MD.

Kiesel, K.B., Underwood, F.B., Mattacola, C.G., Nitz, A.J., Malone, T.R., 2007. A comparison of select trunk muscle thickness change between subjects with low back pain classified in the treatment-based classification system and asymptomatic controls. J Orthop Sports Phys Ther 37, 596–607.

Knapik, J.J., Bauman, C.L., Jones, B.H., Harris, J.M., Vaughan, L., 1991. Preseason strength and flexibility imbalances associated with athletic injuries in female collegiate athletes. Am J Sports Med 19, 76–81.

Lederman, E., 2010. The myth of core stability. J Bodywork Movement Therapies 14, 84–98.

Lee, D., 2003. The Thorax : an integrated approach, 2nd edn. Diane G Lee Physiotherapist Corporation, White Rock, BC.

Lee, D., 2004. The Pelvic Girdle: an approach to the examination and treatment of the lumbopelvic-hip region, 3rd edn. Churchill Living-stone, Edinburgh.

Lee, L.J., Chang, A.T., Coppieters, M.W., Hodges, P.W., 2010. Changes in sitting posture induce multiplanar changes in chest wall shape and motion with breathing. Respir Physiol Neurobiol 170, 236–245.

Macedo, L.G., Latimer, J., Maher, C.G., Hodges, P.W., McAuley, J.H., Nicholas, M.K., et al., 2012. Effect of motor control exercises versus graded activity in patients with chronic nonspecific low back pain: a randomized controlled trial. Phys Ther 92, 363–377.

Macedo, L.G., Latimer, J., Maher, C.G., Hodges, P.W., Nicholas, M., Tonkin, L., et al., 2008. Motor control or graded activity exercises for chronic low back pain? A randomised controlled trial. BMC Musculoskelet Disord 9, 65.

Magee, D., 2006. Orthopedic Physical Assessment, 4th edn. Saunders Elsevier, Philadelphia.

Magill, R.A., 2001. Motor learning: concepts and applications, 6th edn. McGraw–Hill, New York.

Marras, W.S., Ferguson, S.A., Burr, D., Davis, K.G., Gupta, P., 2004. Spine loading in patients with low back pain during asymmetric lifting exertions. Spine J 4, 64–75.

Marshall, P., Murphy, B., 2006. The effect of sacroiliac joint manipulation on feed-forward activation times of the deep abdominal musculature. J Manipulative Physiol Ther 29, 196–202.

McGill, S., Belore, M., Crosby, I., Russell, C., 2010. Clinical tools to quantify torso flexion endurance: normative data from student and firefighter populations. Occup Ergonom 9, 55–61.

McGill, S., Grenier, S., Bluhm, M., Preuss, R., Brown, S., Russell, C., 2003. Previous history of LBP with work loss is related to lingering deficits in biomechanical, physio-logical, personal, psychosocial and motor control characteristics. Ergonomics 46, 731–746.

McGill, S.M., 1992. The influence of lordosis on axial trunk torque and trunk muscle myoelectric activity. Spine 17, 1187–1193.

McGill, S.M., 2007. Low Back Disorders: evidence based prevention and rehabilitation, 2nd edn. Human Kinetics Publishers, Champaign, IL.

McGill, S.M., 2009. Ultimate back fitness and performance, 4th edn. Backfitpro Inc., Waterloo, Canada.

McGill, S.M., Childs, A., Liebenson, C., 1999. Endurance times for low back stabilization exercises: clinical targets for testing and training from a normal database. Arch Phys Med Rehabil 80, 941–944.

McGill, S.M., Hughson, R.L., Parks, K., 2000. Lumbar erector spinae oxygenation during prolonged contractions: implications for prolonged work. Ergonomics 43, 486–493.

McGill, S.M., Karpowicz, A., 2009. Exercises for spine stabilization: motion/motor patterns, stability progressions, and clinical technique. Arch Phys Med Rehabil 90, 118–126.

McGill, S.M., Karpowicz, A., Fenwick, C.M., 2009. Ballistic abdominal exercises: muscle activation patterns during three activities along the stability/mobility continuum. J Strength Cond Res 23, 898–905.

McKenzie, R., May, S., 2003. The lumbar spine, mechanical diagnosis and therapy, 2nd edn. Spinal Publications New Zealand Ltd, Waikanae.

McNair, P.J., Heine, P.J., 1999. Trunk proprioception: enhancement through lumbar bracing. Arch Phys Med Rehabil 80, 96–99.

McNevin, N.H., Shea, C.H., Wulf, G., 2003. Increasing the distance of an external focus of attention enhances learning. Psychol Res 67, 22–29.

Mens, J.M., Vleeming, A., Snijders, C.J., Koes, B.W., Stam, H.J., 2002. Validity of the active straight leg raise test for measuring disease severity in patients with posterior pelvic pain after pregnancy. Spine 27, 196–200.

Mok, N.W., Brauer, S.G., Hodges, P.W., 2007. Failure to use movement in postural strategies leads to increased spinal displacement in low back pain. Spine 32, E537–E543.

Nicholas, M., Siddal, P., Tonkin, L., Beeston, L., 2002. Manage Your Pain. ABC Books, Sydney, NSW.

O'Sullivan, P., 2005. Diagnosis and classification of chronic low back pain disorders: maladaptive movement and motor control impairments as underlying mechanism. Man Ther 10, 242–255.

O'Sullivan, P., Dankaerts, W., Burnett, A., Chen, D., Booth, R., Carlsen, C., et al., 2006. Evaluation of the flexion relaxation phenomenon of the trunk muscles in sitting. Spine 31, 2009–2016.

O'Sullivan, P.B., Beales, D.J., Beetham, J.A., Cripps, J., Graf, F., Lin, I.B., et al., 2002. Altered motor control strategies in subjects with sacroiliac joint pain during the active straight-leg-raise test. Spine 27, E1–E8.

O'Sullivan, P.B., Twomey, L.T., Allison, G.T., 1997. Evaluation of specific stabilizing exercise in the treatment of chronic low back pain with radiologic diagnosis of spondylolysis or spondylolisthesis. Spine 22, 2959–2967.

Panjabi, M.M., 1992. The stabilising system of the spine. Part II. Neutral zone and instability hypothesis. J Spinal Dis 5, 390–397.

Perkins-Ceccato, N., Passmore, S.R., Lee, T.D., 2003. Effects of focus of attention depend on golfers' skill. J Sports Sci 21, 593–600.

Petersen, T., Laslett, M., Thorsen, H., Manniche, C., Ekdahl, C., Jacobsen, S., 2003. Diagnostic classification of non-specific low back pain. A new system integrating patho-anatomic and clinical categories. Physiother Theory Pract 19, 213–237.

Pool-Goudzwaard, A.L., Slieker Ten Hove, M.C., Vierhout, M.E., Mulder, P.H., Pool, J.J., Snijders, C.J., et al., 2005. Relations between pregnancy-related low back pain, pelvic floor activity and pelvic floor dysfunction. Int Urogynecol J Pelvic Floor Dysfunct 16, 468–474.

Remple, M.S., Bruneau, R.M., VandenBerg, P.M., Goertzen, C., Kleim, J.A., 2001. Sensitivity of cortical movement representations to motor experience: evidence that skill learning but not strength training induces cortical reorganization. Behav Brain Res 123, 133–141.

Richardson, C.A., Hodges, P.W., Hides, J.A., 2004. Therapeutic Exercise for Lumbopelvic Stabilisation: a motor control approach for the treatment and prevention of low back pain. Churchill Livingstone, Edinburgh.

Sahrmann, S., 2002. Diagnosis and Treatment of Movement Impairment Syndromes. Mosby, St Louis, MO.

Sapsford, R.R., Hodges, P.W., Richardson, C.A., Cooper, D.H., Markwell, S.J., Jull, G.A., 2001. Co-activation of the abdominal and pelvic floor muscles during voluntary exercises. Neurourol Urodyn 20, 31–42.

Sapsford, R.R., Richardson, C.A., Maher, C.F., Hodges, P.W., 2008. Pelvic floor muscle activity in different sitting postures in continent and incontinent women. Arch Phys Med Rehabil 89, 1741–1747.

Saunders, S.W., Schache, A., Rath, D., Hodges, P.W., 2005. Changes in three dimensional lumbo-pelvic kinematics and trunk muscle activity with speed and mode of locomotion. Clin Biomech (Bristol, Avon) 20, 784–793.

Scholtes, S.A., Gombatto, S.P., Van Dillen, L.R., 2009. Differences in lumbopelvic motion between people with and people without low back pain during two lower limb movement tests. Clinical Biomechanics 24, 7–12.

Scholtes, S.A., Norton, B.J., Lang, C.E., Van Dillen, L.R., 2010. The effect of within-session instruction on lumbopelvic motion during a lower limb movement in people with and people without low back pain. Man Ther 15, 496–501.

Shumway-Cook, A., Woollacott, M., 2006. Motor Control: Translating Research into Clinical Practice, 3rd edn. Lippincott Williams & Wilkins, Philadelphia, PA.

Smith, M.D., Coppieters, M.W., Hodges, P.W., 2007. Postural response of the pelvic floor and abdominal muscles in women with and without incontinence. Neurourol Urodyn 26, 377–385.

Sprague, R., 2001. Differential assessment and mobilisation of the cervical and thoracic spine. In: Donatelli, R., Wooden, M. (eds), Orthopaedic Physical Therapy, 3rd edn. Churchill Livingstone, New York, pp. 108–143.

Stafford, R.E., Ashton-Miller, J.A., Sapsford, R., Hodges, P.W., 2012. Activation of the striated urethral sphincter to maintain continence during dynamic tasks in healthy men. Neurourol Urodyn 31, 36–43.

Stuge, B., Laerum, E., Kirkesola, G., Vollestad, N., 2004. The efficacy of a treatment program focusing on specific stabilizing exercises for pelvic girdle pain after pregnancy: a randomized controlled trial. Spine 29, 351–359.

Sullivan, M.J.L., Bishop, S.R., Pivik, J., 1995. The Pain Catastrophizing Scale: development and validation. Psychol Assess 7, 524–532.

Thacker, M.A., Moseley, G.L., 2012. First-person neuroscience and the understanding of pain. Med J Aust 196, 410–411.

Tsao, H., Galea, M.P., Hodges, P.W., 2010. Driving plasticity in the motor cortex in recurrent low back pain. Eur J Pain 14, 832–839.

Tsao, H., Hodges, P.W., 2007. Immediate changes in feedforward postural adjustments following voluntary motor training. Exper Brain Res 181, 537–546.

Tsao, H., Hodges, P.W., 2008. Persistence of changes in postural control following training of isolated voluntary contractions in people with recurrent low back pain. J Electromyogr Kinesiol 18, 559–567.

Turk, D.C., Flor, H., 2006. The cognitive-behavioural approach to pain management. In: McMahon, S., Koltzenburg, M. (eds), Wall & Melzack's Textbook of Pain. Elsevier, London, pp. 339–348.

Unsgaard-Tondel, M., Lund Nilsen, T.I., Magnussen, J., Vasseljen, O., 2012. Is activation of transversus abdominis and obliquus internus abdominis associated with long-term changes in chronic low back pain? A prospective

study with 1-year follow-up. Br J Sports Med 46, 729–734.

Van Dillen, L.R., Bloom, N.J., Gombatto, S.P., Susco, T.M., 2008. Hip rotation range of motion in people with and without low back pain who participate in rotation-related sports. Phys Ther Sport 9, 72–81.

Van Dillen, L.R., Gombatto, S.P., Collins, D.R., Engsberg, J.R., Sahrmann, S.A., 2007. Symmetry of timing of hip and lumbopelvic rotation motion in 2 different subgroups of people with low back pain. Arch Phys Med Rehabil 88, 351–360.

Van Dillen, L.R., Maluf, K.S., Sahrmann, S.A., 2009. Further examination of modifying patient-preferred movement and alignment strategies in patients with low back pain during symptomatic tests. Man Ther 14, 52–60.

Van Dillen, L.R., Sahrmann, S.A., Norton, B.J., Caldwell, C.A., McDonnell, M.K., Bloom, N., 2003a. The effect of modifying patient-preferred spinal movement and alignment during symptom testing in patients with low back pain: a preliminary report. Arch Phys Med Rehabil 84, 313–322.

Van Dillen, L.R., Sahrmann, S.A., Norton, B.J., Caldwell, C.A., McDonnell, M.K., Bloom, N.J., 2003b. Movement system impairment-based categories for low back pain: stage 1 validation. J Orthop Sports Phys Ther 33, 126–142.

Vasseljen, O., Fladmark, A.M., 2010. Abdominal muscle contraction thickness and function after specific and general exercises: a randomized controlled trial in chronic low back pain patients. Man Ther 15, 482–489.

Vlaeyen, J.W., Linton, S.J., 2000. Fear-avoidance and its consequences in chronic musculoskeletal pain: a state of the art. Pain 85, 317–332.

Voss, D.E., Ionta, M.K., Myers, B.J., 1985. Proprioceptive Neuromuscular Facilitation: patterns and techniques. Lippincott Williams & Wilkins, New York.

Waddell, G., Newton, M., Henderson, I., Somerville, D., Main, C.J., 1993. A Fear-Avoidance Beliefs Questionnaire (FABQ) and the role of fear-avoidance beliefs in chronic low back pain and disability. Pain 52, 157–168.

Whittaker, J.L., Thompson, J.A., Teyhen, D.S., Hodges, P., 2007. Rehabilitative ultrasound imaging of pelvic floor muscle function. J Orthop Sports Phys Ther 37, 487–498.

Woolf, C.J., 2011. Central sensitization: implications for the diagnosis and treatment of pain. Pain 152, S2–S15.

Zazulak, B.T., Hewett, T.E., Reeves, N.P., Goldberg, B., Cholewicki, J., 2007. Deficits in neuromuscular control of the trunk predict knee injury risk: a prospective biomechanical-epidemiologic study. Am J Sports Med 35, 1123–1130.

Index

Page numbers followed by "f" indicate figures, "t" indicate tables, and "b" indicate boxes.

Index

Index

Printed and bound by CPI Group (UK) Ltd, Croydon, CR0 4YY

03/10/2024

01040366-0014